Toward a Science of Clinical Psychology

Cory L. Cobb • Steven Jay Lynn
William O'Donohue
Editors

Toward a Science of Clinical Psychology

A Tribute to the Life and Works of Scott O. Lilienfeld

Springer

Editors
Cory L. Cobb
Department of Human Development
and Family Science
Auburn University
Auburn, AL, USA

Steven Jay Lynn
Department of Psychology
Binghamton University
Binghamton, NY, USA

William O'Donohue
Department of Psychology
University of Nevada
Reno, NV, USA

ISBN 978-3-031-14334-2 ISBN 978-3-031-14332-8 (eBook)
https://doi.org/10.1007/978-3-031-14332-8

This Springer imprint is published by the registered company Springer Nature Switzerland AG
The registered company address is: Gewerbestrasse 11, 6330 Cham, Switzerland

Preface

Dr. Scott O. Lilienfeld was a preeminent scholar who has had a shaping influence on the field of psychological science, particularly clinical science. He inspired and deeply affected the many people close to him: his loving wife, Candice Basterfield, who is a contributor this volume, and the many friends, colleagues, and students whose lives he personally touched. His death, on September 30, 2020, at the age of 59, following a courageous and stoic battle with pancreatic cancer, was an immense loss to the world of psychology and to those people, across the globe, who had the privilege of knowing him, a gift for which we, the editors, will be forever grateful.

For those readers who did not have this special privilege that we were fortunate to have enjoyed, this volume, this tribute and testament to Scott's life and work, will provide somewhat of a feel for what he accomplished professionally and, just as important, for Scott as a person. We feel immensely honored to present this collection of stellar chapters, written by eminent scholars that Scott influenced, as well as students Scott mentored, all of whom he greatly and vocally admired and respected. These chapters cast a spotlight not only on the multifaceted and influential nature of his scientific contributions but also provide warm personal reflections on and details of his journey as a scientist and scholar from his days as an undergraduate student at Cornell University to his academic positions at the University at Albany and later at Emory University and the University of Melbourne prior to his all-too-early death. Along the way, Scott became a friend to many, and his friendship was one of the special joys that life sometimes provides.

As you read this volume, you will find references to Scott's impeccable intellect and keen judgment, curiosity about all things psychology, voracious appetite for learning, and encyclopedic knowledge; his humility, kindness, warmth and empathy, generosity, tireless support of students and junior colleagues, fair-mindedness, humor, and openness to opinions that challenged his own; his indefatigable commitment to combating entrenched myths and misconceptions and pseudoscience in psychology; and his unabashed love of science and devotion to sharing this passion with others. The wide scope of his interests and accomplishments, as well as his collegiality, resulted in a wide range of collaborations with a diverse group of individuals, many of whom are chapter authors in this volume. We editors can say that in our experience of knowing Scott, whatever topic we discussed, he enriched, and whatever intellectual product we collaborated on, he made better; he was a paragon of clear thinking and splendidly lucid writing, and a mensch to boot. Scott also was one of the most intellectually courageous individuals we have known—he fearlessly followed the evidence and the argument and never desisted, even if these led to controversy and perhaps some measure of unpopularity. In short, Scott was imbued with a rare and wonderful combination of qualities; he was at once an intellectual giant and a very special and down-to-earth, caring person.

In compiling the chapters, we thought of Scott frequently and we recalled, with great fondness and at times great feelings of sadness, these and other endearing qualities that we miss so much. We also reflected on how much Scott would have appreciated and enjoyed reading each of the contributions in this book. Taken together, they form a mosaic that we hope readers will find captures Scott's astonishing accomplishments, motivation to make a difference beyond the academy, and the love and respect that he instilled among his peers. We know that Scott would have delighted in the thought that the collective expertise and wisdom presented herein provide a meaningful and substantive platform for pondering and discussing current issues and topics and future directions in clinical psychological science. And perhaps more importantly, we suspect that he would be pleased with the prospect that new generations of students will be turned on to the allure and beauty of psychological science that so moved him to probe an array of topics while never sacrificing depth of inquiry and exactitude of scholarship.

Readers will discover, or appreciate more than ever, that Scott was a leading authority in several substantive areas of clinical science. The multipronged and impactful nature of his work is reflected in his more than 500 articles, chapters, books, and encyclopedia entries that have been cited approximately 45,000 times, as of this writing (April 2022, Google Scholar). Scott could be described as an all-too-rare breed of scientist these days—given the current pressures to specialize in a narrow or singular field of study to attract the grant dollar—"the generalist scientist." Scott made bountiful contributions that spanned psychological diagnosis, personality assessment, psychopathology, evidence-based psychotherapy, and much more. His work influenced the way we think about classifying and assessing mental disorders, sources of comorbidity of psychological conditions, the genesis of dissociative disorders, and the conceptual and empirical links between seemingly disparate disorders such as somatization and psychopathy. The reach of his scholarship stretched far: to forensic psychology and neuroscience, cultural sensitivity and microaggressions, memory and trauma, and beyond. Given his versatility and protean knowledge, Scott was, indeed, the perfect person to serve as one of the editors of the *Encyclopedia of Clinical Psychology*.

Scott is perhaps best known as one of the preeminent scholars in the area of psychopathy, and he was, without question, the foremost authority on pseudoscience in psychology, and how to distinguish the masquerader of science from the real thing. Over three decades, Scott was an articulate and effective public spokesperson for psychology and empirically based clinical practice, and he was our field's staunchest and most dogged critic of pseudoscience: He penned a regular column in

Scientific American, presented a scientific perspective to millions of viewers of prime-time television and radio programs, wrote op-eds for major news outlets, and was interviewed for numerous newspaper and magazine articles. Scott's book, *50 Great Myths of Popular Psychology: Shattering Widespread Misconceptions about Human Behavior* (with Lynn, Ruscio, & Beyerstein, 2010), which has been translated into 20 languages, reached a wide popular and academic audience and provided a much-needed corrective to potentially harmful misinformation propagated by the media and the "pop psych industry." A collection of his columns for *Scientific American Mind*, as a further corrective, was published in a trade book entitled, *Facts and Fictions in Mental Health* (with Arkowitz, 2017). Scott lectured all over the United States and internationally on a vast array of topics relevant to key questions in psychology and to everyday living, making new friends, admirers, and collaborators at stops along the way.

Scott's mission to educate a wide audience regarding the virtues of a scientific mindset and the imperative to teach critical thinking skills was further reflected in highly influential books that he wrote or edited, which have shaped the contours of graduate and undergraduate education and include (a) his widely adopted introductory psychology textbook (*Psychology: From Inquiry to Understanding*, with Lynn & Lohr, 2022), now in its fifth edition, and (b) the treatise, *Science and Pseudoscience in Clinical Psychology* (with Lynn & Lohr, 2nd Ed., 2015), widely read in graduate courses. *The Great Ideas of Clinical Science: The 17 Concepts that Every Mental Health Practitioner and Researcher Should Understand* (with O'Donohue, 2014) brings a broad audience of students, researchers, and clinicians up to speed on issues crucial to appreciating the contributions of psychological science to understanding human thought and action.

Dr. Lilienfeld and his colleagues' (Lilienfeld et al., 2000) critical appraisal of projective testing was featured in *Psychological Science in the Public Interest*, and in a popular book on the subject (Wood et al., 2003). These efforts played an important role in changing the way mainstream clinicians and court systems regard the validity and utility of projective tests. *Brainwashed: The Seductive Appeal of Mindless Neuroscience* (with Satel, 2015), a finalist for the LA Times Book Prize in Science, advances a provocative account of the promise of brain imaging and neuroscience alongside the pitfalls of drawing unwarranted inferences from high-tech methods and the perils of overblown claims. Lilienfeld and his colleagues also did a valuable service in writing critical reviews that counter overblown claims about the effectiveness of eye movement desensitization (EMDR) and facilitated communication for autism, in questioning the validity of the post-traumatic model of dissociation, and in highlighting the potential for the iatrogenic creation of dissociative identity disorder and harmful psychotherapies more generally.

Not surprisingly, Scott valued teaching and was a consummate instructor who was dedicated to providing students with the necessary tools to evaluate arguments and claims in everyday life. His skills on the podium and commitment to students were acknowledged in his selection for the "Great Teachers" Lecturer Series at Emory University, which he regarded as a high honor. Scott valued clarity, a trait that makes someone an effective and popular teacher. Scott often called himself a "workaholic," and part of the long days and weeks Scott spent working was due to his dedication to students—including students whom he had never met and who just wrote him asking for his help or advice. We know of numerous incidents in which Scott spent many hours with a student helping them with their research or careers, even when these students were not in his program or not even in the field of clinical psychology. Scott was generous with his time and expertise and was deeply committed to helping others, something he did frequently and effectively.

Scott's contributions have not gone unnoticed or unappreciated in the professional community. In addition to his prodigious scholarly activity, Scott was honored with the most prestigious awards bestowed by the Association for Psychological Science (APS) and the American Psychological Association (APA), he served as the editor-in-chief of *Clinical Psychological Science* and as the associate editor of *Archives of Scientific Psychology*, and he served on 10 other editorial boards, including the highly regarded *Journal of Abnormal Psychology* (now the *Journal of Psychopathology and Clinical Science*) and the journal *Assessment.* Scott also was elected twice as the President of the Society for a Science of Clinical Psychology and as the President of the Society for the Scientific Study of Psychopathy. Another perhaps less formal recognition, but nonetheless impressive, is that another intellectual giant in our field, Paul Meehl who was one of his mentors at the University of Minnesota, wrote in a letter of recommendation that he learned more from Scott than he believed Scott learned from him.

In closing, we editors feel incredibly fortunate to call Scott our friend and collaborator and to be in a position to honor him with this tribute. We thank all of those who have contributed their time, expertise, and caring for Scott for their participation. It means a lot to us. We also thank Sharon Panulla, at Sage Publishing, for supporting this project. And to you readers, whether you are a student, researcher, teacher, mental health professional, or a curious person with an interest in psychological science, we hope that you enjoy and find value in reading this compendium. We further hope that in your own way, in doing so, you are somehow "better" for your acquaintance with Scott and his important work: We know that we are. Thank you, Scott.

Auburn, AL, USA — Cory L. Cobb
Binghamton, NY, USA — Steven Jay Lynn
Reno, NV, USA — William O'Donohue

References

Arkowitz, H., & Lilienfeld, S. O. (2017). *Facts and fictions in mental health.* Wiley.

Lilienfeld, S. O., Wood, J. M., & Garb, H. N. (2000). The scientific status of projective techniques. *Psychological Science in the Public Interest, 1*(2), 27–66.

Lilienfeld, S. O., Lynn, S. J., Ruscio, J., & Beyerstein, B. L. (2011). *50 great myths of popular psychology: Shattering widespread misconceptions about human behavior.* Wiley.

Lilienfeld, S. O., & O'Donohue, W. T. (Eds.). (2012). *The great ideas of clinical science: 17 principles that every mental health professional should understand.* Routledge.

Lilienfeld, S. O., Lynn, S. J., & Lohr, J. (Eds.) (2015). *Science and pseudoscience in clinical psychology*. Guilford.

Lilienfeld, S. O., Lynn, S. J., & Namy, L. (2022). *Psychology: From inquiry to understanding*. Pearson.

Satel, S., & Lilienfeld, S. O. (2013). *Brainwashed: The seductive appeal of mindless neuroscience*. Basic Civitas Books.

Wood, J. M., Nezworski, M. T., Lilienfeld, S. O., Garb, H. N., & Howard, N. (2003). *What's wrong with the Rorschach. Science confronts the controversial inkblot test.* Jossey-Bass.

Contents

About the Author

Cory L. Cobb is an Assistant Professor at Auburn University in the Department of Human Development and Family Science. Dr. Cobb received his PhD at the University of Central Arkansas in Counseling Psychology followed by two years of postdoctoral training in prevention science using randomized controlled trials at the University of Texas at Austin. His research focuses on the etiology and prevention of mental and behavioral health issues among Latino populations. Dr. Cobb also has interests in refining psychological science, particularly scientific issues related to the study of culture. As an early career psychologist, Dr. Cobb has published upwards of 40 peer-reviewed articles and has served on several editorial boards at top psychology journals. Dr. Cobb is currently an Action Editor at the International Journal of Intercultural Relations.

Part I
Personal Reflections

A Personal Commentary on Scott Lilienfeld

Candice Basterfield

Scott O. Lilienfeld died on September 30, 2020. He was 59 years old. The field of clinical psychology, and psychology more broadly, lost a pioneer, a brilliant scholar, gifted writer and teacher, beloved mentor, colleague, and friend. He was a mensch in every sense of the word. Scott fought a battle against a virulent form of cancer for several months and continued to work up until a few days before he died. In facing his life-threatening diagnosis, Scott found solace in the philosophy of stoicism and in the readings of Marcus Aurelius, a stoic Roman Emperor. Stoicism, an ancient philosophy, stresses that while we may not always have control over the events affecting us, we can have control over how we approach these events (Pigliucci, 2017). Scott faced his impending death as a man of courage and dignity and set an example I hope to follow when my time comes. I became acquainted with Scott's work in graduate school at the University of Melbourne, Australia. During my time in graduate school, I was lucky enough to attend one of his public lectures and got to meet him in Melbourne. We became friends and later we married.

Scott's obituary in the *New York Times* and the *Emory Wheel* captured many of his personal qualities that set him apart from many of us ordinary folk:

> "he helped change the thinking of psychopathy, in a profound way, by focusing on aspects of personality, rather than a list of bad behaviors." (Professor Mark Lenzenweger, Binghamton)
>
> "There was no one like him in his field." (Professor Steven Jay Lynn, Binghamton)
>
> "Scott was the perfect colleague and over the six years I served as chair in psychology, he was the closest thing to the ideal faculty member" …"He was a champion for what is

I would like to thank William O'Donohue, Cory Cobb, and Christopher Patrick for their helpful suggestions on an earlier draft of this chapter.

C. Basterfield (✉)
Department of Psychology, Penn State University, State College, PA, USA

C. L. Cobb et al. (eds.), *Toward a Science of Clinical Psychology*,
https://doi.org/10.1007/978-3-031-14332-8_1

> good and brilliant about psychology and worked tirelessly to make the field better." (Professor Harold Gouzoules, Emory University)
>
> "Dr. Lilienfeld was the best advisor a student could ever have." (Caroline Lee, Emory University student)
>
> Lilienfeld always "made his students feel supported" despite his busy work and global acclaim. (Shauna Bowes, Emory University graduate student)

Scott died at the zenith of his intellectual career, so it is safe to say that none of us will ever know the significance of his contributions that would have followed from his existing work. Therefore, it is only appropriate in this chapter I pay homage to his inestimable contributions to the field of psychology. I hope that this brief review of Scott's educational background and academic work provides readers with an appreciation of the richness of his thinking and effectively highlights some of his contributions to the field of clinical psychology. Admittedly, it is impossible to summarize all of Scott's academic contributions in a single chapter, which would likely require several books to achieve. Therefore, my goal in this chapter is to introduce the brilliant man that served as the primary motivation for this book. Toward this aim, I will highlight a few important milestones in Scott's academic career and share some personal anecdotes along the way.

Early Life and Education

Scott was born and raised in the New York borough of Queens. He grew up in a Jewish household, but from a young age he had his doubts about religion. When he turned 13 years old, he told his parents that he did not want to have a bar mitzvah because he was not sure if he believed in the existence of God. It is clear that Scott was precocious child who possessed a skeptical mindset from a very young age. His father, Ralph, was a radiologist, and his mother, Thelma, was a homemaker. Scott developed an interest in science from an early age, when his father would frequently take him to the American Museum of Natural History in New York City. Growing up, he was fascinated with astronomy and paleontology. Scott succeeded in academics and was the valedictorian of his high school. In his youth, he was an excellent chess player and would compete in chess competitions.

Scott received his bachelor's degree in Psychology from Cornell University in 1982. Although he was initially pre-med and enrolled to study astronomy, he later changed his major to psychology with a concentration in personality and social psychology. One of Scott's intellectual heroes was the late astronomer Carl Sagan, who happened to be teaching at Cornell when Scott was a student there. Scott was lucky enough to have a brief encounter with him at Cornell and later met him formally, at which point he was able to listen to Sagan talk at Cornell University. In an interview with the Association for Psychological Science's (APS) *Observer*, Scott explained how he ended up studying psychology:

> It was a long and circuitous path, especially because my first loves were the natural sciences, paleontology and astronomy in particular (my initial declared major at Cornell

> University, where I did my undergraduate work, was astronomy). I've always loved mysteries, and I know that both of these disciplines satisfied my high score on the investigative sector of Holland's hexagon of interests. For a brief time in college, I was also a premedical student. But—thanks in part to a high school course in psychology that sparked my interests—I decided to take a few psychology courses in my first two years in college, and I was hooked. Although my love for natural science never waned, I eventually fell in love with the mysteries of the internal world—the human mind—even more than those of the external world. (APS, 2010)

Scott went on to graduate studies in the clinical psychology program at the University of Minnesota, with specializations in psychopathology and psychophysiology. For his dissertation, Scott developed and validated a comprehensive measure of psychopathic personality, called the Psychopathic Personality Inventory (PPI), that was designed to assess the core personality dimensions of psychopathy (Latzman & Watts, 2020). In the years since its publication, PPI has become the most widely used and cited self-report measure of psychopathic personality. Minnesota luminary Paul Meehl, another of Scott's intellectual heroes, served as a member of his doctoral committee; Scott kept a letter from Professor Meehl on his office desk:

> From the desk of Paul E. Meehl, 6/11/90
>
> Thesis excellent. You will do yourself and Minnesota ψ proud in career. I've quoted Mike Elliot here: "We know how to select them, and then how to educate them". His insight. PM

Scott received his PhD in Clinical Psychology from the University of Minnesota in 1990 under the joint mentorship of David Lykken and James Butcher. He completed his clinical internship at Western Psychiatric Institute and Clinic in Pittsburgh from 1986 to 1987.

Career as a University Professor

Scott launched his academic career as an assistant professor in the Department of Psychology at SUNY Albany from 1990 through 1994, and then joined the faculty of the psychology department at Emory University. He was promoted to the rank of full professor at Emory in 2008, and also served as a visiting scholar in the School of Psychological Science at the University of Melbourne—Australia.

In addition to him being a top researcher in his field, Scott also made time for administrative and service-related activities. He participated in both departmental and university-related committees and held numerous leadership positions within the field (see Table 1).

Scott was known for being an outstanding reviewer and editor. He founded the *Scientific Review of Mental Health Practice*, a journal devoted to distinguishing science from pseudoscience in clinical psychology and allied fields and served as its Editor-in-Chief from 2000 to 2008. Over the last four years of his life (2016–2020), he served as Editor-in-Chief for the APS journal *Clinical Psychological Science*. He was also an Associate Editor for three other leading journals in the field, the *Journal*

Table 1 Major leadership positions held

2001–2002	Program Chair, Division 12 (Clinical Psychology), American Psychological Association Convention
2002–2003	Chair, Public Education and Media Committee, *Society for a Science of Clinical Psychology*, American Psychological Association, Division 12, Section 3
2002–2003; 2015–2016	President, *Society for a Science of Clinical Psychology*, American Psychological Association, Division 12, Section 3
2004–2008	Associate Editor, *Applied and Preventive Psychology*
2004–2016	Executive Board, *Society for the Scientific Study of Psychopathy*
2005–2016	Regular Columnist, with Hal Arkowitz, *Scientific American Mind* magazine
2010–2020	Executive Board, *Committee for Skeptical Inquiry*
2011–2016	Associate Editor, *Journal of Abnormal Psychology*
2013–2015	President, Society for the *Scientific Study of Psychopathy*
2014–2020	Associate Editor, *Archives of Scientific Psychopathy*
2016–2020	Editor-in-Chief, *Clinical Psychological Science*

of Abnormal Psychology (2011–2016), *Applied and Preventive Psychology* (2004–2008), and *Archives of Scientific Psychology* (2014–2020). Speaking to the depth and breadth of his knowledge of our discipline, Scott also served on the editorial boards of a number of other journals covering a range of subjects including the *Skeptical Inquire*r (1997–2020) and *Scientific American Mind* (2006–2020), to name a few.

A 2014 published survey cited Scott as one of the 350 most eminent psychologists of the modern era (Diener et al., 2014). Prior to this, he was named one of the 50 most productive researchers in United States clinical psychology programs (Stewart et al., 2007). Throughout his distinguished career, Scott has been the recipient of numerous awards for early career and lifetime achievements. Table 2 summarizes the awards and honors he received over the years. In recognition of his many scholarly contributions, APS established the Scott O. Lilienfeld Travel Award, a funding mechanism for graduate students presenting posters at the Society's annual convention.

In addition to his towering intellectual contributions to the field, Scott was a truly exceptional teacher and mentor of students. As an advisor, Scott was dedicated and selfless, continually devoting time to students and junior colleagues in various ways, including serving on master's and dissertation committees, providing career advice, writing letters of recommendation for students working both in and outside of his lab, and corresponding with students from around the globe. As one of Scott's last graduate students noted in a blog post: "Few professors take mentorship as seriously as Scott did in his life. His office door was literally always open to you, whether you were one of his students or not" (Bowes, 2020). A personal anecdote serves to illustrate Scott's generous nature as well as his commitment to his work. While Scott was undergoing chemotherapy, he would frequently provide in-depth emails to colleagues and prospective students in the field. He responded to every person that emailed him, regardless of their being a close colleague or an unfamiliar freshman student. Over time, it became difficult for Scott to type, so I would draft his emails

Table 2 Awards and honors

1998	David Shakow Award for Early Distinguished Contributions to Clinical Psychology, *American Psychological Association*, Division 12
1999	Selected for Emory University's "Great Teachers" Lecture Series (1999)
2004, 2010	*Association for Psychological Science*, "Psychology Superstars" Series
2005	Fellow, *Committee for Skeptical Inquiry*
2007	Fellow, *Association for Psychological Science*
2010	Fellow of the Institute of Science in Medicine
2010	Honorable mention, American Publishers' Awards for Scholarly and Professional Excellence in the Psychology Category for *50 Great Myths of Popular Psychology*
2011	Lifetime Achievement Award, *Connecticut Psychological Association*
2012	James McKeen Cattell Award for Lifetime Contributions to Applied Psychological Science, *Association for Psychological Science*
2013	Article on psychopathy in U.S. presidents named one of the Top 10 articles in psychology/neuroscience that year by *Forbes* magazine
2014	Ernst Hilgard Award for the Integration of Psychology Across Disciplines, *American Psychological Association*, Division 1
2014	David Myers Distinguished Lecturer on the Science and Craft of Teaching, *Association for Psychological Science*
2014	Finalist, Los Angeles Times Book Award, with Sally Satel, for *Brainwashed: The Seductive Appeal of Mindless Neuroscience*
2015	Martin Mayman Award for Distinguished Contributions to the Literature in Personality Assessment, with co-authors Allan R. Harkness and Shannon Reynolds Miles
2019	Robert D. Hare Lifetime Achievement Award, Society for the Scientific Study of Psychopathology
2019	Psychotherapy article of the year from *Journal of Contemporary Psychotherapy* for Meichenbaum, D., & Lilienfeld, S.O. (2018). How to spot hype in the field of psychotherapy: A 9-item checklist. *Professional Psychology: Research and Practice*, *49*, 22–20

as he dictated the thoughts he wished to convey. Although I would tell him it was unnecessary to respond to all messages from every person who wrote to him, given how sick he was, Scott viewed this as an important duty to be fulfilled. I found his determination to continue working productively while undergoing intense chemotherapy treatments and other adversities truly awe-inspiring.

Scott taught a diverse array of courses at Emory University including Personality Assessment, Personality Disorders, Introductory Psychology, Abnormal Psychology, Psychopathology, History of Psychology, and Science and Pseudoscience in Psychology, to name a few. His graduate students also undertook and completed research projects on diverse topics, demonstrating Scott's ability to guide students in whatever directions they wished to pursue (see Table 3 for a list of graduate students). Examples of dissertation titles he supervised include: "Childhood Psychopathic Features and Aggression: A Test of the Fearlessness Hypothesis" (Patrick Sylvers, 2010); "Risky Business: Psychopathy, Risky Decision-Making, and Financial Outcomes" (Sarah Smith, 2016); "The Mixed Effects of Neurological

Table 3 Graduate students

Graduate student	Affiliation
Brian P. Andrews	Ph.D., SUNY Albany (1995)
Tanya Hess	M.A., Emory University (1999)
Alex Morgan	M.A., Emory University (2001)
Stacey Zolondek	M.A., Emory University (2002)
Ellison Cale	Ph.D., Emory University (2003)
Katherine Fowler	Ph.D., Emory University (2007)
Patrick Sylvers	Ph.D., Emory University (2010)
Meredith Jones	Ph.D., Emory University (2011)
Erin Collier	M.A., Emory University (2009)
Joanna Berg	Ph.D., Emory University (2016)
Sarah Francis Smith	Ph.D., Emory University (2016)
Annelore Roose	Ph.D., University of Leuven (2013)
Ashley L. Watts	Ph.D., Emory University (2017)
Brett Murphy	Ph.D., Emory University (2018)
Thomas Costello	M.A., Emory University (2018)
Shauna Bowes	M.A., Emory University (2019)

Information and Brain Images on Perceptions of Psychopathic Wrongdoers" (Julia Marshall, 2015); "Confidence but Clueless?: The Nature and Boundaries of the Link Between Personality Disorder Features and Self-enhancement" (Ashley Watts, 2018); "Expanding the Nomological Network of Intellectual Humility: An Examination of Personality Traits, Cognitive Styles, Critical-Thinking, and Self-Perception" (Shauna Bowes, 2019); "The Varieties of Self-Reported Empathic Tendencies" (Brett Murphy, 2019). These varied dissertation titles illustrate the wide range of themes that occupied Scott and his students, as well as Scott's evolving research interests.

Scientist, Researcher, and Iconoclast

Scott authored, co-authored, and co-edited more than 350 articles and book chapters along with 20 books, including one of the field's most popular introductory textbooks (see Lilienfeld et al., 2018). He published on a wide range of topics including personality disorders, anxiety disorders, dissociative disorders, psychiatric classification, pseudoscience in psychology, teaching of psychology, evidence-based practice (EBP), and intellectual humility. As evidenced by this broad range of interests, Scott was a generalist (Witkowski, 2020), which is incredibly rare in today's hyper-specialist academy. The subsections that follow highlight Scott's contributions in some of his areas of research.

The Etiology and Assessment of Personality Disorders and Personality Traits

Scott's initial work focused on why self-reported measures of psychopathy showed poor agreement, which he concluded was due to the measures' inadequate content coverage of relevant constructs (Lilienfeld & Andrews, 1996). In particular, most measures of psychopathy focused on socially undesirable behaviors (e.g., focus on robbery, arrest, and vandalism), and were largely assessed by overt antisocial and criminal behavior rather than personality traits deemed central to psychopathic personality (Lilienfeld, 1994, 1998). His development of the PPI culminated in a new and comprehensive personality-based measure that filled an important gap in the assessment of psychopathy and was one of the first measures to forge closer research linkages between the disconnected domains of personality and psychopathology (Lilienfeld, 1990, 1998).

Scott also redefined our understanding of personality disorders and psychopathology more broadly. He conceptualized personality disorders as multidimensional and heterogeneous conditions (Lilienfeld et al., 2015a, b, 2019), as opposed to a unitary construct or taxon (a natural category, Meehl & Golden, 1982). In addition, he separated key features of psychopathy into three higher-order dimensions—self-centered impulsivity, cold-heartedness, and fearless dominance (Lilienfeld et al., 2015a, b; Lilienfeld & Windows, 2005). Despite the long-held tradition of linking psychopathic personality to socially undesirable behaviors such as physical aggression (Cale & Lilienfeld, 2006) and substance abuse (Magyar et al., 2011), Scott's research led him to believe that certain psychopathic traits may be linked to prosocial behaviors (i.e., expressed as "successful psychopathy") across a range of real-world domains, such as helping individuals in distress, donating blood, and holding positions of leadership (Lilienfeld, 1994; Lilienfeld et al., 2014a, b, c). In particular, fearless dominance, which reflects fearlessness and social dominance, has been associated with adaptive correlates like successful leadership (Lilienfeld et al., 2012).

Pseudoscientific Practices and Beliefs in Clinical Psychology

Beyond his work in refining key concepts like psychopathy, Scott was also outspoken about the dangers of pseudoscience in clinical psychology. His work challenged the validity of some widespread diagnostic tools and therapies such as pseudoscientific autism therapies, eye movement desensitization and reprocessing (EMDR), projective tests, recovered memory therapy, and lie detectors. Scott pursued some of the most difficult topics in psychology and did so with both intellectual courage and humility. Nevertheless, his work was considered controversial in many corners of academia and, at times, he was criticized for exposing poorly conducted psychological science.

In particular, Scott wrote extensively about projective tests, particularly the Rorschach Test, showing that the test has limited validity for predicting psychiatric conditions and personality traits (Lilienfeld et al., 2001). This work culminated in a popular book, co-authored with colleagues, titled *What's Wrong with the Rorschach?* This book reviewed findings from work using the Rorschach test over the period of half a century and concluded that its clinical use is scientifically questionable (see Wood et al., 2003).

In 2015, Scott, along with Thomas E. Heinzen and Susan A. Nolan, published a popular book called *The Horse That Won't Go Away: Clever Hans, Facilitated Communication, and the Need for Clear Thinking*, which told the story of the horse, Clever Hans, who was supposed to be able to perform difficult arithmetic operations by stomping his right foot. However, it was discovered that the horse was being unconsciously cued to give the right answer by watching his owner, because he was unable to perform mathematical problems when his owner was out of sight. The authors drew parallels between the Clever Hans phenomenon and facilitated communication (FC), and showed how in FC there was unconscious, inadvertent facilitator control over ostensible communications of autistic children (Heinzen et al., 2015; Lilienfeld et al., 2014a, b, c).

Scott was also skeptical about novel treatments claiming to be panaceas. For example, when EMDR came onto the psychotherapeutic scene, it was heralded as a breakthrough in the treatment of anxiety disorders. Commenting on this enthusiasm for EMDR, Scott wrote: "In my experience as an instructor of graduate students in clinical psychology and allied fields for three decades, one of the most widespread thinking errors that I have encountered, among even the best and brightest of students, is what I term "breakthrough-ism" (see Lilienfeld, 2017a about "breakthrough-ism"): the tendency to regard novel interventions as breakthroughs rather than merely as potentially-promising techniques that may be worthy of investigation" (Lilienfeld, 2018).

In 2012, Scott published a thought piece on the topic of public skepticism regarding psychology (Lilienfeld, 2012a), in which he argued that overhyping of novel psychological treatments may backfire and fuel public skepticism toward psychology, because psychologists are not likely able to deliver on overhyped claims. Although EMDR was heralded a breakthrough in the treatment of anxiety disorders, there continues to be no good evidence that EMDR is superior to theoretically established exposure-based treatments, which cognitive–behavioral therapists have been administering for decades (Arkowitz & Lilienfeld, 2012; Lilienfeld, 1996). Nevertheless, Scott was always amenable to change his mind in light of new evidence; for example, he said: "Because of the limited number of controlled studies on EMDR, both practitioners and scientists should remain open to the possibility to its effectiveness" (Lilienfeld, 1996, p. 30). As the late astrophysicist Carl Sagan (1995) noted the capacity to admit when one is mistaken is the hallmark of a genuine scientist.

Evidence-Based Psychological Practice

Scott was also at the forefront of the movement toward evidence-based practice (EBP) in clinical psychology and wrote eloquent conceptual papers on this topic, which have helped our field to think clearly about potentially harmful psychotherapeutic interventions and how we can be fooled into believing these ineffective therapies work. In particular, Scott was especially interested in the application of scientific thinking to clinical psychology and played a major role in distinguishing evidence-based from pseudoscientific practices. In 2007, he published a comprehensive review—which has been cited over 1000 times—of scientific studies showing that certain psychological treatments may cause harm to people they are meant to help (Lilienfeld, 2007). For example, recovered memory techniques, such as repeated therapist prompting of memories and hypnosis, may potentially be harmful and lead to the production of false memories of trauma; in a similar vein, dissociative identity therapy may lead to the production of "alter" personalities through similar suggestive techniques and therapist prompting (Lilienfeld, 2007; Lilienfeld & Arkowitz, 2011). This was followed by an influential book that Scott co-edited, *Science and Pseudoscience in Clinical Psychology*, which reviewed several therapies with the aim of distinguishing scientific from pseudoscientific practices (see Lilienfeld et al., 2015a, b). In a 2013 article on why clinical psychologists are resistant to evidence-based practice, Scott and several colleagues noted that resistance to EBP stems largely from a multitude of sources such as naïve realism and psychological misconceptions, which may make therapists susceptible to rejecting EBP in favor of their clinical intuition (Lilienfeld et al., 2013). A corollary on this topic was followed by another conceptual article on why ineffective psychotherapies appear to work, in which Scott and colleagues highlighted several cognitive errors that can contribute to spurious therapeutic effectiveness, such as naïve realism (e.g., "seeing is believing"), confirmation bias (e.g., the tendency to look for evidence that confirms existing beliefs), and illusory correlation (e.g., perceiving a relationship between variables even when no such relationship exists; Lilienfeld et al., 2014a, b, c).

Heterodox Scholar

More recently, Scott stepped into an ideological battlefield of microaggression research. In 2017, he published a critique of the scientific basis for microaggressions, which have been described subtle snubs, slights, and insults that are directed toward minority-group individuals on an ongoing basis (Lilienfeld, 2017b). In this article, he argued that this concept is inherently subjective in nature and difficult to define (i.e., an "open concept"; see Meehl, 1977, for a discussion), because it does not take into account the motives of the offender or the perceptions of the victim (Lilienfeld, 2017a, b). Although Scott viewed the existing body of research on microaggression to be scientifically problematic, he was always intellectually circumspect, admitting that new research could change his mind and situate the concept on sturdier scientific ground, unlike some of his critics who insisted upon the validity of claims set forth by the microaggression concept. For example, regarding his interpretation of the microaggression research program, Scott stated, "It is entirely possible that future research will alter some of these verdicts" (Lilienfeld, 2017a). This exemplifies Scott's open-mindedness and intellectual humility with regard to the ultimate truth. One can only wish that more people were open to changing their minds in the face of contradictory evidence. In referring to Carl Sagan's book, *The Demon-Haunted World*, Sagan wrote: "Keeping an open mind is a virtue—but, as the space engineer James Oberg once said, not so open that your brains fall out" (1995, p. 187). I like this quotation and think it is particularly germane to Scott's scientific and skeptical mindset, as well as his openness to altering his viewpoint in light of new evidence—the hallmark of a true scientist and scholar.

Scott was not afraid to challenge mainstream psychological assumptions, and his heterodox views often opened the floodgates to hate mail, frequently from people emotionally invested in certain concepts. Scott acknowledged that he had fallen prey at times himself to emotional reasoning when it came to evaluate scientific claims. For example, he said, "I see this kind of reasoning a lot among many students and even among some psychologists. If an idea made me angry or ran counter to my sociopolitical beliefs, I rejected it out of hand" (Zinn, 2010, p. 287). Scott had an insatiable desire to understand complex psychological phenomenon no matter how contentious the topic. Although he received his fair share of hate mail from scholars within the field and individuals in the public at large, he had little concern for political correctness and was guided by a desire to apply psychological science to better humankind.

Scott was concerned about the trend toward ideological uniformity in psychology (Lilienfeld, 2015, 2020), and for this reason was passionate about fostering viewpoint diversity in academia. He was among the first to join Heterodox Academy, a nonpartisan collaboration of professors, administrators, and students committed to "open inquiry, viewpoint diversity, and constructive disagreement in institutions of higher learning." In 2020, he edited a section of the *Archives of Scientific Psychology* on heterodox issues in psychology. His introduction, in the section titled *Embracing Unpopular Ideas: Introduction to the Special Section on Heterodox Issues in Psychology*, discusses the many ways in which heterodox views can facilitate scientific progress by exposing us to different psychological perspectives that contrast with our own, and in the process increase our intellectual humility (Lilienfeld, 2020; see also Lilienfeld, 2007).

Intellectual Humility

Intellectual humility has been defined as being aware of one's intellectual limitations and cognitive biases in order to arrive at a closer approximation of the truth (Lilienfeld & Bowes, 2020; O'Donohue et al., 2017). Scott set an example of what it meant to be intellectually humble. He was open to alternative opinions, encouraged viewpoint diversity, and was able to change his mind when new evidence challenged his initial ideas. For example, his commitment to intellectual humility is embodied in his statement: "Just as I try to model thoughtful uncertainty in my research—taking intellectual risks while acknowledging that I might be wrong—I try to do the same in my teaching. That is, I try to model for students the hybrid stance of the good scientist that Carl Sagan articulated so well—insisting on rigorous evidence for all claims while remaining open to the possibility that these claims might be wrong" (Zinn, 2010, p. 289).

In recent years, Scott was funded by the Templeton Foundation to investigate whether intellectual humility may temper extremism and polarization, and if so, whether it is a skill that can be taught and learned. Although not opposed to external funding, Scott was concerned about the growing trend for psychology departments to expect faculty to acquire external funding in order to secure tenure and promotion. In particular, he believed that the grant culture in academic departments posed problems for the scholarly goals of psychological science (Lilienfeld, 2017c). For example, he was concerned that increased pressure to obtain grants might lead to academic hyperspecialization (Lilienfeld, 2017d). In an article in the *APS Observer*, Scott lamented that big-picture thinkers of the past such as Paul Meehl, Lee J. Cronbach, Donald Campbell, Lloyd Humphreys, Jane Loevinger, and Robyn Dawes have become increasingly rare in academia and may be at risk of extinction in the current grant climate (Lilienfeld, 2017d). In a tongue-in-cheek letter to university administrators, which Scott posted outside his office door, he wrote:

> Dear University or College Administrator: Please do not ask me to engage in fund-raising on behalf of our academic institution. That is your job and that of your fellow administrators, not mine. I am here to contribute to the production and dissemination of scholarship, not to assist you with making money. I will apply for grants to help me conduct my research if and when it is necessary. Asking me to apply for funding (and, in most cases, to take taxpayer dollars) when it is not needed is wasteful, counterproductive and, in some cases, almost certainly unethical. Please do your job, and please allow me to do mine, Now, if you'll kindly excuse me, I have some research, teaching, mentoring, and service to do.

According to his CV, Scott attained approximately nine grants; however, he only had one major grant, from the Templeton Foundation, on which he served as the principal investigator (PI). Despite the fact that he only served as PI on one major grant project, Scott is still regarded as one of the most eminent psychologists of the modern era (Diener et al., 2014). Scott once told me that he was skeptical as to whether he could secure tenure in the current academic climate. It is interesting to think, if Scott were starting out now, whether his career trajectory would have taken the same path in light of increasing pressure to secure external funding. Of note, another big-picture thinker, Paul Meehl, only secured one grant in his academic career (Lilienfeld, 2017d).

Science Communicator and Author

In addition to publishing more than 350 academic journal articles and writing or editing over 20 books, Scott was also deeply committed to disseminating psychological science to the general public. During his 1998 APA Division 12 Early Career Award address, he said "…as academic clinical psychologists we have not done enough to popularize our findings and to communicate the scientific side of our discipline to the general public…we have done little to assist the public with distinguishing those practices within popular psychology that are scientific from those that are not" (Lilienfeld, 2012b, p. 67).

Scott was a phenomenal science communicator and his work was featured in many major public forums including *USA Today*, *Washington Post*, *Los Angeles Times*, *Chronicle of Higher Education*, *New York Times*, and *Science News*, among others. He was especially fond of publishing in the *Skeptical Inquirer*, a periodical devoted to critical thinking and debate, to which he contributed 26 articles. From 2006 to 2015, Scott was also a regular contributor, along with the late Hal Arkowitz, to a column in *Scientific American Mind* magazine titled *Facts and Fictions in Mental Health*, which was later turned into a popular book under the same name. In addition, Scott had a *Psychology Today* column, *The Skeptical Psychologist*, in which he wrote about questionable, controversial, and novel claims in psychology. He also co-authored popular science books including *Brainwashed—The Seductive Appeal of Mindless Neuroscience* (with Sally Satel), which was a finalist for the Los Angeles Times Book Award. In addition, Scott co-authored *50 Great Myths of Popular Psychology*, which was translated into 20 languages. This book examines 50 major misconceptions about human behavior that are prevalent in psychology—such as the notion that opposites attract in romantic relationships, that memory operates like a videotape, that people use only 10% of their brain power, that individuals with schizophrenia have multiple personalities, and that paranormal phenomena like extrasensory perception exist in reality—and challenges these with credible scientific data. The book is a testament to Scott's remarkable breadth and depth of knowledge regarding psychological science and his ability to write about complex psychological concepts with clarity and humility. In response to being asked what his contributions to the field have been, Scott responded:

> That's a difficult question to answer, as I honestly don't know how much of a lasting contribution I've made. I'm well aware that even the most successful of us can hope only to exert a slight impact on how others think. But my hope is that perhaps I can make a small dent in persuading my colleagues that scientific thinking shouldn't merely be a desideratum, but rather an essential component, of psychology courses. In particular, I hope to persuade at least some of them that teaching students to think critically requires one to inculcate in them a sense of their own fallibility and propensity toward error and an

> understanding that scientific methods—although by no means perfect—are essential safeguards against such error. (Zinn, 2010, p. 292)

It is clear that Scott far exceeded his humble expectations of being able to help readers improve their critical thinking skills and in making psychological science accessible to the general public.

Parting Thoughts

Scott was a pioneer and an iconoclast in the field who had the courage to question conventional wisdom in psychological science, and, in the process, situated the field of clinical science on firmer scientific ground. While his work at times touched a nerve, Scott's ultimate goal was always to improve psychological science and make the world a better place. His deep intellectual desire to understand psychological phenomena, coupled with remarkable open-mindedness and humility, led to a number of pioneering contributions. Scott's early research changed the face of how we conceptualize psychopathic personality by situating psychopathy within broader personality domains, and in subsequent ones he advanced understanding in multiple other areas. He had the courage to speak up about ill-conceived harmful psychological treatments such as facilitated communication, multiple personality disorder, and recovered memory therapy, and he played a major role in distinguishing evidence-based from pseudoscientific practices in clinical psychology.

He was an intellectual who stepped into the public sphere to combat pop psychology and fads, and whose books and columns helped people distinguish popular practices within psychology that are scientific from those that are not. In doing so, his work has improved psychology's public image and perception in the media. As one of Scott's heroes, the late civil-rights advocate John Lewis, said: "Never be afraid to make some noise and get in good trouble" (Tweet from June 2018). Scott lived up to those words until the very end.

References

Arkowitz, H., & Lilienfeld, S.O. (2012, August). EMDR: Taking a closer look. *Scientific American, 17*(4s), 10–11. https://www.scientificamerican.com/article/emdr-taking-a-closer-look/

Association for Psychological Science. (2010, October 1). *Champions of psychological science: Scott O. Lilienfeld.* APS Observer. https://www.psychologicalscience.org/observer/scott-o-lilienfeld

Bowes, S. (2020, October 2). Reflecting on the life and legacy of Scott Lilienfeld. *Psychology Today.* https://www.psychologytoday.com/us/blog/dont-believe-everything-you-think/202010/reflecting-the-life-and-legacy-scott-lilienfeld

Cale, E. M., & Lilienfeld, S. O. (2006). Psychopathy factors and risk for aggressive behavior: A test of the "threatened egotism" hypothesis. *Law and Human Behavior, 30*, 51–74.

Carey, B. (2020, October 16). Scott lilienfeld, psychologist who questioned psychology, dies at 59. *New York Times*.
Diener, E., Oishi, S., & Park, J. (2014). An incomplete list of eminent psychologists of the modern era. *Archives of Scientific Psychology, 2*(1), 20–32.
Heinzen, T. E., Lilienfeld, S. O., & Nolan, S. A. (2015). The horse that won't go away: Clever Hans, facilitated communication and the need for clear thinking. New York: Worth Publishers
Huynh, A. (2020, October 7). Emory Community Mourns loss of renowned psychology professor Scott Lilienfeld. *Emory Wheel*. https://emorywheel.com/emory-community-mourns-loss-of-renowned-psychology-professor-scott-lilienfeld/
Latzman, R. D., & Watts, A. L. (2020). In Memoriam: Dr. Scott O. Lilienfeld, 1960–2020. *Journal of Personality Disorders, 34*, 721–722.
Lilienfeld, S. O. (1990). *Development and preliminary validation of a self-report measure of psychopathic personality*. Unpublished doctoral dissertation, University of Minnesota, Minneapolis.
Lilienfeld, S. O. (1994). Conceptual problems in the assessment of psychopathy. *Clinical Psychology Review, 14*, 17–38.
Lilienfeld, S. O. (1996). EMDR treatment. *Skeptical Inquirer, 20*, 25–31.
Lilienfeld, S. O. (1998). Methodological advances and developments in the assessment of psychopathy. *Behaviour Research and Therapy, 36*, 99–125.
Lilienfeld, S. O. (2007). Psychological treatments that cause harm. *Perspectives on Psychological Science, 2*(1), 53–70.
Lilienfeld, S. O. (2012a). Public skepticism of psychology: Why many people perceive the study of human behavior as unscientific. *American Psychologist, 67*, 111–129.
Lilienfeld, S. O. (2012b). Pseudoscience in contemporary clinical psychology: What it is and what we can do about it. In S. O. Lilienfeld & W. T. O'Donohue (Eds.), *Great readings in clinical science: Essential selections for mental health professions* (pp. 66–71). Pearson.
Lilienfeld, S. O. (2015). Lack of political diversity and the framing of findings in personality and clinical psychology. *Behavioral and Brain Sciences, 38*, 1–58.
Lilienfeld, S. O. (2017a). Knowledge of the history of clinical psychology: A partial antidote against "Breakthrough-ism". *Society for the Science of Clinical Psychology*. http://www.sscpweb.org/resources/PDFs/Newsletter/2017/Clinical%20Science%2020(3)%20Fall%20 2017.pdf
Lilienfeld, S. O. (2017b, June). Microaggressions? *Aeon*. https://aeon.co/essays/why-a-moratorium-on-microaggressions-policies-is-needed
Lilienfeld, S. O. (2017c). Psychology's replication crisis and the grant culture: Righting the ship. *Perspectives on Psychological Science, 12*, 660–664.
Lilienfeld, S. O. (2017d, September 29). Seven costs of the money chase: How academia's focus on funding influences scientific progress. *APS Observer*. https://www.psychologicalscience.org/observer/seven-costs-of-the-money-chase-how-academias-focus-on-funding-influences-scientific-progress
Lilienfeld, S. O. (2018). Avoiding the dangers of psychological hype: Studying the history of psychology as a corrective. *Society for the Teaching of Psychology*. https://teachpsych.org/page-1784686/6375500
Lilienfeld, S. O. (2020). Embracing unpopular ideas: Introduction to the special section on heterodox issues in psychology. *Archives of Scientific Psychology, 8*, 1–4.
Lilienfeld, S. O., & Andrews, B. P. (1996). Development and preliminary validation of a self-report measure of psychopathic personality traits in noncriminal population. *Journal of Personality Assessment, 66*, 488–524.
Lilienfeld, S. O., & Arkowitz, H. (2011). Can people have multiple personalities? *Scientific American Mind, 4*, 64–64. https://www.scientificamerican.com/article/can-people-have-multiple-personalities/
Lilienfeld, S. O., & Bowes, S. M. (2020). Intellectual humility: Ten unresolved questions. In P. Graf (Ed.), *The State of the Art in Applied Psychology*. Wiley.

Lilienfeld, S. O., & Windows, M. R. (2005). *Psychopathic personality inventory-revised: Professional manual*. Psychological Assessment Resources.
Lilienfeld, S. O., Wood, J. M., & Garb, H. N. (2001). The scientific status of projective techniques. *Psychological Science in the Public Interest, 1*, 27–66.
Lilienfeld, S. O., Waldman, I. D., Landfield, K., Watts, A. L., Rubenzer, S., & Faschingbauer, T. R. (2012). Fearless dominance and the US presidency: Implications of psychopathic personality traits for successful and unsuccessful political leadership. *Journal of Personality and Social Psychology, 103*, 489–505.
Lilienfeld, S. O., Ritschel, L. A., Lynn, S. J., Cautin, R. L., & Latzman, R. D. (2013). Why many clinical psychologists are resistant to evidence-based practice: Root causes and constructive remedies. *Clinical Psychology Review, 33*, 883–900.
Lilienfeld, S. O., Latzman, R. D., Watts, A. L., Smith, S. F., & Dutton, K. (2014a). Correlates of psychopathic personality traits in everyday life: Results from a large community survey. *Frontiers in Psychology, 5*, 1–11.
Lilienfeld, S. O., Marshall, J., Todd, J. T., & Shane, H. C. (2014b). The persistence of fad interventions in the face of negative scientific evidence: Facilitated communication for autism as a case example. *Evidence-Based Communication Assessment and Intervention, 8*, 62–101.
Lilienfeld, S. O., Ritschel, L. A., Lynn, S. J., Cautin, R. L., & Latzman, R. D. (2014c). Why ineffective psychotherapies appear to work: A taxonomy of causes of spurious therapeutic effectiveness. *Perspectives on Psychological Science, 9*, 355–387.
Lilienfeld, S. O., Lynn, S. J., & Lohr, J. M. (2015a). *Science and pseudoscience in clinical psychology* (2nd ed.).
Lilienfeld, S. O., Watts, A. L., Francis Smith, S., Berg, J. M., & Latzman, R. D. (2015b). Psychopathy deconstructed and reconstructed: Identifying and assembling the personality building blocks of Cleckley's chimera. *Journal of Personality, 83*, 593–610.
Lilienfeld, S. O., Lynn, S. J., & Namy, L. L. (2018). *Psychology: From inquiry to understanding* (4th ed.). Pearson.
Lilienfeld, S. O., Watts, A. L., Murphy, B., Costello, T. H., Bowes, S. M., Smith, S. F., Latzman, R. D., & Tabb, K. (2019). Personality disorders as emergent interpersonal syndromes: Psychopathic personality as a case example. *Journal of Personality Disorders, 33*, 577–622.
Magyar, M. S., Edens, J. F., Lilienfeld, S. O., Douglas, K. S., & Poythress, N. G., Jr. (2011). Examining the relationship among substance abuse, negative emotionality and impulsivity across subtypes of antisocial and psychopathic substance abusers. *Journal of Criminal Justice, 39*, 232–237.
Meehl, P. E. (1977). Specific etiology and other forms of strong influence: Some quantitative meanings. *The Journal of Medicine and Philosophy, 2*(1), 33–53.
Meehl, P. E., & Golden, R. (1982). Taxometric methods. In P. Kendall & J. Butcher (Eds.), *Handbook of research methods in clinical psychology* (pp. 127–181). Wiley.
O'Donohue, W., Casas, J. B., Szoke, D. R., Cheung, D., Hmaidan, R. I., & Burleigh, K. J. (2017). Scientific progress in clinical psychology and epistemically virtuous research. *Behavior and Philosophy, 45*, 44–62.
Pigliucci, M. (2017). *How to be a Stoic: Using ancient philosophy to live a modern life*. Basic Books.
Sagan, C. (1995). *The demon-haunted world: Science as a candle in the dark*. The Random House Publishing Group.
Stewart, P. K., Wu, Y. P., & Roberts, M. C. (2007). Top producers of scholarly publications in clinical psychology PhD programs. *Journal of Clinical Psychology, 63*, 1209–1215.
Witkowski, T. (2020). *Shaping psychology*. Palgrave Macmillan.
Wood, J. M., Nezworski, M. T., Lilienfeld, S. O., & Garb, H. N. (2003). *What's wrong with the Rorschach? Science confronts the controversial inkblot test*. Jossey-Bass.
Zinn, T. E. (2010). The pleasures and lessons of academic mythbusting: An interview with Scott Lilienfeld. *Teaching of Psychology, 37*, 287–293.

Scott Lilienfeld: Friend, Colleague, Champion of Science

Lori Marino

Scott and I met in 1990 at the State University of New York at Albany (SUNY-Albany) and became fast friends. I was a graduate student well on my way toward a PhD in biopsychology, and he had begun his first tenure-track faculty position in clinical psychology. We married in 1992 in upstate New York and, in 1994, moved to Emory University where he was offered an assistant professorship in the Department of Psychology, and I completed my PhD and later became a lecturer in Neuroscience and Behavioral Biology. Although we divorced in 2004, we remained the close friends and colleagues we were always meant to be until his passing on September 30, 2020.

Early in our relationship we discovered that we shared some of the same passions about psychology, science, and the responsibility all scholars have to apply their knowledge to make the world better. In my case, as a neuroscientist and comparative psychologist who has studied dolphins and whales, and also primates, elephants, and farmed animals for many years, I have made it a focus of my career to use my knowledge of these animals to advocate for their protection and well-being. In Scott's case, it was as a clinical psychologist and scholar-advocate for legitimate science in all of its forms. Scott was a trailblazer in using scholarship to protect others from the harms of exploitive clinical practices and pseudoscience claims. We formed a powerful alliance that attests to the unique value of collaboration across disciplines and Scott's broad perspective and interests.

Between 1998 and 2021 we published nine papers together. In two of those papers, we focused on identifying personality characteristics in our closest evolutionary relatives, common chimpanzees. In contrast to the study of personality traits in humans, research on personality in other animals was a late starter. Indeed, up until recently, other animals were denied the capacity for personality and individual

L. Marino (✉)
Kimmela Center for Scholarship-Based Animal Advocacy, Kanab, UT, USA

Whale Sanctuary Project, Kanab, UT, USA

C. L. Cobb et al. (eds.), *Toward a Science of Clinical Psychology*,
https://doi.org/10.1007/978-3-031-14332-8_2

differences. On the other hand, when personality in other animals *was* acknowledged it was often based on claims that were anthropomorphic (in the true sense of the word).

Scott and I collaborated with animal personality expert Sam Gosling (Gosling et al., 2003) to help lay the groundwork for key concepts and definitions of personality, created a framework for evaluating evidence for personality traits in chimpanzees, and set up a list of workable criteria for assessing personality across species. In doing all of this we also discussed criteria for normal and abnormal behavior in other species, and, in particular, other primates. For instance, in Lilienfeld et al. (1999) we developed validation methods for assessing the construct of psychopathy in chimpanzees. This paper was important because it not only showed that chimpanzees shared basic personality characteristics with humans, but that very complex psychopathological personality factors, such as psychopathy, were also shared.

Scott's work in the area of comparative psychology was not limited to the two studies he and I co-authored (see the section below on our work on dolphin-assisted therapy (DAT)). In fact, Scott made substantial contributions to establishing the field of primate personality research with many other collaborations, including Latzman et al. (2016) and Maestripieri and Lilienfeld (2016). In these two papers, Scott and his co-authors addressed conceptual and diagnostic issues of nonhuman primate psychopathology.

Scott's contributions to our understanding of nonhuman primate personality assessment were important for several reasons. First, he helped to bring rigor to the conceptualization and assessment of personality traits in other primate species and, in doing so, moved the study of primate personality and psychopathology into a modern disciplinary framework. Second, through this work he contributed to a shift in how we view other animals, lending credibility and rigor to evidence for personality and individual differences in nonhuman primates. This shift, generally, represented a step forward in ways that go beyond individual papers because our ability to view our primate relatives (and other animals) as individuals with complex personalities and psychologies is vital for advancing our sense of empathy and respect for them. It is also vital for placing human psychology and behavior in an evolutionary perspective.

My own research with another mammal species, bottlenose dolphins, and the ethics of captivity, were brought into direct confrontation when, in 2001, I conducted a research study that showed bottlenose dolphins can recognize themselves in mirrors (Reiss & Marino, 2001). Diana Reiss and I conducted the study with two young dolphins held at the New York Aquarium. Up to that point, only humans and great apes (chimpanzees, bonobos, orangutans, and one gorilla) showed mirror self-recognition. The implications of the findings with dolphins were profound for both science and ethics. The knowledge gained from this study was a major contribution to our understanding of the phenomenon of self-recognition and how it is distributed among species in the animal kingdom. But my work also led me to delve into the backgrounds of the dolphins in my study. And then I learned about the lives of captive dolphins and whales in other facilities around the world. And what I discovered was an industry of exploitation and abuse that led me to give up research with captive dolphins altogether. Instead of exploiting them, I wanted to use my scientific knowledge and experience to advocate for these animals.

Modern-day zoos and aquariums market themselves as places of education and conservation. One paper in 2007 was widely heralded as the first direct evidence that visits to zoos and aquariums produce long-term positive effects on people's attitudes toward other animals, thus contributing to pro-conservation behaviors (Falk et al., 2007). I set about evaluating the validity of this claim and enlisted a team of knowledgeable co-authors. Scott was prominent on that list. I knew that Scott would be able to bring a penetrating assessment to these kinds of questions because of his deep understanding of testing and survey methodology. I understood the animals themselves, but Scott was a virtuoso at analyzing the validity of research claims. And he was always passionate about applying that knowledge to influence the lives and well-being of humans as well as other animals. Scott's incisive critical thinking formed the backbone of that methodological review. We highlighted a major conceptual weakness from the outset. The authors' stated goal was to assess whether zoo and aquarium experiences affect visitors' beliefs and knowledge. With regard to knowledge, however, Falk et al. assessed only what responders said they believed or understood; they administered no direct measures of knowledge. Scott knew that there is copious literature on the inaccuracies associated with self-report measures, and Falk et al. was a textbook example of erroneously using self-report to infer actual changes in knowledge and attitude. We also concluded that Falk et al. (2007) contained at least six more specific major threats to methodological validity that undermined the authors' conclusions (Marino et al., 2010). As such, there remains no compelling evidence for the claim that zoos and aquariums promote attitude change, education, or interest in conservation in visitors, although further investigation of this possibility using methodologically sophisticated designs is warranted.

After that paper and a response from Falk and his colleagues, we published yet another paper—a rejoinder—to Falk's protestations. We concluded, once again, that there was still no evidence to support their claims (Marino et al., 2011).

While a more unforgiving response to the Falk paper may have been justified, Scott's influence elevated our paper and our conclusions in a way that impressed me. Scott was never arrogant and always intellectually humble and, moreover, openhearted in his approach to critiquing scientific and pseudoscientific claims. While he suffered no fools gladly and was clear and direct when he critiqued claims, he did so in a straightforward, unassuming, and also authoritative way that should continue to be a model for all—as it was for me. In our conclusion to the 2011 paper, we wrote:

> …we hope that readers will hold Falk and colleagues to high scholarly standards. Science, as McFall (1996) observed, is about humility— not making assertions that outstrip the data. Regrettably, Falk et al. (2010) violate this cardinal principle by advancing claims regarding the effectiveness of zoo and aquarium visits that are not backed by evidence. We look forward to an appropriate assessment of these claims in adequately designed studies that are free of serious interpretational shortcomings. (Marino et al., 2011, p. 292)

This statement is a prime example of Scott's style of not criticizing for the sake of being correct but for the sake of promoting better science to everyone, including those he disagreed with.

Our collaborations did not always involve applying Scott's expertise in research methodology and psychopathy to animal issues. We also combined my interest and background in evolutionary theory and his in psychopathology to investigate concepts in human psychopathology and its classification in professional psychology manuals like the *Diagnostic and Statistical Manual of Mental Disorders* (APA, 2013). In Lilienfeld and Marino (1995) we took on the work of Jerome Wakefield, the multidisciplinary scholar who proposed a novel idea about the concept of mental disorder. Framing the issue in evolutionary terms, Wakefield said that mental disorder is best conceptualized as a "harmful dysfunction," whereby "harm" is a value judgment regarding the undesirability of a condition, and "dysfunction" is the failure of a system to function as designed by natural selection (Wakefield, 1992a, b, 1993).

We found much to agree with in Wakefield's ideas but argued that there were several problems with his conceptualization of disorder. One of our main criticisms of his stance was that natural selection does not "design" anything and does not produce bright lines in nature. Evolution proceeds through a process of adaptations as well as adaptively neutral exaptations, as put forth by Gould (1991) and many others, for example, Piatelli-Palmarini (1989). And while we acknowledged that Wakefield was not promoting the idea of purposeful design in evolution, we felt that the basic assumption of essentialism did not fit with the dynamic and messy process of natural selection. We went on to discuss how disorders are not always failures of evolved systems. Several recognized disorders, for example, the symptoms of colds, such as sneezing, coughing, and fatigue, are actually highly adaptive. Likewise, the features of many mental disorders (e.g., some phobias, depression) are arguably adaptive in the framework of our evolutionary history but perhaps not so much in modern society. We offered an alternative model to Wakefield's "harmful dysfunction" by proposing that mental and other disorders be defined as a Roschian concept (Rosch, 1973), which, at the time, was widely being applied to definitions of intelligence (Neisser, 1979). Roschian concepts are mental constructions that are typically used to categorize entities in the natural environment (e.g., bird, fruit, mountain), are characterized by unclear boundaries and an absence of defining (i.e., criterial) features, and organized around a hypothetical prototype. We concluded that Wakefield's concept, while not completely without merit, did not correspond to natural processes well enough to be a foundational concept of disorder.

In Lilienfeld and Marino (1999) we revisited these issues with a critique of Wakefield (1999). We discussed the problematic concept of essentialism in nature and proposed 12 conceptual experiments that undermine Wakefield's harmful dysfunction analysis. While a tremendous amount of work in this area has been done since 1999, I am hopeful that our analysis made a substantive contribution to the conversation about definitional issues in psychology and, more broadly, in understanding the nature of biological reality as it relates to human psychology.

Scott and I enjoyed years of discussion, debate, and learning from each other. We did not agree on everything but shared a love of academia with all of its thorns. He never worried about whether his work was politically or philosophically "correct," or even that it was professionally strategic, only that it was sound and empirically based. His desire to help people was based on the principle that the truth (or as close as one can get to it) should form the starting point for any advocacy effort. He had little patience for any attempt to move the goalposts for the sake of belief, personal values, or comfort. He challenged many "third rail" issues such as microaggressions (e.g., Lilienfeld, 2017, 2020), facilitated communication (Lilienfeld et al., 2014; Schlosser et al., 2019), repressed memories (Otgaar et al., 2019), and so many other dubious claims that drew the ire of those who have little respect for empirically based claims and were basing whole cottage industries on assertions that were attractive for emotional and social reasons solely.

One of those claims became the focus of our most substantive and longstanding collaborative effort, which lasted 22 years up until the week before Scott's death. From 1998 to 2021, Scott and I published five papers focused on the global pseudoscience practice known as dolphin-assisted therapy (DAT). DAT is a form of animal-assisted therapy that is based on the claim that swimming or interacting with dolphins has therapeutic value for a wide range of conditions, including autism, developmental delays, palsies, Down's syndrome, and many others, including cancer and infectious disease. It typically involves a patient touching a dolphin, doing a task with a dolphin, or swimming in the water with (or on top of) a dolphin who is being held in a concrete tank. The cost is exorbitant and often involves families bringing young children to places that require flights and hotel stays over several days or weeks in addition to the price of the "therapy" itself. DAT programs are offered across the world, including in Europe, the Middle East, Asia, the United States, the Caribbean, Mexico, Israel, the Bahamas, and South America. There is no professional DAT accreditation.

DAT came to my attention when I was working with captive dolphins, and I soon suspected that it was yet another form of the kind of mythology and quackery that built up around dolphins since the reckless pronouncements of the late neuroscientist John Lilly and his cronies starting in the 1960s about dolphins and lysergic acid diethylamide (LSD), telepathy, angels, and extraterrestrials (Lilly, 1965; Wyllie 1992, 2001). Dolphins had become the ultimate New-Age pseudoscience symbol. As such, people were willing to accept the claim that they have healing powers—the fundamental premise of DAT.

I took my concerns to Scott. Scott did his own literature research on the topic and immediately saw the weaknesses in the claims of DAT proponents. Both of us were stunned and disturbed by the sheer audacity of the industry's promoters, who engaged in pseudoscience, using terms that sounded like science in order to justify charging exorbitant fees. Here was a practice that was not only at odds with evidence-based treatments but was also potentially harmful to both humans and dolphins alike. Desperate parents were being convinced to deplete their financial resources for a supposed antidote for their child's problems. Children and adults were being encouraged to enter the water and interact with a frustrated stressed wild animal (only to be bitten or rammed and sent to the hospital on many occasions). And young dolphins were being kidnapped from their families in the ocean and confined to small barren tanks in order to pull patients around on their dorsal fins in a sham money-making industry.

Scott and I came to realize that both of us would be a formidable team to refute the claims of DAT because of my expertise in dolphins and Scott's in research methodology. We were both convinced that the best way to battle DAT was to point out weaknesses in its scientific validity. So we set about, in 1998, publishing our first in a series of methodological critiques of DAT papers. We did not realize at the time that this would become an ongoing struggle that is not yet finished.

In 1998, we published our first methodological review (Marino & Lilienfeld, 1998) of DAT, focusing upon several peer-reviewed papers by DAT practitioners Dave Nathanson and his colleagues (Nathanson, 1998; Nathanson & de Faria, 1993; Nathanson et al., 1997). (Nathanson was leading the charge as a proponent of DAT at the time.) Scott conceived of a systematic approach to critiquing the DAT claims that was sound, cautious, and rigorous, becoming a model for how we approached all of our later reviews of DAT studies. Scott had suggested we take a very straightforward approach by assessing the validity of each study according to standard criteria put forth by three seminal sources—Cook and Campbell (1979), Kendall and Norton-Ford (1982), and Shaughnessy and Zechmeister (1994)—describing a set of threats to validity that should be avoided in experimental and quasi-experimental research. In later studies we added a fourth source—Shadish et al. (2002). The presence of even one major threat to validity can render a study's findings difficult, or in some cases impossible, to interpret. We assessed Nathanson's work in the area of major threats to several types of internal and external validity. We found that Nathanson's claims about the effectiveness of DAT were weakened by several serious threats to internal and external validity and flawed data analytic methods rendering his findings essentially uninterpretable and his claims unsupportable.

Nine years later, in Marino and Lilienfeld (2007a), we revisited this literature using the same approach by conducting a review of the five DAT papers published between 1998 and 2007. Although we found some improvement in the methodological rigor of some of the studies, we again reported serious threats to validity in all of them. We concluded that the aggregate findings were again difficult to interpret at best.

As we continued to track and respond to the DAT hype through the years, we also published on the weak validity of DAT for autism and other developmental conditions (Marino & Lilienfeld, 2007b, 2019). I was particularly proud to co-author the 2019 piece in the book *Pseudoscience in Child and Adolescent Psychotherapy* by Stephen Hupp because I had become particularly concerned about the use of DAT for children, who were especially vulnerable to severe injuries in swim-with-the-dolphin programs in general.

One of the many ways that Scott and I influenced each other during our collaborations was in mutually enriching and strengthening our sense of empathy. I have always been focused on the well-being of other animals and Scott on that of humans—but *both* were victimized by DAT. And as Scott learned more about the suffering of dolphins in captivity and became increasingly sensitive to the plight of these and other animals, I became more aware and concerned about the profound injustice and risks to people who are preyed upon by the DAT industry. We were both better for having broadened our sphere of concern for other beings—human and nonhuman.

Our last paper on DAT was finished just a week before Scott's death. In Marino and Lilienfeld (2021) we, once again, conducted a systematic review of all of the peer-reviewed DAT papers published since 2007. This time we analyzed six studies in the DAT literature and focused on their merits in the realms of internal and construct validity. While the studies varied in methodological rigor, they all contained serious threats to validity, rendering each of their conclusions questionable and often unwarranted. Hence, the evidence for the efficacy of DAT appeared to be no more compelling than it was in our previous two review articles so many years ago.

When Scott and I set out to write this third paper we were well aware that the practice of DAT persisted across the globe despite the lack of scientific validity, and we were frustrated but not surprised to find that this pseudoscience, like so many others, was so impervious to methodological critique. We showed, repeatedly, that there is absolutely no merit to DAT as a legitimate therapy for any illness. And, to that end, one day when we were chatting about a suitable title for our *third* systematic review, Scott, with his inimitable wit blurted out: "Third times' the charm or three strikes you're out?" We joked about the fact that the title was spot-on but that the journal editor would likely not want to publish such an impertinent title, and we were thrilled when he accepted it. It reflects Scott's humor in so many ways—sharp but with a good-natured warmth. The paper was accepted less than three months after his death and while I know that Scott was proud of this last effort, it remains a bittersweet memory as he never saw it published and it was the last time we would work together.

Our work on this last paper occurred while Scott was fiercely battling the advanced stages of the worst disease imaginable. Yet, during times of extreme difficulty, he was steadfastly the luminous intellect he always was. I will always be grateful to have lobbed one more volley against DAT with Scott, and I know he was proud of our paper and overall effort.

While we still have a long way to go in the battle against DAT, I am intensely dedicated to continuing our work until we see DAT become a thing of the past. On November 17, 2021, I had the pleasure of presenting a live webinar entitled Dolphin Assisted Therapy, Autism, and Pseudoscience with special guest Dr. David Celiberti, Executive Director of the Association for Science in Autism Treatment. We began with a tribute to Scott, acknowledging his seminal scholarship on pseudoscience in psychology and his fearless advocacy for empirical validation for all clinical approaches. It was encouraging to see how much Scott had influenced practitioners like David, who is committed to evidence-based practices in his work with people on the autism spectrum. I am looking forward to working with people like David and others in the clinical psychology community to ensure that the work Scott and I conducted remains an active force for positive change and promoting sound ethical therapy practices.

The collaborative work described above, as substantial as it is, comprises a small part of Scott's overall contributions to psychology. Throughout the almost 30 years I knew him, and especially when we were on the same campus, I observed the way Scott was able to legitimately question the assumptions we all make about human (and nonhuman) psychology. In exposing the weaknesses in his own field he sometimes touched nerves among his own colleagues with his unflinching dedication to evidence-based theory and practice. That is, he not only took on pseudoscientific thinking outside of academia but also within. Scott was fearless, confident, but never mean-spirited and I saw how his professionally mature and respectful approach fostered mutual respect in the face of disagreement. He took the high road, and I never saw him veer from it.

It is difficult to characterize Scott's career in anything but multidimensional terms but Scott was, more than anything, one of the few people I know of who managed the nearly impossible. He was a model of an academic scholar. And he was also an academic rule-breaker. And this is where Scott's character and intellect is singular.

Despite academia's reputation as a bastion of "free thinking," we all know it is far from perfect. The safe way to navigate one's academic career involves a more formulaic approach than some would hope. The "path of least resistance" to tenure and further accolades is paved by a few simple rules. First, be a specialist, and not a generalist, in one's intellectual pursuits and interests. Second, conduct research that brings in high-level grant money as overhead to the university. Third, employ the latest high-tech "sexy" instrumentation and trendy methodology whether it is necessary or not. Fourth, stick to publishing peer-reviewed papers and avoid being a "popularizer." Fifth, steer clear of controversy.

Scott broke all these rules and, at the same time, was a paragon of academic scholarship and success. By his own admission, Scott was a generalist. He contributed to a wide range of areas in psychology (anxiety disorders, psychopathology classification and conceptualization, pseudoscience, of course, and much more) and also became a leading expert in personality disorders and psychopathy, an area in which he had profound knowledge and understanding. He possessed both breadth and depth in his research and writing. Scott was a pure scholar who reveled in the sheer joy of exploring interesting questions. He was driven by what he found fascinating and had no concerns about whether his research was popular, "on-trend," or brought in overhead through grants.

Oftentimes the contingencies of academic grants shape research questions, rather than the other way around. Scott never took that bait. If he needed a grant or support he would avail himself of opportunities but it was never a central component of his work. As such, here too, he broke the mold. Scott's work did not depend upon the latest technological gadgetry. This suited him just fine as he saw no reason to pursue expensive techniques that required huge grants in the first place. His work rested upon good old-fashioned scientific rigor and critical thinking and Scott knew that those qualities were more important than any technical apparatus. In fact, Scott warned against the potential problems with the field's obsession with high-tech brain imaging techniques for drawing conclusions in neuroscience. In Satel and

Lilienfeld (2013), he and co-author Sally Satel brought some sobriety to the wild speculative claims often associated with the use of neuroimaging techniques (fMRI, PET, etc.), as users of these methods can be vulnerable to inferences that go way beyond the capabilities of the methods themselves. In unquestioning hands brain imaging can become a high-tech version of phrenology, reifying such ideas as the "religion" center, the "love" center, the "democrat" center, the "republican" center, the "addiction" center, and so forth. Scott and Satel also sounded a warning bell about new areas of study such as *neuro*politics, *neuro*finance, *neuro*economics, and *neuro*literature. Scott never dismissed any of these new areas of research out of hand and, in fact, co-authored papers based on imaging studies (e.g., Rilling et al. 2007). Although he authored many critiques of reductionistic neuroscience, he also acknowledged the utility of neuroimaging and other neuroscience methods as one tool in the process of understanding human psychology (Schwartz et al., 2016). He was wary of going overboard and of the tendency for anyone to become so giddy about the "bells and whistles" that critical thinking was abandoned. There was never an "agenda" with Scott. It was all about the science.

Scott's work was sometimes controversial—not because he asserted outrageous ideas, but, ironically, because he consistently advocated for sound science, critical thinking, and, most of all, humility. He recognized that everyone, including himself, was prone to influences and biases of all types in their thinking. And he promoted ways to recognize and avoid those pitfalls. His was an examined career. He took on the latest pseudoscience fads without hesitation and, thus, became controversial in circles that prioritized politically correct agendas over empirically based sound practices (e.g., eye movement desensitization and reprocessing, emotional freedom techniques, recovered memories, microaggressions, facilitated communication, and a slew of harmful psychotherapies). He did this because he had a genuine concern for human welfare and the integrity of psychology as a science.

Whereas many in academia see the label of "popularizer" as an epithet, Scott wore the badge with honor. He was dedicated to education in all spheres—in the classroom, as a mentor, as a scientist, and as a human being. He firmly believed that science should be coupled to outreach and advocacy. He was a true scholar-advocate. Like the astronomer Carl Sagan, one of the scientists he admired most, he relished in the idea that science—when handled with caution—can be a path toward a better world for everyone, not just those who resided in the ivory tower. Scott made it his mission to be an educator, mentor, and guide through the potential snags and snares of human psychology. It is no exaggeration to say that through all the years I knew Scott and have been in academia, he was the most dedicated teacher and advisor for his students and for the public I ever knew. He embodied the dignity of being a teacher.

For those of us fortunate enough to have known Scott, we will forever miss him. I never imagined him not in the world. I am heartened by the fact that he influenced so many but, in the end, there is no real solace for such a loss and only a firm commitment to ensuring that he is kept present into a future that he will never know.

References

American Psychiatric Association, D. S., & American Psychiatric Association. (2013). *Diagnostic and statistical manual of mental disorders: DSM-5* (Vol. 5). American Psychiatric Association.

Cook, T. D., & Campbell, D. T. (1979). *Quasi-experimentation: Design and analysis issues for field settings*. Houghton Mifflin.

Falk, J. H., Reinhard, E. M., Vernon, C. L., Bronnenkant, K., Deans, N. L., & Heimlich, J. E. (2007). *Why zoos & aquariums matter: Assessing the impact of a visit to a zoo or aquarium*. Association of Zoos & Aquariums.

Falk, J. H., Heimlich, J., Vernon, C. L., & Bronnenkant, K. (2010). Critique of a critique: Do zoos and aquariums promote attitude change in visitors? *Society and Animals, 18(4)*, 415–419.

Gosling, S., Lilienfeld, S. O., & Marino, L. (2003). Personality. In D. Maestripieri (Ed.), *Primate psychology: The mind and behavior of human and nonhuman primates* (pp. 254–288). University of Chicago Press.

Gould, S. J. (1991). Exaptation: A crucial tool for evolutionary analysis. *Journal of Social Issues, 47*, 43–65.

Kendall, P. C., & Norton-Ford, J. D. (1982). Therapy outcome research methods. In P. C. Kendall & J. N. Butcher (Eds.), *Handbook of research methods in clinical psychology* (pp. 429–460). Wiley.

Latzman, R. D., Drislane, L. E., Hecht, L. K., Brislin, S. J., Patrick, C. J., Lilienfeld, S. O., ... & Hopkins, W. D. (2016). A chimpanzee (Pan troglodytes) model of triarchic psychopathy constructs: development and initial validation. *Clinical Psychological Science, 4*(1), 50–66.

Lilienfeld, S. O. (2017). Microaggressions: Strong claims, inadequate evidence. *Perspectives on Psychological Science, 12*(1), 138–169.

Lilienfeld, S. O. (2020). Microaggression research and application: Clarifications, corrections, and common ground. *Perspectives on Psychological Science, 15*(1), 27–37.

Lilienfeld, S. O., & Marino, L. (1995). Mental disorder as a Roschian concept: A critique of Wakefield's harmful dysfunction analysis. *Journal of Abnormal Psychology, 104*(3), 411–420.

Lilienfeld, S. O., & Marino, L. (1999). Essentialism revisited: Evolutionary theory and the concept of mental disorder. *Journal of Abnormal Psychology, 108(3)*, 400–411.

Lilienfeld, S. O., Gershon, J., Duke, M., Marino, L., & de Waal, F. B. M. (1999). A preliminary investigation of the construct of psychopathic personality (psychopathy) in common chimpanzees (*Pan troglodytes*). *Journal of Comparative Psychology, 113*, 365–375.

Lilienfeld, S. O., Marshall, J., Todd, J. T., & Shane, H. C. (2014). The persistence of fad interventions in the face of negative scientific evidence: Facilitated communication for autism as a case example. *Evidence-Based Communication Assessment and Intervention, 8*(2), 62–101.

Lilly, J. C. (1965). *Man and dolphin*. Doubleday & Company Inc.

Maestripieri, D., & Lilienfeld, S. O. (2016). Using the NIMH Research Domain Criteria (RDoC) in human and nonhuman primate research. *Psychophysiology, 53(3)*, 367–371.

Marino, L., & Lilienfeld, S. O. (1998). Dolphin-assisted therapy: Flawed data, flawed conclusions. *Anthrozoös, 11(4)*, 194–200.

Marino, L., & Lilienfeld, S. O. (2007a). Dolphin assisted therapy: More flawed data, more flawed conclusions. *Anthrozoos, 20*, 239–249.

Marino, L., & Lilienfeld, S. (2007b). Dolphin assisted therapy for autism and other developmental disorders: A dangerous fad. *Psychology in Intellectual and Developmental Disabilities (Division 33). American Psychological Association, 33*(2), 2–3.

Marino, L., & Lilienfeld, S. O. (2019). Does dolphin assisted therapy have healing effects? In S. Hupp (Ed.), *Pseudoscience in child and adolescent psychotherapy* (pp. 37–39). Cambridge Press.

Marino, L., & Lilienfeld, S. O. (2021). Third time's the charm or three strikes you're out? An updated review of the efficacy of dolphin-assisted therapy for autism and developmental disabilities. *Journal of Clinical Psychology*, 1–15. https://doi.org/10.1002/jclp.23110

Marino, L., Lilienfeld, S., Malamud, R., Nobis, N., & Broglio, R. (2010). Do zoos and aquariums promote attitude change in visitors? A critical evaluation of the American Zoo and Aquarium study. *Society and Animals, 18*, 126–138.

Marino, L., Lilienfeld, S. O., Malamud, R., Nobis, N., & Broglio, R. (2011). Strong claims, feeble evidence: A Rejoinder to Falk et al. (2010). *Society and Animals, 19*, 291–293.
McFall, R. M. (1996). Making psychology incorruptible. *Applied and Preventive Psychology, 5(1)*, 9–15.
Nathanson, D. E. (1998). Long-term effectiveness of dolphin-assisted therapy for children with severe disabilities. *Anthrozoos, 11(1)*, 22–32.
Nathanson, D. E., & de Faria, S. (1993). Cognitive improvement of children in water with and without dolphins. *Anthrozoos, 6(1)*, 17–29.
Nathanson, D. E., de Castro, D., Friend, H., & McMahon, M. (1997). Effectiveness of short-term dolphin-assisted therapy for children with severe disabilities. *Anthrozoos, 10(2/3)*, 90–100.
Neisser, U. (1979). The concept of intelligence. *Intelligence, 3*, 217–227.
Otgaar, H., Howe, M. L., Patihis, L., Merckelbach, H., Lynn, S. J., Lilienfeld, S. O., & Loftus, E. F. (2019). The return of the repressed: The persistent and problematic claims of long-forgotten trauma. *Perspectives on Psychological Science, 14*(6), 1072–1095.
Piatelli-Palmarini, M. (1989). Evolution, selection and cognition: From "learning" to parameter setting in biology and in the study of language. *Cognition, 31*, 1–44.
Reiss, D., & Marino, L. (2001). Mirror self-recognition in the bottlenose dolphin: A case of cognitive convergence. *Proceedings of the National Academy of Sciences, 98(10)*, 5937–5942.
Rilling, J. K., Glenn, A. L., Jairam, M. R., Pagnoni, G., Goldsmith, D. R., Elfenbein, H. A., & Lilienfeld, S. O. (2007). Neural correlates of social cooperation and non-cooperation as a function of psychopathy. *Biological Psychiatry, 61*(11), 1260–1271.
Rosch, E. R. (1973). Natural categories. *Cognitive Psychology, 4*, 328–350.
Satel, S., & Lilienfeld, S. O. (2013). *Brainwashed: The seductive appeal of mindless neuroscience*. Basic Civitas Books.
Schlosser, R. W., Hemsley, B., Shane, H., Todd, J., Lang, R., Lilienfeld, S. O., et al. (2019). Rapid prompting method and autism spectrum disorder: Systematic review exposes lack of evidence. *Review Journal of Autism and Developmental Disorders, 6*(4), 403–412.
Schwartz, S. J., Lilienfeld, S. O., Meca, A., & Sauvigné, K. C. (2016). The role of neuroscience within psychology: A call for inclusiveness over exclusiveness. *American Psychologist, 71*(1), 52.
Shadish, W. R., Cook, T. D., & Campbell, D. T. (2002). *Experimental and quasi-experimental designs for generalized causal inference*. Mifflin.
Shaughnessy, J. J., & Zechmeister, E. B. (1994). *Research methods in psychology*. McGraw-Hill.
Wakefield, J. C. (1992a). The concept of mental disorder: On the boundary between biological facts and social values. *American Psychologist, 47*, 373–388.
Wakefield, J. C. (1992b). Disorder as harmful dysfunction: A conceptual critique *of DSM-HI-R's* definition of mental disorder. *Psychological Review, 99*, 232–247.
Wakefield, J. C. (1993). Limits of operationalization: A critique of Spitzer and Endicott's (1978) proposed operational criteria for mental disorder. *Journal of Abnormal Psychology, 102*, 160–172.
Wakefield, J. C. (1999). Evolutionary versus prototype analyses of the concept of disorder. *Journal of Abnormal Psychology, 108*, 374–399.
Wyllie, T. (1992). *Dolphins, ETs & angels: Adventures among spiritual intelligences*. Bear & Co. Publishers.
Wyllie, T. (2001). *Adventures among spiritual intelligences: Angels, aliens, dolphins & shamans*. Wisdom Editions.

Comorbidity, Classification, and Other Adventures in Psychopathology and Psychology: Scott Lilienfeld's Formative Influences and Contributions Through the Lens of Our 40-Year Friendship and Collaboration

Irwin D. Waldman

In this chapter, I offer my perspective on Scott Lilienfeld's contributions to the field of psychology and on his formative influences, through the lens of our long-term collaboration and friendship. In doing so, I hope to illuminate some aspects of Scott's developmental trajectory that contributed to him becoming the person that so many came to know and respect. I was very fortunate to be friends with Scott for 40 years and collaborators for 30 of those. We first met as undergraduates at Cornell University in 1980, as he was a Psychology major and I had just begun majoring in Human Development and Family Studies (HDFS) after winding a circuitous path through various disciplines in the College of Arts and Sciences. As will come as no surprise, I knew of Scott long before I met him. He was a presence on campus, and we all knew just how serious he was about psychology, so much so that my friends and I referred to him as "Young Freud" (back then it could still be construed as a compliment, albeit one mixed with a fair bit of sophomoric sarcasm).

Cornell in the late 1970s and early 1980s was an interesting place to be an undergraduate, intellectually, culturally, and socio-politically. With respect to the last, the political landscape concerning distrust of political figures and the fight for civil rights had quieted substantially relative to the 1970s. It was only 9 years before our arrival at Cornell in 1978 that African-American students had staged a 36-hour takeover of the student union. The students were initially unarmed but after being assaulted by a group of White students who breached the building, the African-American students brandished guns as they eventually emerged from the building upon the takeover's peaceful resolution. Nonetheless, there remained a steady stream of protests befitting a college campus. Culturally, there were many concerts one could attend across a wide variety of genres—ranging from Bruce Springsteen and the Grateful Dead to Chick Corea and Gary Burton. There was a first-class film

I. D. Waldman (✉)
Department of Psychology, Emory University, Atlanta, GA, USA
e-mail: psyiw@emory.edu

C. L. Cobb et al. (eds.), *Toward a Science of Clinical Psychology*,
https://doi.org/10.1007/978-3-031-14332-8_3

club co-led by Terrence Rafferty, a graduate student and lecturer and future New Yorker film critic (Rafferty, 1993), and an intellectual smorgasbord more than adequate for inspiring young minds and honing their developing tastes. Speakers in every imaginable field, including the leading authors of that era's Spanish and Latin American literature, to prominent scientists, and the political and social activist and Yippie founder Abbie Hoffman, graced the campus during our time there. There was no shortage of intellectual heavyweights around campus either, including Nobel Prize winners Hans Bethe in Physics and Roald Hoffman in Chemistry, the eminent historian of foreign policy Walter LaFeber, and the political scientist Theodore Lowi.

But perhaps above all of these in their influence on Scott was the renowned astronomer Carl Sagan. I think what started for Scott as a fascination with the cosmos over time blossomed into an appreciation for the magic of the scientific method and its endless possibilities for nurturing our fascination with and ability to answer questions about the universe. Even more so, what spoke to Scott was the scientific method's unparalleled power for separating science from pseudoscience, a broad consistent thread that would be woven into all of Scott's thinking and work throughout his career, a theme that I'll return to below. Even in his later years, Scott would assign readings by Sagan (e.g., Sagan, 2011) when he guest-lectured in my Freshman seminar on The Nature of Evidence.

The intellectual riches at Cornell characterized psychology as well. Its heavy hitters included the venerable Urie Bronfrenbrenner in Human Development and Family Studies (HDFS) and Ulric Neisser in the Psychology Department. Cornell's Psychology Department was predominantly experimental with concentrations in Cognitive, Psychobiology, and Social, whereas HDFS was highly interdisciplinary and included psychologists, sociologists, economists, and even a historian. There was little emphasis on personality psychology and even less on clinical psychology. Despite this, several of us were considerably interested in pursuing research and coursework in clinical psychology and intended to go on to graduate school to pursue a PhD in clinical psychology. We were able to take a highly idiosyncratic survey course on psychopathology from Ron Mack, who had a distinctly psychodynamic bent (I remember him once commenting on the then-burgeoning neuroscience approaches to psychopathology by asserting that everyone knew there were only three integral parts of the brain—id, ego, and superego); a survey course on child psychopathology from Elaine Walker (with whom I later worked as a Research Assistant); and a course on research in adult psychopathology from Bob Dworkin in which he supplemented our textbook with readings from the primary research literature.

It was against this background that several of us pursued a trajectory that would lead us to gain admission into a clinical psychology PhD program (indeed, Scott and I were preceded in this quest by Mark Lenzenweger a year earlier). It was in this context of pursuing both honors thesis research projects and applying for graduate school in clinical psychology that Scott and I came to know each other and became friends. While I conducted my honors thesis research on an ethological approach to children's dominance hierarchies, Scott conducted his research in the lab of the prominent social psychologist Darryl Bem, who was an iconoclast even then. It seems both highly ironic and somewhat prescient that Scott would work under Bem, given both Bem's later infamous forays into extrasensory perception (ESP) (Bem, 2011) and Scott's later emphases on replicability and Questionable Research Practices (QRPs) (Lilienfeld & Waldman, 2017; Tackett et al., 2017; Waldman & Lilienfeld, 2016). The cosmos has a devilish sense of humor indeed! Bem's idiosyncratic nature apparently extended to his lab as a whole. One morning, Scott came into the lab to test a participant, only to find another undergraduate research assistant asleep on the table in his underwear. Although Scott and I took some of the same classes—Ron Mack's and Bob Dworkin's psychopathology classes, for example—Scott took them before I did. I later learned that this would typify Scott and our collaborations, as he always seemed to be one or more steps ahead of me.

Finally, our time at Cornell was coming to an end. For reasons that I cannot recall, uncharacteristically Scott never completed his Honors Thesis despite running participants and writing much of it. For my part, after a difficult 6 months of writing—surely more difficult for my thesis advisor than for me—I managed to barely finish my thesis and successfully defend it. Regarding our applications to clinical psychology programs, I had only a few interviews and finally was admitted to the University of Waterloo only after another potential student decided at the last minute to go to medical school. In contrast, Scott had his choice of multiple programs and very wisely chose the University of Minnesota, a decision that in many important ways set him on the pathway that was to characterize the remainder of his career. During Scott's time at Minnesota and mine at the University of Waterloo, we kept in touch. Scott's father and step-mother had moved to New Jersey, about 40 min away from where I grew up and where my parents still lived. While home during winter and summer breaks, we would get together in some strip-mall pizza joint—this was New Jersey in the 1980s, after all—one close to either my or his parents' house, and we would share our experiences of being graduate students in a clinical psychology program. We shared what classes we liked and felt we learned from, which we did not care for or thought were rather useless. We also discussed which faculty were intellectually impressive and committed, from whom we learned a great deal, and which faculty seemed kind of irrelevant or like they were just phoning it in. Perhaps most importantly, we also discussed our burgeoning research interests and preoccupations. For Scott, this included topics such as various psychophysiological theories of arousal, the nature of psychopathy, the conceptual and philosophical bases of psychology and psychopathology, and how certain disorders appeared to cluster together both within an individual and within families (more on this below). I think my interests were rather inchoate relative to Scott's, but included the nature of childhood psychopathological conditions such as Attention Deficit Hyperactivity Disorder (ADHD) and aggression and their overlap and neuro- and social-cognitive underpinnings, the burgeoning field of developmental psychopathology, and a growing interest in statistical methods and how they were in many ways opening my eyes to a world of additional research possibilities. For me, it was tremendously helpful to have someone in addition to my fellow graduate students at another top clinical program to bounce ideas off of, mutually develop our scientific knowledge and predilections, and at times just vent. I think Scott must have felt the same way, for this was a pattern that characterized our friendship and collaboration for the next 38 years.

While at Minnesota, Scott was profoundly influenced by many of the senior faculty, including Paul Meehl, Auke Tellegen, Tom Bouchard, and of course his advisor, David Lykken. He also was influenced by a number of junior faculty, including Will Grove, Bill Iacono, and Matt McGue, and by several very bright, capable fellow graduate students, including Steve Gangestaad, Al Harkness, and Niels Waller, the latter two with whom he published several papers while at Minnesota and later as a faculty member. Indeed, these publications were an early reflection of some of the major themes that would characterize Scott's later work. With Niels, Scott investigated commonalities in the underlying structure of and relations between Cloninger's Tridimensional Personality Questionnaire (TPQ) and Tellegen's Multidimensional Personality Questionnaire (MPQ) (Waller et al., 1991), clarifying the nature of the TPQ Harm Avoidance dimension as reflecting neuroticism, in contrast to its name. With Al, Scott described the importance and utility of research on individual differences in personality for treatment planning, highlighting (among other things) the possibility of tailoring treatment approaches based on an individual's personality traits (Harkness & Lilienfeld, 1997). Both of these works reflected Scott's central interests in the underlying nature of personality and the bridge between so-called normal range personality and its abnormal extremes. He also extended this work to the clinical realm of treatment planning.

As impressive as these papers were, they were not Scott's first publications. As an adolescent, Scott was something of a chess prodigy, and at age 16 published his first piece on a chess strategy. Scott completed his predoctoral clinical internship during 1986–1987 at Western Psychiatric Clinic in Pittsburgh, one of the preeminent and most intensive clinical internship programs in North America. While there, in addition to his many clinical responsibilities, Scott managed to also find time to get involved in several research projects with some of Western Psychiatric's most illustrative faculty, including Hagop Akiskal and Sam Turner. The foci of these studies included vestibular dysfunction in panic disorder (Jacob et al., 1989; Lilienfeld et al., 1989a); anxiety sensitivity and the response to hyperventilation (Lilienfeld et al., 1989b), which he'd later reexamine in terms of similarities between anxiety sensitivity and trait anxiety (Lilienfeld et al., 1993); and the relation of histrionic personality disorder to antisocial personality and somatization disorders (Lilienfeld et al., 1986), a topic that he would revisit in later publications in the context of sex differences in the expression of psychopathy and antisocial behavior (Cale & Lilienfeld, 2002a, b; Hamburger et al., 1996; Lilienfeld, 1992). This 1986 paper was not only Scott's first 1st-authored scientific publication, but also it was a harbinger of Scott's interests in comorbidity and classification of psychopathology, a theme that would characterize much of our work together through the years, as I will discuss below.

Rather improbably, in the fall of 1988, I was extraordinarily fortunate to come to Minnesota as a postdoctoral fellow in Behavior Genetics under the supervision of Matt McGue. While there, I worked with several faculty, including Matt, Will Grove, Bill Iacono, Tom Bouchard, Rich Weinberg, and—by extension, given that she was at the University of Virginia but still collaborated with Rich Weinberg—Sandra Scarr. I also benefited from taking classes from and interacting with Paul Meehl, David Lykken, Auke Tellegen, and Bob Cudeck. For those who've never been a student or faculty member there, it is a bit hard to fully convey the unique environment of the University of Minnesota Psychology Department. While not the most warm and fuzzy of places on the surface, faculty—at least those with whom I interacted—were nonetheless supportive in a deep, real, and meaningful way, as reflected by their strong commitment to helping graduate students and postdoctoral fellows develop as critical thinkers and rigorous scientists. For trainees interested in working at the intersection of clinical science, individual differences, and behavior genetics—including Scott, myself, Niels Waller, Al Harkness, and Wendy Slutske—it was an incredibly rich environment, one that helped us all to go on to successful academic careers.

As I mentioned above, it was also a place where collaborations among graduate students and postdocs were encouraged. At the end of my first year as a postdoc, I had collaborated on a publication—one of my first—with Niels Waller on the factor structure of the Wechsler Adult Intelligence Scale-Revised (WAIS-R; Waller & Waldman, 1990). I also began working with Scott on a comprehensive review of the overlap between Attention Deficit Hyperactivity Disorder (ADHD) in childhood and later aggression and antisocial behavior (Lilienfeld & Waldman, 1990). These publications, early as they were in our development, foreshadowed some of the main themes that would characterize our work for much of our careers. Niels and I have continued to use a variety of sophisticated statistical methods in our research—indeed, Niels has been Head of the Quantitative Methods program in Minnesota's Psychology Department for the past 17 years. My publication with Scott directly reflected my strong substantive interest in childhood externalizing disorders and their causes, classification, and sequelae. Although this paper may not seem obvious in its relevance to Scott's interests, it was in many ways an outgrowth of Scott's burgeoning preoccupation with the distinctions and overlap among psychopathological conditions, and their classification more generally. For his Comprehensive Exam paper at Minnesota, Scott reviewed the evidence across numerous domains for the validity of the St. Louis Quartet, a set of conditions that included psychopathy, antisocial behavior, somatization, and histrionic personality disorder. As I recall, Scott reviewed evidence from studies of classification and diagnostic overlap, course and outcome, familiality and available behavior genetic studies, and psychophysiological correlates. This work and our paper were thus early reflections of our shared interest in the classification of psychopathology and the concept of comorbidity that had recently been proposed (Feinstein, 1970) and extended to the realm of psychiatric disorders and was rapidly gaining currency. Before our time together at Minnesota ended, we followed our paper on ADHD and later antisocial behavior with a related publication on the application of diagnostic efficiency indices (i.e., sensitivity, specificity, positive predictive value, and negative predictive value) to examine the overlap and distinctions between ADHD and Oppositional Defiant Disorder (ODD; Waldman & Lilienfeld, 1992), which was my first

1st-authored publication. It also set the stage for our extensive subsequent work on classification and comorbidity, which I will describe further below.

It is interesting and perhaps instructive to think back after all these years about what it was that interested us—and frustrated us—about the term and concept of comorbidity, borrowing part of the title of one of our early papers on this topic (Lilienfeld et al., 1994a). Throughout the history of research on mental disorders, various attempts had been made to classify psychopathology and to grapple with the observation that individual disorders are overlapping, the phenomenon that came to be referred to as "comorbidity." The prototypical way of studying this in the 1970s and 1980s was to examine the overlap among discrete diagnoses, often two at a time. Examples in the literature included Schizophrenia and Bipolar Disorder (Laursen et al., 2009), Major Depressive Disorder (MDD) and Generalized Anxiety Disorder (GAD) (Fava et al., 2000; Kessler et al., 2008), and Attention Deficit Hyperactivity Disorder (ADHD) with Oppositional Defiant Disorder (ODD) and Conduct Disorder (CD) (Biederman et al., 1991). This historical usage of comorbidity was still popular in the late 1980s and early 1990s, as it had not yet been supplanted by the *transdiagnostic* approaches to the classification of psychopathology that began in the 1990s and continues to the present. Given the rampant overlap among diagnostic categories across numerous domains of psychopathology in the late 1980s, what exactly bothered us about the term comorbidity? Well, there were a few things, I suppose.

As we wrote in the abstract of that early paper (Lilienfeld et al., 1994a), most uses of comorbidity "blur the distinction between latent constructs and manifest indicators…We conclude that…application of the term comorbidity to psychopathological syndromes encourages the premature reification of diagnostic entities and arguably has led to more confusion than clarification" (p. 71). We elaborated these issues with the usage of comorbidity to highlight the slippage between overlap among overt symptomatology as opposed to its etiological underpinnings, often leading to great confusion. This paper also was interesting and instructive for us from a career perspective. It appeared as a target article in the very first issue of a fledgling journal called *Clinical Psychology: Science and Practice*. The editor invited commentaries from several luminaries in psychopathology research, including Robert Spitzer (with whom Scott was later to publish several papers) and Sir Michael Rutter. While this was quite exciting for us, given that we were fairly new assistant professors, their comments were really quite negative, to the point that Sir Michael included a slide or two in his talks during that period devoted to refuting our critiques of comorbidity. It was a real "be careful what you wish for" moment!

Its initial reception notwithstanding, we followed this paper with several subsequent publications that continued our work on diagnostic classification and comorbidity, extending it to include examples of how various latent variable models could be used to good effect in investigating issues of classification and construct validity, and perhaps resolve some of the problematic aspects of comorbidity (Lilienfeld & Waldman, 2004; Waldman et al., 1995; Waldman & Lilienfeld, 2001). For my part, I had spent several of my early years as an assistant professor at Emory working with Ben Lahey analyzing data collected through the DSM-IV Field Trials for the

Childhood Disruptive Disorders, which led to a series of publications on various aspects of the classification of child psychopathology (Applegate et al., 1997; Frick et al., 1994; Lahey et al., 1994a, b, 1998; Waldman & Lahey, 1994). As an Assistant Professor at SUNY-Albany, Scott pursued these issues from more of a conceptual and even philosophical vantage point, entering into a spirited and productive debate with Jerome Wakefield over the very conceptualization of mental disorder, in particular the idea of mental disorder as "harmful dysfunction" (Lilienfeld & Marino, 1995, 1999; Wakefield, 1992; Wakefield, 2007). He also interacted closely with several faculty colleagues with particular strengths in quantitative methods, including the statistician Jim Jaccard, the animal behavior geneticist Bruce Dudek, and the Industrial-Organizational psychologists Gene Stone and George Alliger—the last two with whom he published several papers (Alliger et al., 1996; Lilienfeld et al., 1994b, 1995). These colleagues pushed Scott in his knowledge of statistical methods and whetted his appetite to further his learning in this domain.

Of course, Scott characteristically had several parallel lines of research that he simultaneously and seriously pursued. He set about publishing the measure he developed for his dissertation research, the Psychopathic Personality Inventory (PPI; Lilienfeld & Andrews, 1996), which is one of his most cited publications and a testimony to its common use as a tool for assessing multidimensional psychopathic traits in a variety of populations (Poythress et al., 1998). He also continued to conduct studies and write theoretical and conceptual pieces on the nature and correlates of psychopathy (Lilienfeld, 1998; Lilienfeld et al., 1996), well in keeping with his being a graduate student of David Lykken. Another line of research that Scott began to pursue in earnest with his then-wife Lori Marino seemed a bit improbable at the time, at least to me. Lori was a graduate student at SUNY-Albany, working in the lab of the renowned Comparative Psychologist Gordon Gallup. Together, Lori and Scott began to challenge the efficacy of some of the well-intentioned but questionable therapies for serious psychopathological conditions, such as dolphin-assisted therapy for autism and other serious conditions (Marino & Lilienfeld, 1998). At the time this line of research seemed a bit far afield, even for someone with such broad interests as Scott. In hindsight, though, it makes perfect sense, as it coincided with the beginning of a body of research and writings that is among the contributions for which Scott is best known, specifically his challenges of assessment and therapeutic techniques that are lacking evidence, ineffective, or downright harmful.

In the fall of 1994, Scott moved to Emory and joined me as a faculty colleague there for the next 26 years. The Department of Psychology at Emory was in many ways very similar then as it is now, with a few notable exceptions. Our department has been very stable during my 30 years at Emory, with very few faculty leaving other than due to retirements. Two notable exceptions are worth mentioning, however, given the outsized influence they had not only on the department, but also on our field more broadly. These include Ulric (Dick) Neisser and Mike Tomasello. Dick had been at Cornell during my and Scott's time there, and at least Scott was wise enough to take a course from him. Dick is widely considered one of, if not the primary, leaders of the "cognitive revolution" in psychology (Neisser, 1987; Neisser,

2000, 2014), and he was a Woodruff Chaired Professor in psychology at the time of my arrival at Emory in 1991. Mike was a recently tenured associate professor who already had made a significant mark with a diary study of his daughter's very early speech development (Tomasello, 1992, 2009b), a study that has since been emulated and replicated many times. Mike was to go on and make landmark contributions to the parallels and differences between cultural influences on cognition in children and nonhuman primates (Tomasello, 2009a, c; Tomasello et al., 1993, 2005; Tomasello & Call, 1997), as well as studies of behavioral similarities between wolves and dogs from an evolutionary perspective (Hare et al., 2002). In addition, the primatologist Frans de Waal arrived in the department the same year I did. A few years beforehand, Frans had published his landmark book *Chimpanzee Politics* (de Waal & de Waal, 2007). At Emory, he was embarking on many landmark studies of culture and cognition, the nature of empathy, altruism, and equity in nonhuman primates (Brosnan & de Waal, 2003; Preston & de Waal, 2002; de Waal & de Waal, 1996, 2009), and many other seminal works in animal behavior especially (though not exclusively) using nonhuman primates. The prospect and reality of joining a department with three future National Academy of Science members and/or American Association for the Advancement of Science (AAAS) fellows was both very exciting and more than a bit daunting. Life as an Assistant Professor in such a department was challenging, and in most ways these challenges made us stronger as beginning academics.

It was against this background that Scott took the next steps in his career. His work with Lori Marino on animal-assisted therapies soon morphed into a steady stream of studies on assessments and therapies of dubious validity, so much so that they often could be and were harmful. These included the Rorschach inkblot test and other projective tests (Lilienfeld et al., 2001a, b; *The Scientific Status of Projective Techniques – Scott O. Lilienfeld, James M. Wood, Howard N. Garb, 2000*, n.d.; Wood et al., 2000, 2001a, b; Wood & Lilienfeld, 1999), integrity testing in the workplace (Alliger et al., 1996; Lilienfeld et al., 1995), Eye-Movement Desensitization and Reprocessing (EMDR; Herbert et al., 2000; Lohr et al., 1998, 1999; Rosen et al., n.d., 1999), recovered memories (Lilienfeld & Loftus, 1998, 1999), and dissociative identity disorder (commonly referred to as multiple personality disorder) (Lilienfeld et al., 1999). It was also in the mid-1990s that Scott began to write and edit books (Lilienfeld, 1995), because apparently his prolific nature simply could not be contained within the bindings of academic journals and popular magazines such as *Skeptical Inquirer*, *Skeptic*, and *Scientific American*. Tempting as it might be to list and briefly describe his books, this easily would take up a chapter in its own right! Suffice to say, it was only a matter of time before Scott suggested that he and I edit a book together, about which I will say more below.

This line of research and writing on clinical procedures that were ineffective and harmful also blossomed into several other preoccupations, for such was the nature of Scott's intellectual appetites and proclivities. The first of these was with science versus pseudoscience, first within clinical psychology and then extending to psychology in general. Scott delved deeper into the literature on various dubious assessment tools and therapeutic techniques that historically were central to the clinical armamentarium, or that received considerable contemporary attention and grew rapidly in popularity. I suppose it was inevitable that the sense that Scott and I had in graduate school that many of these procedures were lacking in evidence would only be borne out with closer scrutiny. For Scott, this grew into a sub-career in its own right, as he began documenting such problems more deeply and widely. In the company of likeminded colleagues that included James Wood, Howard Garb, Elizabeth Loftus, and Steven Jay Lynn, this work extended beyond questionable assessment methods in clinical psychology to issues in the recovered memory debate and the use of clinical hypnosis (Lilienfeld et al., 2000, 2001a, b; *Science and Pseudoscience in Clinical Psychology, 2nd Ed*, 2015; Lilienfeld & Loftus, 1999; Lynn et al., 2003, 2004).

The second line of research and writing took a bit longer to emerge, but approximately 10 years ago, just after the start of what became widely known as the "replication crisis" in psychology and many domains of science beyond, Scott dove right in. I can still recall the morbid fascination that accompanied our reading of Ed Vul's paper on "voodoo correlations" in neuroscience, which morphed prior to its publication by changing to a more muted title and documenting other related concerns with neuroimaging studies in our field (Vul et al., 2009). Vul's paper inspired subsequent important efforts to reform practices in the neuroscience literature (Button et al., 2013; Poldrack et al., 2017) and in many ways was a precursor to the more general psychological literature on replication and reproducibility that followed.

I also recall sometime afterward our reading of John Ioannidis' seminal paper "Why Most Published Research Findings Are False" (Ioannidis, 2005) and the dramatic impact these papers and many similar others that were to follow had on us (e.g., John et al., 2012; Nelson et al., 2018; Nosek et al., 2015; OPEN SCIENCE COLLABORATION, 2015; Simmons et al., 2011). One impact of this work is that it found its way into my teaching of graduate statistics—particularly my courses on Multiple Regression and the General Linear Model and Latent Variable Modeling. Another is that it inspired in Scott the idea to coedit a book with me centered broadly on issues of research reproducibility and replicability (Lilienfeld & Waldman, 2017). A prelude to exploring some of the ideas that would lay the foundation for this book was a commentary we wrote on issues of reproducibility and replicability in research and in minimizing Questionable Research Practices (QRPs) in psychology (Waldman & Lilienfeld, 2016). But to Scott's dismay, I was quite a tough sell on the idea of editing another book, as I had coedited one a decade before (Flannery et al., 2007) and the aftertaste still lingered. Nonetheless, Scott being Scott, after many long walks in the park on campus that contained the Presidential mansion, Scott finally prevailed. And although I may not have felt this at the time, I am grateful for his tenacity. Predictably, Scott went on to revisit and extend these themes in several subsequent papers, and his commitment to increasing the reproducibility and replicability of research in psychology persisted as a theme until his passing (Aczel et al., 2020; Tackett et al., 2017).

Incredibly, against this background of ever-expanding interests and publications, Scott managed to maintain a consistent focus on the assessment, nature, and correlates of psychopathy. He continued to develop new collaborations across all areas of his research interests, as well as preserve collaborations with longstanding colleagues. Evidence of this can be seen in many quarters, including multiple papers, chapters, and books published with the editors of this volume (Cobb et al., 2020; Lilienfeld & O'Donohue, 2012; Lynn et al., 2012, 2015), as well as with his wife Candice Basterfield (Basterfield et al., 2020; Basterfield & Lilienfeld, 2020; Lilienfeld & Basterfield, 2020). His fostering of his graduate students' careers and varied research programs is the stuff of legend, and I have been fortunate to be a coauthor on several of his students' publications across diverse areas ranging from narcissistic and psychopathic traits among US presidents (Lilienfeld et al., 2012; Watts et al., 2013), to economic decision-making and psychopathic traits (Berg et al., 2013), to most recently the structure and correlates of Left Wing Authoritarianism (Costello et al., 2021). Returning to where I began in this chapter, I feel very fortunate that, against this background of a multitude of other commitments, Scott and I collaborated on many projects, including publications central to our interests on the assessment of psychopathic traits in youth (Poore et al., 2020) and relations between personality traits and psychopathology (Watts et al., 2019), up until just before he passed away. I was ever so lucky to have met Scott on the campus of Cornell University 40 years ago, and I will miss him as a colleague and friend for the rest of my days.

References

Aczel, B., Szaszi, B., Sarafoglou, A., Kekecs, Z., Kucharský, Š., Benjamin, D., Chambers, C. D., Fisher, A., Gelman, A., Gernsbacher, M. A., Ioannidis, J. P., Johnson, E., Jonas, K., Kousta, S., Lilienfeld, S. O., Lindsay, D. S., Morey, C. C., Munafò, M., Newell, B. R., et al. (2020). A consensus-based transparency checklist. *Nature Human Behaviour, 4*(1), 4–6. https://doi.org/10.1038/s41562-019-0772-6

Alliger, G. M., Lilienfeld, S. O., & Mitchell, K. E. (1996). The susceptibility of overt and covert integrity tests to coaching and faking. *Psychological Science, 7*(1), 32–39. https://doi.org/10.1111/j.1467-9280.1996.tb00663.x

Applegate, B., Lahey, B. B., Hart, E. L., Biederman, J., Hynd, G. W., Barkley, R. A., Ollendick, T., Frick, P. J., Greenhili, L., Mcburnett, K., Newcorn, J. H., Kerdyk, L., Garfinkel, B., Waldman, I., & Shaffer, D. (1997). Validity of the age-of-onset criterion for ADHD: A report from the DSM-IV field trials. *Journal of the American Academy of Child & Adolescent Psychiatry, 36*(9), 1211–1221. https://doi.org/10.1097/00004583-199709000-00013

Basterfield, C., & Lilienfeld, S. O. (2020). The history of the early controlled trial: Lessons for contemporary clinical psychologists and students. *PsyArXiv*. https://doi.org/10.31234/osf.io/xqes2

Basterfield, C., Lilienfeld, S. O., Cautin, R. L., & Jordan, D. (2020). Mental illness misconceptions among undergraduates: Prevalence, correlates, and instructional implications. *Scholarship of Teaching and Learning in Psychology*. https://doi.org/10.1037/stl0000221

Bem, D. J. (2011). Feeling the future: Experimental evidence for anomalous retroactive influences on cognition and affect. *Journal of Personality and Social Psychology, 100*(3), 407–425. https://doi.org/10.1037/a0021524

Berg, J. M., Lilienfeld, S. O., & Waldman, I. D. (2013). Bargaining with the devil: Using economic decision-making tasks to examine the heterogeneity of psychopathic traits. *Journal of Research in Personality, 47*(5), 472–482. https://doi.org/10.1016/j.jrp.2013.04.003

Biederman, J., Newcorn, J., & Sprich, S. (1991). Comorbidity of attention deficit hyperactivity disorder with conduct, depressive, anxiety, and other disorders. *The American Journal of Psychiatry, 148*(5), 564–577. https://doi.org/10.1176/ajp.148.5.564

Brosnan, S. F., & de Waal, F. B. M. (2003). Monkeys reject unequal pay. *Nature, 425*(6955), 297–299. https://doi.org/10.1038/nature01963

Button, K. S., Ioannidis, J. P. A., Mokrysz, C., Nosek, B. A., Flint, J., Robinson, E. S. J., & Munafò, M. R. (2013). Power failure: Why small sample size undermines the reliability of neuroscience. *Nature Reviews Neuroscience, 14*(5), 365–376. https://doi.org/10.1038/nrn3475

Cale, E. M., & Lilienfeld, S. O. (2002a). Histrionic personality disorder and antisocial personality disorder: sex-differentiated manifestations of psychopathy? *Journal of Personality Disorders, 16*(1), 52–72. https://doi.org/10.1521/pedi.16.1.52.22557

Cale, E. M., & Lilienfeld, S. O. (2002b). Sex differences in psychopathy and antisocial personality disorder: A review and integration. *Clinical Psychology Review, 22*(8), 1179–1207. https://doi.org/10.1016/S0272-7358(01)00125-8

Cobb, C. L., Lilienfeld, S. O., Schwartz, S. J., Frisby, C., & Sanders, G. L. (2020). Rethinking multiculturalism: Toward a balanced approach. *The American Journal of Psychology, 133*(3), 275–293. https://www.jstor.org/stable/10.5406/amerjpsyc.133.3.0275

Costello, T. H., Bowes, S. M., Stevens, S. T., Waldman, I. D., Tasimi, A., & Lilienfeld, S. O. (2021). Clarifying the structure and nature of left-wing authoritarianism. *Journal of Personality and Social Psychology*. https://doi.org/10.1037/pspp0000341

de Waal, F. B. M., & de Waal, F. (1996). *Good natured: The origins of right and wrong in humans and other animals*. Harvard University Press.

de Waal, F., & de Waal, F. B. M. (2007). *Chimpanzee politics: Power and sex among apes*. JHU Press.

de Waal, F. B. M., & de Waal, F. B. M. (2009). *Peacemaking among primates*. Harvard University Press.

Fava, M., Rankin, M. A., Wright, E. C., Alpert, J. E., Nierenberg, A. A., Pava, J., & Rosenbaum, J. F. (2000). Anxiety disorders in major depression. *Comprehensive Psychiatry, 41*(2), 97–102. https://doi.org/10.1016/S0010-440X(00)90140-8

Feinstein, A. R. (1970). The pre-therapeutic classification of co-morbidity in chronic disease. *Journal of Chronic Diseases, 23*(7), 455–468. https://doi.org/10.1016/0021-9681(70)90054-8

Flannery, D. J., Vazsonyi, A. T., & Waldman, I. D. (2007). *The Cambridge handbook of violent behavior and aggression*. Cambridge University Press.

Frick, P. J., Lahey, B. B., Applegate, B., Kerdyck, L., Ollendick, T., Hynd, G. W., Garfinkel, B., Greenhill, L., Biederman, J., Barkley, R. A., McBURNETT, K., Newcorn, J., & Waldman, I. (1994). DSM-IV field trials for the disruptive behavior disorders: Symptom utility estimates. *Journal of the American Academy of Child & Adolescent Psychiatry, 33*(4), 529–539. https://doi.org/10.1097/00004583-199405000-00011

Hamburger, M. E., Lilienfeld, S. O., & Hogben, M. (1996). Psychopathy, gender, and gender roles: Implications for antisocial and histrionic personality disorders. *Journal of Personality Disorders, 10*(1), 41–55. https://doi.org/10.1521/pedi.1996.10.1.41

Hare, B., Brown, M., Williamson, C., & Tomasello, M. (2002). The domestication of social cognition in dogs. *Science, 298*(5598), 1634–1636. https://doi.org/10.1126/science.1072702

Harkness, A. R., & Lilienfeld, S. O. (1997). Individual differences science for treatment planning: Personality traits. *Psychological Assessment, 9*(4), 349–360. https://doi.org/10.1037/1040-3590.9.4.349

Herbert, J. D., Lilienfeld, S. O., Lohr, J. M., Montgomery, R. W., O'Donohue, W. T., Rosen, G. M., & Tolin, D. F. (2000). Science and pseudoscience in the development of eye movement desensitization and reprocessing: Implications for clinical psychology. *Clinical Psychology Review, 20*(8), 945–971. https://doi.org/10.1016/S0272-7358(99)00017-3

Ioannidis, J. P. A. (2005). Why most published research findings are false. *PLoS Medicine, 2*(8), e124. https://doi.org/10.1371/journal.pmed.0020124

Jacob, R. G., Lilienfeld, S. O., Furman, J. M. R., Durrant, J. D., & Turner, S. M. (1989). Panic disorder with vestibular dysfunction: Further clinical observations and description of space and motion phobic stimuli. *Journal of Anxiety Disorders, 3*(2), 117–130. https://doi.org/10.1016/0887-6185(89)90006-6

John, L. K., Loewenstein, G., & Prelec, D. (2012). Measuring the prevalence of questionable research practices with incentives for truth telling. *Psychological Science, 23*(5), 524–532. https://doi.org/10.1177/0956797611430953

Kessler, R. C., Gruber, M., Hettema, J. M., Hwang, I., Sampson, N., & Yonkers, K. A. (2008). Comorbid major depression and generalized anxiety disorders in the national comorbidity survey follow-up. *Psychological Medicine, 38*(3), 365–374. https://doi.org/10.1017/S0033291707002012

Lahey, B. B., Applegate, B., McBurnett, K., Biederman, J., Greenhill, L., Hynd, G. W., Barkley, R. A., Newcorn, J., Jensen, P., Richters, J., Garfinkel, B., Kerdyk, L., Frick, P. J., Ollendick, T., Perez, D., Hart, E. L., Waidman, I., & Shaffer, D. (1994a). DMS-IV field trials for attention deficit hyperactivity disorder in children and adolescents. *The American Journal of Psychiatry, 151*(11), 1673–1685. https://doi.org/10.1176/ajp.151.11.1673

Lahey, B. B., Applegate, B., Barkley, R. A., Garfinkel, B., McBurnett, K., Kerdyk, L., Greenhill, L., Hynd, G. W., Frick, P. J., & Newcorn, J. (1994b). DSM-IV field trials for oppositional defiant disorder and conduct disorder in children and adolescents. *The American Journal of Psychiatry, 151*(8), 1163–1171. https://doi.org/10.1176/ajp.151.8.1163

Lahey, B. B., Loeber, R., Quay, H. C., Applegate, B., Shaffer, D., Waldman, I., Hart, E. L., Mcburnett, K., Frick, P. J., Jensen, P. S., Dulcan, M. K., Canino, G., & Bird, H. R. (1998). Validity of DSM-IV subtypes of conduct disorder based on age of onset. *Journal of the American Academy of Child & Adolescent Psychiatry, 37*(4), 435–442. https://doi.org/10.1097/00004583-199804000-00022

Laursen, T. M., Agerbo, E., & Pedersen, C. B. (2009). Bipolar disorder, schizoaffective disorder, and schizophrenia overlap: A new comorbidity index. *The Journal of Clinical Psychiatry, 70*(10), 1432–1438. https://doi.org/10.4088/JCP.08m04807

Lilienfeld, S. O. (1992). The association between antisocial personality and somatization disorders: A review and integration of theoretical models. *Clinical Psychology Review, 12*(6), 641–662. https://doi.org/10.1016/0272-7358(92)90136-V

Lilienfeld, S. O. (1995). *Seeing both sides: Classic controversies in abnormal psychology*. Wadsworth Publishing Company.

Lilienfeld, S. O. (1998). Methodological advances and developments in the assessment of psychopathy. *Behaviour Research and Therapy, 36*(1), 99–125. https://doi.org/10.1016/S0005-7967(97)10021-3

Lilienfeld, S. O., & Andrews, B. P. (1996). Development and preliminary validation of a self-report measure of psychopathic personality traits in noncriminal population. *Journal of Personality Assessment, 66*(3), 488–524. https://doi.org/10.1207/s15327752jpa6603_3

Lilienfeld, S. O., & Basterfield, C. (2020). Reflective practice in clinical psychology: Reflections from basic psychological science. *Clinical Psychology: Science and Practice, 27*(4), e12352. https://doi.org/10.1111/cpsp.12352

Lilienfeld, S. O., & Loftus, E. F. (1998). Repressed memories and World War II: Some cautionary notes. *Professional Psychology: Research and Practice, 29*(5), 471–475. https://doi.org/10.1037/0735-7028.29.5.471

Lilienfeld, S. O., & Loftus, E. F. (1999). A step backward in the recovered memory debate. *Professional Psychology: Research and Practice, 30*(6), 623–623. https://doi.org/10.1037/0735-7028.30.6.623.b

Lilienfeld, S. O., & Marino, L. (1995). Mental disorder as a Roschian concept: A critique of Wakefield's "harmful dysfunction" analysis. *Journal of Abnormal Psychology, 104*(3), 411–420. https://doi.org/10.1037/0021-843X.104.3.411

Lilienfeld, S. O., & Marino, L. (1999). Essentialism revisited: Evolutionary theory and the concept of mental disorder. *Journal of Abnormal Psychology, 108*(3), 400–411. https://doi.org/10.1037/0021-843X.108.3.400

Lilienfeld, S. O., & O'Donohue, W. T. (2012). *The great ideas of clinical science: 17 principles that every mental health professional should understand.* Routledge.

Lilienfeld, S. O., & Waldman, I. D. (1990). The relation between childhood attention-deficit hyperactivity disorder and adult antisocial behavior reexamined: The problem of heterogeneity. *Clinical Psychology Review, 10*(6), 699–725. https://doi.org/10.1016/0272-7358(90)90076-M

Lilienfeld, S. O., & Waldman, I. D. (2004). Comorbidity and Chairman Mao. *World Psychiatry, 3*(1), 26–27. https://www.ncbi.nlm.nih.gov/pmc/articles/PMC1414658/

Lilienfeld, S. O., & Waldman, I. D. (Eds.). (2017). *Psychological science under scrutiny.* Wiley Blackwell.

Lilienfeld, S. O., Van Valkenburg, C., Larntz, K., & Akiskal, H. S. (1986). The relationship of histrionic personality disorder to antisocial personality and somatization disorders. *The American Journal of Psychiatry, 143*(6), 718–722. https://doi.org/10.1176/ajp.143.6.718

Lilienfeld, S. O., Jacob, R. G., & Furman, J. M. (1989a). Vestibular dysfunction followed by panic disorder with agoraphobia. *Journal of Nervous and Mental Disease, 177*(11), 700–701. https://doi.org/10.1097/00005053-198911000-00009

Lilienfeld, S. O., Jacob, R. G., & Turner, S. M. (1989b). Comment on Holloway and McNally's (1987) "Effects of anxiety sensitivity on the response to hyperventilation". *Journal of Abnormal Psychology, 98*(1), 100–102. https://doi.org/10.1037/0021-843X.98.1.100

Lilienfeld, S. O., Turner, S. M., & Jacob, R. G. (1993). Anxiety sensitivity: An examination of theoretical and methodological issues. *Advances in Behaviour Research and Therapy, 15*(2), 147–183. https://doi.org/10.1016/0146-6402(93)90019-X

Lilienfeld, S. O., Waldman, I. D., & Israel, A. C. (1994a). A critical examination of the use of the term and concept of comorbidity in psychopathology research. *Clinical Psychology: Science and Practice, 1*(1), 71–83. https://doi.org/10.1111/j.1468-2850.1994.tb00007.x

Lilienfeld, S. O., Andrews, B. P., Stone-Romero, E. F., & Stone, D. (1994b). The relations between a self-report honesty test and personality measures in prison and college samples. *Journal of Research in Personality, 28*(2), 154–169. https://doi.org/10.1006/jrpe.1994.1013

Lilienfeld, S. O., Alliger, G., & Mitchell, K. (1995). Why integrity testing remains controversial. *American Psychologist, 50*(6), 457–458. https://doi.org/10.1037/0003-066X.50.6.457

Lilienfeld, S. O., Hess, T., & Rowland, C. (1996). Psychopathic personality traits and temporal perspective: A test of the short time horizon hypothesis. *Journal of Psychopathology and Behavioral Assessment, 18*(3), 285–303. https://doi.org/10.1007/BF02229050

Lilienfeld, S. O., Kirsch, I., Sarbin, T. R., Lynn, S. J., Chaves, J. F., Ganaway, G. K., & Powell, R. A. (1999). Dissociative identity disorder and the sociocognitive model: Recalling the lessons of the past. *Psychological Bulletin, 125*(5), 507–523. https://doi.org/10.1037/0033-2909.125.5.507

Lilienfeld, S. O., Wood, J. M., & Garb, H. N. (2000). The scientific status of projective techniques. *Psychological Science in the Public Interest, 1*(2), 27–66. https://doi.org/10.1111/1529-1006.002

Lilienfeld, S. O., Wood, J., & Garb, H. N. (2001a). The Rorschach Inkblot Test: A debate. The Rorschach Test is scientifically questionable. *The Harvard Mental Health Letter, 18*(6), 5–6.

Lilienfeld, S. O., Wood, J. M., & Garb, H. N. (2001b). What's wrong with this picture? *Scientific American, 284*(5), 80–87. https://www.jstor.org/stable/26059212

Lilienfeld, S. O., Waldman, I. D., Landfield, K., Watts, A. L., Rubenzer, S., & Faschingbauer, T. R. (2012). Fearless dominance and the U.S. presidency: Implications of psychopathic personality traits for successful and unsuccessful political leadership. *Journal of Personality and Social Psychology, 103*(3), 489–505. https://doi.org/10.1037/a0029392

Lilienfeld, S. O., Lynn, S. J., & Lohr, J. M. (Eds.). (2015). *Science and pseudoscience in clinical psychology* (2nd ed., pp. xxvii, 548). The Guilford Press.

Lilienfeld, S. O., Turner, S. M., & Jacob, R. G. (n.d.). *De´ja Vu all over again: Critical misunderstandings concerning anxiety sensitivity and constructive suggestions for future research* (p. 12).

Lohr, J. M., Tolin, D. F., & Lilienfeld, S. O. (1998). Efficacy of eye movement desensitization and reprocessing: Implications for behavior therapy. *Behavior Therapy, 29*(1), 123–156. https://doi.org/10.1016/S0005-7894(98)80035-X

Lohr, J. M., Lilienfeld, S. O., Tolin, D. F., & Herbert, J. D. (1999). Eye movement desensitization and reprocessing: An analysis of specific versus nonspecific treatment factors. *Journal of Anxiety Disorders, 13*(1), 185–207. https://doi.org/10.1016/S0887-6185(98)00047-4

Lynn, S. J., Lock, T., Loftus, E. F., Krackow, E., & Lilienfeld, S. O. (2003). The remembrance of things past: Problematic memory recovery techniques in psychotherapy. In *Science and pseudoscience in clinical psychology* (pp. 205–239). Guilford Press.

Lynn, S. J., Knox, J. A., Fassler, O., Lilienfeld, S. O., & Loftus, E. F. (2004). Memory, trauma, and dissociation. In *Posttraumatic stress disorder: Issues and controversies* (pp. 163–186). Wiley. https://doi.org/10.1002/9780470713570.ch9

Lynn, S. J., Lilienfeld, S. O., Merckelbach, H., Giesbrecht, T., & van der Kloet, D. (2012). Dissociation and dissociative disorders: Challenging conventional wisdom. *Current Directions in Psychological Science, 21*(1), 48–53. https://doi.org/10.1177/0963721411429457

Lynn, S. J., Krackow, E., Loftus, E. F., Locke, T. G., & Lilienfeld, S. O. (2015). Constructing the past: Problematic memory recovery techniques in psychotherapy. In *Science and pseudoscience in clinical psychology* (2nd ed., pp. 210–244). The Guilford Press.

Marino, L., & Lilienfeld, S. O. (1998). Dolphin-assisted therapy: Flawed data, flawed conclusions. *Anthrozoös, 11*(4), 194–200. https://doi.org/10.2752/089279398787000517

Neisser, U. (1987). Cognition and reality. 認知の構図. https://ci.nii.ac.jp/naid/10013492242/

Neisser, U. (2000). *Memory observed: Remembering in natural contexts*. Macmillan.

Neisser, U. (2014). *Cognitive psychology: Classic edition*. Psychology Press.

Nelson, L. D., Simmons, J., & Simonsohn, U. (2018). Psychology's renaissance. *Annual Review of Psychology, 69*, 511–534. https://doi.org/10.1146/annurev-psych-122216-011836

Nosek, B. A., Alter, G., Banks, G. C., Borsboom, D., Bowman, S. D., Breckler, S. J., Buck, S., Chambers, C. D., Chin, G., Christensen, G., Contestabile, M., Dafoe, A., Eich, E., Freese, J., Glennerster, R., Goroff, D., Green, D. P., Hesse, B., Humphreys, M., et al. (2015). Promoting an open research culture. *Science, 348*(6242), 1422–1425. https://doi.org/10.1126/science.aab2374

OPEN SCIENCE COLLABORATION. (2015). Estimating the reproducibility of psychological science. *Science, 349*(6251), aac4716. https://doi.org/10.1126/science.aac4716

Poldrack, R. A., Baker, C. I., Durnez, J., Gorgolewski, K. J., Matthews, P. M., Munafò, M. R., Nichols, T. E., Poline, J.-B., Vul, E., & Yarkoni, T. (2017). Scanning the horizon: Towards transparent and reproducible neuroimaging research. *Nature Reviews Neuroscience, 18*(2), 115–126. https://doi.org/10.1038/nrn.2016.167

Poore, H. E., Watts, A. L., Lilienfeld, S. O., & Waldman, I. D. (2020). Construct validity of youth psychopathic traits as assessed by the Antisocial Process Screening Device. *Psychological Assessment, 32*(6), 527–540. https://doi.org/10.1037/pas0000809

Poythress, N. G., Edens, J. F., & Lilienfeld, S. O. (1998). Criterion-related validity of the Psychopathic Personality Inventory in a prison sample. *Psychological Assessment, 10*(4), 426–430. https://doi.org/10.1037/1040-3590.10.4.426

Preston, S. D., & de Waal, F. B. M. (2002). Empathy: Its ultimate and proximate bases. *Behavioral and Brain Sciences, 25*(1), 1–20. https://doi.org/10.1017/S0140525X02000018

Rafferty, T. (1993). *The thing happens: Ten years of writing about the movies* (1st ed.). Grove Press.

Rosen, G. M., McNally, R. J., & Lilienfeld, S. O. (1999). Eye movement magic. *Skeptic (Altadena, CA), 7*(4), 66–66. https://go.gale.com/ps/i.do?p=AONE&sw=w&issn=10639330&v=2.1&it=r&id=GALE%7CA60898895&sid=googleScholar&linkaccess=abs

Rosen, G. M., Mcnally, R. J., Lohr, J. M., Herbert, J. D., & Lilienfeld, S. O. (n.d.). *Four points to consider before you buy EMDR products: A reply to Shapiro et al.*

Sagan, C. (2011). *The Demon-Haunted world: Science as a candle in the dark* (Reprint ed.). Ballantine Books.

Simmons, J. P., Nelson, L. D., & Simonsohn, U. (2011). False-positive psychology: Undisclosed flexibility in data collection and analysis allows presenting anything as significant. *Psychological Science, 22*(11), 1359–1366. https://doi.org/10.1177/0956797611417632

Tackett, J. L., Lilienfeld, S. O., Patrick, C. J., Johnson, S. L., Krueger, R. F., Miller, J. D., Oltmanns, T. F., & Shrout, P. E. (2017). It's time to broaden the replicability conversation: Thoughts for and from clinical psychological science. *Perspectives on Psychological Science, 12*(5), 742–756. https://doi.org/10.1177/1745691617690042

The Scientific Status of Projective Techniques—Scott O. Lilienfeld, James M. Wood, Howard N. Garb, 2000. (n.d.). Retrieved December 9, 2021, from https://journals.sagepub.com/doi/abs/10.1111/1529-1006.002

Tomasello, M. (1992). *First verbs: A case study of early grammatical development.* Cambridge University Press.

Tomasello, M. (2009a). *Why we cooperate.* MIT Press.

Tomasello, M. (2009b). *Constructing a language.* Harvard University Press.

Tomasello, M. (2009c). *The cultural origins of human cognition.* Harvard University Press.

Tomasello, M., & Call, J. (1997). *Primate cognition.* Oxford University Press.

Tomasello, M., Kruger, A. C., & Ratner, H. H. (1993). Cultural learning. *Behavioral and Brain Sciences, 16*(3), 495–511. https://doi.org/10.1017/S0140525X0003123X

Tomasello, M., Carpenter, M., Call, J., Behne, T., & Moll, H. (2005). Understanding and sharing intentions: The origins of cultural cognition. *Behavioral and Brain Sciences, 28*(5), 675–691. https://doi.org/10.1017/S0140525X05000129

Vul, E., Harris, C., Winkielman, P., & Pashler, H. (2009). Puzzlingly high correlations in fmri studies of emotion, personality, and social cognition. *Perspectives on Psychological Science, 4*(3), 274–290. https://doi.org/10.1111/j.1745-6924.2009.01125.x

Wakefield, J. C. (1992). Disorder as harmful dysfunction: A conceptual critique of DSM-III-R's definition of mental disorder. *Psychological Review*, 232–247.

Wakefield, J. C. (2007). The concept of mental disorder: Diagnostic implications of the harmful dysfunction analysis. *World Psychiatry, 6*(3), 149–156. https://www.ncbi.nlm.nih.gov/pmc/articles/PMC2174594/

Waldman, I. D., & Lahey, B. B. (1994). Design of the DSM-IV disruptive behavior disorder field trials. *Child and Adolescent Psychiatric Clinics of North America, 3*(2), 195–208. https://doi.org/10.1016/S1056-4993(18)30496-6

Waldman, I. D., & Lilienfeld, S. O. (1992). Diagnostic efficiency of symptoms for oppositional defiant disorder and attention-deficit hyperactivity disorder. *Journal of Consulting and Clinical Psychology, 59*(5), 732. https://doi.org/10.1037/0022-006X.59.5.732

Waldman, I. D., & Lilienfeld, S. O. (2001). Applications of taxometric methods to problems of comorbidity: Perspectives and challenges. *Clinical Psychology: Science and Practice, 8*(4), 520–527. https://doi.org/10.1093/clipsy.8.4.520

Waldman, I. D., & Lilienfeld, S. O. (2016). Thinking about data, research methods, and statistical analyses: Commentary on Sijtsma's (2014) "Playing with Data". *Psychometrika, 81*(1), 16–26. https://doi.org/10.1007/s11336-015-9447-z

Waldman, I. D., Lilienfeld, S. O., & Lahey, B. B. (1995). Toward construct validity in the childhood disruptive behavior disorders. In T. H. Ollendick & R. J. Prinz (Eds.), *Advances in clinical child psychology* (pp. 323–363). Springer. https://doi.org/10.1007/978-1-4757-9044-3_8

Waller, N. G., & Waldman, I. D. (1990). A reexamination of the WAIS—R factor structure. *Psychological Assessment: A Journal of Consulting and Clinical Psychology, 2*(2), 139–144. https://doi.org/10.1037/1040-3590.2.2.139

Waller, N. G., Lilienfeld, S. O., Tellegen, A., & Lykken, D. T. (1991). The tridimensional personality questionnaire: Structural validity and comparison with the multidimensional personality questionnaire. *Multivariate Behavioral Research, 26*(1), 1–23. https://doi.org/10.1207/s15327906mbr2601_1

Watts, A. L., Lilienfeld, S. O., Smith, S. F., Miller, J. D., Campbell, W. K., Waldman, I. D., Rubenzer, S. J., & Faschingbauer, T. J. (2013). The double-edged sword of grandiose narcissism: Implications for successful and unsuccessful leadership among U.S. Presidents. *Psychological Science, 24*(12), 2379–2389. https://doi.org/10.1177/0956797613491970

Watts, A. L., Poore, H. E., Lilienfeld, S. O., & Waldman, I. D. (2019). Clarifying the associations between Big Five personality domains and higher-order psychopathology dimensions in youth. *Journal of Research in Personality, 82*, 103844. https://doi.org/10.1016/j.jrp.2019.07.002

Wood, J. M., & Lilienfeld, S. O. (1999). The Rorschach Inkblot Test: A case of overstatement? *Assessment, 6*(4), 341–351. https://doi.org/10.1177/107319119900600405

Wood, J. M., Lilienfeld, S. O., Garb, H. N., & Nezworski, M. T. (2000). Limitations of the Rorschach as a diagnostic tool: A reply to Garfield (2000), Lerner (2000), and Weiner (2000). *Journal of Clinical Psychology, 56*(3), 441–448. https://doi.org/10.1002/(SICI)1097-4679(200003)56:3<441::AID-JCLP19>3.0.CO;2-Q

Wood, J. M., Lilienfeld, S. O., Nezworski, M. T., & Garb, H. N. (2001a). Coming to grips with negative evidence for the comprehensive system for the Rorschach: A comment on Gacono, Loving, and Bodholdt; Ganellen; and Bornstein. *Journal of Personality Assessment, 77*(1), 48–70. https://doi.org/10.1207/S15327752JPA7701_04

Wood, J. M., Nezworski, M. T., Garb, H. N., & Lilienfeld, S. O. (2001b). Problems with the norms of the Comprehensive System for the Rorschach: Methodological and conceptual considerations. *Clinical Psychology: Science and Practice, 8*(3), 397–402. https://doi.org/10.1093/clipsy.8.3.397

Part II
Science and Pseudoscience in Clinical Psychology

The Limitations of Science: The Importance of Rationalism in Clinical Science

William O'Donohue, Kylie A. Baer, Jorge A. Cao-Noya, Kieffer Christianson, Natalia Duda, Brandon T. Hunley, Haylee Lafrentz, and Stephanie R. Reyes

The Limitations of Science: The Importance of Rationalism

There have been canonical publications regarding the relationship between science and clinical psychology. Hans Eyensck's (1952) review indicating the poor methodological quality of psychotherapy outcome studies, and thus the lack of actual scientific support for the efficacy of then current therapies, might be one good candidate for such a pivotal publication. B.F. Skinner's (1953) publications, particularly his *Science and Human Behavior*, might be another. Paul Meehl's (1954) body of work, particularly on actuarial vs clinical prediction, would also be an important one. Gordon Paul's (1969) elucidation of the complexity of outcome research is another reasonable candidate. Steven Haynes's (Haynes et al., 1984) work on understanding the complexities of clinical measurement and psychometrics is perhaps another. Richard McFall's (1991) *Manifesto for a Science of Clinical Psychology* is one of the more recent canonical publications on this issue. There is certainly a myriad of other publications over the past 70 years or so, but these are some particularly influential writings.

Importantly, there has been little counterargument against science serving as the basic epistemic approach in applied psychology. That is, there has been no significant movement advancing the notion that science ought not be the principal epistemic approach to the growth of knowledge in clinical psychology. It is another set of questions, however, regarding the extent to which a general commitment to science has resulted in high-quality science (see, for example, O'Donohue et al., in press), or optimal progress in the growth of knowledge, or even the extent to which this general commitment to science has resulted in consistent science-based practice.

W. O'Donohue (✉) · K. A. Baer · J. A. Cao-Noya · K. Christianson · N. Duda · B. T. Hunley
H. Lafrentz · S. R. Reyes
University of Nevada, Reno, NV, USA
e-mail: wto@unr.edu

C. L. Cobb et al. (eds.), *Toward a Science of Clinical Psychology*,
https://doi.org/10.1007/978-3-031-14332-8_4

Part of the gap between the overall commitment to science and problematic practice may be due to a lack of a clear understanding of science itself. For example, O'Donohue and Halsey (1997) found that diverse psychologists such as Freud, Skinner, Carl Rogers, and Albert Ellis all thought their therapeutic approach was scientific. However, each of these scholars also advanced radically different notions of what exactly they thought science was. Important and fundamental questions remain in clinical science about what science is and thus what clinical science is. Such questions include: What properties constitute science? What is pseudoscience? What are the limits of science? Regarding the last question, if science does have limits, then an important question becomes: How can epistemic progress be made outside the limits of science? That is, if there are content domains or questions that science for some reason cannot address, are there other ways of making progress in these areas?

This chapter will address these last two questions. We will argue that science is limited in at least eight major ways: (1) Although science is a form of rationality, there are rational methods that can generate knowledge that are not themselves scientific; (2) Ethical questions are generally outside the scope of science (Hempel, 1965); (3) The singularity of the individual and the resultant personal knowledge are generally beyond the scope of science (Houts, 2009); (4) Metaphysical statements transcend the scope of science but can still influence science (Popper, 1959); (5) Existence claims cannot be falsified, and if science is viewed as an epistemic process attempting to root out error by seeking falsifications (Popper, 1959), then existence claims are beyond the scope of science; (6) Logic and mathematics produce truths but are beyond the scope of science; (7) Scientific regularities are underdetermined by science (i.e., asserting belief in a scientific law or regularity goes beyond scientific evidence); and (8) Power affects science, and this is seen by postmodernists as a limit to science (O'Donohue, 2013).

It is important for clinical scientists to understand the limits of science for at least two reasons. First, a lack of understanding regarding how the limits of scientific epistemology can lead to *scientism* (i.e., an irrationally positive view of science that erroneously asserts that it has characteristics or abilities that in fact science does not). Someone embracing scientism might informally be thought of as a "true believer" in science. There has been too little concern about scientism within clinical science as the emphasis has been on increasing acceptance and use of science, which is understandable given the use of rational belief formation strategies by many psychologists that are problematic. However, there has been relatively little scholarly work on ensuring that the legitimate scope of science is not misconstrued or exaggerated. This paper will attempt to describe the legitimate scope of science. Second, this paper will argue that just because science has limitations does not mean that knowledge cannot be gained outside these limits.

This paper adopts Bartley's (1984) pan-critical rationalism as this is a general approach to defining and understanding rationalism and rational knowledge generation both within and outside the limits of science. Bartley was a student of Sir Karl Popper and advocated an approach to rational belief formation that is based on maximizing criticism to identify and modify error. Bartley argued that justificationist approaches to knowledge, such as confirmationist approaches in which some kinds or amounts of evidence are viewed as warranting/confirming/justifying a belief, are logically problematic. For Bartley, justificationism either leads to an infinite regress in which any proffered justification for some claim would in turn need its own justification; or the other fork of the dilemma is to end this regress by dogmatically accepting some knowledge claims to be basic and thus in no need of justification themselves. To escape this dilemma, Bartley suggested an approach that he called pan-critical rationalism in which all statements are open to criticism, including the claims of pan-critical rationalism itself. Rationality, in this approach, becomes a thoroughgoing critical enterprise in which one attempts to identify error in beliefs by maximizing criticism. The beliefs that best survive the most severe criticism, especially with respect to their competitors, are regarded as the most rational. Science, if done correctly, becomes one tool in this arsenal of criticism—beliefs are subjected to severe tests, usually empirical tests, and those that best survive this testing are regarded as the most rational. However, it must be remembered that further criticism including future empirical testing may subsequently falsify these beliefs. Criticism is an ongoing process.

The late Professor Scott Lilienfeld of Emory University was one of the most influential scholars in the past few decades in the role of criticism in science and rationality. He published influential papers on the problematic scientific status of projective testing (Wood et al., 2011), on the scientific status of psychotherapies such as Eye Movement Desensitization and Reprocessing (Herbert et al., 2000) and dolphin-assisted therapy (Marino & Lilienfeld, 2007), on iatrogenesis in psychotherapy (Lilienfeld, 2007), on pseudoscience in clinical psychology (Lilienfeld et al., 2014), on scientifically unsupported popular myths regarding psychology (Lilienfeld et al., 2011), on hyperbole associated with neuroscience (Satel & Lilienfeld, 2013), on hyperbole associated with psychotherapy and bibliotherapy (Meichenbaum & Lilienfeld, 2018; Rosen & Lilienfeld, 2016), on science in the courtroom (Skeem et al., 2009), on questionable research practices (O'Donohue et al., in press), and on the scientific status of problematic and poorly defined constructs in psychology such as microaggressions (Lilienfeld, 2017). These publications would not exist without a significant degree of intellectual courage—this skeptical and critical attitude might not be as fully appreciated when it is turned on someone's favored beliefs.

A good part of Lilienfeld's work can be construed as an attempt to understand science and what might interfere with good science, as well as to apply this understanding to real-world problems. To understand any limit of science, one must first understand what science is. Lilienfeld approached the relationship between meta-science and clinical science in three primary ways, which correspond to three major influences upon his views. To understand Lilienfeld's view of science, it is useful to understand his influences. First, he was influenced by meta-scientists such as Carl Sagan (1995) and Sir Karl Popper (1959). Second, he was influenced by important work on the role of science in countering cognitive limitations reflected in heuristics such confirmation bias. Third, he developed his own approach highlighting the importance of intellectual humility (Bowes et al., 2020).

Meta-Scientists: Carl Sagan and Sir Karl Popper

Carl Sagan (1983) was not trained as a philosopher of science but rather was an astronomer at Cornell University, Lilienfeld's undergraduate alma mater. Scott would often quote Sagan in his papers on meta-science. Sagan was one of the most widely recognized popularizers of science, especially astronomy and cosmology. One of Sagan's priorities was the use of science as a corrective to our cognitive errors, particularly errors associated with the way we would like the world to be or the way that some tradition has taught us how the world is. A key pillar of Sagan's (1983) general view of science is found in his book, *Cosmos*: "Science has taught us that, because we have a talent for deceiving ourselves, subjectivity may not freely reign" (p. 333). However, Sagan emphasized that skepticism alone was insufficient for the growth of knowledge in science. Scientists, according to Sagan (1983), also need to be open and creative:

> At the heart of science is an essential tension between two seemingly contradictory attitudes—an openness to new ideas, no matter how bizarre or counter-intuitive they may be, and the most ruthless skeptical scrutiny of all ideas, old and new. This is how deep truths are winnowed from deep nonsense … (p. 17)

Scott certainly embodied this openness—he was always ready to consider new data, new arguments, and new possibilities. However, these needed to pass critical muster.

Sagan (1995, p. 116), in his "The Fine Art of Baloney Detection," provided some details of how this critical method could be practiced:

- Wherever possible there must be independent confirmation of the "facts."
- Encourage substantive debate on the evidence by knowledgeable proponents of all points of view.
- Arguments from authority carry little weight — "authorities" have made mistakes in the past. They will do so again in the future. Perhaps a better way to say it is that in science there are no authorities; at most, there are experts.
- Spin more than one hypothesis. If there's something to be explained, think of all the different ways in which it could be explained. Then think of tests by which you might systematically disprove each of the alternatives.
- Try not to get overly attached to a hypothesis just because it's yours. It's only a way station in the pursuit of knowledge. Ask yourself why you like the idea. Compare it fairly with the alternatives. See if you can find reasons for rejecting it. If you don't, others will.
- If whatever it is you're explaining has some measure, some numerical quantity attached to it, you'll be much better able to discriminate among competing hypotheses. What is vague and qualitative is open to many explanations.
- If there's a chain of argument, *every* link in the chain must work (including the premise)—not just most of them.
- Occam's Razor. This convenient rule-of-thumb urges us when faced with two hypotheses that explain the data *equally well* to choose the simpler. Always ask whether the hypothesis can be, at least in principle, falsified…. You must be able

> to check assertions out. Inveterate skeptics must be given the chance to follow your reasoning, to duplicate your experiments and see if they get the same result.

Finally, Sagan (1980, p. 333), like many others such as W.V.O. Quine, Sir Karl Popper, and psychologist Donald Campell (see O'Donohue, 2013), linked epistemology with evolution, in essence naturalizing epistemology by viewing humans' proclivity toward science as a byproduct of natural selection:

> There is no other species on Earth that does science. It is, so far, entirely a human invention, evolved by natural selection in the cerebral cortex for one simple reason: It works. It is not perfect. It can be misused. It is only a tool. But it is by far the best tool we have, self-correcting, ongoing, applicable to everything. It has two rules. First: there are no sacred truths, all assumptions must be critically examined; arguments from authority are worthless. Second: whatever is inconsistent with the facts must be discarded or revised. We must understand the Cosmos as it is and not confuse how it is with how we wish it to be.

Lilienfeld also had a deep appreciation for the work of Sir Karl Popper (1959). Popper argued that because there was no such thing as an ampliative (roughly, content increasing) inductive logic, and because *modus tollens* was a valid deductive logical inference rule, for science to be undergirded by logic it ought to seek falsification of favored beliefs. *Modus tollens* can be expressed as:

1. If Theory A, then Observation B
2. *Not Observation B*
3. Therefore, Not Theory A

Popper claimed that science was problem-solving (as is evolution). Popper thought science progressed according to the following schema:

$$\text{Problem} \rightarrow \text{Tentative Solution} \rightarrow \text{Error Elimination Attempt} \rightarrow$$
$$\text{Problem 2} \rightarrow \text{Tentative Solution 2} \ldots \text{and so on.}$$

Popper advocated proposing theories as tentative solutions that have high empirical content. The empirical content of a claim is the number of potential empirical states of affairs that the theory rules out (i.e., is inconsistent with). For example, the proposition, "All males drink water" rules out fewer states of affairs than "All humans drink water" because the first claim doesn't rule out females not drinking water, while the former does. Thus, the latter claim is easier to falsify—an observation of a woman who does not drink water only falsifies the latter. Beyond the extension of the subject of a claim, increased precision in the claim also rules out more states of affairs. The statement "All humans drink exactly 42 ounces of water" rules out more states of affairs than any of the prior statements due to its precision.

The final component of Popper's philosophy of science that will be reviewed here is his view that the quality of scientific research could be partially captured by the severity of its tests. For Popper, tests of some belief vary in severity—as some tests are easier to pass than others. Popper's view is that if the scientist is sincerely attempting to efficiently find if his or her beliefs contain error, then the wise scientist would use severe testing to more quickly discover if his or her beliefs are indeed false. Severe tests attempt to examine the states of affairs that are inconsistent with the belief that have the highest probability of occurring. Imagine if one wants to test the claim, "Religious leaders do not swear." A less severe test of this would be to examine whether they swear during their sermons, or when they are teaching religious classes for children. A more severe test would be to examine situations in which swearing is generally more common (e.g., after stubbing their toes, when they are angry, or when someone cuts them off in traffic, and so on). Popper advocated that the best science involves proposing solutions that have high empirical content and then severely testing these.

Cognitive Limitations

Lilienfeld emphasized that antecedently held biases as well as problematic cognitive shortcuts, both, could bias the clinical judgment of psychologists (e.g., in making a diagnosis): and knowing these heuristic errors, striving to identify them, and correcting them was a key activity of the clinical scientists (Bowes et al., 2020). Lilienfeld stated:

> To the extent that one crucial element of wisdom is an awareness of one's fallibilities and a sense of humility concerning the limits of one's knowledge, debiasing the general public against confirmation bias and related biases may be an essential step toward a wiser—and perhaps ultimately safer—world. Psychologists would be wise to make this effort a priority. (Lilienfeld et al., 2009, p. 395)

Probably the best-known heuristic error, and one that science particularly combats, is confirmation bias—the tendency to seek, value, and emphasize information that confirms or is consistent with one's prior beliefs. Lilienfeld also wrote about blindspot bias, a bias that one does not see one's own biases (Bowes et al., 2020). However, other biases were also relevant such as the representativeness heuristic, base rate neglect, and illusory correlation, among others.

Intellectual Humility

Finally, Lilienfeld became interested in the epistemic virtue called intellectual humility during the last decade or so of his life. Intellectual humility has been defined in various ways but basically is a meta-cognitive stance toward being open to reexamine one's beliefs, especially in the light of new evidence or arguments. Arrogance and closed-mindedness would be its antonyms (Bowes et al., 2020; Bowes et al., this volume).

Now that we understand some of what Lilienfeld correctly took to be characteristics of science, we turn now to the questions of its limits and how knowledge can be obtained outside these limits.

1. Rationality as Subsuming Science But Not Co-Extensive

Science is viewed as part of rationalism; however, it is not the entirety of rational discourse (Popper, 1959). The essential feature of rationalism for Popper is criticism, particularly maximizing a wide variety of severe criticism—and criticism can be applied to any claim or argument. For example, although arguments for the comparative advantages of science over intuition, or over the use of astrology, are not themselves scientific, however, these can nevertheless produce valuable increments in knowledge. Arguments about what constitutes good science also generally are not the products of science but again fall under the general umbrella of rationalism. Arguments about what reputable scientists such as Newton, Darwin, or Einstein discovered are, again, not science but rather can be rational arguments (subject to the kind of thoroughgoing criticism described by Bartley) from an accurate reading of the historical record.

Thus, there are many nonscientific questions that are meaningful and even important surrounding the practice of science that are not scientific but that can still be addressed rationally.

2. Ethics

Science produces "*is* statements," both descriptive claims (e.g., "The delta variant of COVID-19 is more contagious than the omicron variant") and causal claims ("Heat is the cause of expansion in metals"). Ethics is a branch of philosophy investigating moral questions. Ethics involves what someone *ought* to do or ought not to do. Ponder the classic trolley example (Thomson & Parent, 1986). You are the driver of a trolley whose breaks have just failed. The trolley is already heading down one path, on which it will kill five people. You do not have time to get off the track, but you are able to turn the trolley to head down a second path, containing one person. If you direct the trolley down the second path, you will kill one person; if you do nothing, five people will die. What *ought* you do in this situation? This question is not asking for an answer expressed as an *is* statement, that is, a statement describing some state of affairs of the world.

Hume was the philosopher who first introduced the *is-ought* distinction—"*ought* cannot be derived from *is*" (Hume, 1737). This became known as Hume's Law—that, as a matter of logic, conclusions involving *ought* claims cannot be validly derived from premises containing only *is* statements (Cohon, 2018). Thus, one cannot draw ethical conclusions from the premises produced by scientific statements.

The early twentieth century philosopher G.E. Moore presented another argument: that the *is* statements of science are not sufficient for properly defining moral constructs (Moore, 1903). Moore advanced the "naturalistic fallacy": a logical fallacy in which there is some attempt to define what is *good* by only using naturalistic properties, such as *desirable* or *pleasant*. This argument, which also has been called the "the open-question argument," attempts to demonstrate that *good* is a simple, unanalyzable quality. The argument consists of taking any proposed naturalistic definition of *good* and turning it into a question. For example, if the proposed definition is, "Good means whatever leads to pleasure," then it can be asked, "Is whatever leads to pleasure good?" The issue is not whether the answer to this question is "yes" or "no." Moore suggests that if this latter query is at all meaningful—for example, if a negative answer is not obviously self-contradictory—then the proposed definition of *good* simply cannot be correct, because a sound definition must preserve the meaning of the term that is being defined. If it does preserve the meaning, then this question would be absurd as it would be asking something that is obvious. It would be similar to asking the question, "Do all triangles have three sides?" Thus, the open-question argument is taken to demonstrate that naturalistic definitions, such as those found in *is* statements from science, do not comprehensively capture all that is ordinarily meant by the moral concept of *good*.

The philosopher of science, Carl Hempel (1965), also agreed with this *is-ought* distinction and that this distinction indicated that science alone is not capable of answering ethical questions. Utilizing Laplace's demon—a placeholder for a perfect scientific intelligence who knows all scientific laws that will ever exist (Laplace, 1902)—Hempel offered a situation in which an individual can consult with Laplace's demon when faced with an ethical decision. The demon would be able to inform the individual, Hempel argued, of the consequences of any decision with absolute precision throughout all space and time. Once the demon offered a complete description of the world for each possible action, however, his task would be complete. This task would still leave the moral agent to choose which course of action is morally best. Considering every possible scenario, what *ought* the individual do, remains unanswered by this complete account of empirical matters.

> Let us assume, then, that faced with a moral decision, we are able to call upon the Laplacean demon as a consultant. What help might we get from him? Suppose that we have to choose one of several alternative courses of action open to us and that we want to know which of these we ought to follow. The demon would then be able to tell us, for any contemplated choice, what its consequences would be for the future course of the universe, down to the most minute detail, however remote in space and time. But, having done this for each of the alternative courses of action under consideration, the demon would have completed this task; he would have given us all the information that an ideal science might provide under the circumstances. And yet he would not have resolved our moral problem, for this requires a decision as to which of the several alternative sets of consequences mapped out by the demon as attainable to us is best; which of them we ought to bring about. And the burden of the decision would still fall upon our shoulders; it's we who would have to commit ourselves to an unconditional (absolute) judgment of value by singling out one of the set of consequences as superior to the alternatives. (Hempel, 1965, pp. 88–89)

In sum, propositions involving what *is* and propositions involving what *ought* to be done are regarded as two distinct kinds of claims. While science can answer questions from the domain of descriptive ethics (i.e., *is* questions pertaining to empirical matters regarding ethics, such as, What percentage of individuals believe abortion is morally permissible?), it cannot resolve the underlying normative ethical question, Is abortion moral or immoral?

How, then, are these normative, *ought* ethical questions addressed? One contender again is Bartley's (1984) account, which aims to advance moral knowledge and solve ethical problems by separating criticism—the expression of disapproval of something based on perceived faults—from justification—the showing of something to be correct or reasonable. Bartley claimed that the approximations to truth (what he calls, "verisimilitude") can be reached if propositions and arguments, including those regarding ethical matters, are open to criticism by anyone on a variety of grounds. (Note that the question of the legitimacy or illegitimacy of the grounds is even open to criticism in this approach, hence, "pan-critical.") In utilizing this approach, individuals engage in a dialogue of perpetual criticism designed to identify errors and the arguments that best survive this criticism process will best approach truth about ethical matters. Bartley's pan-critical rationalism may be the best method for reconciling the divergence between ethical and scientific questions—it employs a systematic approach (analogous to science) for solving the questions that cannot be answered by science (i.e., ethical *ought* questions).

3. Radical Ideography and the Personal Knowledge of Jerusalem

Another question is whether there is a "second demarcation" problem; specifically, are there essential differences between the physical sciences and the human/psychological sciences, perhaps because of some unique properties of humans such as each individual's radical ideography and unique personal life history (O'Donohue et al., 2019)? And if so, do these unique properties limit the scientific scope of the social sciences in particular and create the need for a distinct framework and method for psychological inquiry?

The physical sciences have discovered many quantifiable universal laws while psychology has not. Psychology has generally only uncovered nonquantifiable and probabilistic regularities such as the statistical relationship between depression and suicide—and even in this relationship, there is little consensus regarding how that ought to be properly quantified (Sher et al., 2001). Additionally, the field of psychology is currently in a replicability crisis in which key studies are not replicating (O'Donohue et al., in press; Wiggins & Christopherson, 2019; Watts, Poore et al., 2019). The lack of generation of universal laws in the field of psychology coupled with the current replicability crisis may also point to a second demarcation problem. Popper himself appeared to agree with this demarcation in that he argued that the social sciences should proceed differently and that one should instead regularly use the rationality principle to explain human behavior (O'Donohue, 2013). Simply stated, the rationality principle proposes that people always act appropriately to their perceptions of the situation they are in. Further, Meehl (1978) also seemed to agree with this second demarcation problem as he argued that the "soft" psychological sciences fail to progress in a cumulative manner in the same way as the physical sciences.

O'Donohue et al. (2019) discussed how the unique individuality of each human being engenders distinctive problems for psychological science. Every human has innumerable unique life experiences, each of which contributes to the development of their unique personality, the unique content of their memories, as well as their subsequent unique behavior. People are not fungible—if we should lose our mothers, they cannot be replaced with identical mothers. Human individuals are a singularity. This singularity presents a problem when attempting to understand human behavior. Scientists attempt to generalize across large groups; how reliable can generalizations be when everyone is unique?

The same kind of radical individuality simply does not exist in the physical sciences, which may inherently limit the science of psychology from progressing at the rate of the physical sciences. For example, each atom of some element is the same and is only individually characterized by differences in spatial position. O'Donohue et al. (2019) argued that this "radical ideography," which describes unique individuals, cannot be captured in the abstract constructs of psychological science. These individual particularities may be so important that science will ignore important details about the individual's unique history. Psychology commonly attempts to develop constructs such as "borderline personality disorder," which, as a generalized category, abstracts by proposing key shared definitional features. However, in doing so, ignores (many) other particular details related to the singularity of an individual who is being diagnosed. To illustrate further, the Maddahi et al. (2012) finding that being raised by "authoritative" parents is correlated with the personality trait "openness" is an example of this generalization across abstract categories. Pithily calling attention to this "radical ideography" of humans, Leo Tolstoy states in his novel *Anna Karenina* (1877/2008, p. 15) that "Happy families are all alike; every unhappy family is unhappy in its own way."

Biographies can more fully capture this individuality and particularity (O'Donohue et al., 2019). This approach to knowledge allows the inclusion of rich individualistic detail about the person including much of their history, the unique details of their environment, and the unique psychological characteristics across their distinctive journey through time (which is also a unique era).

However, even with approaches that can capture more unique detail, there are still potential problems, such as feasibility and costs of idiographic data collection given the number of data points that would be required to capture such individuality accurately and comprehensively. Finally, even though idiographic data may better account for the person's individuality, without data points representing every moment of a person's life, the full picture of individuality will remain incompletely described.

Houts (2009) also pointed to the limits of traditional scientific psychological investigation. Within this analysis, Houts makes a distinction between the "knowledge of Athens" and the "knowledge of Jerusalem." Houts (2009) stated:

> From the standpoint of the [protestant] tradition, an argument for God is like a bake sale for Bill Gates. This is a succinct way of highlighting the stark difference between the biblical and the Greek traditions regarding the place of rationality and logic, where in the latter tradition logic is the supreme arbiter of what is rational and what is not. From the culture of Athens, we have inherited the traditions of critical reflection and the use of rational argument to settle points of disagreement. From the dialogues of Socrates to the *Principia Mathematica* of Russell and Whitehead (Whitehead & Russell, 1910), rationality and its bedrock, logic, have been the central force of western philosophy as well as a chief ingredient in synthesizing theological expositions. In contrast to this rational emphasis on reasoned argument and the well-crafted treatise, the biblical traditions featured illustrative stories, recitation of great moments for decision and action, poetry, riddles, grand fantastic visions, and prophesy. At various times in the history of western culture, the conflict between these

> two very different modes of thought and expression has erupted in solitary thinkers and even in the culture at large. (p. 268)

Science is an exemplar of the knowledge of Athens, developed through reason, and that knowledge is expressed with the use of abstract categories (such as "intelligence" and "self-esteem") and emotional detachment. Ultimately, the knowledge of Athens, embedded in science, attempts to reveal universal regularities such as "All copper conducts electricity." In the Athenian view, detachment attempts to minimize emotional biases to arrive at pure and objective knowledge that is cleansed from any influence from personal bias.

The Mertonian (Merton, 1877) value of universalism aligns here with Houts' description of the knowledge of Athens. Universalism is the idea that scientific knowledge is general, of wide scope, and is not localized to the particular—truths are discovered about all matter, not the matter that Sally currently has in her top drawer; this universalism, however, comes at the cost of particularity (Macfarlane & Cheng, 2008). Conversely, the knowledge of Jerusalem is derived through personal experience (including canonically, through some unique religious experience) that may result in important and unique personal knowledge.

The contrast is evident. Instead of using reason and abstraction as in the Athenian manner, Jerusalem knowledge, in its origins, is acquired through specific experiences (such as the experience of being born again) and subsequent engagement with the world through the lens of the experience. For example, in the story of *The Tower of Babel*, a city falls at a particular time in history due to certain sins such as the pride of its people's attempt to build a particular tower to reach heaven. The story describes the specific construction materials for the tower such as "brick for stone and bitumen for the mortar" (Gen. 11:3, New American Bible Revised Edition). While this type of story can have multiple instructional lessons, followers can perhaps have a specific personal experience and personal reaction to this story. From this reaction, they may perhaps learn from it a personal lesson to apply to their lives about the danger of pride and the importance for them to remain humble during their individual circumstances. The moral of the story can then further reveal itself in the individual's life by engendering a form of personal experiential knowledge. By engaging with these experiences, people can encounter and experience the world, which can potentially discover important personal truths. For example, these truths may include ways to live in their world or important personal moral messages more successfully; these truths may be gained through experiences such as personal tragedies or important moments in life like falling in love or losing a loved one.

Additionally, the relevance of this type of knowledge can be seen in secular clinical contexts. For example, listening to unique experiences told by trauma victims in a trauma support group, the therapist can help other victims work through their own unique traumatic experiences. The victim detailing an event can include all the particularity of their individual life experience (e.g., the perpetrator was their cocaine-addicted stepfather who was tall and had long black hair). By hearing stories of those who have been through similar events, with all the particularity of the events included, other victims can perhaps relate and, through empathy, experience somewhat the unique world of the speaker.

Houts' Jerusalem-Athenian distinction has emerged recently in certain claims that the unique personal experiences of minority members in a prejudicial society can only be expressed and understood on a personal experiential level, but ought to be given epistemic legitimacy and perhaps even epistemic priority (Ceci & Williams, 2018). For example, students at Middlebury College, discussing views on their lived experiences, stated in a group document that "[they] contend that experiences and emotions are valid ways to see the world, and that the hegemony of rational thought-based perspectives often found in a university setting limit [the] collective creativity, health, and potential" (Brockelman et al., 2017, para. 8). These students, and others espousing similar ideas, believe that their unique experience as minority group members is exclusive to them and engenders knowledge that a majority group member cannot understand because they do not share the minority group member's lived experience. As discussed above, fully discounting this type of felt and lived experience in favor of only Athenian scientific and rational arguments may lead to an incomplete picture of someone's individual experience of prejudice.

However, although attempting to understand an individual's lived experience can provide knowledge that scientific Athenian knowledge may not capture, it is important to understand that one must be cautious when accepting another's lived experience as a truth statement (Ceci & Williams, 2018). Individuals may distort, exaggerate, minimize, or leave out important details of a lived experience. From the Athenian perspective, there are well-known validity problems to self-report of private experience. Research has shown that biases such as selective perception, blind-spot bias, and my-side bias can distort the reality of a self-report and call into question the validity of the self-report. Research on my-side bias, for example, shows that people are much more likely to accumulate information that confirms their side and rate it as more positively than another's viewpoint (Ceci & Williams, 2018). While experiential knowledge has shown to offer insight, it is also clear that it may be necessary to exercise caution due to potential issues of validity. Again, consistent with Bartley's pan-critical rationalism, these statements as well as their epistemic defense should be critically scrutinized.

Due to the unique history and the extreme individuality of every person, the methods currently used in psychological science are limited in their ability to understand individuality. Idiographic methods with a greater focus on individuality might offer a partial solution to this limitation, but it is unlikely that we will ever be able to fully account for each person's unique life history and particularities, if only for practical barriers of gathering some voluminous information even for one individual. Finally, because of the subjectivity of personal experience, personal knowledge is difficult for researchers to fully understand further limiting the scope of psychological science.

4. Underdetermination of Scientific Regularities

The underdetermination thesis maintains that scientific evidence is always insufficient to logically entail the tested hypothesis or theory (Turnbull, 2017). Thus, the logic of the argument is invalid—the conclusion does not logically follow from the evidence contained in the premises. Scientific theories, laws, and hypotheses are therefore always underdetermined by empirical evidence. Popper (1959) argued that because all possible tests for a theory can never be feasibly conducted, it is possible that one of the unconducted tests may falsify a theory (O'Donohue, 2013). Popper expressed this in an equation:

$$\frac{\textit{Tests conducted}}{\textit{All possible tests}} = 0$$

Thus, even in the falsificationist view scientific claims are always underdetermined. As an example, the empirical claim "All copper conducts electricity" is underdetermined by evidence as not every piece of copper in existence throughout the universe has been tested to determine if in fact all copper always conducts electricity. In addition, all empirical evidence to date supports another scientific law (i.e., "All copper conducts electricity until March 1, 2030, and then none will"). Thus, the evidence for the conclusion is not unequivocal—it supports multiple claims that are inconsistent with one another.

Additional issues with theory testing are problems in drawing valid conclusions about which claims in the logic of the research are false in the face of conflicting evidence. Holist underdetermination, also known as either confirmational holism or the Quine-Duhem thesis (Quine, 1975), posits that theories can only be tested in association with a (often large) number of auxiliary assumptions, and thus are never tested in isolation (Stanford, 2017). The following logic summarizes the holist underdetermination argument (O'Donohue, 2013):

1. If Theory, and Aux_1, and Aux_2, and Aux_3, …, and Aux_n, then Observation
2. *Not Observation*
3. *Therefore, Not (Theory, and* Aux_1*, and* Aux_2*, and* Aux_3*, …, and* Aux_n*)*
4. Therefore, Not Theory or not Aux_1 or not Aux_2 or not Aux_3 or not Aux_n

The logic above demonstrates that when conflicting evidence emerges, such as prediction failures, logic alone does not indicate where the error lies and thus where modifications must be made to the scientist's web of beliefs (Quine & Ullian, 1978). However, the choice of where to direct the arrows of *modus tollens* is underdetermined both by logic and by the evidence available. One is free to attach blame for the prediction failure to any claim in one's web of belief. In fact, Quine (1951) further stated:

> The totality of our so-called knowledge or beliefs, from the most casual matters of geography and history to the profoundest laws of atomic physics or even of pure mathematics and logic, is a man-made fabric which impinges on experience only along the edges. Or, to change the figure, total science is like a field of force whose boundary conditions are experience. A conflict with experience at the periphery occasions readjustments in the interior of the field. … But the total field is so underdetermined by its boundary conditions, experi-

ence, that there is much latitude of choice as to what statements to reevaluate in the light of any single contrary experience. No particular experiences are linked with any particular statements in the interior of the field, except indirectly through considerations of equilibrium affecting the field as a whole. (pp. 39–40)

Quine states that a scientist is free to portion blame to any belief in the face of contradictory evidence but suggests that scientists employ a pragmatic criterion to make this choice. The criterion includes the following five virtues (Quine & Ullian, 1978):

Virtue 1: *Conservatism* asserts that theories or hypotheses created to explain an event may conflict with previous beliefs and the less conflict the better.

Virtue 2: *Modesty* states that a hypothesis is more modest than another hypothesis "if the events that it assumes to have happened are of a more usual and familiar sort, hence more to be expected" (p. 41).

Virtue 3: *Simplicity* focuses on hypotheses that are more parsimonious and more likely to occur than others. Simpler hypotheses are more likely to be adopted.

Virtue 4: *Generality* concerns "the wider range of application of a hypothesis" (p. 45).

Virtue 5: *Refutability* refers to "the cost of retaining the hypothesis in the face of imaginable events" (p. 48) and the sacrifice one must make to save a hypothesis when one needs to reject previously cherished beliefs.

Underdetermination continues to limit science as there is insufficient evidence to guide decision-making when accepting or rejecting hypotheses and theories, changing personal beliefs, and drawing valid conclusions. Thus, any scientific claim can be criticized as going beyond the evidence and as possibly being falsified by future tests.

5. Existence Claims

Popper (1959) also argued that because scientists are not capable of observing the universe all places simultaneously, existence claims are pragmatically impossible to falsify. According to this principle, claims of existence such as, "There is a Santa Claus," are not falsifiable, as we cannot observe all possible space–time points simultaneously. The existence of multiple personality disorder and repressed memories are other examples of such existence claims. According to Popper, it is not possible to falsify such claims as it is always possible that these exist at some unexamined space–time point.

6. Metaphysics

The word "metaphysics" literally translates as "after the *Physics*" because Aristotle's writing on the subject followed his writing on his views about physics. While the philosophers Rene Descartes and Immanuel Kant considered the role of metaphysics in scientific knowledge, the logical positivists attempted to eliminate it as they thought that metaphysical claims were meaningless. Metaphysics can be defined as an interest in questions regarding "being as such" (modern ontology); with categories of existence ("Do abstract properties like redness actually exist?");

with questions of meaning (e.g., "What is the meaning of life?"); and with philosophical questions such as freedom vs determinism, and with first causes (such as God). Note that even denying the existence of God is a metaphysical statement. Satre said, "I do not think myself any less a metaphysician in denying the existence of God than Leibniz was in affirming it" (1949, p. 139).

O'Donohue (1989) has argued that metaphysics, although not a part of science, often influences science. Metaphysics can be involved in conducting science given its role in hypothesis generation and in evaluating the plausibility of the plausible rival hypothesis. First, science can attempt to answer questions that come from metaphysics (e.g., What kinds of entities exist?). Second, the hypothesis generation process traditionally begins with what is scientifically known but is typically constrained by metaphysical assumptions or claims about what exists and what does not exist. Scientific hypotheses generally don't involve entities such as angels and demons because, in general, our metaphysical commitments are such that these are not considered as existents. Metaphysics also plays a key role in assessing plausibility in judgments in research design with attempts to control for "plausible" rival hypotheses. Metaphysics dictates what can be determined as a *plausible* rival hypothesis (e.g., one does not control or match for astrological sign as the scientist's metaphysical world view typically excludes the legitimacy of astrological entities and claims).

A key metaphysical distinction in psychology is the possible distinction between the material brain and the mental, which generally is considered to involve two distinct kinds of entities: a physical brain and a nonphysical mind. Mental events, unlike physical events, are generally considered to have a temporal location but not a physical one. For example, my thought of chocolate occurred at 1 pm, but no one can point to the location of the thought. Thus, the intersection between the limits of science and metaphysics also can be observed in the modern distinction between the mind and brain. Descartes pioneered dualism in the sixteenth century by distinguishing the immaterial mind from the material body. Few contemporary neuroscientists are likely to self-identify as dualists, and yet this Cartesian dualism persists today (Bennett & Hacker, 2003). Modern neuroscience recognizes this distinction in that it is the empirical study of the brain, not the immaterial mind. The direct experience of the mental, sometimes called *qualia*, is distinct from variables found in neuroscience such as processing speed and working memory capacity. While some self-identified materialists refute the mind as being separate from the brain, the predominant perspective across the multiple subfields of science involves studying the brain while largely ignoring the mind (Churchland, 1986; Thibaut, 2018).

7. Mathematics and Logic

Mathematics typically plays an essential role in parts of science, particularly in the natural sciences. Universal laws such as Newton's laws of motion are expressed and calculated with the use of mathematics. Similarly, logic contributes to justifying both in mathematics and in science as there can be both a logic of research (*modus tollens* according to Popper) and its use in formulating and critiquing arguments in scientific papers. In general, the view is that the good scientist ought to constrain him or herself to valid inference rules and sound reasoning (Wong & O'Donohue, in press), without which no sound arguments in science would be made, such as the predictive entailments of theories.

However, an important clarification should be made about these disciplines: mathematics and logic are not products of science. The claims of math and logic are not the result of empirical investigations. Empirical measurements of the lengths of a large sample of triangles are not necessary to prove the Pythagorean Theorem (Maor, 2019). The statement "The proposition A implies A" did not need to be empirically tested under multiple conditions to establish that it is a valid inference.

8. Postmodernism and the Limits of Science

Before examining the implications of postmodernism for the limitations of clinical science, we need to describe postmodernisms' central claims. O'Donohue (2013) summarized the central ideas of postmodernism as the following:

- Postmodernism rejects the modern (post-Enlightenment) perspective of the world as objectively describable through the use of science and also questions the idea that this scientific approach has produced progress.
- Postmodernism supports the idea that what we know as scientific language is inextricably linked to ethics and politics.
- Human knowledge does not reflect reality but rather creates a construction of it that is influenced by ideologies, cultures, traditions, and race. Scientific constructs are thus considered social constructions.
- Knowledge claims are considered, in part, as an attempt to control others, as these privilege some people and not others.
- *Deconstruction* is an important intellectual project and its goals are to expose the influences of prejudices, problematic frames of reference, or political motivations in the development and use of scientific constructs. Deconstruction consists of identifying the distinction between language and meaning, it marks out places where the function of the text works against its apparent meaning, and describes the influences that can play a role on its interpretation (Aylesworth, 2015).
- Meaning of words and sentences is complex and shows multivocality.
- Postmodernism involves a radical critique of the culture of science and its manifold relationship to power; texts are seen as possibly related, implicitly or explicitly, to cultural hegemony, violence, and exclusion. Michel Foucault (1975), for example, stated "language is oppression."
- Key concepts, especially dichotomies or "binaries," such as male vs female or gay vs straight or white vs black, are problematic as these are influenced by historical contingency, power, and hierarchy (they are not "found" or "discovered" in nature) and can have multiple problematic political uses.
- The assumptions in science of universality, consensus, and reality are rejected and considered to relate to "authority" and are substituted by more personal and aesthetic ways of knowing. They defend the idea of epistemic pluralism; they state that there are multiple ways of knowing, and science should not have a monopoly that oppresses other ways of knowing.

- Scientists never know reality; instead, scientists as well as others have readings of experience that are true for us individually but not necessarily for others. *Hermeneutics* is the process of interpretation of these readings.
- An important philosopher in this tradition, Jacques Lyotard, stated that the central notion of postmodernism is the incredulity toward all meta-narratives (Lyotard, 1984). Lyotard attempts to dissolve master narratives like "progress" and "history" by exposing the contingent and constructed ideologies involved in these. "Progress," "reason," and the power of modern medicine would be considered failed master narratives or failed "big stories."
- Discoveries are simply considered human inventions, as they have a particular history that will reveal their contingency. Scientific discoveries are artificial and ought to be seen as *human artifacts*, as artificial as a skyscraper, instead of discoveries that mirror the world.
- Postmodernism seeks to expose the "*late-capitalistic*" *ideology* in the contemporary consumerist culture. If examined properly (through deconstruction), the West's claims of prosperity and freedom are empty promises and failed narratives that reflect militarism, cultural hegemony, and oppression. These also denigrate *local tribal ways of knowing and wisdom* that is communicated through myths and legends.
- Aesthetic and value judgments, such as those involved in the construct of social justice, are considered more important than truth. Scientists are insufficiently attentive toward social justice and too concerned with truth.

The idea that scientific knowledge is constructed and influenced by multiple forces as well as power and financial interests has had some influence in the past several decades. Concepts such as cultural sensitivity (Sue, 1983), including unique cultural knowledge as well as even unique cultural epistemologies, point to these power differentials such as systemic racism. This analysis has helped to describe and begin to attempt to resolve ways of oppression that can be found in science that had been largely unnoticed or understated within clinical science for decades (Lilienfeld, 2017). The recognition of the role that financial forces can play in clinical research has drawn us to demand the disclosure of any possible conflict of interest influencing our studies. This may be considered as one example of how power relationships may exert as a limitation of science in multiple levels, as well as their influence on both scientific interpretations and divulgation of results, highlighting the need for the study of those.

However, parsing these power relationships and their actual effects on clinical science can be difficult. Postmodernists may assume that all minorities, because they have all been victims of forces of oppression, will have the same conception of privilege. However, a White woman may see all men as privileged, regardless of their race, whereas a Black man may see all White people as privileged, regardless of their gender.

Thus, postmodernism consistent with Bartley represents several radical critiques of science and thus clinical science. It is beyond the scope of this chapter to scrutinize each of these—but again, Bartley's (1984) pan-critical rationalism ought to be used to investigate the merits of these critiques.

Conclusions

Science has considerable abilities for assisting in problem-solving and knowledge generation. However, this paper argues that science is not without boundaries but has several important limits that have been poorly recognized in the clinical science literature. The limitations of science need not be a cause for concern or despair, unless one holds that science is the only method of knowledge generation. That science has the monopoly on problem solving and knowledge generation is a type of scientism that needs to be avoided in sound clinical science.

What can be done to create knowledge outside the bounds of science? Bartley's (1984) pan-critical rationalism provides a method. Bartley, a student of Popper, argued that there is an important distinction between justificationist and critical approaches to knowledge generation. Bartley argued that justification approaches inevitably fail because any attempt to justify a claim inevitably results in a dilemma of either an infinite regress or an irrational dogmatic commitment. Bartley argued that this dilemma can be avoided because it is possible to hold all beliefs to criticism and reexamination. Bartley (1984, p. 19) describes the dilemma that the justificationist approach leads to:

> The dilemma of infinite regress versus dogmatism arises like this: if a belief claims validation by a supporting argument, what justifies that argument? If a critic persists in asking for further supporting statements, when and how does the chain of justification stop? An infinite regress (that is, an endless sequence of questions, without hope of a final answer) can be forced by anyone who keeps on asking, 'Why do you believe that? How do you justify that claim?' …It appears that it can only be avoided by a dogmatic or arbitrary decision to break the chain at some stage and settle on a belief at that point.

However, Bartley points out this stopping point—in which an arbitrary decision is made not to pursue any additional justification—then renders the justificatory enterprise to be dogmatic. One has found a stopping point to the regress, but this comes at the cost of adopting this foundation in a dogmatic, uncritical, and irrational manner. Thus, Bartley advocates abandoning such justificational attempts for our beliefs and instead replacing this approach with a *critical epistemology* (i.e., the view that although no position can be definitively justified, yet some beliefs will turn out to be better than others because they hold up better to critical appraisal and tests). Thus, rationality, both within science and beyond the limits of science, becomes maximizing severe criticism of beliefs and then adopting the position that has best stood up to this criticism. It is important that a critical component of this process also is self-critical (i.e., this critical process ought to occur with respect to one's critical processes—how can we become better critics?).

Thus, the conventional justification notions of science held by clinical psychologists need to be replaced by one that emphasizes criticism, and one good candidate is Bartley's (1984) pan-critical rationalism. In this view, a good clinical scientist is a person who holds all beliefs open to criticism and admits only the positions best surviving this criticism process. This criticism process can be instantiated both by severe testing of beliefs to see if their low probability consequences obtain, and by any other method of critical examination of beliefs. For example, ethical matters were argued in this chapter to be outside the domain of science. However, ethical matters are not outside the domain of rationality: Ethical proposals can be criticized rationally on grounds such as their internal consistency, soundness of their positive arguments, whether they lead to undesirable or obviously false entailments, as well as how their competitors do on these and other dimensions of criticism.

Professor Scott Lilienfeld was a master at this criticism process. He knew how to criticize severely but fairly. He applied criticisms based on methodological weaknesses, absence of key data, psychometric limitations, problematic statistical analyses, problems in definition, use of heuristics and other cognitive biases, inconsistency with or ignoring findings from other relevant research, gaps in arguments, and so on. Yet, he criticized with a sense of openness and intellectual humility, as well as a genuine interest in solving problems. He will be missed, but it is hoped that his example will continue to be an inspiration for others.

References

Anna Karenina. (1877). The Floating Press.

Aylesworth, G. (2015). "Postmodernism". In Edward N. Zalta (Ed.), *The Stanford Encyclopedia of Philosophy (Spring 2015 Edition)*. https://plato.stanford.edu/archives/spr2015/entries/postmodernism/

Bartley, W. W. (1984). *The retreat to commitment* (2nd ed.). Open Court.

Bennett, M. R., & Hacker, P. M. S. (2003). *Philosophical foundations of neuroscience*. Wiley.

Bowes, S. M., Ammirati, R. J., Costello, T. H., Basterfield, C., & Lilienfeld, S. O. (2020). Cognitive biases, heuristics, and logical fallacies in clinical practice: A brief field guide for practicing clinicians and supervisors. *Professional Psychology: Research and Practice, 51*, 435–445. https://doi.org/10.1037/pro0000309.

Brockelman, A., Bliska, E., Carlson, A., Pandya, J., Haight, O., Ramachandran, V., … Bazemore, M. (2017, March 12). *Broken inquiry on campus: A response by a collection of Middlebury students [Blog post]*. Retrieved from https://brokeninquiryblog.wordpress.com/

Ceci, S. J., & Williams, W. M. (2018). Who decides what is acceptable speech on campus? Why restricting free speech is not the answer. *Perspectives on Psychological Science, 13*, 299–323. https://doi.org/10.1177/1745691618767324

Churchland, P. S. (1986). *Neurophilosophy: Toward a unified science of the mind-brain*. MIT Press.

Cohon, R. (2018). Hume's moral philosophy. In E. N. Zalta (Ed.), *The Stanford Encyclopedia of Philosophy*. https://plato.stanford.edu/archives/fall2018/entries/hume-moral/

Foucault, M. (1975). *Discipline and Punish: The Birth of the Prison*.

Haynes, S., Chavez, R. E., & Samuel, V. (1984). Assessment of marital communication and distress. *Behavioral Assessment, 6*, 315–321.

Hempel, C. G. (1965). Science and human values. In C. G. Hempel (Ed.), *Aspects of scientific explanation*. Free Press.

Herbert, J. D., Lilienfeld, S. O., Lohr, J. M., Montgomery, R. W., O'Donohue, W. T., Rosen, G. M., & Tolin, D. F. (2000). Science and pseudoscience in the development of eye movement desensitization and reprocessing: Implications for clinical psychology. *Clinical Psychology Review, 20*, 945–971. https://doi.org/10.1016/s0272-7358(99)00017-3. PMID: 11098395.

Houts, A. (2009). Reformed theology is a resource in conflicts between psychology and religious faith. In N. Cummings, W. O'Donohue, & J. Cummings (Eds.), *Psychology's war on religion* (pp. 257–311). Tucker & Theisen, Inc..

Hume, D. (1737). *An inquiry into human understanding*. Oxford University Press.
Laplace, P. S. (1902). *A philosophical essay on probabilities*. J. Wiley; Chapman & Hall. http://archive.org/details/philosophicaless00lapliala
Lilienfeld, S. O. (2007). Psychological treatments that cause harm. *Perspectives on Psychological Science, 2*, 53–70.
Lilienfeld, S. O. (2017). Microaggressions: Strong claims, inadequate evidence. *Perspectives on Psychological Science, 12*, 138–169. https://doi.org/10.1177/1745691616659391
Lilienfeld, S. O., Lynn, S. J., Ruscio, J., & Beyerstein, B. (2011). *50 great myths of popular psychology*. Wiley-Blackwell.
Lilienfeld, S. O., Lynn, S. J., & Lohr, J. (2014). *Science and pseudoscience in clinical psychology*. The Guilford Press.
Lilienfeld, Lynn, S. J., Ruscio, J., & Beyerstein, B. L. (2009). *50 great myths of popular psychology: shattering widespread misconceptions about human behavior*. Wiley.
Lyotard, J. F. (1984). *The postmodern condition: A report on knowledge* (Vol. 10). U of Minnesota Press.
Macfarlane, B., & Cheng, M. (2008). Communism, universalism and disinterestedness: Re-examining contemporary support among academics for Merton's scientific norms. *Journal of Academy of Ethics, 6*, 67–78. https://doi.org/10.1007/s10805-008-9055-y
Maddahi, M. E., Javidi, N., Samadzedeh, M., & Amini, M. (2012). The study of relationship between parenting styles and personality dimensions. *Indian Journal of Science and Technology, 5*, 3332–3336.
Maor, E. (2019). *The Pythagorean theorem: A 4,000-year history*. Princeton University Press.
Marino, L., & Lilienfeld, S. O. (2007). Dolphin-assisted therapy: More flawed data and more flawed conclusions. *Anthrozoos: A Multidisciplinary Journal of The Interactions of People & Animals, 20*, 239–249. https://doi.org/10.2752/089279307X224782
McFall, R. M. (1991). Manifesto for a science of clinical psychology. *The Clinical Psychologist, 44*, 75–88.
Meehl, P. E. (1954). *Clinical versus statistical prediction: A theoretical analysis and a review of the evidence*. University of Minnesota Press. https://doi.org/10.1037/11281-000
Meehl, P. E. (1978). Theoretical risks and tabular asterisks: Sir Karl, Sir Ronald, and the slow progress of soft psychology. *Journal of Consulting and Clinical Psychology, 46*, 806–834.
Meichenbaum, D., & Lilienfeld, S. O. (2018). How to spot hype in the field of psychotherapy: A 19-item checklist. *Professional Psychology: Research and Practice, 49*, 22–30. https://psycnet.apa.org/doi/10.1037/pro0000172.
Moore, G. E. (1903). *Principia ethica*. CreateSpace.
O'Donohue, W. (1989). The even bolder model—The clinical psychologist as metaphysician-scientist-practitioner. *The American Psychologist, 44*, 1460–1468. https://doi.org/10.1037/0003-066X.44.12.1460
O'Donohue, W. (2013). *Clinical psychology and the philosophy of science*. Springer. https://doi.org/10.1007/978-3-319-00185-2
O'Donohue, W. T., & Halsey, L. B. (1997). The substance of the scientist-practitioner relation: Freud, rogers, skinner and Ellis. *New Ideas in Psychology, 15*, 35–53.
O'Donohue, W. T., Burleigh, K., & Kinzler, A. (2019). Capturing the unique nature of the human sciences: The second demarcation problem. *Behavior and Philosophy, 47*, 15–33.
O'Donohue, W. T., Masuda, A., & Lilienfeld, S. O. (in press). *Clinical psychology and questionable research practices*. Springer.
Paul, G. L. (1969). Behavior modification research: Design and tactics. In C. M. Franks (Ed.), *Behavior therapy: Appraisal and status* (pp. 29–62). McGraw-Hill.
Popper, K. (1959). *The logic of scientific discovery*. Basic Books.
Quine, W. V. O. (1951). Main trends in recent philosophy: Two dogmas of empiricism. *The Philosophical Review, 60*(1), 20–43. https://doi.org/10.2307/2181906
Quine, W. V. O. (1975). On empirically equivalent systems of the world. *Erkenntnis, 9*, 313–328. https://doi.org/10.1007/BF00178004

Quine, W. V. O., & Ullian, J. S. (1978). *The web of belief.* McGraw Hill.
Robert K. Merton. (1877). *The normative structure of science*. Retrieved from https://www.panarchy.org/merton/science.html
Rosen, G. M., & Lilienfeld, S. O. (2016). On the failure of psychology to advance self-help: Acceptance and commitment therapy (ACT) as a case example. *Journal of Contemporary Psychotherapy: On the Cutting Edge of Modern Developments in Psychotherapy, 46*(2), 71–77. https://doi.org/10.1007/s10879-015-9319-y
Sagan, C. (1980). *Cosmos*. Random House.
Sagan, C. (1983). *Cosmos*. Random House.
Sagan, C. (1995). *The demon-haunted world: Science as a candle in the dark*. Random House.
Satel, S., & Lilienfeld, S. O. (2013). *Brainwashed: The seductive appeal of mindless neuroscience*. Basic Books.
Sher, L., Oquendo, M. A., & Mann, J. J. (2001). Risk of suicide in mood disorders. *Clinical Neuroscience Research, 1*(5), 337–344.
Skeem, J., Douglas, & Lilienfeld, S. O. (2009). *Psychological science in the courtroom: Consensus and controversy*. The Guilford Press.
Skinner, B. F. (1953). *Science and human behavior*. Free Press.
Stanford, K. (2017, October 12). *Underdetermination of scientific theory.* Stanford Encyclopedia of Philosophy. https://plato.stanford.edu/entries/scientific-underdetermination/
Sue, S. (1983). Ethnic minority issues in psychology: A reexamination. *American Psychologist, 38*, 583.
Thibaut, F. (2018). The mind-body Cartesian dualism and psychiatry. *Dialogues in Clinical Neuroscience, 20*(1), 3–3. https://doi.org/10.31887/DCNS.2018.20.1/fthibaut
Thomson, J. J., & Parent, W. (1986). *Killing, letting die, and the trolley problem.* Harvard University Press.
Turnbull, M. G. (2017). Underdetermination in science: What it is and why we should care. *Philosophy Compass, 13*, e12475. https://doi.org/10.1111/phc3.12475
Watts, Poore, H. E., Lilienfeld, S. O., & Waldman, I. D. (2019). Clarifying the associations between Big Five personality domains and higher-order psychopathology dimensions in youth. *Journal of Research in Personality, 82*, 103844–. https://doi.org/10.1016/j.jrp.2019.07.002
Whitehead, A. N., & Russell, B. (1910). *Principia Mathematica*. University Press.
Wiggins, B., & Chrisopherson, C. D. (2019). The replication crisis in psychology: An overview for theoretical and philosophical psychology. *Journal of Theoretical and Philosophical Psychology, 39*, 202–217.
Wood, J., Nezworski, M. T., Lilienfeld, S. O., & Garb, H. (2011). *What's wrong with the Rorschach?* Jossey Bass.

When Clinical Judgment and Science Conflict, How Does One Decide? The Epistemological Status of Learning from Experience vs. Science

David Faust and Austin Furman

A Tribute to Scott Lilienfeld

We were honored to contribute to this book, especially given Scott's esteemed status. We imagine that various chapter writers will address Scott's many lasting academic contributions and his championship of science as the leading means for acquiring knowledge. Thus, in this tribute, we wish to focus on his fundamental decency and generosity of spirit.

Scott's admirable qualities were captured in his response to a request from one of my (the first author's) students, who sought Scott's input on a questionnaire this student was developing on pseudo-science. Scott barely knew this individual, and, as I happened to know, he was incredibly busy with a broad scope of activities when the request was made. Nevertheless, Scott not only was kind and encouraging, but he then volunteered to review the questionnaire in detail and address certain difficult psychometric challenges. Scott spent considerable time writing numerous helpful and constructive recommendations and possible suggestions for revising items. The student was astounded (as was I) with the time and effort Scott put into this work and the quality of his advice.

D. Faust (✉)
Department of Psychology, Ryan Institute of Neuroscience, University of Rhode Island, Kingston, RI, USA

Department of Psychiatry and Human Behavior, Warren Alpert Medical School of Brown University, Providence, RI, USA
e-mail: faust@uri.edu

A. Furman
Odenton, MD, USA

C. L. Cobb et al. (eds.), *Toward a Science of Clinical Psychology*,
https://doi.org/10.1007/978-3-031-14332-8_5

I mention this anecdote because I saw it reenacted on multiple other occasions, showing a quality of character that equaled Scott's impressive scholarly prowess. It also demonstrated something else. Those who may have felt the heat of Scott's criticisms or read his penetrating (and some might say biting) commentary, may have formed misimpressions about his character or motivations. However, it seems clear that Scott's acts of kindness and generosity instantiated his deep humanity and caring, his genuine distress at practices that may have compromised the care of those in need, and an unwavering commitment to enhancing human welfare. Thus, we applaud both Scott's scientific accomplishments and his inherent goodness, and, in equal parts, miss him terribly and appreciate his remarkable, enduring scientific achievements.

The Moment of Truth

All clinicians eventually find themselves at the moment of truth in which their clinical experience and judgment lead them in one direction, but scientific evidence suggests a contrasting alternative. Perhaps the clinician is pondering whether a patient is likely to act out violently if discharged from a controlled setting, and hence what action to take next. One's clinical experience and internal reasoning suggest that the risks are unacceptably high, but pertinent scientific evidence suggests that the risks are low and that extending inpatient treatment will likely do more harm than good. Here and in other situations, one can be faced with deciding between incompatible and directly contrary actions, for example, discharge or do not discharge, do or do not refer to a particular specialist, or do or do not accept the individual as a client as opposed to referring out to someone else who might be better qualified to render the type of treatment that is needed. In such situations, clinicians may be forced to decide whether to go with their clinical judgment or instead defer to what the science seems to indicate.

At times, there is no easy or feasible way to combine conclusions that scientifically-validated decision procedures signal versus those reached through clinical judgment as the two can lead to directly contradictory courses of action. In contrast, in some circumstances, accuracy may not make much difference. For example, one might be choosing between two well-established treatment approaches that are both likely to be effective, although perhaps with minor differences in efficacy. However, in other situations, accuracy can make all the difference, such as when one is consulting to an airline and the main issue is a pilot's readiness to return to flying commercially. Mental health professionals are faced with many choice points or provide input in many high-stakes situations, such as suicide prevention, propensity to act out violently, detection of disorders with high levels of morbidity, or decisions to possibly transfer adolescents to adult court.

If one's experience and judgment lean strongly in one direction, and science in another, how can one determine which of the two will most likely be correct? Limitations in the science or gaps in one's experience can make choices between alternatives, or which to elevate over the other, agonizing conundrums. Nevertheless, inaction may not be a viable option and a choice may be required. It is this very type of dilemma and worthy subject that occupied much of Scott Lilienfeld's thought and work and that makes up the main topic of our chapter.

Finding Common Ground for Comparing the Merits of Clinical Judgment and Science

Considerable evidence suggests that when science and clinical judgment conflict, the latter is often elevated over the former (e.g., see Boisvert & Faust, 2003, and further below). Many debates about the relative merits of clinical judgment and science, regardless of the side one prefers, are characterized as much, or more, by their vehemence than by anything else. Strong feelings are understandable given what may be at stake for clients, practitioners, and the profession. However, overly extreme views and emotionalism often do not advance knowledge and only harden positions. At times, criticisms rest on false stereotypes or exaggerated views about the positions of those with opposing views.

For example, is the typical psychologist who argues for greater implementation of science a hardcore, extreme empiricist who believes that science delivers the truth with a capital T, and that scientists comprise a valorous elite who retain nearly pure objectivity and are minimally swayed by personal values or cultural context? Or, conversely, are most individuals who generally defer to clinical judgment and experience over science given limits in what science has delivered to practitioners in the trenches to date, muddle-headed obscurantists who believe that all knowledge claims have equal merit and that science has nothing to offer beyond other methods for acquiring knowledge?

It is one thing to argue, as we will, that in various circumstances, well-conducted and corroborated science is the best knowledge game in town or has advantages over impressionistic judgment, but this is a far cry from arguing that clinical judgment in the mental health field has little to offer. There is a difference between asserting, for example, that scientifically-derived knowledge can have an edge, and sometimes a sizeable one, over clinical judgment, as opposed to arguing that clinical judgment is all but useless, the latter of which is certainly not our view.

For example, across the numerous studies on clinical judgment and statistical decision making, many comparisons generate similar levels of validity. If clinical judgment was so bad, how could that be the case? Also, most studies on clinical judgment (e.g., see AEgisdóttir et al., 2006; Grove et al., 2000) have shown significant contributions to enhancing accuracy, at times reducing error by about one-third to one-half in comparison to chance levels or mere guessing. Although one might wish for higher accuracy levels, there may be good reasons to rely on clinical judgment and recognize its contributions to enhancing decision accuracy.

Research dating back decades shows that information gathered by clinicians through structured and unstructured interviews can enhance accuracy when combined with formal methods for integrating and combining information, such as validated interpretive procedures (see Sawyer, 1966; Dawes et al., 1989). Clinical observation and judgment have also proven invaluable in identifying applied problems that merit investigation, and in the discovery process.

In many clinical circumstances, critical scientific knowledge is lacking, such as literature that would closely tie psychological assessment results to treatment design and choice, and thus there is little option other than to rely on clinical judgment. In other cases, it is very difficult to connect scientific studies to applied clinical activities, such as when treatment studies eliminate very common co-occurring disorders and other complicating factors that are present in most cases. Other studies use extreme groups to diminish ambiguities in group assignment (e.g., those who are and are not malingering), but end up with clear-cut cases that provide help where it is not needed and have a very questionable application to clinical cases in which help is needed most. Research may also provide little guidance to help determine whether outcomes with one group generalize to other individuals with widely differing cultural backgrounds and life experiences. Studies may also use weak methodology, rest on highly questionable assumptions, or generate frequently conflicting and ever-changing outcomes. Hence, in our opinion, it is a mistake to reflexively dismiss reliance on clinical judgment or experience as anti-scientific or ill-advised.

We do not condone broad disregard of science or dismissals of scientific research with the wave of a hand or some highly questionable rationale, for example, the studies are conducted by ivory tower psychologists who have little appreciation for clinical realities (despite many of these researchers also being active care providers). There are certainly a growing number of areas in which well-founded research can make a real difference in clinical effectiveness and merit integration into practice. We simply want to acknowledge that questions and doubts about the value of research may be fair-minded and balanced and that deferring to clinical judgment and experience over science in some circumstances can be founded on carefully considered positions and realistic appraisals of limits in the scientific knowledge base.

Likewise, some advocates for deferring to science above all else can be overly extreme and narrow-minded. Hence, there are worthwhile issues to examine here, and some vexing problems that can lead to difficult choices. Such disagreements need not devolve into divisiveness, disparagement, or dogmatism. Our main intent here is to compare the methodological or epistemological status of learning through clinical experience as opposed to learning through well-conducted scientific methodology and to consider where that awareness might lead to when deciding which source of knowledge should trump the other when they yield conflicting conclusions and one must make important clinical choices.

Context of Discovery Versus Verification

Some of the nonproductive debates between the merits of clinical or impressionistic judgment versus scientific methodology stem from insufficient consideration of whether one is primarily in a stage of generating ideas versus testing knowledge claims. Consequently, it can be useful to distinguish between the context of discovery and the context of justification or verification, or as a rough equivalent, generating versus testing hypotheses. The distinction is often attributed to Reichenbach (1938) (although the differentiation he made was actually somewhat different). In many cases, relaxing evidentiary standards when generating new ideas can avoid rejecting them too quickly, especially ideas that may turn out to have a major value, although one can go too far. Turning hypothesizing into a complete free-for-all beyond an early point can lead to major inefficiencies and wasted effort. Nonetheless, innovative ideas are often the main drivers of scientific breakthroughs and should not be discouraged too readily.

Distinguishing between the context of discovery versus justification can avoid unwarranted criticisms. For example, when confronting novel situations and problems, initially loosening evidentiary standards may prove productive. However, there are often critical differences between approaches that are most effective for generating ideas as opposed to testing them. When standards for evidence or evaluation are not adjusted in line with the applicable context, problems and disagreements frequently arise. Someone who applies relaxed standards across both contexts and undervalues more rigorous methods to test new ideas will almost inevitably make too many errors. Conversely, applying overly strict standards of evidence in the context of discovery may lead one to miss critical opportunities to uncover potentially fruitful ideas. Thus, if case conferences or a single case study become a basis for generating ideas, and less so to test them, impugning these efforts due to insufficient rigor is probably unfounded, just as someone who does not apply more rigorous methods for testing the ideas that result from such activities has likely made the opposing error. Methods for generating ideas are often limited or insufficient means for testing ideas, and thus applying equivalent standards across the two contexts will likely prove unproductive and can lead to unwarranted criticisms directed at individuals who modify the level of rigor in relation to context. We believe that many arguments about the use of clinical judgment or impressionistic methods versus scientific findings could benefit from distinguishing between generating and testing ideas, or discovery versus verification.

Both authors of the current chapter believe that a major aim of science is verisimilitude (i.e., truthlikeness), or to approximate truth as closely as possible. (Note the use of the lower case *t* here in truthlikeness.) As such, we align in part with scientific realists in believing that an external world exists independent of us or our perceptions and that a key aim of science is to come as close as possible to capturing the external world accurately, much as the concept of verisimilitude conveys. Our views do *not* align with extreme relativism or extreme empiricism, and we recognize that a myriad of background factors and biases can derail scientific efforts and thinking. To acknowledge that scientists, in common with individuals from all walks of life, are susceptible to the limits and fallibilities of human judgment, is not to argue that all ideas, thinkers, and decision-making processes are equally sound. Rather, we take the seemingly noncontroversial position that evidence counts, and that statements like, *because I say so and believe so*, by themselves, do little to establish true knowledge credentials.

When Sound Science Has a Decided Advantage Over Impressionistic Judgment: Covariation Analysis as an Exemplar

In a range of circumstances, learning from science has considerable advantages over learning from personal experience or clinical practice, regardless of the intelligence and acumen of practitioners. For example, personal experience may not provide access to critical information or to necessary comparisons. As an illustration, evaluating the relative merits of a treatment (e.g., back surgery) by considering its success rate does not allow one to determine how it stacks up against no treatment or another treatment if one lacks comparison data. One would not say that someone missing the needed comparison information is responsible for falling short in some way, but rather that the problem originates in being placed at this serious methodological or informational disadvantage.

In this section, rather than addressing a broad range of methodological or informational situations, we will narrow down to a rudimentary determination that cuts across many decision tasks: appraising the presence or absence of an association between variables, and, when an association is present, determining the strength of that association. Such judgments may be involved, for example, in formulating a diagnosis or prediction. Practitioners are in the prediction business, although we might not always realize it, because some predictions are explicit, but many others are implicit and not even necessarily thought of as predictive tasks. For example, an explicit prediction might involve assessing the likelihood of violent behavior, whereas an implicit prediction might involve treatment selection or referral to a specialist. Presumably, treatment selection or referrals to specialists rest, among other things, on beliefs about the likelihood of a successful outcome or improvement in the client's status. In turn, selecting a treatment or making an explicit or implicit prediction often rests substantially on presumed associations between the selected treatment and outcome. In the following discussion, we begin by considering the association between a single variable (e.g., a symptom) and an outcome (e.g., the presence of a certain disorder), although the same fundamental principles apply whether we are considering one or a combination of variables on either the input or outcome end, such as combining multiple pieces of information to formulate a prediction.

By *covariation*, we are referring to the association or correlation between variables—that is, how variables may or may not change together. Association, of course, does not necessarily establish causation. The rooster crowing does not cause the sun to rise. Arkes provides the following example (Faust et al., 2022): The number of pigs in the United States in a specific year covaries with the amount of pig iron produced in that same year. Of course, the birth of pigs does not cause pig-iron production to increase, nor does the level of pig-iron production increase pig birth. Rather, a third variable, economic growth or decline, impacts both factors. Hence, association is a cue to causation, and sometimes a strong one, but co-occurrence may also be due to the operation of a third or other variables. However, if two things are not correlated, then except under unusual conditions, they cannot be causally linked.

For a diagnostic sign, psychological test, or other predictive variable to be useful, it must covary with some outcome or diagnosis of interest. Thus, covariation analysis is basic to almost any diagnostic or predictive task in psychology. In turn, proper covariation analysis requires two fundamental conditions. First, the necessary steps for achieving accurate covariation analysis must be performed. As we will discuss, those needed steps are often not intuitively obvious or performed correctly. Second, the needed information must be available. To fulfill this second condition, the available information must be sufficient to generate trustworthy results, a requirement that can be very difficult to meet experientially or in the course of clinical practice.

Procedures for Performing Accurate Covariation Analysis

As can be seen in Table 1, covariation tables contain four cells. The formatting for Table 1 designates the upper-left cell as the *true positive* (present-present) cell, or Cell A. This initial cell represents instances in which a sign or diagnostic indicator is present and a condition is present, although one may be looking at other types of predictive variables (e.g., a test score, some type of manifested behavior or mood state) or outcomes (e.g., response to a therapeutic intervention, violent acting out). This is the *true positive* cell because both the sign and the condition are present. The upper-right cell is the *false positive* (present-absent) cell, or Cell B, because the symptom is present but the disorder is absent. The lower-left entry is the *false negative* (absent-present) cell, or Cell C, because the symptom is absent but the disorder is present; and the lower-right entry is the *valid negative* (absent-absent) cell, or Cell D, because the symptom is absent and the disorder is absent. Again, covariation

Table 1 Four cells of a covariation table with letter designations

		Disorder present	
		Yes	No
Symptom X present?	Yes	Cell A (32)	Cell B (52)
	No	Cell C (8)	Cell D (13)

tables do not have to list symptoms or disorders and can be used to look at potential associations between other types of variables. In addition, covariation analysis captures the essentials for evaluating the association between variables, although, as is well known, there are various other procedures for appraising relations between variables.

To perform accurate covariation analysis, one must consider all four cells of Table 1. Research shows, however, that laypersons and highly skilled professionals alike may misperceive the presence of an association due to incomplete covariation analysis (e.g., Smedslund, 1963; Ganguly & Hammersley, 2009). Many laypersons and professionals focus mainly on Cell A (the present-present cell), or cells A and B (the present-present and present-absent cells). Thus, especially when a condition or outcome occurs with relatively high frequency when a symptom is present, there is a tendency to assume the two are related, even when the frequency of the outcome is as great (or even greater) when the sign or symptom is absent.

For example, assume a practitioner is considering an important condition, such as progressive cognitive decline. The clinician has been taught that substantial scatter or variation between high and low test scores is an indicator of brain dysfunction, which seems to accord with that clinician's experience. Assume also that the true diagnosis is known. It may seem like the figures in Table 1 suggest an association between scatter (the symptom) and neuropsychological dysfunction (the disorder), but they do not. When the disorder is present, extreme scatter occurs 80% of the time (32/40). However, this same 80% rate of extreme scatter occurs when the disorder is absent (52/65). One must take all four cells of a covariation table into account to make this determination (ratio of disorder present when the sign is present versus ratio of disorder present when the sign is absent). If a condition occurs no more or no less often when a symptom is present than when it is absent, the symptom is not associated with the disorder—they do not covary with one another.

If one does not consider all four cells in Table 1, but rather focuses primarily on the first column (cases in which the disorder is present), the high frequency with which those with the disorder show the symptom could lead to a false conclusion about a positive association between the symptom and disorder. However, as research shows, normal individuals often demonstrate levels of variability across tests similar to the levels obtained among individuals with brain disorders. Nevertheless, over-interpretation of scatter as indicative of abnormality has been common among neuropsychologists for decades, likely because of an overemphasis on Cell A (see Faust & Ahern, 2012). If wide variation is common among individuals with and without brain impairments, then wide variation will be present among individuals who undergo neuropsychological evaluation, even if it has little or no diagnostic value.

Note that the sheer number of entries is not the issue, but rather the proportion of occurrence when the symptom is present versus when it is absent. Even if the numbers in the four cells in Table 1 ran into the thousands but the proportions among the cells were the same, the analysis or comparison of the ratios would yield exactly the same result. When the sample size increases, it may be easy to pile up large numbers in various cells, such as Cell B (people who smoke and do not develop lung cancer), and potentially promote a false impression. Alternatively, excessive focus on the false-negative cell, or Cell C, might lead one to conclude mistakenly that magnetic resonance imaging is of limited or no value because it failed to identify thousands of cases of brain tumors.

There are numerous examples in psychology in which a primary focus on Cell A, or failure to consider all four cells, has fostered questionable or inaccurate conclusions among both the public and professionals. For example, despite epidemiological evidence indicating that the overall rate of violent behavior is similar across individuals with and without major psychological disorders (with isolated exceptions), many individuals believe that such disorders are linked to violence. Highly publicized and dramatic cases (e.g., Jeffrey Dahmer, Ted Bundy) that fall within Cell A (major pathology present-violence present) can lead to misperceptions or false associations. Moreover, clinicians may not direct sufficient attention to the frequency with which signs or indicators assumed to be potentially strong indicators of pathology occur among normal individuals (cells B and D). Other examples include insufficient recognition of the overlap in symptoms or problems reported by healthy individuals and individuals who have experienced concussions; various supposed indicators of physical or sexual abuse; and the frequency of abnormal scores on cognitive measures (e.g., Cook et al., 2019; Binder et al., 2009; Schretlen et al., 2008; Voormolen et al., 2019).

Suppose instead one was interested in a possible association between an intervention and an outcome. Although positive results may follow treatment in a certain percentage of cases, determining how that rate compares to outcomes with another treatment, or even without treatment, also requires proper covariation analysis. A 65% success rate does not demonstrate treatment efficacy if one achieves similar rates without treatment. In contrast, even relatively low rates of positive outcomes with treatment-resistant conditions may still exceed the rate of positive outcomes without treatment or with alternative treatments.

Other individuals focus primarily on comparing cells A and B, or on instances in which the symptom and disorder do and do not coincide. For example, if the positive–positive instances in Cell A outnumber the positive–negative instances in Cell B, a positive association may be assumed to be present. The result might be to believe, for example, that a potential marker of suicidal risk has value, even if the indicator has minimal utility or *decreases* predictive accuracy (especially when compared to the best predictive variables).

Access to the Needed Information and Quality of Information

Accurate covariation analysis depends not only on following the necessary steps but also on gathering needed information of sufficient quality. This latter requirement often sets limits on how far one can get by depending primarily on clinical experience, regardless of how much experience one might have or one's level of intellectual and clinical abilities. When appraising the quality of information, some dimensions are clear cut. For example, one must have information for all four cells. If that condition is not met, covariation analysis will be enfeebled. Other dimensions of quality are matters of degree, such as sample sizes for the four cells.

One also needs representative samples from each cell. For example, if the cells containing individuals with one or another condition are comprised primarily of extreme cases or atypical cases in some respect (e.g., especially unskilled and extreme cases of feigned disorder), then outcomes may generalize poorly to more typical clinical cases. Also, if one intends to apply results in clinical settings for specific differentiations, then the closer the match between the groups studied and the to-be-differentiated groups the better. For example, to identify effective indicators for distinguishing between those with posttraumatic stress disorder (PTSD) versus those with generalized anxiety disorder (GAD), then covariation analysis comparing individuals with PTSD to normal individuals may have little or no utility. One also needs to assign individuals to cells without too much error. For example, if a sizeable percentage of individuals assigned to the PTSD (disorder present) cell or cells do not have the condition, then there may be too much error in outcomes to be of much clinical utility. Often, if the proper procedures are applied, then some error in group assignment will not overly compromise results and corrective steps can be taken (Dawes & Meehl, 1966; Jewsbury & Bowden, 2014), and sometimes trying to reduce error in group assignment to an absolute minimum creates overly extreme groups that compromise generalization or utility even more (see Faust et al., 2021).

In some circumstances, for example, when comparing new or alternative treatments, or treatment to no treatment, random assignment to the varying conditions may be essential and provide major advantages. In contrast, assignment that might be based on client preferences or treatment failure with other interventions under study may produce hopelessly confounded results. Other helpful or important steps might include various procedures to attenuate biases, such as single- or double-blinding. We certainly appreciate that in many practice settings, random assignment would not be appropriate or feasible, and we are merely pointing out differences in the potential to obtain outcome data that facilitate interpretability.

Although robust associations between variables are often desirable, even relatively small incremental improvements (such as a 5% gain in predictive accuracy or treatment outcomes), especially when accumulated across a lifetime of clinical cases, can make important differences. Contrary to the great breakthroughs commonly depicted in the media, treatment advances often proceed in small steps, which slowly cumulate to create meaningful differences.

Covariation Analysis in Naturalistic Conditions

We can now return to the original inquiry comparing conclusions or decisions founded on clinical experience to those founded on well-conducted scientific study. As probably is apparent, various conditions that must be met or that increase the quality of information are highly impractical or all but precluded in naturalistic treatment settings, especially when providers' personal resources are often already stretched to the limit in addressing pressing client needs. Not to be farcical, but imagine if during an intake with a sobbing patient tormented by feelings of remorse after the sudden death of a spouse, the therapist stated, "Because random assignment can improve conditions for scientific learning, we'll be selecting a treatment approach for you by chance in order to learn whether or how well it works." Creating conditions in, say, a private practice setting that approaches the quality of information obtained in a well-funded and carefully designed study is often unrealistic.

Examination of covariation analysis provides insight into some of the potential advantages of well-conducted science across various circumstances for testing hypotheses and acquiring knowledge in comparison to relying primarily on clinical judgment and experience. Again, we do not question the benefits of experience for learning certain things or generating new ideas, but it also comes with substantial limitations and hindrances in a range of important situations. In treatment settings, it is often the same person/therapist who "assigns" individuals to cells (i.e., selects the intervention used) and who judges the outcome. For this and other reasons, it may not be feasible to obtain representative samples across the cells. What candidates for intervention might the clinician place in a no-treatment control group and insist they not seek treatment elsewhere to keep that control group intact? How could one ask therapists to implement treatments they believe are not the best available option for their clients? Would the therapist providing the treatment assign an independent party to evaluate the outcome, and how could conflicting appraisals between an independent evaluator and the clinician's own, salient impressions, possibly keep from influencing the clinician's ultimate conclusions about client status or response to treatment? If the therapist wished to obtain long-term outcome data, how could the clinician ensure that clients with positive and negative reactions responded with similar frequency to inquiries?

With covariation analysis, accurate and representative data from all four cells are essential. A treater's personal experience is unlikely to provide such information. For example, individuals who are faring well are less likely to seek clinical services than those experiencing serious psychological challenges. Additionally, if a therapist consistently uses a particular intervention for certain symptoms or difficulties, the therapist does not know what would have occurred had a different approach been used. Consequently, the therapist typically lacks a comparison or control group. A control group is arguably the closest solution thus far developed for addressing the philosopher's counterfactual inquiry: What would have happened had one done otherwise? In contrast, in clinical practice, one might have information about the A and B cells (specific information about the percentage of individuals who do and do not do well), but not about the other two cells, essentially precluding proper covariation analysis. The specific intervention used might have been maximally effective, but without an alternative treatment group, how could that determination be made?

Typical treatment settings create substantial obstacles to obtaining the needed information to perform proficient covariation analysis and cannot be expected to match the methodological advantages gained by conducting a large-scale randomized controlled trial or series of trials. Thus, when trying to learn certain things based primarily on clinical experience, there will almost always be major gaps in the available information, which, in the case of covariation analysis, puts the practitioner at a sizeable disadvantage.

One might object that many clinicians have broad knowledge about scientific studies and integrate it with their clinical impressions. We do not question that, but wish to circle back to the current chapter's essential inquiry: When clinical judgments or impressions and scientific findings conflict, and one must select one or the other (as commonly occurs in situations requiring dichotomous choices), what are the knowledge credentials of these different sources of guidance and how does one decide?

Some Advantages of Scientific Methods

Covariation analysis is being used here as an exemplar, although a fundamental and critical one. Science can provide considerable advantages over personal experience in obtaining the type and quality of information needed to appraise possible associations among variables. How can even the most astute clinician, operating on the basis of experience, compare relative frequencies in the A and B cells to those in the C and D cells if that practitioner lacks representative information from the C and D cells, or has barely any information at all? No matter one's capabilities, trying to determine whether the ratio of A:B differs from the ratio of C:D without the needed information to proceed proficiently does not speak to one's intelligence.

Although we have thus far emphasized the quality of data and certain methods for attenuating bias, we have directed minimal attention to the potential advantages of scientific methods over impressionistic judgment for combining or integrating information. Such advantages include the use of advanced quantitative methods that can offer powerful means for managing large or massive databases; detecting modest or small differences that may nevertheless make meaningful impacts (for example, in clinical interventions, or that may signal important phenomena); integrating complex sources of information through such methods as meta-analysis; separating statistical fact and artifact; determining effect sizes; combining quantitative and qualitative information; and applying increasingly sophisticated methods for identifying and mapping causal pathways.

One can acknowledge the potential value of clinical impressions and observations in adding to the database (which is one reason we referred to qualitative information above), but here we are emphasizing methods that provide advantages for combining and analyzing information (see further below). Without dogmatically placing science above all other methods of knowing across all situations, it is important to identify circumstances in which science brings epistemological or methodological advantages that can elevate it beyond personal experience, and assist considerably in extending the limits of personal observation.

The Boundaries of Clinical/Impressionistic Judgment and Experiential Learning

Research provides important insights into the strengths and limits of clinical or impressionistic judgment and the comparison to other means for generating and integrating information. As we will describe, such research includes studies on *illusory correlations,* investigations on the relation between experience and judgmental accuracy, and studies comparing different methods for combining and integrating information. Research on human decision making has a constructive intent, which is to clarify what we do well and not so well, and how we can use this knowledge to do better. This research sometimes generates favorable outcomes for clinical decision making, but at other times raises doubts about widely held beliefs.

Chapman and Chapman and Illusory Correlations

Loren and Jean Chapman (1967, 1969) conducted seminal studies on diagnostic processes. In an initial series of experiments, they studied the interpretation of human figure drawings, based partly on their curiosity about the regular use (at that time) of a method that had generated predominantly negative research on its accuracy. It was commonly assumed that clients with various symptoms tend to draw" pictures of people that demonstrate particular features. For example, persons with paranoid thinking purportedly drew pictures of people with large eyes, and persons who were overly passive drew pictures of people with their hands behind their back. In other words, clinicians tended to *perceive* covariation between certain psychological difficulties and the pictures that those individuals drew, despite research raising serious doubts about various such associations. How might these mistaken beliefs have been formed?

In their 1967 study, the Chapmans collected drawings produced from clients at an inpatient setting, and then randomly paired drawing characteristics with personality descriptions. For example, for drawings with accented eyes, some might be paired with statements about suspiciousness, but an equal number with completely different descriptions. Thus, there were no systematic relationships between the drawing characteristics and the personality descriptions. They then asked different groups, psychologists included, what they observed after reviewing the drawings and the respective personality descriptions. Respondents tended to overestimate the frequency of supportive cases and to believe, incorrectly, that systematic relationships were present in the data. Their conclusions coincided with prior beliefs they held about such associations. Thus, they "saw" supportive evidence in the data that did not exist by over-attending to positive evidence over negative evidence. These prior beliefs aligned with common social beliefs or stereotypes (e.g., that accented eyes in drawings reflected paranoid tendencies).

The Chapmans characterized these misperceptions of associations between variables as *illusory correlations*. In follow-up studies, the Chapmans' (1969) obtained similar results when examining Rorschach interpretations, and additionally found that illusory beliefs interfered with the detection of valid relationships. Detection of valid relations required data that supported such associations nearly without exception, or a percentage of confirming instances that exceeded the levels one would expect for even robust variables.

Various other studies and commentary have addressed illusory correlations (e.g., Herman, 2005; Kurtz & Garfield, 1978; Lueger & Petzel, 1979; Nickerson, 2004). This research shows how difficult it can be to appraise associations between variables using clinical or impressionistic judgment, and how belief in illusory correlations, once formed, are often maintained even in the face of contrary evidence and passed on to other generations of clinicians. Even mixed evidence or evidence that is disconfirming overall will often still contain some "confirming" instances, and disproportionate attention to positive cases may make it seem like one's beliefs are supported. Even individuals without serious emotional disorders can be impulsive, reckless, hostile, moody, and apathetic at times. Hence, for one expecting to see pathology, instances of supportive evidence will often be present.

Experience Is Not Always the Best Teacher

Benjamin Franklin is often quoted as saying something like, "Experience is a dear teacher…" In the old English of the time, "dear" did not mean highly valued, but costly, which might explain the completion of the sentence with, "…and fools learn from no other," or something similar. A large body of research has examined the relation between clinical experience and diagnostic and predictive accuracy. This research generally fails to support common assumptions that clinical experience produces large gains in proficiency. Rather, some studies show modest to small effect sizes, and other studies show little or no impact, and a point of diminishing returns that may come fairly early, or before a great deal of experience has been acquired (e.g., Faust & Faust, 2012; Garb et al., 2012; Lichtenberg, 2009; Spengler et al., 2009; Spengler & Pilipis, 2015; Volmer et al., 2013). Research also indicates that experience often leads to a greater increase in confidence than in accuracy, with the level of confidence surpassing accuracy to an increasing degree. Overconfidence in judgmental accuracy carries a host of risks and problems (see further below).

Experience and practice can be invaluable tools for skill development and self-improvement in wide-ranging areas. Experience may also foster remarkably fruitful ideas and hypotheses that may subsequently be verified. However, for improving performance on certain types of tasks, such as the judgments often called on when making explicit and implicit clinical predictions or identifying disorders, experience often has restricted value, and in some situations may be plainly misleading. Much like difficulties performing covariation analysis due to deficiencies in data and the typical conditions of clinical practice, limited gains through experience often come down to similar factors that sheer intellectual power cannot overcome directly or without accessing other informational sources. As discussed later, the conditions of clinical practice often create so-called *wicked* learning environments. Fortunately, we often have access to additional means, methods, and knowledge, which can help us overcome certain boundaries in experiential learning, such as well-conducted scientific studies that fill informational gaps. Rather than viewing limits in experiential learning attributable to naturalistic conditions as reflecting negatively on human abilities, one might focus more on the other side of the coin, or how the development of methods to overcome such barriers reflects human ingenuity, aptitude, and sometimes true genius.

Also, although we might perceive a clear demarcation between personal experience and research, research data provide a means for acquiring large amounts of empirical/experiential information and organizing it in condensed and orderly forms. (We are using the term *empirical* here to refer to its original formal meaning, as referring to observational data, and not as synonymous with experimental or research evidence.) For example, an investigator who collects 10,000 MMPI-2 profiles may have created a database that far exceeds a clinician's personal exposure to such information during a lifetime of practice. What should count as experiential (or empirical) information is not always as clear-cut as it might seem; the researcher's compilation of MMPI-2 profiles comprises a wealth of empirical information. We appreciate that research data cannot capture various elements of direct experience. However, direct experience frequently is accompanied not only by potential advantages but also by potential limitations and misleading elements. For example, the salience of information in a clinical session may have a sizeable impact on judgment yet show limited relation to informational value.

Clinical Versus Statistical Data Integration

Framing the Issue and Definition of the Two Methods

Meehl (1954, 1986, 1996) is often credited with introducing the topic of clinical and statistical decision methods to a broad audience of psychologists, and given this and the clarity of his thinking, we will take his lead in framing the issue and defining the contrasting methods. Although some stereotyped Meehl as anti-clinician, he was a practicing therapist for many years and openly described the benefits he obtained from his own therapy. Meehl diligently considered and described potential advantages of clinical judgment over statistical methods, with almost half of his seminal 1954 book covering that topic.

Unfortunately, certain misconceptions about clinical and statistical decision methods arise often and lead to nonproductive cross-talk, and thus we will attempt to be as clear as we can. The core issue is the relative accuracy of contrasting methods for combining or integrating information when both rely on the same information, and thus neither method has an informational edge. Note that the primary inquiry involves methods for integrating or interpreting information, as opposed to the type of data or information being integrated. These data may be "objective," such as test scores, but may also rest solely or additionally on other informational sources, including subjective impressions (e.g., a clinician's sense that a client has flat affect or is socially awkward).

The two fundamental approaches being compared are the *clinical* method and the *statistical* (or termed *actuarial*) method. The term *clinical* is not ideal because it does not necessarily refer to a clinician. For example, a basketball coach may rely heavily on clinical judgment when scouting a college prospect. Rather, clinical judgment refers to data integration in one's head, or using subjective or impressionistic methods. The college coach may use various sources of information, including detailed quantitative analyses, such as measurements of height and vertical leap. Ultimately, however, the combination or interpretation of whatever information is gathered is through subjective mental processes.

In the statistical method, as per Meehl, two conditions must be met. First, data combination must be fixed or standardized, or to state this in another way, given the same data, the method always produces the same result. Once developed, the statistical method itself does not depend on clinical judgment. That does not mean one must uniformly accept the outcome, but rather that in proceeding from the data to the outcome, subjective judgment plays no part.

Second, the conclusion or output must rest on empirically established relations. For example, if the height of a basketball player is being considered for inclusion, there must be an empirical basis that establishes an association between that variable and the outcome or outcomes of interest. When developing statistical decision procedures, a range of variables may be examined for potential utility, but if a variable turns out to lack predictive utility, it will (should) be excluded from the statistical decision method. Further, when multivariate methods are used to develop statistical decision procedures, as is common, then given the propensity of such methods to capitalize on chance and consequently produce inflated results, further validation or cross-validation should usually be conducted before comparing the accuracy of the statistical decision procedure to clinical judgment.

Fulfilling only one of the two conditions is not sufficient to meet the definition being used here for statistical decision methods. For example, computerized interpretive programs are automated or unvarying, but they may be designed to reproduce an expert's judgments; and that expert's interpretations may be founded, at least partly, on clinical judgment as opposed to empirically established relationships. Various other judgment approaches may be developed or proposed, such as efforts to combine clinical and statistical methods, but given space limits we will primarily address the two basic decision methods.

Research Outcomes

When the first edition of Meehl's (1954) book on clinical and statistical decision methods appeared, limited comparative studies were available. That literature showed that clinical and statistical methods achieved similar accuracy rates in a number of comparisons. However, when there was a difference, the statistical method consistently outperformed the clinical method, thereby suggesting that the statistical method was superior overall. At that point, many important questions remained to be addressed, such as whether highly skilled clinicians might gain an advantage by detecting patterns in data that statistical methods failed to identify. The hundreds of studies that followed addressed this and various other issues. Although certain questions could still benefit from further research, the fundamental findings have been supported or strengthened over time (AEgisdóttir et al., 2006; Grove et al., 2000; Sawyer, 1966).

Sawyer's (1966) review covered about 50 studies, which provided 75 comparisons between clinical and statistical decision methods. It might be noted here that statistical methods can incorporate interview or qualitative information, as long as it is coded, for example, flat affect can be coded as: 1 = judged as present, 0 = judged as absent, thus making it possible to compare not only conclusions based on testing, but also conclusions based on interviews, or interviews and testing. Although a considerable percentage of the comparisons demonstrated ties (i.e., no statistically significant differences between methods), when a difference was present, the statistical method exceeded the clinical method on every occasion, a level of consistency in research outcomes unusual in psychology. In addition, even when studies went outside Meehl's stated conditions for a fair comparison, but instead provided more information to clinical judges than the statistical method, the latter still always equaled or exceeded the clinical method.

Sawyer also examined a condition in which clinicians were provided with the outcomes of statistical decision methods and could use or disregard them at their discretion. For example, if a dichotomous decision was required and the clinician's conclusion and the statistical decision method's outcome conflicted, the clinician could retain the original conclusion or defer to the statistical method. One can see how closely this condition approximates the main question posed in this chapter, which is when to go with one's clinical judgment as opposed to an alternative method or conclusion when the two conflict. If properly designed statistical decision procedures can be placed within the body of science (seemingly an appropriate categorization), then these lines of inquiry are directly related, although not all encompassing or dispositive.

Meehl had previously described circumstances that might call for one to reject the results of a statistical decision method as *broken leg* examples, relating them to situations in which a certain outcome or behavior is expected, but an unusual event occurs that upends expectations. Infrequent or rare events are often unaccounted for by statistical methods, making the identification of potential exceptions a key concern. Even when statistical prediction methods surpass clinical judgment, they may still generate errors in an unsettling percentage of cases. For example, clinical predictions might be correct 65% of the time (or generate a 35% error rate) and statistical predictions correct 75% of the time (or generate a 25% error rate). Error reduction is desirable, but if a potentially serious matter is at issue, such as possible homicidal behavior, being wrong one in four times is far from satisfactory. Hence, if exceptions to statistical predictions can be identified with sufficient regularity, error rate could be further reduced.

Studies on countervailing, although somewhat limited in scope and number, show that clinicians given access to statistical decision methods countervail them often (e.g., 25% of the time or more), with one study obtaining a rate exceeding 70% (Schmidt et al., 2016). Countervailing only becomes an option when the outcome of clinical judgment and statistical decision procedures conflict, thus making these rates higher or considerably higher than the absolute percentages suggest.

Further, study outcomes show that countervailing statistical decision methods (as opposed to following them uniformly), *at best*, does not increase accuracy, but at least does not reduce it. However, the impact of countervailing is usually not neutral, but rather to diminish accuracy. The decrease may be small to modest, but can be substantial, even reducing accuracy rates from relatively good levels to chance levels (Guay & Parent, 2018; Krauss et al., 2004; Schmidt et al., 2016; Storey et al., 2012; Wormith et al., 2012). Stated in another way, for every incorrect statistically-based conclusion corrected by countervailing, there is at least one, and often more than one, correct statistically-based decision that is spoiled or changed into an error. This is a simple matter of math, not a philosophical proposition. We are not suggesting that clinicians uniformly or mindlessly defer to statistical decision methods, but only that countervailing occurs too frequently and that greater caution is warranted.

Following Sawyer's review, hundreds of subsequent studies in psychology have compared clinical judgment to the statistical method. Both AEgisdóttir et al. (2006) and Grove et al. (2000) performed comprehensive meta-analyses. AEgisdóttir et al.'s meta-analysis focused on literature from the mental health field, whereas Grove et al.'s meta-analysis also incorporated studies from medicine, although the number of medical studies made up a relatively small proportion of the overall body of research. A summary of results appears in Table 2, which was compiled based on these two meta-analyses. The table only includes studies that reported hit rates, which did make up the large majority of investigations, and for Grove et al.'s meta-analysis, medical studies were excluded. The studies cover wide-ranging judgment tasks, including diagnosis, prognosis, length of treatment, and evaluation of suicide risk.

Both meta-analyses align with Sawyer's (1966) much earlier review and demonstrate the potential advantages of statistical decision methods in increasing overall accuracy. For example, looking at the highest category for level of accuracy in Table 2 and across the two meta-analyses, one sees that the statistical method achieves this uppermost level considerably more often than clinical judgment methods. Conversely, examining the lowest level of accuracy listed in Table 2, the respective percentages for the clinical method versus the statistical method is about two times greater in the Grove et al. meta-analysis and about four times greater in the AEgisdóttir et al. meta-analysis. Taken together, these differences in overall accuracy might not seem all that great examined one case at a time, but when

Table 2 Outcomes across studies for which Grove et al. (2000) and AEgisdóttir et al. (2006) provided hit rates

Level of accuracy	Percentage of studies	
	Clinical method	Statistical method
Grove et al. (2000)		
0.80–0.99	6%	17%
0.60–0.79	60%	58%
0.50–0.59	19%	17%
0.49 or lower	15%	8%
AEgisdóttir et al. (2006)		
0.80–0.99	3%	20%
0.60–0.79	60%	61%
0.50–0.59	29%	17%
0.49 or lower	9%	2%

accumulated across a lifetime of cases, they result in many more accurate decisions and many fewer mistakes. It may be disturbing to be equaled or exceeded in certain domains by an algorithm or statistical formula. However, the efficacy of statistical decision procedures is hardly a threat to most central activities clinicians perform, such as forming curative, empathic connections with clients. The use of statistical decision methods also requires the oversight of mental health professionals. Most importantly, improved diagnostic and predictive accuracy can help us deliver better services in important domains and thereby improve client outcomes.

The meta-analyses, however, do not support the mistaken or overblown claim sometimes heard that statistical methods almost always, or always, surpass clinical judgment. There are many ties in the literature. Rather, *when there is a difference*, the statistical method almost always surpasses the clinical method, justifying its description as a better method *overall*, but certainly not as consistently exceeding clinical judgment.

AEgisdóttir et al. (2006) also examined whether clinicians performed at higher levels when they had access to information collected in their own practice settings. The analysis is important because in many judgment studies, clinicians evaluate information drawn from settings other than their own; hence, inaccessibility of direct experience with their own clientele and local knowledge could place practitioners at an unfair disadvantage. However, access to information from the clinicians' own settings did not generate more favorable outcomes for clinical judgment.

I Don't Believe It; Underuse and Undervaluation of Science

Given the potential advantages of science and such methods as statistical decision procedures, Scott and many others have advocated passionately for greater utilization of science in applied psychology. After briefly reviewing literature on the use or underuse of science, we then examine powerful factors that are nearly omnipresent in applied settings, and that understandably and compellingly can bend appraisals of the relative benefits of science versus personal experience and judgment in a counterproductive direction.

Underuse and Undervaluation of Science

Over the years, many commentators have expressed concerns about practitioners' tendencies to underutilize research in their practices (e.g., Barlow, 1981; Boisvert & Faust, 2003; Kazdin, 2008; Lilienfeld et al., 2013; Nathan, 2000; Stricker, 1992). Survey research often supports these concerns, such as results indicating that clinicians rely more on experience with clients than on research to guide their psychotherapy practices (e.g., Morrow-Bradley & Elliot, 1986; Stewart & Chambless, 2007). In an early study on test selection, Wade and Baker (1977) concluded that survey respondents were "indifferent to negative research evidence because their opinions of a test's value derive principally from their personal experience with the test" (p. 879). Later surveys have reported similar results (e.g., Watkins et al., 1995; Kranzler et al., 2020), thereby suggesting that in the domain of psychological assessment, clinical experience may often be prioritized over scientific knowledge.

Other surveys show that clinicians underuse well-established science or scientifically-based procedures, such as statistical judgment methods (Furman, 2005; Vrieze & Grove, 2009), hold beliefs that are inconsistent with scientific findings, or seem to reject the value of science as a whole (e.g., Boisvert & Faust, 2006; Kranzler et al., 2020; Rock, 1994; Lilienfeld et al., 2018; Wade & Baker, 1977). Meyer's (2015) survey on scientific and pseudo-scientific beliefs provides multiple startling examples of broad rejection of various fundamental scientific and mathematical principles, such as the relation between the frequency of events (i.e., base rates) and the frequency of false-negative and false-positive errors. Furman's (2005) survey shows broad rejection of formal decision aids and a high frequency of false beliefs about clinical and statistical decision methods. Where quality studies have consistently yielded similar outcomes and the resultant knowledge is directly applicable to important clinical decisions and issues, then underuse suggests that science is being rejected too frequently in favor of something else, presumably clinical experience and judgment when the two conflict. Of course, "relying" on science when it accords with one's beliefs and rejecting it when it does not is often functionally equivalent to not relying on science at all.

Factors Leading to Potential Underuse and Undervaluation of Science

There can be a reflexive tendency to reject science when it conflicts with one's perceptions or experiences. Experience is highly salient, whereas science may seem abstract and removed from the challenges and messiness of applied settings. One of science's greatest values is to test belief, but when research generates counterintuitive findings or contradicts human phenomenology, those findings often must compete with impressions hardened through seeming confirmation across numerous instances and multiple years. Changing a belief is often much harder than forming a belief in the first place, especially if the original belief seems strongly supported by personal observation and the contrary belief rests on such sources as bland statistics and pages of a journal. Additionally, because even the best decision procedures may be wrong 10% or 20% of the time or more often, it can be easy to point to errors that seemingly override these methods' advantages. Even individuals inclined to use statistical decision methods are more likely to reject such procedures after becoming aware that they made an error (Dietvorst et al., 2016), a reaction that seems to disregard overall accuracy.

Naturalistic Conditions Are Likely to Create Overconfidence in One's Judgmental Proficiency

Research on the accuracy of decision methods, such as statistical decision procedures, generates outcomes showing how often they are and are not correct. In contrast, evaluating one's judgmental accuracy can be a considerably more challenging or ambiguous undertaking. Furthermore, as we will describe, conditions are often present in naturalistic or applied settings that make it appear that one's level of accuracy exceeds one's true rate of accuracy. Consequently, suppose studies show that a statistical decision procedure achieves 70% accuracy, and naturalistic practice conditions make it appear that one's accuracy is 80% or higher (rather than actually falling, say, at about 60%). In such circumstances, one can easily see why practitioners would elevate their judgments over the statistical decision procedure. Therefore, to the extent naturalistic settings contain compelling features that inflate confidence even among highly skilled and rational individuals, the result will often be to elevate clinical judgment over statistical decision methods as well as other scientifically derived procedures that may also seem like inferior choices. Charges of irrationality that may appear in writings on the science-practice divide might sometimes be better directed toward errors that are difficult to avoid in naturalistic environments when attempting to calibrate one's level of confidence.

Many individuals in many walks of life are more confident than is warranted, including mental health professionals. One survey found that the average clinician believed their treatment effectiveness fell at the 80th percentile, with one-quarter placing that level at the 90th percentile (Walfish et al., 2012). *Not a single respondent* believed they performed below the 50th percentile. Along related lines, studies show that psychologists are often overconfident in their judgmental accuracy (e.g., Oskamp, 1965; Wedding, 1983; Faust et al., 1988), or demonstrate a relatively low association between confidence and accuracy (e.g., Goldberg, 1959; Nadler et al., 1994; Desmarais et al., 2010). Miller et al.'s (2015) meta-analysis found a small (although statistically significant) correlation between confidence and accuracy. However, if confidence is often greater than accuracy, as studies commonly indicate, a researcher may still find a correlation between the two, even though confidence is not well calibrated (i.e., matched with accuracy). The association between confidence and accuracy needs to be distinguished from calibration. For example, if an individual is generally overconfident by 20 or 30%, one may well find a correlation between confidence and accuracy, yet at the same time systematic overconfidence.

We can briefly review a series of factors that inflate confidence (for greater detail see Faust et al., 2022). First, in treatment settings, it is difficult to avoid what is alternatively referred to as *treatment effects*, *self-fulfilling prophecies*, or *channeling effects*. Here, the clinicians' assumptions or judgments impact clients' behavior in a manner that tends to confirm their initial beliefs. For example, clients may agree with clinicians' impressions, whether they are actually accurate or inaccurate. A neuropsychologist who conducts an extensive assessment and who provides feedback that the client's memory concerns reflect normal human failings may well be believed, with client agreement perceived as providing some level of confirmation for the conclusion. Alternatively, however, the client may well have also agreed if the clinician indicated that the results fell outside normal limits. If both conclusions cannot be correct but a client might agree in either case, then the rate of client agreement across cases may well exceed the practitioner's judgmental accuracy, and thereby inflate confidence. Alternatively, a clinician who feels very optimistic about a client's prospects for a positive treatment outcome, even without realizing it, may offer greater encouragement than might occur for a client whose treatment prospects seem poor, and thus may unintentionally foster the predicted outcome.

Numerous studies have examined the tendency to believe that outcomes, once known, seem more predictable in hindsight than is actually the case in advance or in foresight (e.g., Arkes et al., 1988; Hastie et al., 1999; LeBourgeois et al., 2007; Nickerson, 1998). Given the ingenuity of the human mind to formulate causal explanations for events, an outcome that would have been difficult to predict in advance might start to seem more predictable than was actually the case, or almost inevitable. In addition, given the reconstructive elements of memory and this same propensity to formulate explanations for outcomes, individuals tend to recall their original predictions as more consistent with outcomes than was actually the case. Such reconstruction may explain an exchange like the following between two individuals who originally made different predictions. Upon later learning what happened, one may insist, "I told you so," with the other retorting, "No, as *I* told *you* so!" If individuals tend to recall their predictions as more consistent with outcomes than is actually the case, the seeming frequency of confirmation for one's predictions will exceed the true rate of accuracy and promote overconfidence.

As the Chapmans' (1967, 1969) studies show, and as a large body of subsequent research on what is often termed *confirmatory bias* also indicates, laypersons and professionals with pre-existing beliefs who review information that does not support their hypotheses, may nevertheless over-attend to and overweight confirming instances and under-attend to and underweight negative instances (see Faust & Ahern, 2012). The result may well be to believe their initial hypotheses were confirmed or to over-appraise the strength of the evidence. Professionals in these studies are not merely trying to prove their point (especially when their results are anonymous). Even when individuals are highly motivated to reach accurate conclusions, tendencies to be overly swayed by supportive evidence and less impacted by negative evidence commonly skew their judgments in favor of their initial beliefs. Again, given the tendency to overestimate and overweight instances that seem to confirm initial judgments, the seeming frequency of confirming instances will exceed their true rate, and potentially inflate confidence.

Various other factors could be discussed, such as nonrepresentative feedback (e.g., clients with more favorable progress are more likely to remain in treatment than clients who are dissatisfied), and research suggesting that experts may have a tendency, as time passes and memory capacities are strained, to forget case facts that diverge from their diagnoses or conclusions and to mis-recall signs or symptoms congruent with their original case formulations as having been present. Recognizing that memory is a reconstructive process, extensive familiarity with diagnostic conditions may lead to a subtle reshaping of recall consistent with expected case features. Such shifts in recall can make it more difficult to recognize subsequent diagnostic errors, again promoting the belief that accuracy is greater than is truly the case. When one considers all of these mechanisms, which often seem to occur outside of awareness, one can see how difficult it can be to avoid overconfidence. The end result may be a sincere, but often inaccurate, belief that accuracy rates reported for statistical decision procedures and other scientifically-validated methods fall short of what the clinician usually achieves, and consequently are inferior choices.

It is also worth considering the quality of evidence for self-appraising one's accuracy, which often depends largely on subjective impressions. Relying primarily on subjective impressions (one's own and others) often reduces or eliminates the opportunity to use various research methods that could attenuate potential biases, such as single- or double-blind appraisal. Additionally, to refer back to covariation analysis, such attempts at self-appraisal also lack a comparison group, and thus one does not know what outcomes would have occurred had one made other decisions or judgments. Perhaps a favorable client outcome signifies a superior treatment choice, but one is not in a position to determine if a comparable or better outcome would have occurred with another selection. Overall, for these and additional reasons covered earlier in the section on covariation, the quality of evidence one uses to appraise one's judgmental accuracy impressionistically often falls well short of the quality of evidence produced by well-conducted research and, when available, meta-analyses. One might believe one regularly beats statistical decision procedures, but how well do such subjective impressions match up to, say, the 300+ studies on clinical versus statistical decision making? Hence, if practitioners claim or believe they are exceptions, it is reasonable to inquire about the quality of evidence supporting the contrary belief. It seems clear where the burden of proof should lie.

Rather than depending mainly on subjective impressions about our decision accuracy, a critical additional source of information may be available and provide a better guide: credible research on the effectiveness of the methods one uses, preferably obtained in research settings similar to one's practice and with similar clients. At times there will be a sizeable body of literature that has demonstrated consistent, or at least fairly consistent, results. These research outcomes should offer evidence that is likely to be considerably stronger than one's subjective impressions. This assumes that the clinician uses evaluative or predictive methods as designed, because if they are modified, then little may be known about how well they work, likely making the clinician's beliefs highly speculative. Further, research on countervailing suggests that, if anything, such modifications will degrade accuracy.

What's So Bad About Being Overconfident?

Overconfidence creates a range of problems with potentially serious consequences (see Faust et al., 2022). Overconfident decision-makers often reach conclusions too quickly, before essential information has been obtained, and are susceptible to making overly extreme or risky decisions. For example, they may feel more certain than is warranted that a client will follow through on a therapeutic contract. In addition, overconfident practitioners are more likely to miss errors and to overlook or reject needed corrective actions than those with better calibrated confidence levels. Further, overconfidence is associated with reduced use of potentially helpful decision aids and research innovations.

Factors Impacting Experiential Learning: Kind and Wicked Learning Environments

The distinction is sometimes made between *kind* (or *high validity*) learning environments and *wicked* learning environments, or between circumstances that tend to promote, versus impede, learning from experience (Hogarth et al., 2015; Kahneman & Klein, 2009). Some of the differences are a matter of degree, and thus involve the extent to which conditions tend to favor experiential learning.

Kind learning environments are characterized by such features as rapid, explicit feedback with minimal error, or feedback that rarely misleads (Arkes, 2001; Dawes, 1989; Fischhoff & Broomell, 2020.) Thus, when one is correct, the feedback consistently indicates so; and likewise, when errors occur, the feedback consistently indicates such. Additionally, one obtains comprehensive and representative feedback of outcomes as a whole. For example, if 80% of clients who receive a certain treatment improve and 20% do not, outcome data reflect or approximate that proportion. Likewise, if 60% receiving another treatment improve and 40% do not, feedback on that intervention would also be accurate and allow one to compare the success of the alternative intervention. These and other features of kind learning environments help explain why randomized control trials (RCTs), which contain all of these elements, can be so useful.

By contrast, in wicked learning environments, which are common in clinical settings, one major obstacle to experiential learning is that feedback often contains significant noise or error. If the feedback one receives is incomplete or ambiguous at times, outcome information about the method might suggest a higher (or lower) error rate than is actually the case, or be misleading in a fairly high percentage of cases. To the extent feedback is probabilistic rather than deterministic, or contains a significant error component, learning from experience is likely to be reduced or seriously compromised (Dawes, 1989; Witteman, 2018). As Hogarth (2015, p. 379) stated, "Intuitions acquired in wicked environments are likely to be mistaken."

A somewhat abstract example, but one with parallels to other forms of concept learning and identification, can be used to illustrate difficulties caused by error in feedback, especially in situations in which one is trying to appraise categories or constructs (e.g., a clinical presentation suggesting the occurrence of child abuse). Suppose capital letters are presented one at a time, and one tries to figure out the concept underlying their classification. "A" is presented, one guesses the letter does not represent the category, and one is told one is correct. "B" is presented, one guesses it does represent the category, and are again told one is correct. "C" follows, one guesses it falls within the category, but one is told one is incorrect. Thus, if the concept one was considering is letters with curves, feedback on the letter "C" would seem to disconfirm the hypothesis. Assume for the subsequent presentations of the letters "D," "E," and "F," the responses are all "no's," and the feedback given is that one is correct each time. Although many respondents would likely be at a loss at this point, suppose the concept was indeed letters with curved lines. However, what is occurring, parallel to a method that is correct 7 of 10 times, is that the feedback contains about a 30% error rate. The error in the feedback would make what would otherwise likely be learning a simple concept considerably more difficult.

Suppose further, as is the case with many key concepts in psychology, one had to learn more complex concepts or identifiers, such as every other letter with curves, or an ascending sequence, such as the first letter with curves, the third letter with curves, the fifth letter with curves, or something even more complex or involving more dimensions simultaneously. Wicked learning environments often contain considerable error in feedback, and thus can make learning from experience or in naturalistic environments exceedingly difficult. In a clinical setting, if the clinician is regularly appraising the risk of dangerous behavior or other events with low frequencies, even poor methods will often be correct if they tend to predict nonoccurrence, potentially making them seem like effective tools even if they have poor accuracy in positive cases.

In wicked learning environments, one often lacks comparison groups and often falls considerably short of obtaining complete feedback. For example, if a client drops out of treatment, should the clinician conclude that the intervention resolved problems and the client felt that treatment was no longer needed, or that the intervention was likely unsuccessful? Additionally, many false-negative assessment errors (e.g., missing child abuse, intimate partner violence, or an eating disorder) may never be detected due to client nondisclosure, and thus it will not be apparent or known when errors occur. Alternatively, when positive client changes are observed during treatment, it may sometimes be hard to determine whether other factors, such as spontaneous remission or occurrences largely unrelated to the therapy might have played a substantial role (Faust & Faust, 2012; Lilienfeld et al., 2013; Witteman, 2018).

Contrary to Common Assumptions, Complex Data Integration Can Be Extremely Difficult

Writings on psychological assessment across decades commonly include statements about integrating extensive information, which are often presented as all but givens. For example, in her 1983 text, Muriel Lezak, a widely recognized neuropsychologist, stated that:

> For the examination to supply answers to many of the diagnostic questions and most of the treatment and planning questions *requires integration of all of the data* [emphasis added] –from tests, observations made in the course of the examination, and the history of the problem (p. 162).

In the fifth edition of her text nearly 30 years later, Lezak did not change this statement at all (Lezak et al., 2012, p. 177). Other examples of similar statements can be found in Exner (1974, pp. 6–7) and Mitrushina et al. (2005, pp. 3–4, 6).

These types of statements and guidance call for gathering extensive information and then integrating much or all of it, attending closely to data patterns or configural relationships. In principle, the emphasis on configural relationships seems compelling. Many phenomena in nature show patterns or interaction effects, and thus accounting for them may provide a significant predictive advantage. Many of the most compelling examples in which deep knowledge of complex interrelationships has been captured successfully originate from scientific areas in which advanced knowledge has been achieved. These developments often rest on exacting measurement tools, comprehensive understanding of the major factors that influence outcome, and advanced theories with well-established scientific foundations.

When we lack advanced knowledge and theories, but rather try to integrate complex information based primarily on mental processes or impressionistic judgment, how well do we do? Exemplar statements on combining information suggest that our powers of information integration have remarkable reach and proficiency. However, how can even leading intellects in the mental health field integrate most or all of the data successfully when one may be dealing with hundreds or even thousands of data points (e.g., numerous test responses, an array of behavioral observations, various events in an individual's life history, and more). Are there potential benefits to appraising our capacities accurately and potential costs to misappraisals?

In almost every instance, assertions about extraordinary data integration capacities are not accompanied by citations to studies that have examined such capacities and confirmed their existence, which is of particular interest because there is extensive research on the topic. Instead, the primary basis for these beliefs seems to be compelling subjective impressions that these activities have and can be performed successfully (perhaps along with positive clinical outcomes being offered as a form of verification). Rather than limiting the evaluation of such beliefs to subjective impressions, we can turn to the available body of literature on the topic.

Research on Complex Data Integration Capacities

At least three major lines of research have examined complex data integration capacities: (1) studies on amount of information and judgmental accuracy, (2) direct examination of complex concept formation, and (3) modeling studies of human judgment. Space limitations require a truncated summary of this research, with more detailed coverage available in other sources (e.g., Faust et al., 2022).

Various studies show that beyond a surprisingly small amount of information—perhaps as little as two or three of the most valid and least redundant variables—and especially when clinical judgment is used to integrate information, further information often does little or nothing to increase diagnostic or predictive accuracy, or may even reduce accuracy (e.g., Dana et al., 2013; Dawes, 1971; Oskamp, 1965; Wedding, 1983). How can such research outcomes be explained?

Clinical settings often provide potential access to multiple or numerous informational sources. The predictive utility of differing information will often vary widely, and some of the information may seem to be helpful but may actually have negligible value. Other key factors, such as the level of overlap or redundancy across informational sources may alter the relative value of variables considerably, yet determining such things as comparative level of validity and redundancy is very challenging to accomplish without formal decision aids, quantification, or the needed research basis. Thus, discerning what should and should not be used, or optimal combinations of variables, is daunting to perform subjectively, and an admonishment to integrate all of the data is almost certain to stray from maximally effective judgmental practices.

A better guide than integrating all of the available information is to prioritize *incremental validity*, or the impact of adding additional information to the best information that is already available. Adding additional information may: (1) increase accuracy, (2) not alter accuracy (thus making its use unnecessary and a potential waste of resources), or (3) decrease accuracy. Unfortunately, as research shows, the emphasis on integrating as much information as possible and the extreme challenges of subjective data integration result in the second or third outcome far too often.

A second line of research has directly examined the capacity to form or identify complex concepts. That research (e.g., Makridakis et al., 2009; Ruscio, 2003) runs contrary to the belief that individuals can come close to performing the type of extraordinary data integration commonly described or presumed.

A final line of studies addresses the capacity to model or reproduce decision makers' conclusions (e.g., Goldberg, 1970; Armstrong, 2001). Case scenarios are developed that are usually based primarily on information decision makers identify as critical in reaching conclusions, for example, diagnostic determinations, treatment selection, or the prediction of behavior, such as whether violent acts are likely to occur. Across the case scenarios, cues or variables are altered one at a time (e.g., flat affect), in order to study whether, or the extent to which, change in those variables impacts decision making. In turn, mathematical analyses of judges' decisions allow researchers to build models that are intended to duplicate judges' decisions in new cases.

This extensive research on modeling shows that to the degree decision makers are consistent (i.e., reach the same conclusions given the same data), models can often reproduce their decisions in a considerable percentage of cases, such as 75–85% of the time. Further, simple models often reproduce decisions successfully by simply adding a few variables together, and without needing to account for patterns or potential interactions among variables. For example, Goldberg (1970) found that psychologists' MMPI test interpretations, which the clinicians believed involved complex data integration, could often be reproduced by models that placed little reliance on configural judgments or pattern analysis and merely added up three variables and subtracted two other variables. Finally, modeling studies often reveal wide disparities between subjective impressions about the use of information and the outcome of formal means for measuring the impact of variables on decision makers' conclusions. For example, variables believed to impact judgments considerably may have little impact, and vice versa; and contrary to common subjective beliefs, only a few variables, rather than a considerable number, may have impacted conclusions substantially.

Obstacles to the Integration of Complex Information

The biggest reason we struggle to integrate complex information in our heads is likely because it is often exceedingly difficult. The bounds of our working memory, or how much information we can keep in mind simultaneously, is a key factor limiting our capacity to integrate complex information. In addition, the subject matter in psychology, which thus far often escapes precise measurement, makes it vexing to identify the full range of influential factors, and tends to place heavy demands on inferential thinking, creates its own heightened challenges. Maximizing the integration of large, complex data sets also necessitates determining the presence and strength of association between variables accurately, and preferably with precision, the degree of overlap or redundancy among variables, and at times the relative weights to assign to predictive variables.

In contrast to the prototypical statements (such as Lezak's above), which seem to assume that incredible acts of data integration can be achieved given the needed combination of training and experience, Meehl's (1986) classic comment on this matter offers a clear contrast:

> Surely we all know that the human brain is poor at weighting and computing. When you check out at the supermarket, you don't eyeball the heap of purchases and say to the clerk, "Well, it looks to me as if it's about $17.00 worth; what do you think?" The clerk adds it up. There are no strong arguments…from empirical studies…for believing that human beings can assign optimal weights to equations subjectively or that they apply their own weights optimally. (p. 372)

To which Dawes et al. (1989) later added:

> It might be objected that this analogy, offered not probatively but pedagogically, presupposes an additive model that a proponent of configural judgment will not accept. Suppose instead that the supermarket pricing rule were, "Whenever both beef and fresh vegetables are involved, multiple the logarithm of .78 of the meat price by the square root of twice the vegetable price"; would the clerk and customer eyeball that any better? Worse, almost certainly. When human judges perform poorly at estimating and applying the parameters of a simple or component mathematical function, they should not be expected to do better when required to weight a complex composite of these variables (p. 1672).

Implications of Research on Complex Data Integration

Various lines of research demonstrate limits in aspects of human cognition under certain conditions. These studies show that our capabilities have upper bounds that do not approach common assumptions about our ability to integrate hundreds or thousands of data points effectively or at exceptionally high levels. There is no shame in falling short of unrealistic expectations. Rather, it is these faulty expectations that seem most in need of revision. The various factors that foster overconfidence and subjective impressions about the ability to perform complex data analysis are often barriers to resetting expectations and taking corrective actions. Using clinical judgment to integrate extensive information and discern what may be complex patterns can be extremely challenging, especially when measurement is imprecise, and feedback is delayed, only partial, and ambiguous or frankly misleading at times, conditions that often characterize clinical and naturalistic settings.

Bad News or Good News?

Should we bemoan limits in unaided human judgment, or instead embrace the creation of methods that extend our capacities, permit us to do better, and show the remarkable things we can accomplish when faced with challenges? Human aptitude and at times outright brilliance have led to the creation of various helpful methods that often go a long way toward countering or overcoming the bounds of unaided human judgment. These developments can be framed as showing more about what we can do and not about what we cannot do. Scientific method, quantification, ingenious research, and the development of helpful decision aids (e.g., statistical decision methods), if used properly, serve to supplement and extend our judgmental capacities and increase the contributions we can make to society and to client care.

Examples of invaluable decision methods or guides that can assist in patient care, to name a few, include statistical decision methods, use of base rates or frequency of occurrence, and evaluation of incremental validity (see Faust et al., 2022, for an extensive discussion about applied uses of these and other decision aids). Often, the best predictor of diagnostic and predictive accuracy in the mental health field is meticulous adherence to the best-validated methods, including the use of statistical decision procedures when available and validated for the tasks at hand. Although it is sometimes claimed that such procedures are often lacking, there are literally thousands of statistical decision procedures available in applied psychology (see Chapter 8 of Faust et al., 2022). Incorporating base rates into decision making can often realize a considerable gain in judgmental accuracy, especially when low- or high-frequency events are at issue. For example, as often should be done, combining the diagnosticity of predictive signs or indicators with base rates may increase accuracy rates by twofold or more. Finally, we previously referred to incremental validity, or results achieved by combining new predictive variables with the best previously available predictors, as a far better guide for determining whether to seek or include new information than integrating all of the available information. Analysis of incremental validity may show that the potential addition increases accuracy, make no difference, or even reduces accuracy. It obviously is bad practice to include a variable that makes things worse, as can easily happen if one believes all the data should be combined.

Closing Comment

We return to the moment of truth and the conflict that regularly arises between conclusions based on clinical judgment and experience as opposed to science (as the two commonly diverge). It seems evident that across a range of circumstances, conclusions indicated by science are more likely to be correct. Practices that never or always defer to science are almost certainly too extreme, but the more common problematic tendency seems to be to value clinical judgment and experience above, or far beyond, science. In either case, whether choosing between clinical judgment or science when the two dictate opposing courses of action, errors may still result, and precautions to prevent disastrous outcomes may need to be implemented. Decisions in applied settings are often difficult and agonizing, given what may be at stake. It might seem too colloquial to say one makes one's bets and takes one's chances, but of course, the person with the most to gain or lose is often the client, whose welfare can rest substantially in the clinician's hands. Thus, we need to choose wisely, stepping back as much as we can from dogma, and collecting and integrating the highest quality information with the best methods within our grasp.

References

AEgisdóttir, S., White, M. J., Spengler, P. M., Maugherman, A. S., Anderson, L. A., Cook, R. S., et al. (2006). The meta-analysis of clinical judgment project: Fifty-six years of accumulated research on clinical versus statistical prediction. *The Counseling Psychologist, 34*(3), 341–382.

Arkes, H. R. (2001). Overconfidence in judgmental forecasting. In J. S. Armstrong (Ed.), *Principles of forecasting: A handbook for researchers and practitioners* (pp. 495–515). Springer.

Arkes, H. R., Faust, D., Guilmette, T. J., & Hart, K. (1988). Eliminating the hindsight bias. *Journal of Applied Psychology, 73*(2), 305–307.

Armstrong, J. S. (2001). Judgmental bootstrapping: Inferring experts' rules for forecasting. In J. S. Armstrong (Ed.), *Principles of forecasting: A handbook for researchers and practitioners* (pp. 171–192). Springer.

Barlow, D. H. (1981). On the relation of clinical research to clinical practice: Current issues, new directions. *Journal of Consulting and Clinical Psychology, 49*(2), 147–155.

Binder, L. M., Iverson, G. L., & Brooks, B. L. (2009). To err is human: "Abnormal" neuropsychological scores and variability are common in healthy adults. *Archives of Clinical Neuropsychology, 24*(1), 31–46.

Boisvert, C. M., & Faust, D. (2003). Leading researchers' consensus on psychotherapy research findings: Implications for the teaching and conduct of psychotherapy. *Professional Psychology: Research and Practice, 34*(5), 508–513.

Boisvert, C. M., & Faust, D. (2006). Practicing psychologists' knowledge of general psychotherapy research findings: Implications for science-practice relations. *Professional Psychology: Research and Practice, 37*(6), 708–716.

Chapman, L. J., & Chapman, J. P. (1967). Genesis of popular but erroneous psychodiagnostic observations. *Journal of Abnormal Psychology, 72*(3), 193–204.

Chapman, L. J., & Chapman, J. P. (1969). Illusory correlation as an obstacle to the use of valid psychodiagnostic signs. *Journal of Abnormal Psychology, 74*(3), 271–280.

Cook, N. E., Karr, J. E., Brooks, B. L., Garcia-Barrera, M. A., Holdnack, J. A., & Iverson, G. L. (2019). Multivariate base rates for the assessment of executive functioning among children and adolescents. *Child Neuropsychology, 25*(6), 836–858.

Dana, J., Dawes, R. M., & Peterson, N. (2013). Belief in the unstructured interview: The persistence of an illusion. *Judgment and Decision Making, 8*(5), 512–520.

Dawes, R. M. (1971). A case study of graduate admissions: Application of three principles of human decision making. *American Psychologist, 26*(2), 180–188.

Dawes, R. M. (1989). Experience and validity of clinical judgment: The illusory correlation. *Behavioral Sciences & the Law, 7*(4), 457–467.

Dawes, R. M., & Meehl, P. E. (1966). Mixed group validation: A method for determining the validity of diagnostic signs without using criterion groups. *Psychological Bulletin, 66*(2), 63–67.

Dawes, R. M., Faust, D., & Meehl, P. E. (1989). Clinical versus actuarial judgment. *Science, 243*(4899), 1668–1674.

Desmarais, S. L., Nicholls, T. L., Read, J. D., & Brink, J. (2010). Confidence and accuracy in assessments of short-term risks presented by forensic psychiatric patients. *Journal of Forensic Psychiatry and Psychology, 21*(1), 1–22.

Dietvorst, B. J., Simmons, J. P., & Massey, C. (2016). Overcoming algorithm aversion: People will use imperfect algorithms if they can (even slightly) modify them. *Management Science, 64*(3), 1155–1170.

Exner, J. E., Jr. (1974). *The Rorschach: A comprehensive system* (Vol. 1). Wiley.

Faust, D., & Ahern, D. C. (2012). Clinical judgment and prediction. In D. Faust (Ed.), *Coping with psychiatric and psychological testimony* (6th ed., pp. 147–208). Oxford University Press.

Faust, D., & Faust, K. A. (2012). Experts' experience and diagnostic and predictive accuracy. In D. Faust (Ed.), *Coping with psychiatric and psychological testimony* (6th ed., pp. 131–146). Oxford University Press.

Faust, D., Guilmette, T. J., Hart, K., Arkes, H. R., Fishburne, F. J., & Davey, L. (1988). Neuropsychologists' training, experience, and judgment accuracy. *Archives of Clinical Neuropsychology, 3*(2), 145–163.

Faust, D., Gaudet, C. E., Ahern, D. C., & Bridges, A. J. (2021). Assessment of malingering and falsification: Continuing to push the boundaries of knowledge in research and clinical practice. In A. M. Horton & C. R. Reynolds (Eds.), *Detection of malingering during head injury litigation* (3rd ed., pp. 1–156). Springer.

Faust, D., Arkes, H. R., & Gaudet, C. (2022, in press). Doing better: Applying decision research to improve psychological assessment, prediction, and clinical outcomes. Oxford University Press.
Fischhoff, B., & Broomell, S. B. (2020). Judgment and decision making. *Annual Review of Psychology, 71*, 331–355.
Furman, A. L. (2005). *Clinicians' knowledge and use of decision-making research.* (Unpublished master's thesis). University of Rhode Island.
Ganguly, A. R., & Hammersley, J. S. (2009). Covariation assessments with costly information collection in audit planning: An experimental study. *Auditing: A Journal of Practice & Theory, 28*(1), 1–27.
Garb, H. N., Lilienfeld, S. O., & Fowler, K. A. (2012). Psychological assessment and clinical judgment. In J. E. Maddux & B. A. Winstead (Eds.), *Psychopathology: Foundations for a contemporary understanding* (pp. 121–144). Routledge/Taylor & Francis Group.
Goldberg, L. R. (1959). The effectiveness of clinicians' judgments: The diagnosis of organic brain damage from the Bender-Gestalt Test. *Journal of Consulting Psychology, 23*(1), 25–33.
Goldberg, L. R. (1970). Man versus model of man: A rationale, plus some evidence, for a method of improving on clinical inferences. *Psychological Bulletin, 73*(6), 422–432.
Grove, W. M., Zald, D. H., Lebow, B. S., Snitz, B. E., & Nelson, C. (2000). Clinical versus mechanical prediction: A meta-analysis. *Psychological Assessment, 12*(1), 19–30.
Guay, J. P., & Parent, G. (2018). Broken legs, clinical overrides, and recidivism risk: An analysis of decisions to adjust risk levels with the LS/CMI. *Criminal Justice and Behavior, 45*(1), 82–100.
Hastie, R., Schkade, D. A., & Payne, J. W. (1999). Juror judgments in civil cases: Hindsight effects on judgments of liability for punitive damages. *Law and Human Behavior, 23*(5), 597–614.
Herman, S. (2005). Improving decision making in forensic child sexual abuse evaluations. *Law and Human Behavior, 29*(1), 87–120.
Hogarth, R. M., Lejarraga, T., & Soyer, E. (2015). The two settings of kind and wicked learning environments. *Current Directions in Psychological Science, 24*(5), 379–385.
Jewsbury, P. A., & Bowden, S. C. (2014). A description of mixed group validation. *Assessment, 21*(2), 170–180.
Kahneman, D., & Klein, G. (2009). Conditions for intuitive expertise: A failure to disagree. *American Psychologist, 64*(6), 515–526.
Kazdin, A. E. (2008). Evidence-based treatment and practice: New opportunities to bridge clinical research and practice, enhance the knowledge base, and improve patient care. *American Psychologist, 63*(3), 146–159.
Kranzler, J. H., Maki, K. E., Benson, N. F., Eckert, T. L., Floyd, R. G., & Fefer, S. A. (2020). How do school psychologists interpret intelligence tests for the identification of specific learning disabilities? *Contemporary School Psychology, 24*(4), 445–456.
Krauss, D. A., Lieberman, J. D., & Olson, J. (2004). The effects of rational and experiential information processing of expert testimony in death penalty cases. *Behavioral Sciences & the Law, 22*(6), 801–822.
Kurtz, R. M., & Garfield, S. L. (1978). Illusory correlation: A further exploration of Chapman's paradigm. *Journal of Consulting and Clinical Psychology, 46*(5), 1009–1015.
LeBourgeois, H. I., Pinals, D. A., Williams, V., & Appelbaum, P. S. (2007). Hindsight bias among psychiatrists. *The Journal of the American Academy of Psychiatry and the Law, 35*(1), 67–73.
Lezak, M. D. (1983). *Neuropsychological assessment* (2nd ed.). Oxford University Press.
Lezak, M. D., Howieson, D. B., Bigler, E. D., & Tranel, D. (2012). *Neuropsychological assessment* (5th ed.). Oxford University Press.
Lichtenberg, J. W. (2009). Effects of experience on judgment accuracy. *The Counseling Psychologist, 37*(3), 410–415.
Lilienfeld, S. O., Ritschel, L. A., Lynn, S. J., Cautin, R. L., & Latzman, R. D. (2013). Why many psychologists are resistant to evidence-based practice: Root causes and constructive remedies. *Clinical Psychology Review, 33*(7), 883–900.
Lilienfeld, S. O., Mckay, D., & Hollon, S. D. (2018). Why randomised controlled trials of psychological treatments are still essential. *The Lancet Psychiatry, 5*(7), 536–538.

Lueger, R. J., & Petzel, T. P. (1979). Illusory correlation in clinical judgment: Effects of amount of information to be processed. *Journal of Consulting and Clinical Psychology, 47*(6), 1120–1121.
Makridakis, S., Hogarth, R. M., & Gaba, A. (2009). Forecasting and uncertainty in the economic and business world. *International Journal of Forecasting, 25*(4), 794–812.
Meehl, P. E. (1954). *Clinical versus statistical prediction: A theoretical analysis and a review of the evidence*. University of Minnesota Press.
Meehl, P. E. (1986). Causes and effects of my disturbing little book. *Journal of Personality Assessment, 50*(3), 370–375.
Meehl, P. E. (1996). *Clinical versus statistical prediction: A theoretical analysis and a review of the evidence* (Revised ed.). Jason Aronson.
Meyers, J. F. (2015). *Development and psychometric evaluation of a clinical beliefs questionnaire for licensed psychologists*. [Unpublished doctoral dissertation]. University of Rhode Island.
Miller, D. J., Spengler, E. S., & Spengler, P. M. (2015). A meta-analysis of confidence and judgment accuracy in clinical decision making. *Journal of Counseling Psychology, 62*(4), 553–567.
Mitrushina, M., Boone, K. B., Razani, J., & D'Elia, L. F. (2005). *Handbook of normative data for neuropsychological assessment* (2nd ed.). Oxford University Press.
Morrow-Bradley, C., & Elliot, R. (1986). Utilization of psychotherapy research by practicing psychotherapists. *American Psychologist, 41*(2), 188–197.
Nadler, J. D., Mittenberg, W., DePiano, F. A., & Schneider, B. A. (1994). Effects of patient age on neuropsychological test interpretation. *Professional Psychology: Research and Practice, 25*(3), 288–295.
Nathan, P. E. (2000). The Boulder model: A dream deferred—or lost? *American Psychologist, 55*(2), 250–252.
Nickerson, R. S. (1998). Confirmation bias: A ubiquitous phenomenon in many guises. *Review of General Psychology, 2*(2), 175–220.
Nickerson, R. S. (2004). *Cognition and chance: The psychology of probabilistic reasoning*. Lawrence Erlbaum Associates.
Oskamp, S. (1965). Overconfidence in case-study judgments. *Journal of Consulting Psychology, 29*(3), 261–265.
Reichenbach, H. (1938). *Experience and prediction: An analysis of the foundations and the structure of knowledge*. The University of Chicago Press.
Rock, D. L. (1994). Clinical judgment survey of mental-health professionals: An assessment of opinions, ratings, and knowledge. *Journal of Clinical Psychology, 50*(6), 941–950.
Ruscio, J. (2003). Comparing Bayes's theorem to frequency-based approaches to teaching Bayesian reasoning. Teaching of Psychology, 30(4), 325–328.
Sawyer, J. (1966). Measurement and prediction, clinical and statistical. *Psychological Bulletin, 66*(3), 178–200.
Schmidt, F., Sinclair, S. M., & Thomasdóttir, S. (2016). Predictive validity of the youth level of service/case management inventory with youth who have committed sexual and non-sexual offenses: The utility of professional override. *Criminal Justice and Behavior, 43*(3), 413–430.
Schretlen, D. J., Testa, S. M., Winicki, J. M., Pearlson, G. D., & Gordon, B. (2008). Frequency and bases of abnormal performance by healthy adults on neuropsychological testing. *Journal of the International Neuropsychological Society, 14*(3), 436–445.
Smedslund, J. (1963). The concept of correlation in adults. *Scandinavian Journal of Psychology, 4*(1), 165–173.
Spengler, P. M., & Pilipis, L. A. (2015). A comprehensive meta-reanalysis of the robustness of the experience-accuracy effect in clinical judgment. *Journal of Counseling Psychology, 62*(3), 360–378.
Spengler, P. M., White, M. J., AEgisdóttir, S., Maugherman, A. S., Anderson, L. A., Cook, R. S., et al. (2009). The meta-analysis of clinical judgment project: Effects of experience on judgment accuracy. *The Counseling Psychologist, 37*(3), 350–399.
Stewart, R. E., & Chambless, D. L. (2007). Does psychotherapy research inform treatment decisions in private practice? *Journal of Clinical Psychology, 63*(3), 267–281.

Storey, J. E., Watt, K. A., Jackson, K. J., & Hart, S. D. (2012). Utilization and implications of the Static-99 in practice. *Sexual Abuse, 24*(3), 289–302.

Stricker, G. (1992). The relationship of research to clinical practice. *American Psychologist, 47*(4), 543–549.

Volmer, S., Spada, H., Caspar, F., & Burri, S. (2013). Expertise in clinical psychology. The effects of university training and practical experience on expertise in clinical psychology. *Frontiers in Psychology, March, 2013*(4), Article 141.

Voormolen, D. C., Cnossen, M. C., Polinder, S., Gravesteijn, B. Y., Steinbuechel, N. V., Real, R. G., & Haagsma, J. A. (2019). Prevalence of post-concussion-like symptoms in the general population in Italy, the Netherlands, and the United Kingdom. *Brain Injury, 33*(8), 1078–1086.

Vrieze, S. I., & Grove, W. M. (2009). Survey on the use of clinical and mechanical prediction methods in clinical psychology. *Professional Psychology: Research and Practice, 40*(5), 525–531.

Wade, T. C., & Baker, T. B. (1977). Opinions and use of psychological tests: A survey of clinical psychologists. *American Psychologist, 32*(10), 874–882.

Walfish, S., McAlister, B., O'Donnell, P., & Lambert, M. J. (2012). An investigation of self-assessment bias in mental health providers. *Psychological Reports, 110*(2), 639–644.

Watkins, E. C., Campbell, V. L., Nieberding, R., & Hallmark, R. (1995). Contemporary practice of psychological assessment by clinical psychologists. *Professional Psychology: Research and Practice, 26*(1), 54–60.

Wedding, D. (1983). Clinical and statistical prediction in neuropsychology. *Clinical Neuropsychology, 5*(2), 49–55.

Witteman, C. L. M. (2018). Concluding commentary: Clinical decision making. *Clinical Psychological Science, 6*(2), 266–270.

Wormith, J. S., Hogg, S., & Guzzo, L. (2012). The predictive validity of a general risk/needs assessment inventory on sexual offender recidivism and an exploration of the professional override. *Criminal Justice and Behavior, 39*(12), 1511–1538.

Intellectual Humility: Definitions, Questions, and Scott O. Lilienfeld as a Case Example

Shauna M. Bowes, Adele Strother, Rachel J. Ammirati, and Robert D. Latzman

> *Given that an awareness of one's biases is a key barometer of wisdom and perhaps a protective factor against ideological extremism, few scientific endeavors would appear to be more pressing for the forthcoming generation of psychologists.* (Lilienfeld & Bowes, 2018)

Human beings are notoriously unaware of the pervasiveness of their own cognitive biases. Generally referred to as bias blind spot, most individuals are quick to identify biased cognitive processes in others, yet they remain dubious of manifesting these same biases themselves (e.g., Pronin et al., 2002). In recent decades, there has been growing interest in the ubiquity of cognitive biases and our impoverished ability to recognize our own biases. Numerous studies illustrate the broad-ranging deleterious consequences of cognitive biases for decision-making, including inaccurate psychiatric diagnoses (e.g., Mendel et al., 2011) and endorsement of ineffective bias management strategies in the legal domain (e.g., MacLean et al., 2019), to name a few. This neglect to evaluate and/or reflect upon our biases contributes to unjustified belief certainty and belief polarization (e.g., Hall & Raimi, 2018; Lilienfeld et al., 2009). Given the potentially far-reaching and dangerous implications of unchecked cognitive bias in society, it is essential to consider psychological correlates of cognitive bias and bias blind spot that may protect against, or confer risk for, committing cognitive errors in decision-making contexts.

One potential remedy for the problem of bias blind spot is intellectual humility (IH). IH broadly refers to the tendency to reflect upon the veracity of one's opinions and update one's views in accordance with compelling evidence (e.g., Leary et al., 2017). Herein, we describe conceptualizations of IH and review its emerging

S. M. Bowes (✉) · A. Strother
Department of Psychology, Emory University, Atlanta, GA, USA

R. J. Ammirati
Emory University School of Medicine, Druid Hills, GA, USA

R. D. Latzman
Georgia State University, Atlanta, GA, USA

C. L. Cobb et al. (eds.), *Toward a Science of Clinical Psychology*,
https://doi.org/10.1007/978-3-031-14332-8_6

nomological network in the psychological domain. Moreover, we discuss open questions surrounding work on IH, and its potential applications to psychological science, clinical practice, and education. Throughout this chapter, we delve into why IH is an important, albeit still nascent, construct in psychology and emphasize its potential value for improving critical thinking. We conclude our chapter with an exemplar of IH, namely Dr. Scott O. Lilienfeld. Lilienfeld recognized the critical need to understand cognitive biases and their implications, and that is one major reason why he dedicated his career to promoting scientific psychology (Lilienfeld, 2010) and the study of individual differences (i.e., stable, enduring characteristics that meaningfully differ across people) writ large. Accordingly, in this chapter, we explain why Lilienfeld considered the study of IH crucial, particularly as it pertains to cognitive bias proneness and its impact on the future of psychological science.

Conceptualizing Intellectual Humility

Intellectual humility (IH) has long been of interest in philosophy, as it is theorized to be a character virtue that ultimately promotes rational thinking (see Whitcomb et al., 2017, for a review).[1] In the philosophical domain, IH has been defined in various ways. For instance, some maintain that IH is a multifaceted construct comprising the tendency to accurately self-assess one's knowledge, be mindful of one's ego, and remain open to new information (e.g., Tangney, 2000). Others emphasize that IH entails holding accurate, "proper" beliefs based on a sound evaluation of the available evidence (e.g., Church & Samuelson, 2017; Hazlett, 2012). Dovetailing with these accounts of IH, other accounts advance the perspective that IH reflects a proper attentiveness to the limitations of one's views and a willingness to acknowledge such limitations (Whitcomb et al., 2017). Still others define IH as the inverse of epistemic vices (i.e., thinking styles that impede or prevent forming accurate beliefs and pursuing truth), including but not limited to vanity, arrogance, and self-complacency (e.g., Roberts & Wood, 2018).

In addition to conceptualizing IH as a standalone construct, some contend that IH is a specific instantiation of general humility in the context of one's values, attitudes, and beliefs (e.g., Van Tongeren et al., 2019). General humility reflects a decreased tendency to be arrogant and manipulative and an increased tendency to view oneself in a balanced, and hence accurate, light (Lee & Ashton, 2018; McElroy et al., 2019). One of the most commonly used indices of general humility is the honesty-humility subscale from *HEXACO Personality Inventory-Revised* (HEXACO

[1] IH is sometimes referred to as epistemic humility. Although these two terms can be used interchangeably to some extent, they are not isomorphic. Epistemic humility is an intellectual virtue that (a) fosters rational beliefs, (b) is rooted in scientific methods and attitudes, and (c) is founded upon the notion that most bodies of knowledge are characterized by uncertainty and human bias (see Lilienfeld et al., 2017). Hence, epistemic humility is typically more closely tied to philosophies of science than IH.

PI-R; Lee & Ashton, 2018), which assesses four personality facets: modesty, sincerity, greed-avoidance, and fairness. Although IH certainly aligns with honesty-humility, lending credence to hypotheses that IH is a manifestation of general humility, evidence suggests that IH measures (described below) account for significant variance in certain outcomes, such as open-mindedness (Davis et al., 2016), after controlling for honesty-humility. Such results indicate that IH predicts unique variance in constructs of interest and is certainly not isomorphic to general humility.

Definitional debates have carried forward into psychological research on IH. For example, there are 20 distinct measures drawing on different definitions of humility (McElroy-Heltzel et al., 2019). There has been an explosion of self-report measures of IH, with at least four different measures identified in a recent review (McElroy-Heltzel et al., 2019). For a description of several commonly used IH measures, refer to Table 1. These different measures of IH have unique theoretical underpinnings and illustrate the variety of definitions used in the literature.

Although there are several IH measures rooted in different definitions, there is some consensus on the key features of IH within the psychological domain. Specifically, all self-report measures of IH include metacognitive characteristics, such as the tendency to self-reflect and the propensity to be open-minded (e.g., Krumrei-Mancuso & Rouse, 2016). Nevertheless, there is disagreement in the literature surrounding the extent to which IH is also characterized by relational or interpersonal features. For instance, some scholars contend that IH is primarily metacognitive, as it "fundamentally reflects people's private assessments of their beliefs" (Leary et al., 2017, p. 793). According to these perspectives, IH may bear downstream implications for interpersonal characteristics, such as being more respectful or tolerant, but these interpersonal characteristics are not integral to IH. As such, measures assessing metacognitive definitions, such as the *General Intellectual Humility Scale* (Leary et al., 2017), almost exclusively measure tendencies to be open-minded and reflect on one's intellectual limitations.

In contrast, other scholars contend that IH comprises both metacognitive and relational features, the latter of which includes the tendency to be respectful toward others, regulate emotions in the face of cognitive dissonance, maintain a low concern for personal intellectual status, recognize others for their intellectual strengths, and admit to intellectual limitations (Alfano et al., 2018; Krumrei-Mancuso & Rouse, 2016; McElroy-Heltzel et al., 2014; Porter & Schumann, 2018). Accordingly, IH is "fundamentally relational in nature" (McElroy-Heltzel et al., 2014, p. 20). Thus, relational features may not encompass the entirety of IH, but they are key to it. Interpersonally oriented conceptualizations of IH align with the social-oil hypothesis of humility, which maintains that humility buffers against relational tension in situations of conflict (Van Tongeren et al., 2019).

Not surprisingly, measures including both intrapersonal and interpersonal features of IH tend to be multidimensional. One measure (McElroy et al., 2014) yields two dimensions, Intellectual Openness ("I am open to competing ideas") and Intellectual Arrogance ("I make fun of people with different viewpoints"). A separate measure, the *Limitations-Owning Intellectual Humility Scale* (Haggard et al., 2018), yields the following three dimensions: Appropriate Discomfort with

Table 1 Overview of intellectual humility measures

	Definition	Dimensions	Example items
McElroy-Heltzel et al. (2014)	"Having (a) insight about the limits of one's knowledge, marked by openness to new ideas; and (b) regulating arrogance, marked by the ability to present one's ideas in a non-offensive manner and receive contrary ideas without taking offense"	Intellectual openness; intellectual arrogance (reversed)	"I often become angry when my ideas are not implemented" (reversed); "I am open to competing ideas"
Krumrei-Mancuso & Rouse (2016)	"A nonthreatening awareness of one's intellectual fallibility"	Independence of intellect and ego; openness to revising one's viewpoint; respect for other's viewpoints; lack of intellectual overconfidence	"I am willing to change my position on an important issue in the face of good reasons"; "I can respect others, even if I disagree with them in important ways"
Hoyle et al. (2016)	"The recognition that a particular personal view may be fallible, accompanied by an appropriate attentiveness to limitations in the evidentiary basis of that view and to one's own limitations in obtaining and evaluating information relevant to it."	–	"My views about X are just as likely to be wrong as other views"; "my sources for information about X might not be the best"
Leary et al. (2017)	"Recognizing that a particular personal belief may be fallible, accompanied by an appropriate attentiveness to limitations in the evidentiary basis of that belief and to one's own limitations in obtaining and evaluating relevant information"	–	"I question my own opinions, positions, and viewpoints because they could be wrong"; "I reconsider my opinions when presented with new evidence"
Porter & Schumann (2018)	"Being aware of one's intellectual fallibility… [and] a willingness to appreciate others' intellectual strengths"	–	"I am willing to admit it if I don't know something"; "I like to compliment others on their intellectual strengths"
Haggard et al. (2018)	"A proper recognition of the impact of intellectual limitations and a motivation to overcome them"	Love of learning; appropriate discomfort with limitations; limitations-owning	"When I don't understand something, I try hard to figure it out"; "I am quick to acknowledge my intellectual limitations"

(continued)

Table 1 (continued)

	Definition	Dimensions	Example items
Alfano et al. (2018)	A constellation of "cognitive, affective, behavioral, and motivational" characteristics pertaining to self-reflection and interpersonal interactions"	Open-mindedness, intellectual modesty; engagement, corrigibility	"I feel no shame learning from someone who knows more than me"; "I appreciate being corrected when I make a mistake"
Krumrei-Mancuso et al. (2020)	An "awareness of the limits of one's knowledge… [in addition to] confidence in the knowledge one possesses"	Know-it-all (reversed); intellectual openness	"My intellectual ideas are usually superior to others' ideas" (reversed); "I can learn from other people"

Note. This table does not reflect an exhaustive review of the literature

Limitations ("I tend to get defensive about my intellectual limitations and weaknesses" [reversed]), Limitations-Owning ("I feel comfortable admitting my intellectual limitations"), and Love of Learning ("I care about truth"). Other measures yield four dimensions, although these four dimensions vary across measures. For the self-report inventory created by Alfano et al. (2018), the four dimensions are Open-mindedness ("I feel no shame learning from someone who knows more than me"), Intellectual Modesty ("Being smarter than other people is not especially important to me"), Corrigibility ("I appreciate being corrected when I make a mistake"), and Engagement ("I enjoy reading about the ideas of different cultures"). For the *Comprehensive Intellectual Humility Scale* (Krumrei-Mancuso & Rouse, 2016), the four dimensions are Independence of Intellect and Ego ("I feel small when others disagree with me on topics that are close to my heart" [reversed]), Openness to Revising One's Viewpoint ("I am willing to change my position on an important issue for good reasons"), Respect for Others' Viewpoints ("I can have great respect for someone, even when we don't see eye-to-eye on important topics"), and Lack of Intellectual Overconfidence ("My ideas are usually better than other people's ideas" [reversed]).

Hence, even within perspectives on IH in psychology, there is still considerable heterogeneity regarding which relational and/or metacognitive characteristics are central to IH. For instance, as just described, some measures contain a dimension dedicated to learning (e.g., Haggard et al., 2018) whereas others do not assess stances toward learning (e.g., McElroy et al., 2014). Along these lines, some measures assess emotional reactions to disagreement (e.g., Krumrei-Mancuso & Rouse, 2016), whereas others assess metacognitive stances toward disagreement (e.g., Haggard et al., 2018). There is not only debate surrounding the extent to which IH is relational but also surrounding the relational building blocks themselves.

Most existing measures of IH are domain-general and decontextualized, as IH appears to be dispositional and thus is likely to be relatively consistent across different situations (Krumrei-Mancuso & Rouse, 2016). Nevertheless, in line with longstanding person-situation debates in personality psychology (see Epstein & O'Brien, 1985), IH may vary, and perhaps even vary considerably, across situations or belief domains (e.g., religion, politics, science). Put differently, even those who score high on measures of domain-general IH may hold views they are unwilling to revise or update, and consequently score low on certain domain-specific measures of IH (Hoyle et al., 2016). For instance, politics-specific IH appears to be a stronger negative correlate of political outcomes, such as affective polarization (i.e., tendencies to not only disagree with but also dislike political outgroup members; Bowes et al., 2020a, b, c) and political myside bias (i.e., tendencies to systematically favor one's political party over the other when interacting with political information; Bowes et al., 2021), than domain-general IH. Such results are consistent with broader findings in personality psychology that contextualized, domain-specific traits (e.g., openness to experience in the workplace) are more robust predictors of certain outcomes (e.g., work performance) than decontextualized, domain-general personality traits (e.g., Swift & Peterson, 2019). Still, domain-general IH and measures of specific IH tend to manifest medium to large positive intercorrelations (r ranges from to 0.24 to 0.63; Bowes et al., 2020a, b, c, 2021; Hoyle et al., 2016).

In aggregate, there is no universally accepted definition of IH. However, there is considerable consensus that IH comprises, to some degree, metacognitive characteristics that contribute to open-mindedness, appropriate and balanced self-reflections, and a willingness to accept that one's views may be incorrect. There is still disagreement over whether IH also comprises interpersonal characteristics, such as admiring others' intellectual strengths and respecting views that differ from one's own views. Even though there is disagreement regarding the interpersonal piece of the proverbial puzzle, most, if not all, scholars agree that IH bears implications for interpersonal outcomes (e.g., respectfulness, tolerance of difference, willingness to forgive in a disagreement). Moreover, IH can be assessed as a domain-general trait (i.e., how intellectually humble are you in general?) and as a domain-specific trait (i.e., how intellectually humble are you about your political views?), which affords more nuanced and richer examinations of IH.

Intellectual Humility's Preliminary Nomological Network

Parallel to increasing interest in defining and measuring intellectual humility (IH), scholars also have grown increasingly interested in IH's nomological network (i.e., understanding IH's relation with key psychological constructs to generate a conceptual, integrative framework). Based on existing definitions of IH, it should be positively related to constructs akin to epistemic virtues, including orientation to accuracy and truth, thoughtfulness, and open-mindedness. In contrast, IH should be negatively related to constructs akin to epistemic vices, including arrogance, self-centeredness, and irrationality. Given these possibilities, scholars have examined the relations among measures of IH and a range of potentially relevant outcomes, including personality traits, cognitive styles, decision-making abilities, and belief polarization.

Regarding personality traits, domain-general IH tends to exhibit moderate positive associations with honesty-humility, agreeableness, openness, and conscientiousness (e.g., Alfano et al., 2018; Davis et al., 2016; Krumrei-Mancuso & Rouse, 2016; Porter & Schumann, 2018). Research on domain-general IH and extraversion and neuroticism is more mixed in comparison. Some studies report that extraversion is moderately positively associated with IH (Alfano et al., 2018; Meagher et al., 2015), whereas others report that it is negligibly associated (Porter & Schumann, 2018) and perhaps even negatively related (Leary et al., 2017). Two studies suggest that emotional stability, often conceptualized as reversed neuroticism, positively predicts domain-general IH (Porter & Schumann, 2018; Meagher et al., 2015), whereas one study indicated that emotional stability was negligibly associated with IH (Leary et al., 2017). Although there is no apparent reason as to why these results vary across studies, it could be that they are mixed as a function of the IH measure used.

In addition to general personality traits, scholars have found that the relation between domain-general IH and total scores on narcissism self-report inventories is generally negative (e.g., Bak & Kutnik, 2021). In contrast, domain-general IH is positively related to self-esteem (e.g., Bak & Kutnik, 2021), indicating that it is associated with a healthy sense of self and less pathological pride. Preliminary research also suggests that domain-general IH is negatively related to total scores on depression and anxiety self-report inventories (Hill et al., 2021). Taken together, IH may entail or relate to a constellation of adaptive dispositional features, including high honesty-humility, high agreeableness, high conscientiousness, high openness to experience, and low neuroticism. IH also seems to be related to positive self-regard that is not overly inflated (i.e., low narcissism), or self-regard that is overly negative (i.e., high levels of depression and anxiety). Painting with a broad brush, IH appears, in many ways, to reflect "healthy" personality.

Similarly, researchers have also examined the relations between IH and a variety of cognitive styles. Consistent with definitions of IH that it comprises balanced self-reflection, domain-general IH tends to be positively related to need for cognition, objectivism, intellectual curiosity, open-minded thinking, preferences for balanced (as opposed to one-sided) arguments (in the religious domain), and a willingness to question one's existential beliefs (e.g., Davis et al., 2016; Krumrei-Mancuso et al., 2020; Leary et al., 2017). Moreover, it manifests moderate-to-large positive relations with both cognitive and affective empathy as well as valuing benevolence and universalism (e.g., Krumrei-Mancuso, 2017). Perhaps unsurprisingly, domain-general IH tends to be negatively related to tendencies to overclaim one's knowledge, dogmatism, intolerance of ambiguity, self-righteousness, and intellectual arrogance (e.g., Deffler et al., 2016; Leary et al., 2017; Meagher et al., 2021). Collectively, this burgeoning corpus of research indicates that IH is related to desiring complexity and accuracy in one's thinking, striving to be objective and open-minded, valuing others' perspectives, and possessing an ability to perspective-take. These results additionally indicate that IH reflects low needs for closure, low unjustified belief certainty, and low psychological entitlement.

IH is positively related not only to valuing accuracy but also to objective accuracy in decision-making paradigms. Domain-general IH manifests small-to-medium positive correlations with intelligence, cognitive flexibility, cognitive reflection, metamemory, science literacy, and the ability to parse strong from weak evidence (e.g., Bowes et al., 2021; Deffler et al., 2016; Haggard et al., 2018; Leary et al., 2017). In addition, researchers (Porter et al., 2020) found that even in the face of potential failure (i.e., provided as sham feedback), domain-general IH was positively related to wanting to learn more about a task and choosing to learn more about the task. Domain-general IH is also positively related to engaging in more investigative behaviors when presented with fake news headlines but not when presented with real news headlines, indicating an increased discrimination between fake and real information (Koetke et al., 2021).

Research thus far has made important inroads for understanding IH. Collectively, IH appears to be related to adaptive personality features, cognitive styles pertaining to flexibility and open-mindedness, increased decision-making accuracy, and the ability to discern fake news from real news. In response to these findings, Dr. Scott O. Lilienfeld and other research teams grew interested in leveraging research on the nomological network of IH to conduct "risky tests" (i.e., studies that bear on theory such that results may put the theory at risk; see Zachar, 2015) that continue to advance research on IH. He and others sought to evaluate potentially core aspects of IH and determine whether theories of IH hold when subjected to empirical scrutiny. For instance, most definitions of IH and research are based on the premise that it comprises or gives rise to enhanced accuracy motives and in turn to holding accurate beliefs. According to this view, IH should be related to holding fewer misinformed beliefs and more informed beliefs.

One study co-authored by Lilienfeld examined the relations between IH and conspiratorial ideation (Bowes et al., 2020b). Domain-general IH was found to be correlated negatively with conspiratorial ideation, providing preliminary evidence that IH is related to holding fewer misinformed beliefs. Other studies, including one co-authored by Lilienfeld, also indicate that (a) both politics-specific IH and domain-general IH are related to holding more accurate beliefs, as they are positively correlated with support for anthropogenic global warming, and (b) domain-general IH is also related to favorable vaccine attitudes and intentions to be vaccinated (Bowes et al., 2021; Huynh & Senger, 2021; Senger & Huynh, 2020).

Consistent with the notion of "risky tests," Lilienfeld and others also examined the relations between IH and belief polarization. Whether conceptualizing IH from a metacognitive or relational perspective, IH should be related to less belief polarization. If IH is not found to be related to less belief polarization, then perhaps it possesses less practical utility than originally presumed and/or it does not help people remain open-minded about cherished beliefs. Both possibilities would require scholars to revisit definitions of IH and measurement strategies.

Most studies of IH have focused squarely on two belief domains: religion and politics, which mirrors contemporary issues pervading American and international societies. Deadly wars are repeatedly fought in the name of religious disputes, and, at a less lethal level, certain religious groups are strongly disparaged and ostracized within certain communities (e.g., atheists in America; see Gervais, 2013). Moreover, the tendency to not only disagree with but dislike political opponents (i.e., affective polarization; Iyengar et al., 2019) has steadily increased over the last few decades. Increases in affective polarization impede much-needed bipartisanship in American politics and foster potentially dangerous attitudes toward political outgroup members (e.g., lethal partisanship; Kalmoe & Mason, 2019).

Research suggests that IH indeed appears to be a fruitful path for lessening both religious and political polarization. For example, in one study, religion-specific IH was positively related to religious tolerance in a sample of Christian pastors, even after controlling for known covariates such as political ideology and religious commitment (Hook et al., 2017). Additionally, religion-specific IH is positively related to forgiveness of a potential religious offense (Hook et al., 2015; Zhang et al., 2018) and the perceived credibility of opposing religious viewpoints (Rodriguez et al., 2017). When evaluating religious information, intellectually humble individuals (a) report less certainty that their religious views are correct and superior to other religious views and (b) manifest less religious bias when evaluating the authors of opposing religious views (Leary et al., 2017).

Results from studies examining the relations between political polarization and IH mirror those from studies examining religious polarization. For instance, in two studies co-authored by Lilienfeld and in other recent studies, both domain-general and politics-specific IH were related to less affective polarization and less susceptibility to same-party cues when evaluating political information (Bowes et al., 2020a, b, c, 2021; Krumrei-Mancuso & Newman, 2020; Leary et al., 2017). Domain-general and politics-specific IH are also positively related to more open-mindedness when encountering politically incongruent information, an increased willingness to seek out politically disconfirmatory information, and an increased willingness to forgive potential political transgressions (Bowes et al., 2021; Hodge et al., 2020; Porter & Schumann, 2018; Stanley et al., 2020). Hence, it appears that IH may temper religious and political extremity, increase openness to diversity, and lessen polarization and bias.

Implications of Intellectual Humility for Psychological Science, Practice, and Education

Just as intellectual humility (IH) bears implications for belief polarization and decision-making, it is relevant to psychological science, practice, and education. In fact, we can think of IH as the fuel required to drive scientific inquiry. Science is a critical safeguard against human error and confirmation bias, but it must be properly used and applied (e.g., O'Donohue et al., 2012). IH leads us to re-evaluate our favored theories, conduct disconfirmatory rather than confirmatory analyses, remain open-minded to new evidence, and generate conclusions based on good evidence rather than intuition. Indeed, "science, including clinical science, is fundamentally a prescription for our intellectual humility, as it reminds us that we can all be fooled by ourselves and be fooled by others" (Meichenbaum & Lilienfeld, 2018, p. 27). Below, we will describe the relevance of IH to psychological science, specifically focusing on the replication crisis, clinical practice, and psychological education.

The field of psychological science has undergone numerous transformations in recent history. The so-called replication crisis has forced the field to confront the fact that many of the findings from the past several decades do not withstand independent replication efforts (e.g., Nosek et al., 2015). The replication crisis gained attention in the 2010s when researchers began to use the term to describe a troubling phenomenon—when experiments were repeated, rather than reproducing the effects observed in the original work, the results often failed to replicate (in a review by Nosek et al., 2015 only 39% of the original effects were successfully replicated; see also Ioannidis, 2005). These results are alarming for several reasons, perhaps chief among them being that they call into question the very nature of scientific discovery and the integrity of psychology as a discipline. Since the start of the replication crisis, several research teams have compiled evidence that unchecked biases and other questionable research practices (QRPs) have contributed to researchers drawing faulty conclusions (e.g., Shrout & Rodgers, 2018). In essence, the replication crisis arose due to a widespread neglect to interrogate one's results and approaches and effectively use the scientific method to evaluate the reliability of findings. IH provides an impetus to confront and contend with this crisis.

While the replication crisis was and is sobering, Lilienfeld reminded us that "the replication crisis highlights the operation of psychological science at its best, as it reflects our growing humility" (Lilienfeld, 2017, p. 660). The decision to question previously established findings and to act on the challenging evidence uncovered in the process requires objectivity and integrity characteristic of IH. IH helps us take a step back and consider the evidence thoroughly, even if it means revising or abandoning previously "established" theories or questioning past findings absent replication. Without IH, the replication crisis may have continued unchallenged for years to come, damaging the integrity of the field of psychological science and thus harming the people it serves. Moreover, science rests on the presumption that we must continuously examine our techniques to produce accurate and credible evidence. This self-reflection is a necessary and important safeguard against future crises; without a continued exercise of IH, we risk falling victim to the same biases and QRPs indefinitely (see Lilienfeld et al., 2017).

In addition to helping combat the replication crisis, Lilienfeld viewed IH, coupled with a solid knowledge of the philosophy of science and methods, as a safeguard against implementing ineffective and even harmful therapeutic interventions. Currently, a plethora of questionable psychotherapies are promoted as solutions to a range of mental health concerns; nevertheless, many of these therapies remain untested and consequently lack the evidence requisite for justifying their use (e.g., emotional freedom techniques) whereas others have been demonstrated to be harmful (e.g., facilitated communication for autism spectrum disorders) (e.g., see Lack, 2018; Lilienfeld, 2007, 2012). Importantly, cognitive biases, such as confirmation bias, bias blind spot, and overconfidence, may be at the heart of the continued use of untested, ineffective, and otherwise harmful therapies (see Bowes et al., 2020b; Lilienfeld et al., 2014). All too often we overly rely on our gut hunches and intuitions rather than double-checking the facts and data at hand (see Bowes et al., 2020b). Given that IH may mitigate bias in other areas, such as religion and politics, and that it generally promotes accurate thinking, IH may be equally if not more important in the domain of clinical reasoning. IH may provide at least a partial solution to overhyped and unsubstantiated claims, inviting clinicians and researchers alike to take a critical look at the way these therapies are marketed, evaluated, and applied (e.g., Meichenbaum & Lilienfeld, 2018). By systematically checking our biases (e.g., consider-the-opposite, use of checklists and semi-structured interviews; see Bowes et al., 2020b), we can "plant the seeds of healthy self-doubt in practitioners and trainees… to help to nurture in them a sense of humility in treatment selection and delivery" (Meichenbaum & Lilienfeld, 2018, p. 24).

One major avenue for planting these important seeds of self-doubt and fostering IH is graduate-level education in psychological science. Yet survey findings are not promising in this regard, as they collectively suggest that clinicians may not be routinely receiving foundational clinical training in cognitive biases. For example, a recent survey of practicing clinicians in forensic settings revealed that a substantial percentage of those surveyed held erroneous perceptions of effective bias management strategies and claimed to be familiar with at least one nonexistent bias (e.g., Sutter effect; MacLean et al., 2019). Additionally, a survey of American Psychological Association (APA) accredited clinical psychology doctoral programs indicated that less than 15% offered formal coursework on statistical prediction and merely 5% provided formal training on clinical decision-making (Harding, 2007).

One potential path for providing consistent education at the graduate level on cognitive biases and clinical decision-making procedures is to use IH as the bedrock of all coursework (Lilienfeld et al., 2017). A training model that prioritizes IH "makes explicit that the distinguishing feature of the scientist is not conducting research, but holding a scientific attitude. The heart of this attitude, in turn, is the awareness that we are all susceptible to information-processing biases and that scientific methods are the best means of compensation for them" (Lilienfeld et al., 2017, p. 9). Emphasizing IH across all aspects of graduate-level education may help trainees to work toward the epistemic and ethical duty "to know," and more specifically, to know the limits of their knowledge both in research and clinical pursuits. The model for training programs should be centered on the pursuit of scientific methods, deep self-reflection, and a focus on genuinely pursuing truth as opposed to signaling that one values truth for the sake of social acceptance or status.

Scott O. Lilienfeld: A Case Example of Intellectual Humility in Psychological Research

The most one can do or hope for as an instructor is to change people's lives in some small way and maybe make them get to think about their life and their worlds just a little bit differently—Dr. Scott O. Lilienfeld

In this chapter, we have reviewed definitions of intellectual humility (IH), its preliminary nomological network, and its implications for a few key areas in psychological science. We believe that we would be remiss not to conclude with an exemplar of an intellectually humble individual. In other words, what does it look like to be an intellectually humble person, even in fields or spaces where it is especially difficult to self-reflect and admit to one's limitations? In our opinion, Dr. Scott O. Lilienfeld was the embodiment of the intellectually humble scholar. For a selection of his publications focusing on IH or reflecting on his own IH, refer to Table 2.

Throughout his impressive and prolific career, Lilienfeld continuously delineated the importance of IH in psychological science. Even when he did not explicitly use the phrase "intellectual humility," most of his research and scholarship were connected to important aspects of IH. To name a few of the many instances of his emphasis on IH, he advocated for the importance of embracing heterodox ideas that challenge prevailing scientific "truths" (Lilienfeld, 2020b), detailed harmful and ineffective therapies and scientific practices (e.g., Lilienfeld, 2007), emphasized the importance of acknowledging fundamental limitations of human cognition (e.g., Lilienfeld et al., 2009), and pushed for science to be open and available to those outside of the ivory tower through his many contributions to popular press outlets (e.g., *Scientific American*) and popular press books (e.g., *Brainwashed: The seductive appeal of mindless neuroscience*).

When discussing science with a lay audience, it's not uncommon to encounter the criticism that science is inaccessible, inflexible, and often irrelevant to the average citizen. The field of psychology enjoys a unique brand of criticism, with both recent and historical data suggesting that public trust in the discipline is low (e.g.,

Table 2 Ten selected Dr. Scott O. Lilienfeld publications that reflect (a) IH scholarship and/or (b) his own IH

	Summary of publication's relevance to IH
Bowes et al. (2020a, b, c)	An examination of the relations between IH and affective polarization
Bowes et al. (2020b)	An examination of the relations between IH and conspiratorial ideation
Bowes et al. (2021)	An examination of the relations between IH and political myside bias
Costello et al. (2021)	An examination of the relations between left-wing authoritarianism and IH
Lilienfeld et al. (2009)	A discussion of the need for more research on combatting confirmation bias and promoting welfare
Lilienfeld (2010)	A discussion of whether psychology is a science and, if not, how it can become one
Lilienfeld (2016)	A discussion of how the skepticism movement can improve itself and advance its scientific aims
Lilienfeld et al. (2017b)	A discussion of how epistemic humility can be the foundation for clinical psychology programs
Lilienfeld & Bowes (2018)	An overview of IH, focusing on its definitions and future directions
Lilienfeld & Bowes (in press)	A discussion of ten unresolved questions in research on IH

Fearon et al., 2020). Lilienfeld was one of the first to admit that these arguments are not without merit; rather than being dismissive, he insisted that the field be held responsible for its shortcomings. Indeed, he once wrote that "all is not well in the field of psychology" (Lilienfeld, 2010, p. 283). Lilienfeld dedicated significant time and effort to advancing science communication, advancing skepticism, and engaging in critical debates across various scientific domains. As a regular contributor to the *New York Times*, *Psychology Today*, *Skeptical Inquirer*, and *Scientific American*, Lilienfeld worked to distribute knowledge to those in and outside of academia. For instance, Lilienfeld served as an author or co-author on at least 23 *Skeptical Inquirer articles* and 50 *Scientific American* articles. In addition, he published, to our knowledge, at least 45 separate publications that were reviews, commentaries, responses, rejoinders, and/or letters to the editor, with some of these pieces being cited nearly 1000 times (e.g., Lilienfeld, 2013, 2020; Lilienfeld et al., 2016; Lilienfeld & Thames, 2009). These works collectively demonstrate his intellectual engagement with the field and openness to debate, both of which reflect dimensions of IH (e.g., Alfano et al., 2018).

Lilienfeld also directly modeled what it means to be an intellectually humble scholar. For example, he opened one of his academic articles with a list of his own misguided and misinformed beliefs about psychological science, noting that "at the time, it never occurred to me that some of these beliefs were not only poorly supported, but contradictory" (Lilienfeld, 2010, p. 281). In describing these misinformed beliefs and his failure to recognize them as misinformed earlier in his career, he embodied the limitations-owning account of IH (Haggard et al., 2018). Even as an expert in personality psychology and the science behind clinical practice, he still made sure to evaluate his views and acknowledge his limitations to others in his field. On balance, Lilienfeld was a critical and vocal member of the skeptic's movement throughout most of his career. As a member of this movement, Lilienfeld encouraged the field to address its shortcomings and scholars to evaluate their own biases. In a characteristic display of insight and IH, Lilienfeld included himself in this conversation: "I have on occasion detected more than a whiff of arrogance among some of us in the skeptical movement, and I have no doubt fallen prey to this tendency myself from time to time" (Lilienfeld, 2016). In addition to pointing out times when he personally neglected IH, he modeled humility in his scholarship, openly inviting pushback. For example, in a paper he coauthored, the authors noted that "in the spirit of our own humility, we provide this list [of psychotherapy hype warning signs] merely as a first approximation, and we welcome suggestions and constructive criticisms from readers" (Meichenbaum & Lilienfeld, 2018, p. 24).

Moreover, Lilienfeld "practiced what he preached," particularly concerning embracing heterodox ideas in psychological science. Lilienfeld emphasized the threat that ideological uniformity often poses in research science, as it can easily turn into a bulwark that impedes scientific advancement and fosters unchecked biases (Lilienfeld, 2020). Not only did Lilienfeld encourage the promotion and evaluation of heterodox ideas, but he examined heterodox ideas in his own research. He challenged the wide-scale usage of popular, albeit scientifically unsound, assessments (e.g., projective tests; Lilienfeld et al., 2000) and pushed for evidence-based definitions and examinations of social psychological processes (e.g., microaggressions; Lilienfeld, 2017b). He helped to operationalize overlooked and understudied psychological phenomena (e.g., left-wing authoritarianism; Costello et al., 2021). He argued against grantsmanship for the sake of grantsmanship in psychological science (e.g., Lilienfeld, 2017). And he was committed to teaching and disseminating psychological knowledge to broad audiences (e.g., *50 Great Myths of Popular Psychology*).

Lilienfeld strove to advance psychological science with an open mind and respectful voice. His writings and efforts reflect the imperative to question "conventional wisdom" and maintain a stance of being open to findings that falsify our cherished beliefs. The heterodox movement in psychology, he argued, can "help us to better appreciate psychological perspectives that differ sharply from our own, thereby ideally increasing our IH and willingness to tolerate ideological diversity" (Lilienfeld, 2020, p. 2). Along these lines, Lilienfeld's work reflects the difference between IH and diffidence—to be intellectually humble, one does not have to abandon one's views. Instead, one can be intellectually humble and have strong convictions; what makes an individual intellectually humble is a thoughtful, pragmatic willingness to update and revise one's opinions when new evidence comes to light (e.g., Alfano et al., 2018).

Much more can be written about Lilienfeld's work on IH and his commitment to IH in his own scholarship, and this book is a testament to these claims. We believe that Lilienfeld was and will continue to be a model of IH in academia and specifically in psychological science. He embodied the metacognitive and relational characteristics of IH, as he was curious, open to disconfirmation, engaged, respectful, tolerant, and able to separate his ego from his scholarship. He strove to acknowledge his limitations and share them with the field in the service of encouraging debate. He also demonstrated that one can be intellectually humble and still hold strong convictions. As described earlier, IH is not isomorphic with diffidence or apathy. Instead, IH reflects how people *engage* with their beliefs as opposed to how *strongly* they feel about their beliefs (Alfano et al., 2018; Krumrei-Mancuso & Rouse, 2016). In fact, Lilienfeld felt strongly about the importance of IH and debiasing efforts, yet he made his case with thoughtful deliberation and supported it with evidence. We share his sentiments that now, perhaps more than ever, it is crucial to self-reflect as scientists and to promote research on factors that mitigate bias and extremism. In his words,

> To the extent that one crucial element of wisdom is an awareness of one's fallibilities and a sense of humility concerning the limits of one's knowledge, debiasing the general public against confirmation bias and related biases may be an essential step toward a wiser—and perhaps ultimately safer—world. Psychologists would be wise to make this effort a priority. (Lilienfeld et al., 2009, p. 395).

We could not agree more.

References

Alfano, M., Iurino, K., Stey, P., Robinson, B., Christen, M., Yu, F., & Lapsley, D. (2018). Development and validation of a multi-dimensional measure of intellectual humility. *PLoS One, 12*, 1–28.

Bak, W., & Kutnik, J. (2021). Domains of intellectual humility: Self-esteem and narcissism as independent predictors. *Personality and Individual Differences, 177*. Advance online publication.

Bowes, S. M., Blanchard, M. C., Costello, T. H., Abramowitz, A. I., & Lilienfeld, S. O. (2020a). Intellectual humility and between-party animus: Implications for affective polarization in two community samples. *Journal of Research in Personality, 88*. Advanced online publication.

Bowes, S. M., Ammirati, R. J., Costello, T. H., Basterfield, C., & Lilienfeld, S. O. (2020b). Cognitive biases, heuristics, and logical fallacies in clinical practice: A brief field guide for practicing clinicians and supervisors. *Professional Psychology: Research and Practice, 51*, 435–445.

Bowes, S. M., Costello, T. H., Ma, W., & Lilienfeld, S. O. (2020c). Looking under the tinfoil hat: Clarifying the personological and psychopathological correlates of conspiracy beliefs. *Journal of Personality*. Advance online publication.

Bowes, S. M., Costello, T. H., Lee, C., McElroy-Heltzel, S., Davis, D. E., & Lilienfeld, S. O. (2021). *Stepping outside the echo chamber: Is intellectual humility associated with less political myside bias?*. Personality and Social Psychology Bulletin. Advance online publication.

Church, I. M., & Samuelson, P. L. (2017). *Intellectual humility: An introduction to the philosophy and science*. Bloomsbury.

Costello, T. H., Bowes, S. M., Stevens, S. T., Waldman, I. D., & Lilienfeld, S. O. (2021). *Clarifying the structure and nature of left-wing authoritarianism*. Journal of Personality and Social Psychology: Personality Processes and Individual Differences.

Davis, D. E., Rice, K., McElroy, S., DeBlaere, C., Choe, E., Van Tongeren, D. R., & Hook, J. N. (2016). Distinguishing intellectual humility and general humility. *The Journal of Positive Psychology, 11*, 215–224.

Deffler, S. A., Leary, M. R., & Hoyle, R. H. (2016). Knowing what you know: Intellectual humility and judgments of recognition memory. *Personality and Individual Differences, 96*, 255–259.

Epstein, S., & O'Brien, E. J. (1985). The person–situation debate in historical and current perspective. *Psychological Bulletin, 98*, 513–537.

Fearon, P. A., Götz, F. M., & Good, D. (2020). Pivotal moment for trust in science-don't waste it. *Nature, 580*, 456–457.

Gervais, W. M. (2013). In godlessness we distrust: Using social psychology to solve the puzzle of anti-atheist prejudice. *Social and Personality Psychology Compass, 7*, 366–377.

Haggard, M., Rowatt, W. C., Leman, J. C., Meagher, B., Moore, C., Fergus, T., et al. (2018). Finding middle ground between intellectual arrogance and intellectual servility: Development and assessment of the limitations-owning intellectual humility scale. *Personality and Individual Differences, 124*, 184–193.

Hall, M. P., & Raimi, K. T. (2018). Is belief superiority justified by superior knowledge? *Journal of Experimental Social Psychology, 76*, 290–306.

Harding, T. P. (2007). Clinical decision-making: How prepared are we? *Training and Education in Professional Psychology, 1*, 95–104.

Hazlett, A. (2012). Higher-order epistemic attitudes and intellectual humility. *Episteme, 9*, 205–223.

Hill, P. C., Lewis Hall, M. E., Wang, D., & Decker, L. A. (2021). Theistic intellectual humility and well-being: Does ideological context matter? *The Journal of Positive Psychology, 16*, 155–167.

Hodge, A. S., Mosher, D. K., Davis, C. W., Captari, L. E., Hook, J. N., Davis, D. E., & Van Tongeren, D. R. (2020). Political humility and forgiveness of a political hurt or offense. *Journal of Psychology and Theology, 48*, 142–153.

Hook, J. N., Davis, D. E., Van Tongeren, D. R., Hill, P. C., Worthington, E. L., Jr., Farrell, J. E., & Dieke, P. (2015). Intellectual humility and forgiveness of religious leaders. *The Journal of Positive Psychology, 10*, 499–506.

Hook, J. N., Farrell, J. E., Johnson, K. A., Van Tongeren, D. R., Davis, D. E., & Aten, J. D. (2017). Intellectual humility and religious tolerance. *The Journal of Positive Psychology, 12*, 29–35.

Hoyle, R. H., Davisson, E. K., Diebels, K. J., & Leary, M. R. (2016). Holding specific views with humility: Conceptualization and measurement of specific intellectual humility. *Personality and Individual Differences, 97*, 165–172.

Huynh, H. P., & Senger, A. R. (2021). A little shot of humility: Intellectual humility predicts vaccination attitudes and intention to vaccinate against COVID-19. *Journal of Applied Social Psychology*. Advance online publication.

Ioannidis, J. P. (2005). Why most published research findings are false. *PLoS Medicine, 2*.

Iyengar, S., Lelkes, Y., Levendusky, M., Malhotra, N., & Westwood, S. J. (2019). The origins and consequences of affective polarization in the United States. *Annual Review of Political Science, 22*, 129–146.

Kalmoe, N. P., & Mason, L. (2019). *Lethal mass partisanship: Prevalence, correlates, and electoral contingencies*. Paper presented at the NCAPSA American Politics Meeting.

Koetke, J., Schumann, K., & Porter, T. (2021). *Intellectual humility predicts scrutiny of COVID-19 misinformation*. Social Psychological and Personality Science. Advanced online publication.

Krumrei-Mancuso, E. J. (2017). Intellectual humility and prosocial values: Direct and mediated effects. *The Journal of Positive Psychology, 12*, 13–28.

Krumrei-Mancuso, E. J., & Newman, B. (2020). Intellectual humility in the sociopolitical domain. *Self and Identity*, 1–28.

Krumrei-Mancuso, E. J., & Rouse, S. V. (2016). The development and validation of the comprehensive intellectual humility scale. *Journal of Personality Assessment, 98*, 209–221.

Krumrei-Mancuso, E. J., Haggard, M. C., LaBouff, J. P., & Rowatt, W. C. (2020). Links between intellectual humility and acquiring knowledge. *The Journal of Positive Psychology, 15*, 155–170.

Lack, C. (2018, November 14). *Energy psychology: An APA-endorsed pseudoscience.* Center for Inquiry. https://centerforinquiry.org/blog/energy-psychology-an-apa-endorsed-pseudoscience/.

Leary, M. R., Diebels, K. J., Davisson, E. K., Jongman-Sereno, K. P., Isherwood, J. C., Raimi, K. T., et al. (2017). Cognitive and interpersonal features of intellectual humility. *Personality and Social Psychology Bulletin, 43*, 793–813.

Lee, K., & Ashton, M. C. (2018). Psychometric properties of the HEXACO-100. *Assessment, 25*, 543–556.

Lilienfeld, S. O. (2007). Psychological treatments that cause harm. *Perspectives on Psychological Science, 2*, 53–70.

Lilienfeld, S. O. (2010). Can psychology become a science? *Personality and Individual Differences, 49*, 281–288.

Lilienfeld, S. O. (2012). Public skepticism of psychology: Why many people perceive the study of human behavior as unscientific. *American Psychologist, 67*, 111–129.

Lilienfeld, S. O. (2013). Is psychopathy a syndrome? Commentary on Marcus, Fulton, and Edens. *Personality Disorder: Theory, Research, and Treatment, 4*, 85–86.

Lilienfeld, S. O. (2016). How can skepticism do better? *Skeptical Inquirer, 40*. Online publication.

Lilienfeld, S. O. (2017). Psychology's replication crisis and the grant culture: Righting the ship. *Perspectives on Psychological Science, 12*, 660–664.

Lilienfeld, S. O. (2017b). Microaggressions: Strong claims, inadequate evidence. *Perspectives on Psychological Science, 12*, 138–169.

Lilienfeld, S. O. (2020). Microaggression research and application: Clarifications, corrections, and common ground. *Perspectives on Psychological Science, 15*, 27–37.

Lilienfeld, S. O. (2020b). Embracing unpopular ideas: Introduction to the special section on heterodox issues in psychology. *Archives of Scientific Psychology, 8*, 1–4.

Lilienfeld, S. O., & Bowes, S. M. (2018). Intellectual humility: A key priority for psychological research and practice. *Psynopsis (Canadian Psychological Association), 3*, 20–21.

Lilienfeld, S. O., & Thames, A. D. (2009). Review of correcting fallacies about educational and psychological testing [Review of the book *Correcting fallacies about educational and psychological testing*, by R. P. Phelps, Eds.]. *Archives of Clinical Neuropsychology, 24*, 631–633.

Lilienfeld, S. O., & Bowes, S. M. (in press). Intellectual humility: Ten unresolved questions. In P. Graf (Ed.), *Current breakthroughs in applied psychology*. Springer.

Lilienfeld, S. O., Wood, J. M., & Garb, H. N. (2000). The scientific status of projective techniques. *Psychological Science in the Public Interest, 1*, 27–66.

Lilienfeld, S. O., Ammirati, R., & Landfield, K. (2009). Giving debiasing away: Can psychological research on correcting cognitive errors promote human welfare? *Perspectives on Psychological Science, 4*, 390–398.

Lilienfeld, S. O., Lynn, S. J., Ruscio, J., & Beyerstein, B. L. (2010). 50 great myths of popular psychology: Shattering widespread misconceptions about human behavior. Wiley-Blackwell.

Lilienfeld, S. O., Ritschel, L. A., Lynn, S. J., Cautin, R. L., & Latzman, R. D. (2014). Why ineffective psychotherapies appear to work: A taxonomy of causes of spurious therapeutic effectiveness. *Perspectives on Psychological Science, 9*, 355–387.

Lilienfeld, S. O., Smith, S. F., & Watts, A. L. (2016). The perils of unitary models of the etiology of mental disorders—The response modulation hypothesis of psychopathy as a case example: Rejoinder to Newman and Baskin-Sommers. *Psychological Bulletin, 142*, 1394–1403.

Lilienfeld, S. O., Lynn, S. J., O'Donohue, W. T., & Latzman, R. D. (2017). Epistemic humility: An overarching educational philosophy for clinical psychology programs. *Clinical Psychologist, 70*, 6–14.

MacLean, N., Neal, T., Morgan, R. D., & Murrie, D. C. (2019). Forensic clinicians' understanding of bias. *Psychology, Public Policy, and Law, 25*, 323–330.

McElroy, S. E., Rice, K. G., Davis, D. E., Hook, J. N., Hill, P. C., Worthington, E. L., Jr., & Van Tongeren, D. R. (2014). Intellectual humility: Scale development and theoretical elaborations in the context of religious leadership. *Journal of Psychology and Theology, 42*, 19–30.

McElroy-Heltzel, S. E., Davis, D. E., DeBlaere, C., Worthington, E. L., Jr., & Hook, J. N. (2019). Embarrassment of riches in the measurement of humility: A critical review of 22 measures. *The Journal of Positive Psychology, 14*, 393–404.

Meagher, B. R., Leman, J. C., Bias, J. P., Latendresse, S. J., & Rowatt, W. C. (2015). Contrasting self-report and consensus ratings of intellectual humility and arrogance. *Journal of Research in Personality, 58*, 35–45.

Meagher, B. R., Leman, J. C., Heidenga, C. A., Ringquist, M. R., & Rowatt, W. C. (2021). Intellectual humility in conversation: Distinct behavioral indicators of self and peer ratings. *The Journal of Positive Psychology, 16*, 417–429.

Meichenbaum, D., & Lilienfeld, S. O. (2018). How to spot hype in the field of psychotherapy: A 19-item checklist. *Professional Psychology: Research and Practice, 49*, 22–30.

Mendel, R., Traut-Mattausch, E., Jonas, E., Leucht, S., Kane, J. M., Maino, K., Kissling, W., & Hamann, J. (2011). Confirmation bias: Why psychiatrists stick to wrong preliminary diagnoses. *Psychological Medicine, 41*, 2651–2659.

Nosek, B. A., Aarts, A. A., Anderson, J. E., Kappes, H. B., & Open Science Collaboration. (2015). Estimating the reproducibility of psychological science. *Science, 349*.

O'Donohue, W. T., Lilienfeld, S. O., & Fowler, K. A. (2012). Science is an essential safeguard against human error. In *The great ideas of clinical science* (pp. 33–58). Routledge.

Porter, T., & Schumann, K. (2018). Intellectual humility and openness to the opposing view. *Self and Identity, 17*, 139–162.

Porter, T., Schumann, K., Selmeczy, D., & Trzesniewski, K. (2020). Intellectual humility predicts mastery behaviors when learning. *Learning and Individual Differences, 80*, 101888.

Pronin, E., Lin, D. Y., & Ross, L. (2002). The bias blind spot: Perceptions of bias in self versus others. *Personality and Social Psychology Bulletin, 28*, 369–381.

Roberts, R. C., & Wood, W. J. (2018). Understanding, humility, and the vices of pride. In *The Routledge handbook of virtue epistemology* (pp. 363–376). Routledge.
Rodriguez, C. G., Moskowitz, J. P., Salem, R. M., & Ditto, P. H. (2017). Partisan selective exposure: The role of party, ideology and ideological extremity over time. *Translational Issues in Psychological Science, 3*, 254–271.
Satel, S. L., & Lilienfeld, S. O. (2013). *Brainwashed: The seductive appeal of mindless neuroscience*. Basic Books.
Senger, A. R., & Huynh, H. P. (2020). Intellectual humility's association with vaccine attitudes and intentions. *Psychology, Health & Medicine*, 1–10.
Shrout, P. E., & Rodgers, J. L. (2018). Psychology, science, and knowledge construction: Broadening perspectives from the replication crisis. *Annual Review of Psychology, 69*, 487–510.
Stanley, M. L., Sinclair, A. H., & Seli, P. (2020). Intellectual humility and perceptions of political opponents. *Journal of Personality*, 1–21.
Swift, V., & Peterson, J. B. (2019). Contextualization as a means to improve the predictive validity of personality models. *Personality and Individual Differences, 144*, 153–163.
Tangney, J. P. (2000). Humility: Theoretical perspectives, empirical findings and directions for future research. *Journal of Social and Clinical Psychology, 19*, 70–82.
Van Tongeren, D. R., Davis, D. E., Hook, J. N., Witvliet, & van Oyen, C. (2019). Humility. *Current Directions in Psychological Science, 28*, 463–468.
Whitcomb, D., Battaly, H., Baehr, J., & Howard-Snyder, D. (2017). Intellectual humility: Owning our limitations. *Philosophy and Phenomenological Research, 94*, 509–539.
Zachar, P. (2015). Popper, Meehl, and progress: The evolving concept of risky test in the science of psychopathology. *Psychological Inquiry, 26*, 279–285.
Zhang, H., Hook, J. N., Farrell, J. E., Mosher, D. K., Van Tongeren, D. R., & Davis, D. E. (2018). The effect of religious diversity on religious belonging and meaning: The role of intellectual humility. *Psychology of Religion and Spirituality, 10*, 72–78.

Combating Pseudoscience in Clinical Psychology: From the Scientific Mindset, to Busting Myths, to Prescriptive Remedies

Steven Jay Lynn, Damla Aksen, Fiona Sleight, Craig Polizzi, Luciana S. Moretti, and Leonardo Adrián Medrano

Scott Lilienfeld passed away on September 30, 2020, after a valorous struggle with pancreatic cancer. The resultant loss to the field of psychology is beyond measure. One of many reasons why his legacy already borders on legendary is that, in addition to his prolific contributions well-represented in this volume, Scott was a seeker, never content to settle for the status quo—there were always more questions to puzzle; more to learn, discover, and communicate to others. His innumerable and expansive undertakings were guided by his unquenchable curiosity and his immense respect for—truly his love for—the beguiling beauties of science. Each of the authors of this chapter was influenced to be a better scientist by Scott's perpetual quest to address challenging problems, better society via the dissemination of accurate information, and his dedicated efforts to make a difference in people's lives. Scott was, is, and will continue to be a role model extraordinaire.

Scott's vision and influence extended far beyond his impact on friends and collaborators to the frontiers of psychology and clinical psychological science, in particular. Scott regarded psychological science as a precious gift, one that carried with it an obligation for its fruits to be shared not only with the professional community but with the general public as well. He took delight in sharing this gift with humility, grace, and courage, and he fully embraced doing so as his passion and mission.

We have known people to comment that Scott was "courageous" in challenging entrenched beliefs and insisting that they withstand the most searching scrutiny and

S. J. Lynn (✉)
Binghamton University (SUNY), Binghamton, NY, USA

Psychology Department, Binghamton University, Binghamton, NY, USA

D. Aksen · F. Sleight · C. Polizzi
Binghamton University (SUNY), Binghamton, NY, USA

L. S. Moretti · L. A. Medrano
Siglo 21 University, Córdoba, Argentina

C. L. Cobb et al. (eds.), *Toward a Science of Clinical Psychology*,
https://doi.org/10.1007/978-3-031-14332-8_7

disputation. Yet he neither regarded himself as heroic nor brave. Rather, he believed that healthy skepticism should be the calling of any person who considers themselves to be a scientist and an informed clinical practitioner. Inspired by the former Supreme Court justice Louis Brandeis's maxim that sunlight is the best disinfectant, Scott exposed the all-too-often ignored or shrouded dark side of psychotherapy, which revealed that psychotherapy could potentially harm as well as heal and warned that pseudoscience and misinformation about psychology could exact a dear price as well.

In this chapter, we distill a large corpus of literature that Scott produced with his colleagues on science vs. pseudoscience, distinguishing myths and misconceptions and fact and fiction in psychology, the virtues of evidence-based clinical practice, and teaching scientific thinking skills. All these endeavors are critical to becoming not only an active clinical psychological scientist but also an informed citizen in an increasingly media-driven and technological society rife with fake news and bogus information.

The Scientific Mindset

Our discussion is framed by the overarching mindset regarding scientific inquiry that Scott championed, including his call for greater awareness of cognitive biases and logical fallacies that promote overconfidence and mistaken inferences on a quotidian and professional basis. While scientific thinking is surely not a panacea, it is also surely our best safeguard against errors in clinical judgment and vital to shaping the perspective and activities of clinical psychological scientists (O'Donohue et al., 2012).

Scott vociferously and persuasively advocated for a scientific attitude variously called epistemic or intellectual humility (see Chap. 6 for an in-depth discussion) that encompassed constructive questioning of a claim, healthy self-doubt, and open-minded skepticism. Writing with Donald Meichenbaum (Meichenbaum & Lilienfeld, 2018), Scott stated, "Humility should be our watchword" and called attention to Carl Sagan's (1995) remark that the best scientists hear "a little voice in our heads that repeatedly intones, You might be mistaken. You've been wrong before" (p. 39). Lilienfeld et al. (2022) thus viewed psychological science as a prescription for humility and endorsed the Nobel Prize-winning physicist Richard Feynman's stance that good scientists bend over backward to prove themselves wrong: We should be flexible and open enough in our thinking to change our minds when evidence contradicts our beliefs, whether they relate to assessment, psychopathology, psychotherapy, or our favored theory.

Lilienfeld et al. (2022) appreciated the need to distinguish skepticism from cynicism. He voiced discomfort with being labeled a "debunker" for his persistent and effective efforts to challenge prevalent myths and misconceptions about psychology. Rather, he greatly preferred to be perceived as a skeptic and served proudly as both the author of the *Psychology Today* blog, *The Skeptical Psychologist,* and a consulting editor of the *Skeptical Inquirer* magazine. Scott contended that the scientific skeptic evaluates all claims with an open mind but insists on persuasive evidence before accepting them. In sharp contrast, the cynic dismisses claims before they have been evaluated adequately (Lilienfeld et al., 2022; Sagan, 1995). He cautioned that we should not be overly zealous to dismiss new psychotherapies as ineffective prior to their rigorous evaluation (Beutler & Harwood, 2001). Such therapies could be considered "nonscientific," as evidence has not yet accrued to judge their effectiveness, and thus they lack scientific support that may in the future be forthcoming or not.

Yet we should not be too quick to jump on the bandwagon of a newly hyped psychotherapy (e.g., Primal Scream Therapy, Janov, 1970). Scott dubbed this tendency "breakthroughism" (Lilienfeld, 2017), and he contended that training graduate students to avoid the seductive allure of therapeutic hype is among our foremost responsibilities as teachers (Lilienfeld, 2015). The necessity of this perspective is underscored by the fact that promising interventions do not consistently bear up to the tests of time or replication, and initial scientific conclusions are often premature, flat-out wrong, or require revision (e.g., EMDR: Lilienfeld, 2017; Lilienfeld et al., 2022). A scientific approach could have helped to side-step notorious errors and harmful interventions in the history of clinical psychology and psychiatry. These include insulin coma therapy, surgical removal of organs, phrenology, prefrontal lobotomy, and, more recently, facilitated communication for autism and blatantly suggestive recovered memory techniques.

As Scott (Lilienfeld, 2015) keenly observed, placebo effects warrant that hope can be helpful (Kirsch, 2005), but false hope can prove detrimental and even cruel to patients and their loved ones when their hopes are quashed. We certainly cannot rely on the popular media to serve as a watchdog for interventions that promise far more than they deliver. After all, sensational and seeming breakthrough developments are what grab headlines and serve as clickbait, whereas failures to replicate are typically not deemed "newsworthy," relegated to no more than a footnote, or garner scant attention. Media coverage can also reduce complex events and explanations to simplistic, either-or accounts, over-estimate the frequency of sensational events, and underestimate the frequency of less sensational events (Lilienfeld et al., 2022).

The scientific mindset (a) demands that whether the claim is dramatic or not, the burden of proof of a claim always falls on the claimant (Shermer, 2002) and (b) calls for limits to "open-mindedness." In this context, Scott's was particularly fond of quoting James Oberg's pithy and playful dictum that maintaining an open mind is a virtue, "just not so open that your brains fall out" (as cited in Sagan, 1995, p. 187). Scott cautioned that when the theoretical basis for a psychological intervention is dubious or contradicts what we know, we would do well to set a higher standard for convincing research evidence than if the theoretical basis of the treatment is well established. This Bayesian way of thinking converges with astronomer Carl Sagan's (1995) contention that extraordinary claims require extraordinary evidence (Lilienfeld, 2011).

Contrary to the facile notion that science is best construed as a monolithic, lockstep prescriptive method or as a mere conglomeration of facts and figures, Scott, instead, regarded science as a systematic *approach* to knowledge that helps shield against errors in inference. More specifically, science is a ceaseless process of reflection, self-correction, and updating of extant knowledge that mitigates everyday cognitive biases in information processing. Still, systematic errors can fool even the most discerning among us. We humans are subject to intransigent biases, even to the point that we are biased to not be aware of our own biases, even though they may be starkly apparent to us in other people (bias blind spot; Pronin et al., 2002). Perforce, there are limits to which introspection and reflection can eliminate biases (Lilienfeld & Basterfield, 2020). Nevertheless, we can employ principles of critical thinking, acknowledge our cognitive limitations, monitor what we know and do not know, and look to science as a vehicle to compensate for tunnel vision and thereby be better equipped to identify errors in our beliefs (Bensley & Lilienfeld, 2017; Meichenbaum & Lilienfeld, 2018).

Principles of Critical Thinking

Lilienfeld et al. (2022) recognized the importance of teaching well-delineated principles of scientific thinking as early as students' first formal exposure to psychology in introductory psychology classes. In their textbook, *Psychology: From Inquiry to Understanding* 5th edition, Scott and his colleagues Steven Jay Lynn and LauraNamy (Lilienfeld et al., 2022) form the crux of their teaching mission around such principles to assist in evaluating claims regarding human nature. The value of doing so is one of the backbone premises of their text that pivots around the following six scientific thinking principles: ruling out rival hypotheses, not confusing correlation with causation, the importance of falsifiability, the value of replication, generalizability, and extraordinary claims require extraordinary evidence. Knowledge of these principles can be invaluable to members of the public as well as students and professionals at all levels.

The first principle, ruling out rival hypotheses, challenges students to consider and rule out plausible rival hypotheses that could account for a particular finding in support of a claim. Learning to generate and explore alternative explanations can be an effective means to counteract common biases, such as confirmation bias, that we will review (Lewandowsky et al., 2012).

The second principle, correlation is not causation, cautions against assuming that because two variables are correlated, it should not be understood to signify that one necessarily causes the other (related to the correlation-causation fallacy mentioned below). Causal relations are best tested using longitudinal designs and well-controlled randomized controlled trials, and students should also be alert to the possibility that the association between two variables could be accounted for by a third or more variables.

The third principle, falsifiability, is based on the observations of Sir Karl Popper (1959) who argued that a theory must be capable of being falsified for it to be scientific. That is, scientifically minded students should question whether the theory can be tested and disproved and whether the proponents of the theory specify in advance what evidence would qualify not only in support of the theory but against the theory as well. Another consideration is whether the claim is so broad that any finding would be deemed supportive; in the latter case, the theory would not be amenable to falsification.

The fourth principle, replicability, refers to the ability to reproduce findings consistently. Not much stock should be invested in a psychological finding until it has been replicated by independent researchers (Lilienfeld et al., 2022; O'Donohue et al., in press). This caution is especially resonant in light of the so-called "replication crisis" in psychology spurred by the inability of scientists to replicate influential results on a consistent basis, with as many as 40% of the original findings failing to hold up (Fiedler & Prager, 2018). Still, we should not be too cavalier about dismissing the original findings, insofar as even minor variations in the methodology of the research or the population sampled, for example, could account for variability across studies. Moreover, a failure to replicate does not necessarily represent a blanket falsification of the validity of the construct, only that it failed to duplicate one particular test of the hypothesis (O'Donohue, 2021). Nevertheless, we cannot take the reliability of positive findings for granted, especially in cases in which failures to replicate are the product of less-than-optimal scientific practices. Lilienfeld and Strother (2020; see also Lilienfeld & Waldman, 2017; Wiggins & Christopherson, 2019) suggest that questions about replicability have engendered (a) needed self-reflection and self-correction in the field and (b) scrutiny of potential causes of failures to replicate that originate in questionable research practices (e.g., p-hacking, not publishing failures to replicate, failure to register study methods and hypotheses in advance).

To be a literate and critical consumer of psychological knowledge, it is important to appreciate the fifth principle—generalizability—which highlights the need to ask whether research findings and conclusions reflect the vast diversity of the human experience in terms of variables such as sex, gender, age, race, ethnicity, religion, socioeconomic status, sexual orientation, and cultural values and differences. To underscore the importance of this principle, Henrich et al. (2010) published a paper with the intriguing title, "The Weirdest People in the World?" "WEIRD," in this context, is an acronym for Western Educated Industrialized Rich Democratic societies. The authors warned against assuming that findings based on people from these privileged societies will apply to highly diverse populations, as they contended that 99% of published psychology research is not only conducted by Western researchers, but more than two-thirds of those studies focus exclusively on college undergraduate students. Tellingly, people from WEIRD cultures not infrequently deviate from individuals from other cultures in their responses that range from perceptual illusions to decision-making in psychology studies (Lilienfeld et al., 2022).

The final sixth principle underscores the proviso that extraordinary claims require extraordinary evidence. Accordingly, the more a claim contradicts extant knowledge, the more the scientist is obligated to provide convincing evidence, and the more the informed consumer should demand such evidence.

Cognitive Biases and Logical Fallacies

To arm students with additional scientific thinking tools, Scott (Lilienfeld et al., 2022) and his colleagues introduced readers to the science of heuristics and biases that represent mental shortcuts. These shortcuts are adaptive insofar as our brains are predisposed to fabricate order out of disorder, find sense in nonsense, and negotiate the often-perplexing world in which we live (Alcock, 1995). Doing so constrains the endless cascades of information that we neither have the time nor mental bandwidth to process (Lilienfeld et al., 2022). For example, the representativeness heuristic (the shortcut by which we judge the probability of an occurrence by its similarity to a prototype) and the availability heuristic (the shortcut by which we judge the probability of an occurrence by the ease with which it comes to mind) are generally adaptive in everyday life and in clinical settings, and they can play a formative role in generating hypotheses. Yet, this adaptive tendency can also misguide us when we perceive nonexistent yet seemingly meaningful patterns and contribute to biases if applied uncritically (Lilienfeld et al., 2022; Stanovich, 2018).

In addition to maintaining awareness of these ubiquitous heuristics, clinicians would do well to be especially cognizant of at least eight biases that are indispensable in evaluating claims: (1) confirmation bias (favoring evidence that supports our hypotheses, to deny, dismiss or distort evidence that does not; can induce belief perseverance), (2) hindsight bias (overestimating the predictability of an outcome after it happens than it was before it happened), (3) illusory correlation (perceiving a correlation where none exists or overestimating the strength of the association), (4) emotional reasoning (using emotions as sole or primary guides for evaluating the validity of a claim), (5) gender and race biases (drawing inaccurate inferences based on gender or race), (6) overconfidence in the accuracy of a judgment or decision, (7) the clinician's illusion (overestimating the chronicity of a psychological condition such as substance use disorders, Bowes et al., 2020), and (8) bias blind spot. The pervasiveness of these biases is reflected in findings that scientists are as prone to confirmation bias as nonscientists (Griggs & Ransdell, 1986; Mahoney & DeMonbreun, 1977) and that highly intelligent people are as prone to bias blind spot as are other individuals tested (West et al., 2012).

Additionally, numerous logical fallacies can impact the ability to evaluate claims, most notably post hoc, ergo propter hoc reasoning (because an event B, followed event A, event B must be caused by event A), confusing correlation with causation, bandwagon fallacy (assuming a claim is correct just because many people believe it), argument from authority (accepting a claim merely because an authority figure endorses it), either-or fallacy (framing a question as though it can be answered in only one of two extreme ways), genetic fallacy (confusing the correctness of a belief with its origin or genesis), ad hominem fallacy (demeaning the person who proposed an argument rather than addressing the merits of an argument), golden mean fallacy (concluding that an argument is valid when it represents the middle ground between two opposing positions), argument from antiquity (concluding that a claim is valid just because it has been around for a long time), and argument from personal incredulity fallacy (concluding that a claim is unbelievable, so it must be false or improbable) (Pope & Vasquez, 2016; see also Meehl, 1973).

Debiasing and misinformation corrective efforts may succeed to the extent that they steer cognitive processing from a heuristic automatic mode of thinking to a more flexible, meta-aware, controlled mode of cognition (Kahneman, 2003; Stanovich & West, 2000). Educational efforts to correct memory misconceptions have produced long-term changes in beliefs tested 18 months later (Sauerland & Otgaar, 2021).

Critical thinking skills and awareness of our cognitive biases afford some protection against *naïve realism* (Ross & Ward, 1995), the intuitively appealing but erroneous assumption that we can always trust our sensory impressions (i.e., "seeing is believing") and that we passively and objectively absorb the "real" world, just as it is, through our sensory portals. Lilienfeld et al. (2014) have described how research procedures of various kinds, including controlled psychotherapy outcomes and process methods, can help to protect us against naïve realism. An assortment of causes of spurious therapeutic effectiveness may lead us to the wrong conclusion that therapy is responsible for positive outcomes after treatment when other causes are operative. Such causes include placebo effects, regression to the mean (e.g., people embark on therapy when they experience symptom exacerbations; they are "at their worst"), multiple treatment interference (e.g., starting an exercise program), natural fluctuations in the course of a psychiatric condition, positive life experiences, and demand characteristics that can bias self-reports.

Science and Pseudoscience

Yet another key to avoid falling prey to naïve realism is the ability to recognize pseudoscience and indicators that distinguish a pseudoscientific from a scientific approach and to appreciate the costs and harms that pseudoscience can impose on psychotherapy consumers and the general public. Lilienfeld et al. (2022) have characterized pseudoscience as an imposter or masquerader of science that fundamentally lacks the safeguards against both confirmation bias and belief rigidity that mark science. No sharp dividing line of features cleanly demarcates science from pseudoscience. Yet, as Lilienfeld (2005) observes, whereas the differences between science and pseudoscience are neither absolute nor clear-cut, they are neither arbitrary nor subjective either.

In fact, the following set of "warning signs" or rules of thumb are useful in identifying pseudoscientific claims and disciplines (Bensley & Lilienfeld, 2015; Lilienfeld, 2005; Lilienfeld et al., 2015, 2022), with more indicia providing greater confidence that the claim warrants skepticism: (a) excessive reliance on anecdotes and personal testimony rather than empirical evidence to buttress claims; (b) a tendency to place the burden of proof on skeptics, not proponents of claims; (c) an absence of self-correction and replication; (d) an emphasis on confirmation rather than refutation; (e) an absence of "connectivity"; that is, inadequate linkages with existing areas of scientific knowledge and constructs; (f) the use of impressive-sounding jargon (i.e., "psychobabble") that confuses rather than clarifies and lends claims a facade of scientific credibility; (g) a lack of boundary conditions; that is, a failure to specify the settings and circumstances under which claims do and do not hold; (h) a lack of ability to falsify claims; (i) a tendency to invoke ad hoc hypotheses; that is, "escape hatches" or loopholes, which protect claims from falsification; and (j) evasion of peer review.

Lilienfeld et al. (2008, pp. 21–22) described an additional eight symptoms of psychological pseudoscience as follows: (1) promises of simple, rapid, and dramatic cures for longstanding and complex problems; (2) exaggerated claims of treatment success based on a meager or nonexistent research base; (3) promoting and marketing novel techniques before supportive scientific studies have been conducted; (4) the erroneous assumption that untested interventions are helpful or at worst harmless; (5) failure to consider alternative explanations for apparent positive treatment effects; (6) failure to attend to well-established scientific findings; (7) cavalier dismissal of negative scientific results on flimsy or illogical grounds; and, finally, (8) the "Rasputin effect," named after the Russian monk who somehow survived multiple attempts to slay him: namely, the tendency of questionable techniques to live on in the face of overwhelming disconfirming evidence (e.g., facilitative communication).

To this list, we would add warnings compiled by Meichenbaum and Lilienfeld (2018) of "hype" in psychotherapy that complement and round out the signs of pseudoscience already mentioned: (1) inadequate scientific support for the intervention; (2) heavy reliance on endorsements from presumed experts; (3) use of salesmanship and extensive promotional efforts, including sale of paraphernalia; (4) tendency of advocates to be defensive and dismiss critics; (5) claims that treatment "fits all"; (6) claims that treatment is "evidence-based" on the basis of informal clinical observations; and (7) no proposed scientific basis for change mechanisms (David et al., 2018; Rosen & Davison, 2003).

Clearly, there are many grounds for considering an intervention to be pseudoscientific that merit attention by clinical practitioners, researchers, and the general public. The distinction between science and pseudoscience is neither insubstantial nor absent real-world consequences: Ineffective pseudoscientific interventions carry opportunity costs such that consumers neglect to seek or avail themselves of truly effective treatments (Lilienfeld et al., 2013) and incur needless financial costs from participating in useless interventions. For example, Lilienfeld et al. (2022) cite troubling data (Layard & Clark, 2014) that more than a third of people with major depression, who are at heightened risk for suicide, receive no treatment at all. Additionally, most treatment seekers receive interventions with little or no scientific support for depression such as lengthy psychoanalysis, herbal remedies, and so-called energy therapies rather than empirically supported methods such as cognitive-behavioral therapy (David et al., 2018). Generally, the longer people refrain from receiving effective treatment for a psychological condition, the poorer the treatment outcome (Marshall et al., 2005).

Even direr in consequence, Lilienfeld (2007, 2016; Lilienfeld et al., 2022; Meichenbaum & Lilienfeld, 2018) cautioned that pseudoscientific treatments have been implicated in direct psychological and physical harm and even death (see also Chap. 16 this volume), as in the tragic case of Candace Newmaker who participated in rebirthing therapy. Candace died in 2000 while reenacting her supposed birth trauma (the purported cause of her psychological problems and attachment difficulties) in which her therapist wrapped her in a blanket, squeezed her repeatedly, sat on her, and ignored her pleas that she couldn't breathe and was going to die. Sadly, she did not emerge from the blanket alive (Mercer et al., 2003). Another example of harm would be the effects of memory recovery therapies in which false memories of childhood abuse engender negative personal repercussions that can extend to family members who are falsely accused as perpetrators or cases in which suggestive psychotherapies create the belief that a client possesses "multiple personalities."

In his landmark article on therapies that harm, cited well over 1000 times (Google Scholar), Scott (Lilienfeld, 2007) earmarked potentially harmful interventions that included scared straight programs, critical incident stress debriefing, facilitated communication, dissociative-identity oriented therapy, peer group interventions for conduct disorder, attachment therapies (e.g., rebirthing therapy), and relaxation for panic-prone individuals. In a recent meta-analysis of randomized controlled trials of additional methods, which Scott (Lilienfeld, 2007) also identified as potentially harmful, Williams et al. (2021) found the most evidence of harm for critical incident stress debriefing to assist emergency responders and others exposed to a severe stressor and for scared straight programs geared to deter future criminal behavior. The reviewers found more ambiguous evidence for the iatrogenic effects of grief counseling, boot camp for conduct disorder, DARE programs, and expressive-experiential psychotherapies, due in some measure to the poor methodological quality of the research reviewed (e.g., over-reliance on no-treatment comparison groups, randomization inconsistencies). Notably, ambiguous evidence is not an indication of the absence of harm but rather of the need for better and more concerted research (see Chap. 16), as the rate of client deterioration subsequent to psychotherapy may approximate 10% (Boisvert & Faust, 2003). The absence of systematic research and information regarding the harms of psychological interventions renders it problematic for consumers, clinicians, and policymakers to make informed and optimal decisions regarding treatments to recommend or pursue (Halfond et al., 2021).

Lilienfeld et al. (2005) also highlighted other more indirect but nevertheless invidious consequences of pseudoscience that extend beyond individual psychological treatments to eroding public confidence in the profession of psychology, including the credibility of potentially effective interventions (Lilienfeld, 2012). Additionally, as Lilienfeld (2002, p. 9) comment: "By continuing to ignore the imminent dangers posed by questionable mental health techniques, we send an implicit message to our students that we are not deeply committed to anchoring our discipline in scientific evidence or to combating potentially unscientific practices."

Myths of Psychology: The Dangers of Psychomythology

Scott's project to contain and spotlight such practices becomes all the more salient when considered in view of the explosion of myths of psychology that are channeled through media venues including the Internet, films, magazines, podcasts, blogs, and self-help books. Over the past few decades, the popular psychology industry has bombarded the public with an incessant flow of misinformation, along with dispensing the occasional kernel of useful, accurate, and science-based information. In 2019 alone, publishers sold nearly 19 million copies of self-help books, with the vast majority never evaluated systematically (Arkowitz & Lilienfeld, 2006; see also Rosen et al., 2015). Whereas some experts are reliable advocates for psychological science, other self-proclaimed "experts," with minimal or no scientific credentials, are highly visible in popular media as purveyors of pseudoscience who keep alive, resuscitate, or actively foment prevalent myths of psychology. These deleterious developments, in isolation and combination, pose a threat to the scientific foundations of psychology (Lilienfeld et al., 2003a, b).

One gauge of the wide sweep of Scott's contributions can be measured in his success in busting some of the most prevalent myths across the sprawling landscape of psychology and, more pertinent to the current book, clinical psychology. His efforts to do so are not only reflected in his book for a general audience, *50 Great Myths of Popular Psychology: Shattering Widespread Misconceptions about Human Behavior* (Lilienfeld et al., 2010a); his graduate textbook, *Science and Pseudoscience in Clinical Psychology* (Lilienfeld et al., 2013); and his introduction to psychology textbook (Lilienfeld et al., 2022), as well as other books (Lilienfeld et al., 2008; Lilienfeld & Waldman, 2017; Lynn et al., 2014; O'Donohue & Lilienfeld, 2012, 2013; Satel & Lilienfeld, 2013); many articles in journals and magazines; and in the regular column in Scientific American that he and Hal Arkowitz contributed for many years.

Scott used the term "psychomythology" to refer to the immense aggregate body of misinformation about psychology. Psychological misconceptions, in turn, can be defined as false beliefs that often originate from informal sources (e.g., Internet, news and entertainment media, informal conversations) and are commonly held but are inconsistent with or contradict established research in psychology (Bensley & Lilienfeld, 2015; DiSessa, 2006). Misconceptions can take on "mythic" proportions when they become widely prevalent and regarded as commonsense, givens, and received knowledge and evade careful examination. Lilienfeld and colleagues (Lilienfeld et al., 2010b) believed no one was immune from the innate human tendency to be fooled because so many of the falsehoods inherent in psychomythology "dovetail with our intuitions, hunches, and experiences" (p. 42).

As we have argued, scientific thinking tools can be deployed to assist in evaluating the viability and strength of claims and in identifying those that are more moored in pseudoscience than science. Yet many myths are rarely questioned given they are often heavily sculpted by the media and the socio-cultural containers in which they have incubated. Scott, therefore, maintained that it was crucially important to identify misconceptions, as they exert potent influence in the field of clinical psychology, in our everyday lives, and how we educate citizens and clinical psychologists.

Psychological myths not only impede or compete with accurate knowledge but also discourage people from seeking and acquiring professional help or engender other harms. Consider the following five cases selected from among many myths and misconceptions we could use as examples:

1. The mistaken belief that diagnostic labels—rather than people's behaviors—are stigmatizing (Basterfield et al., 2020; 86% of undergraduates endorse the myth) may discourage individuals with serious psychological problems from help-seeking for fear of being labeled in pejorative terms.
2. Misinformation can affect treatment decisions, such as whether to receive pharmacological treatment for depression, because it is believed to be more effective than evidence-based cognitive-behavioral treatment (CBT), when this is not the case (Basterfield et al., 2020; 81% of people endorse this myth). In actuality, CBT can be more effective in preventing relapse than antidepressant medication and is at least equally effective as pharmacological intervention in alleviating depression (Lilienfeld et al., 2022).
3. The notion that human memory works like a video recorder and accurately records the events we have experienced, alongside the notion that individuals commonly repress memories of traumatic events, could lend credence to recovered (and inaccurate) memories unearthed by suggestive procedures such as hypnosis or leading questions (Lynn et al., 1997). As many as 90% of respondents endorse a belief in repressed memory (e.g., Dodier et al., 2019; Houben et al., 2019; Patihis et al., 2014).
4. The myth that asking people about suicide increases the likelihood that they will kill themselves may dissuade caring and concerned people from supporting the potentially suicidal person by discussing depression and suicidal thoughts, which could thereby reduce the probability of suicide or encourage the depressed person to get help. More than 80% of undergraduates concur with this misconception (Basterfield et al., 2020; 81% endorse the myth).
5. The popular idea that it is better to express anger to others than to hold it in (Brown, 1983; 66% of undergraduates endorsed this myth) does not accord with research indicating that emotional catharsis of anger can increase rather than decrease aggression (Bushman et al., 1999; Littrell, 1998).

Concerns and Prescriptive Remedies

David Shakow, widely acknowledged as the architect of contemporary clinical psychology (Cautin, 2006), argued that clinical psychologists should be psychologists first and clinical psychologists second. Specifically, competent and ethical psychotherapists ought to possess a broad and deep understanding of basic psychological science, including social psychology, personality, health psychology, affect, perception, genetics, memory, learning, psychometrics, and neuroscience (Lilienfeld & O'Donohue, 2012; Sechrest & Smith, 1994). For example, effective psychotherapists should be prepared to implement social psychological principles of persuasion (Cialdini & Cialdini, 2007; Pratkanis, 2011) to overcome client reactance to changing their ingrained patterns of behavior and confront anxieties in finding adaptive ways to respond to stressful situations.

Lilienfeld et al. (2017) amended the Shakow model to argue that clinical psychologists should be scientists first, psychologists second, and clinical psychologists third. These priorities would go some way toward narrowing the so-called science-practice gap that refers to the sizable gulf between research on the (a) efficacy of psychological interventions and the validity of assessment measures and (b) implementing these techniques in clinical practice. More broadly, evidence-based practice encompasses research evidence, clinical experiences, and client preferences/values and thus marries clinical science and practice to optimize clinical decision-making and outcomes. Just as science is best construed as an approach rather than a monolithic method, experience-based practice refers not to a corpus of empirically supported interventions but instead to a systematic approach to evaluating scientific evidence and implementing it in practice. Still, O'Donohue and Lilienfeld (2012) argued that one goal of evidence-based practice accords with a broader vision: "the systematic use of quality improvement in behavioral health care" (p. 51).

Scott strongly believed that psychological scientists have a responsibility to not stand idly by when myths and misconceptions are propagated, pseudoscientific interventions are passed off as scientific, opportunities to educate new generations of students are ignored or not implemented, and professional organizations such as the American Psychological Association fail to impose quality control over what is taught in workshops that offer continuing education credit. Scott and his colleagues initiated a campaign to advance ideas regarding how scientific thinking could be taught and myths busted in the classroom, with the principles in his introduction to psychology textbook representing just one way this could be done. For example, Lilienfeld et al. (2010c) provided concrete recommendations for teaching psychology in which they touted the value of an *activation approach* that juxtaposes facts and fictions of psychology and misconceptions and then rebuts misconceptions directly and respectfully with accurate information (Kowalski & Taylor, 2009).

This approach appears to be more effective than the standard one of merely presenting factual information alongside misconceptions and yields reductions in the latter on the order of 50% or more among undergraduates (Bensley & Lilienfeld,

2017; Kowalski & Taylor, 2009). Nevertheless, the activation approach can be counterproductive in cases when "misconceptions are repeated multiple times during refutation, leading people to confuse familiarity with veracity (*the familiarity backfire effect*), and when prior beliefs and preferences lead people to strongly endorse misconceptions, producing the *worldview backfire effect*" (Bensley & Lilienfeld, 2017, p. 380; Lewandowsky et al., 2012). We suggest that encouraging critical thinking skills in relation to specific myths, reflection on their accuracy and implications, and warnings about backfire effects can perhaps mitigate their influence. Even if myths are challenging to eradicate in their entirety, they, nevertheless, provide fodder to train students in scientific thinking, cognitive errors, and bias mitigation.

Scott was deeply committed to promulgating a vision of graduate training in clinical science, as reflected in his placing a strong emphasis on scientific thinking and healthy skepticism in the curriculum. Bensley et al. (2022) reported that scientific skepticism negatively predicted both paranormal and conspiracy theory belief. Lilienfeld et al. (2001) went so far as to provide a model syllabus for teaching science and pseudoscience that included a general introduction to science and the scientific method, the differences between science and pseudoscience, the fallibility of human reasoning processes, and tying-in scientific thinking with specific topics and myths of psychology.

Lilienfeld et al. (2013) described a top-down model of psychotherapy education they called the protocol-based approach in which students learn about evidence-based interventions with the greatest weight of empirical support and how to administer them. However, Lilienfeld et al. (2019) argued that this approach should be supplemented with a *rationale-based approach* that is akin to the activation approach in that it counters initial exposure to the sorts of common errors in causal inference we reviewed with knowledge of how EBP helps to compensate for these errors.

Many of Scott's prescriptive proposals, whether they target professional or educational issues, were explicitly intended to (a) foster EBP and raise awareness of pseudoscience, and (b) advocate for accrediting bodies (APA, PCSAS) to require formal training in a scientific mindset and coverage of key topics such as cognitive biases, philosophy of science, judgment and prediction, research methods, human genetics, and philosophy of science (O'Donohue, 1989; the "philosopher-scientist-practitioner model") that constitute basic elements of a critical thinking core curriculum (Lilienfeld et al., 2017). Lilienfeld also advocated for the following:

1. a list of interventions lacking in empirical support and potentially harmful. We would add that the list should also distinguish among therapies that are devoid of support for positive clinical outcomes and theorized mechanisms of change (David et al., 2018). Such a list would be subject to periodic revision.
2. Professional organizations such as APA should assume greater oversight in monitoring science-based content in approving continuing education workshops in order to stem the tide of pseudoscientific and/or harmful practices and encourage workshop development and proliferation of science-based programs.
3. Lilienfeld et al. (2005, p. 214) also called for professional organizations (APA, APS, state and provincial licensing boards) to "impose meaningful sanctions on

practitioners who provide clinical services that are devoid of scientific support or that have been shown to be potentially harmful…" and to revise the code of ethics "to make more explicit the responsibilities of mental health professionals to be familiar with the scientific evidence regarding the costs and potential dangers of their services."

Scott and his colleagues are by no means alone in encouraging a movement toward science-based psychology. Recent developments at APA are encouraging, as exemplified by the appointment of Mitchell Prinstein as a vocal and effective advocate for psychological science as APA's Chief Science Officer. APA has (a) expanded its science directorate and increased the visibility of psychological research in pitching stories to the media based on research in APA journals, (b) facilitated link-ups of experts with media outlets, (c) sponsored scientifically oriented podcasts ("Speaking of Psychology"), (d) advanced recommendations to government entities in support of key issues germane to psychological scientists, and (e) conducted surveys of directors of clinical programs in psychology to determine ways that APA can support science-based initiatives and graduate training in clinical psychology. Time will tell whether and to what extent these endeavors will meet with success.

We suggest that future efforts by the APA and other professional organizations, such as APS, be directed toward correcting erroneous claims prevalent in popular media via developing coordinated networks of media contacts and experts to educate the public and promote effective psychological interventions. We also recommend that greater attention be devoted to evidence-based supervision that shapes the development of clinical scientists in graduate training programs (Barrett et al., 2020).

The expansion of accreditation of clinical psychology doctoral programs by the Psychological Clinical Science Accreditation System (PCSAS) is a welcome development given its emphasis on producing graduates who are well-versed in research skills and succeed in securing careers in research settings. Yet the "epistemic humility model" that Lilienfeld et al. (2017) advocated prizes training in the scientific mindset above attaining a research-oriented professional position. Rather, this mindset equips graduates to think like scientists regardless of the relative balance in their careers as "researchers" or "clinicians" and promises to bridge the science-practice gap in a wide range of helping professions (e.g., psychiatry, social work, mental health counseling) and clinical settings.

Conclusion

We hope that readers will appreciate the impact of Scott's efforts to combat pseudoscience and disseminate the nature and value of a scientific mindset. We further hope that readers will assume the mantle of Scott's herculean efforts to extend the reaches of clinical psychological science to students, the general public, and ultimately to consumers of psychological services. In the past two decades, important strides have carried us some distance in this regard. Yet, as we are certain Scott would agree, "There's work to be done."

References

Alcock, J. E. (1995). The propensity to believe. *Annals of the New York Academy of Sciences, 775*(1), 64–78.

Arkowitz, H., & Lilienfeld, S. O. (2006). Do self help books help. *Scientific American Mind, 17*(5), 90–91.

Barrett, J., Gonsalvez, C. J., & Shires, A. (2020). Evidence-based practice within supervision during psychology practitioner training: A systematic review. *Clinical Psychologist, 24*(1), 3–17. https://doi.org/10.1111/cp.12196

Basterfield, C., Lilienfeld, S. O., Cautin, R. L., & Jordan, D. (2020). Mental illness misconceptions among undergraduates: Prevalence, correlates, and instructional implications. *Scholarship of Teaching and Learning in Psychology.* Advance online publication. https://doi.org/10.1037/stl0000221

Bensley, D. A., & Lilienfeld, S. O. (2015). What is a psychological misconception? Moving toward an empirical answer. *Teaching of Psychology, 42*(4), 282–292. https://doi.org/10.1177/0098628315603059

Bensley, D. A., & Lilienfeld, S. O. (2017). Psychological misconceptions: Recent scientific advances and unresolved issues. *Current Directions in Psychological Science, 26*(4), 377–382.

Bensley, D. A., Watkins, C., Lilienfeld, S. O., Masciocchi, C., Murtagh, M. P., & Rowan, K. (2022). Skepticism, cynicism, and cognitive style predictors of the generality of unsubstantiated belief. *Applied Cognitive Psychology, 36*, 83–99. https://doi.org/10.1002/acp.3900

Beutler, L. E., & Harwood, T. M. (2001). Antiscientific attitudes: What happens when scientists are unscientific? *Journal of Clinical Psychology, 57*(1), 43–51.

Boisvert, C. M., & Faust, D. (2003). Leading researchers' consensus on psychotherapy research findings: Implications for the teaching and conduct of psychotherapy. *Professional Psychology: Research and Practice, 34*(5), 508–513. https://doi.org/10.1037/0735-7028.34.5.508

Bowes, S. M., Ammirati, R. J. J., Costello, T. H., Basterfield, C., & Lilienfeld, S. O. (2020). Cognitive biases, heuristics, and logical fallacies in clinical practice: A brief field guide for practicing clinicians and supervisors. *Professional Psychology: Research and Practice, 51*(5), 435–445. https://doi.org/10.1037/pro0000309

Brown, L. T. (1983). Some more misconceptions about psychology among introductory psychology students. *Teaching of Psychology, 10*(4), 207–210.

Bushman, B. J., Baumeister, R. F., & Stack, A. D. (1999). Catharsis, aggression, and persuasive influence: Self-fulfilling or self-defeating prophecies?. *Journal of Personality and Social Psychology, 76*(3), 367. https://doi.org/10.1037/0022-3514.76.3.367

Cautin, R. L. (2006). David Shakow: Architect of modern clinical psychology. In D. A. Dewsbury, L. T. Benjamin, & M. Wertheimer (Eds.), *Portraits of pioneers in psychology* (pp. 207–221). American Psychological Association/Lawrence Erlbaum Associates Publishers.

Cialdini, R. B., & Cialdini, R. B. (2007). *Influence: The psychology of persuasion* (Vol. 55, p. 339). Collins.

David, D., Lynn, S. J., & Montgomery, G. H. (Eds.). (2018). *Evidence-based psychotherapy: The state of the science and practice*. Wiley-Blackwell.

diSessa, A. A. (2006). A history of conceptual change research: Threads and fault lines. In R. K. Sawyer (Ed.), *The Cambridge handbook of the learning sciences* (pp. 265–281). Cambridge University Press.

Dodier, O., Patihis, L., & Payoux, M. (2019). Reports of recovered memories of childhood abuse in therapy in France. *Memory, 27*(9), 1283–1298.

Fiedler, K., & Prager, J. (2018). The regression trap and other pitfalls of replication science—Illustrated by the report of the Open Science Collaboration. *Basic and Applied Social Psychology, 40*(3), 115–124. https://doi.org/10.1080/01973533.2017.1421953

Griggs, R. A., & Ransdell, S. E. (1986). Scientists and the selection task. *Social Studies of Science, 16*(2), 319–330.

Halfond, R. W., Wright, C. V., & Bufka, L. F. (2021). The role of harms and burdens in clinical practice guidelines: Lessons learned from the American Psychological Association's guideline development. *Clinical Psychology: Science and Practice, 28*(1), 19–28. https://doi.org/10.1111/cpsp.12343

Henrich, J., Heine, S. J., & Norenzayan, A. (2010). Most people are not WEIRD. *Nature, 466*(7302), 29–29.

Houben, S. T., Otgaar, H., Roelofs, J., Wessel, I., Patihis, L., & Merckelbach, H. (2019). Eye movement desensitization and reprocessing (EMDR) practitioners' beliefs about memory. *Psychology of Consciousness: Theory, Research, and Practice, 8(3)*, 258–273.

Janov, A. (1970). *The primal scream: Primal therapy: The cure for neurosis.* G P Putnam's Sons.

Kahneman, D. (2003). A perspective on judgment and choice: Mapping bounded rationality. *American Psychologist, 59*(9), 697–720.

Kowalski, P., & Taylor, A. K. (2009). The effect of refuting misconceptions in the introductory psychology class. *Teaching of Psychology, 36*, 153–159.

Kirsch, I. (2005). Placebo psychotherapy: Synonym or oxymoron?. *Journal of Clinical Psychology, 61*(7), 791–803. https://doi.org/10.1002/jclp.20126

Layard, R., & Clark, D. M. (2014). Thrive: The power of evidence-based psychological therapies. Penguin UK.

Lewandowsky, S., Ecker, U. K., Seifert, C. M., Schwarz, N., & Cook, J. (2012). Misinformation and its correction continued influence and successful debiasing. *Psychological Science in the Public Interest, 13*, 106–131.

Lilienfeld, S.O. (2002). Our raison d'Etre. The Scientific Review of Mental Health Practice, 1(1), 1–5.

Lilienfeld, S. O. (2005). The 10 commandments of helping students distinguish science from pseudoscience in psychology. *APS Observer, 18*(9). https://www.psychologicalscience.org/observer/the-10-commandments-of-helping-students-distinguish-science-from-pseudoscience-in-psychology?science%3Fof%3Fself%3Freport

Lilienfeld, S. O. (2007). Psychological treatments that cause harm. *Perspectives on Psychological Science, 2*, 53–70.

Lilienfeld, S. O. (2011). Distinguishing scientific from pseudoscientific psychotherapies: Evaluating the role of theoretical plausibility, with a little help from Reverend Bayes. *Clinical Psychology: Science and Practice, 18*(2), 105. https://doi.org/10.1111/j.1468-2850.2011.01241.x

Lilienfeld, S. O. (2012). Public skepticism of psychology: Why many people perceive the study of human behavior as unscientific. *American Psychologist, 67*(2), 111.

Lilienfeld, S. O. (2017). Psychology's replication crisis and the grant culture: Righting the ship. *Perspectives on Psychological Science, 12*, 660–664.

Lilienfeld, S. O., & Basterfield, C. (2020). Reflective practice in clinical psychology: Reflections from basic psychological science. *Clinical Psychology: Science and Practice, 27*(4), e12352.

Lilienfeld, S. O., & O'Donohue, W. T. (Eds.). (2012). *The great ideas of clinical science: 17 principles that every mental health professional should understand.* Routledge.

Lilienfeld, S. O., Ritschel, L. A., Lynn, S. J., Cautin, R. L., & Latzman, R. D. (2013). Why many clinical psychologists are resistant to evidence-based practice: Root causes and constructive remedies. *Clinical Psychology Review, 33*(7), 883–900. https://doi.org/10.1016/j.cpr.2012.09.008

Lilienfeld, S. O. (2015). Introduction to special section on pseudoscience in psychiatry. *The Canadian Journal of Psychiatry, 60*(12), 531–533

Lilienfeld, S. O., Sauvigné, K. C., Lynn, S. J., Cautin, R. L., Latzman, R. D., & Waldman, I. D. (2015). Fifty psychological and psychiatric terms to avoid: a list of inaccurate, misleading, misused, ambiguous, and logically confused words and phrases. *Frontiers in Psychology,* 1100. https://doi.org/10.3389/fpsyg.2015.01100

Lilienfeld, S. O., & Strother, A. N. (2020). Psychological measurement and the replication crisis: Four sacred cows. *Canadian Psychology/Psychologie Canadienne, 61*(4), 281.

Lilienfeld, S. O., & Waldman, I. D. (Eds.). (2017). *Psychological science under scrutiny: Recent challenges and proposed solutions.* Wiley.

Lilienfeld, S. O., Lohr, J. M., & Morier, D. (2001). The teaching of courses in the science and pseudoscience of psychology: Useful resources. *Teaching of Psychology, 28*(3), 182–191.

Lilienfeld, S. O., Lynn, S. J., & Lohr, J. (2003a). Science and pseudoscience in clinical psychology: Initial thoughts, reflections, and considerations. In S. O. Lilienfeld, J. M. Lohr, & S. J. Lynn (Eds.), *Science and pseudoscience in clinical psychology.* Guilford Press.

Lilienfeld, S. O., Lynn, S. J., & Lohr, J. (2003b). Science and pseudoscience in clinical psychology: Concluding thoughts and constructive remedies. In S. O. Lilienfeld, J. M. Lohr, & S. J. Lynn (Eds.), *Science and pseudoscience in clinical psychology.* Guilford Press.

Lilienfeld, S. O., Fowler, K., Lohr, J., & Lynn, S. J. (2005). Pseudoscience, nonscience, and nonsense in clinical psychology: Dangers and remedies. In N. Cummings & G. Koocher (Eds.), *Destructive trends in mental health: The well-intentioned road to hell.* Brunner/Routledge.

Lilienfeld, S. O., Ruscio, J., & Lynn, S. J. (Eds.). (2008). *Navigating the mindfield: A guide to separating science from pseudoscience in mental health.* Prometheus Books.

Lilienfeld, S. O., Lynn, S., Ruscio, J., & Beyerstein, B. L. (2010a). *50 great myths of popular psychology: Shattering widespread misconceptions about human behavior.* Wiley-Blackwell.

Lilienfeld, S. O., Lynn, S. J., Ruscio, J., & Beyerstein, B. (2010b). The top ten myths of popular psychology. *Scientific American Mind.* (Invited).

Lilienfeld, S. O., Lynn, S. J., Ruscio, J., & Beyerstein, B. L. (2010c). Mythbusting in introductory psychology courses: The whys and the hows. *Excellence in Teaching, Chapter, 11*, 55–61.

Lilienfeld, S. O., Lynn, S. J., O'Donohue, W. T., & Latzman, R. D. (2017). Epistemic humility: An overarching educational philosophy for clinical psychology programs. *Clinical Psychologist, 70*, 6–14.

Lilienfeld, S. O., Ritschel, L. A., Lynn, S. J., & Latzman, R. D. (2019). The insufficiently appreciated raison d'être of evidence-based practice. In S. Dimidjian (Ed.), *Evidence-based practice in action: Bridging clinical science and intervention* (pp. 43–63). The Guilford Press.

Lilienfeld, S., Lynn, S. J., & Namy, L. (2022). *Psychology: From inquiry to understanding* (5th ed.). Pearson Higher Education.

Littrell, J. (1998). Is the reexperience of painful emotion therapeutic?. *Clinical Psychology Review, 18*(1), 71–102. https://doi.org/10.1016/S0272-7358(97)00046-9

Lynn, S. J., Lock, T. G., Myers, B., & Payne, D. G. (1997). Recalling the unrecallable: Should hypnosis be used to recover memories in psychotherapy? *Current Directions in Psychological Science, 6*(3), 79–83.

Lynn, S. J., William, T. O., & Lilienfeld, S. O. (Eds.). (2014). *Health, happiness, and well-being: Better living through psychological science.* SAGE.

Mahoney, M. J., & DeMonbreun, B. G. (1977). Psychology of the scientist: An analysis of problem-solving bias. *Cognitive Therapy and Research, 1*, 229–238.

Marshall, M., Lewis, S., Lockwood, A., Drake, R., Jones, P., & Croudace, T. (2005). Association between duration of untreated psychosis and out-come in cohorts of first-episode patients: A systematic review. *Archives of General Psychiatry, 62*, 975–983. https://doi.org/10.1001/archpsyc.62.9.975

Meehl, P. E. (1973). Why I do not attend case conferences. In P. E. Meehl (Ed.), *Psychodiagnosis: Selected papers* (pp. 225–302). University of Minnesota Press.

Meichenbaum, D., & Lilienfeld, S. O. (2018). How to spot hype in the field of psychotherapy: A 19-item checklist. *Professional Psychology: Research and Practice, 49*, 22–30.

Mercer, J., Sarner, L., & Rosa, L. (2003). *Attachment therapy on trial: The torture and death of Candace Newmaker.* Greenwood Publishing Group.

O'Donohue, W. (1989). The (even) bolder model: The clinical psychologist as metaphysician-scientist-practitioner. *American Psychologist, 44*(12), 1460.
O'Donohue, W. (2021). Are psychologists appraising research properly? Some Popperian notes regarding replication failures in psychology. *Journal of Theoretical and Philosophical Psychology, 41*(4), 233–247. https://doi.org/10.1037/teo0000179
O'Donohue, W. T., & Lilienfeld, S. O. (2012). Professional issues and evidence-based practice: The quality problem in behavioral health care. In *Handbook of evidence-based practice in clinical psychology* (Vol. 1, pp. 51–72). Wiley.
O'Donohue, W. T., & Lilienfeld, S. O. (Eds.). (2013). *Case studies in clinical psychological science: Bridging the gap from science to practice*. Oxford University Press.
O'Donohue, W. T., Lilienfeld, S. O., & Fowler, K. A. (2012). Science is an essential safeguard against human error. In *The great ideas of clinical science* (pp. 33–58). Routledge.
O'Donohue, W. T., Masuda, A., & Lilienfeld, S. O. (Eds.). (in press). *Questionable research practices and clinical psychology*. Springer.
Patihis, L., Ho, L. Y., Tingen, I. W., Lilienfeld, S. O., & Loftus, E. F. (2014). Are the "memory wars" over? A scientist-practitioner gap in beliefs about repressed memory. *Psychological Science, 25*(2), 519–530.
Popper, K. (1959). The logic of scientific discovery. Routledge Classics.
Pope, K., & Vasquez, M. (2016). *Common logical fallacies in psychology: 26 types & examples*. Retrieved from: http://kspope.com/fallacies/fallacies
Pratkanis, A. R. (Ed.). (2011). *The science of social influence: Advances and future progress*. Psychology Press.
Pronin, E., Lin, D. Y., & Ross, L. (2002). The bias blind spot: Perceptions of bias in self versus others. *Personality and Social Psychology Bulletin, 28*, 369–381.
Rosen, G. M., & Davison, G. C. (2003). Psychology should identify empirically supported principles of change (ESPs) and not credential trademarked therapies or other treatment packages. *Behavior Modification, 27*, 300–312. https://doi.org/10.1177/0145445503027003003
Rosen, G. M., Glasgow, R. E., Moore, T. E., & Barrera, M., Jr. (2015). Self-help therapy: Recent developments in the science and business of giving psychology away. In S. O. Lilienfeld, S. J. Lynn, & J. M. Lohr (Eds.), *Science and pseudoscience in clinical psychology* (pp. 245–274). The Guilford Press.
Ross, L., & Ward, A. (1995). Naive realism: Implications for misunderstanding and divergent perceptions of fairness and bias. *Values and Knowledge*, 103–135.
Sagan, C. (1995). *The demon-haunted world: Science as a candle in the dark*. Random House.
Satel, S., & Lilienfeld, S. O. (2013). *Brainwashed: The seductive appeal of mindless neuroscience*. Basic Civitas Books.
Sauerland, M., & Otgaar, H. (2021). Teaching psychology students to change (or correct) controversial beliefs about memory works. *Memory, 30*(6)1–10. https://doi.org/10.1080/09658211.2021.1874994
Sechrest, L., & Smith, B. (1994). Psychotherapy is the practice of psychology. *Journal of Psychotherapy Integration, 4*, 1–29.
Shermer, M. (2002). *Why people believe weird things: Pseudoscience, superstition, and other confusions of our time*. Holt.
Stanovich, K. E. (2018). Miserliness in human cognition: The interaction of detection, override and mindware. *Thinking & Reasoning, 24*, 423–444. https://doi.org/10.1080/13546783.2018.1459314
Stanovich, K. E., & West, R. F. (2000). Individual differences in reasoning: Implications for the rationality debate? *Behavioral and Brain Sciences, 23*(5), 645–665.
West, R. F., Meserve, R. J., & Stanovich, K. E. (2012). Cognitive sophistication does not attenuate the bias blind spot. *Journal of Personality and Social Psychology, 103*(3), 506.

Wiggins, B. J., & Christopherson, C. D. (2019). The replication crisis in psychology: An overview for theoretical and philosophical psychology. *Journal of Theoretical and Philosophical Psychology, 39*(4), 202.

Williams, A. J., Botanov, Y., Kilshaw, R. E., Wong, R. E., & Sakaluk, J. K. (2021). Potentially harmful therapies: A meta-scientific review of evidential value. *Clinical Psychology: Science and Practice, 28*(1), 5–18. https://doi.org/10.1111/cpsp.12331

Part III
Assessment and Psychopathology

Clinical and Personality Assessment: An Essay in the Honor of Scott O. Lilienfeld

Martin Sellbom, Yossef S. Ben-Porath, and Robert D. Latzman

Introduction

Assessment of personality is part of human nature. As social animals, human beings have an intrinsic need to assess and predict others' behavior to both maximize survival benefit and have a sense of social order, including development of norms and conventions. Such informal assessment is an integral component of social interaction. Individuals evaluate their peers (friends and enemies) on a variety of dimensions, including (but not limited to) friendliness, trustworthiness, emotional stability, and dangerousness, in an effort to determine who will constitute a potential threat versus who might become part of the social "herd" (or friend group) for protection, security, and in some cases, mating. Of course, this form of personality assessment is unsystematic; most people would likely not characterize their instinctive social evaluations as a form of assessment.

Clinical psychologists, including scholars and practitioners, rely on more formal approaches to personality assessment. Specifically, in this context, personality assessment refers to a systematic effort to identify an individual's personality characteristics. This information is used to describe and/or make predictions about the individual's behavior and psychological functioning. Such assessments can be idiographic or nomothetic, with the former being tailored specifically to an individual's unique attributes, whereas nomothetic assessments are conducted in reference to a group of peers. Nomothetic approaches in particular require standardized

M. Sellbom (✉)
Department of Psychology, University of Otago, Dunedin, New Zealand
e-mail: martin.sellbom@otago.ac.nz

Y. S. Ben-Porath
Kent State University, Kent, OH, USA

R. D. Latzman
Takeda Pharmaceuticals, Cambridge Massachusetts, Cambridge, USA

C. L. Cobb et al. (eds.), *Toward a Science of Clinical Psychology*,
https://doi.org/10.1007/978-3-031-14332-8_8

procedures, which are needed to generalize normative data comparisons of an individual to a larger group. This requirement is particularly relevant to psychological testing, which is an ingredient of a formal clinical assessment; tests have uniform rules about administration scoring and interpretation.

Assessment and testing are terms often used interchangeably, but need to be differentiated in important ways (American Educational Research Association [AERA], American Psychological Association [APA], & National Council on Measurement in Education [NCME], 2014). Assessment refers to the process of using scientifically grounded methods to collect, interpret, integrate, and report data pertaining to various aspects of psychological functioning. Testing, on the other hand, is the process of administering, scoring, and interpreting scientifically grounded, standardized procedures for measuring psychological constructs. Tests are typically part of a broader assessment.

The aim of the current chapter is to provide an introduction to clinical personality assessment. We will cover historical precursors to assessment psychology and discuss important issues pertaining to the clinical assessment process. Because psychological testing is a critical ingredient in the assessment process, and the assessment of personality is particularly important to the late Scott Lilienfeld's scholarly legacy, we will cover such testing with particular emphasis. We will provide a basic introduction to scale construction, including how one particular approach resulted in one of Lilienfeld's major contributions in the personality assessment area. We will also describe basic psychometric principles of reliability and construct validity, which are critical to evaluating psychological tests.

A Brief History of Personality Assessment

Ben-Porath and Butcher (1991) identified three primary personality assessment techniques and differentiated between them based on the means and sources used for data collection. Behavioral observations include methods in which personality is assessed by systematically recorded observations of an individual's behavior. Examples include Cattell's (1965, 1979) T (systematic experimentation) and L (behavioral observation) data. Somatic examinations consist of techniques that rely on some form of physical measurement as the basis for assessing psychological functioning. Examples include various psychophysiological measures (e.g., Keller et al., 2000). Verbal examinations rely on verbalizations (oral, written, or a combination of the two) produced by the individual being assessed or another person who presumably knows the assessment target. Self-report inventories and projective or performance-based assessment techniques (e.g., the Rorschach Inkblot Method about which Lilienfeld had much to say; e.g., Lilienfeld et al., 2000) also fall under this definition. Because verbal examinations, and in particular self-report inventories (SRIs), have evolved as the primary methods of clinical personality assessment, we focus on this mode of personality assessment in our historical overview.

Ben-Porath and Butcher (1991) traced the early origins of verbal examinations to an elaborate system of competitive examinations (described in detail by Dubois, 1970) used for over 3000 years to select personnel for the Chinese civil service. Candidates for government positions were tested (and retested every three years) to determine their suitability for these prestigious appointments. Examinees were required to write essays for hours at a time, over several successive days. The essays were used (among other purposes) to gauge the candidates' character and fitness for office (DuBois, 1970), portending modern employment-related applications of clinical personality assessment.

In the modern era, Sir Francis Galton was the first to suggest and try out systematic procedures for measuring psychological variables based on verbalizations (as well as some novel approaches to behavioral observations). Influenced heavily by the writings of his cousin, Charles Darwin, Galton was interested in devising precise methods for measuring individual differences in mental traits he believed were the product of evolution. Laying the foundations for quantitative approaches to personality assessment, Galton wrote:

> We want lists of facts, every one of which may be separately verified, valued, and revalued, and the whole accurately summed. It is the statistics of each man's conduct in small everyday affairs that will probably be found to give the simplest and most precise measure of his character. (Galton, 1884, p. 185)

Most of Galton's efforts to elicit such information through verbalizations focused on devising various associative tasks, some of which evolved into modern sentence completion inventories.

The Dutch scholars Heymans and Wiersma (1906) were the first to devise a questionnaire for personality assessment. They constructed a 90-item rating scale and asked some 3000 physicians to use the scale to describe people with whom they were well acquainted. Based upon correlations they found among the trait ratings, Heymans and Wiersma, in essence, developed a crude, hierarchical, factor-analytically generated personality model. They proposed that individuals may be described in terms of their standing on eight lower-order traits: Amorphous, Apathetic, Nervous, Sentimental, Sanguine, Phlegmatic, Choleric, and Impassioned. These traits consisted, in turn, of various combinations of three higher-order traits labeled Activity, Emotionality, and Primary versus Secondary Function. This structure bears substantial similarity to Eysenck's three-factor (Extraversion, Neuroticism, and Psychopathy) personality model (Eysenck & Eysenck, 1975) and the three higher-order factors of Tellegen's (1982; Tellegen & Waller, 2008) Multidimensional Personality Questionnaire.

Hoch and Amsden (1913) and Wells (1914) provided further elaboration on the Heymans and Wiersma (1906) model's utility for personality description and assessment by adding to it various psychopathology symptoms. Their work, in turn, laid the foundations for the first systematic effort to develop a self-report personality questionnaire, Woodworth's (1920) Personal Data Sheet. Woodworth developed the Personal Data Sheet to assist in identifying psychoneurotic individuals who were unfit for duty in the US military during World War I. This need arose because of the large number of combat personnel who had developed "shell shock" during the conflict. The questionnaire was to be used as a screening instrument so that recruits who exceeded a certain threshold would be referred for follow-up examinations.

DuBois (1970) reported that Woodworth initially compiled hundreds of "neurotic" items from various sources as candidates for inclusion on his questionnaire. Candidate items were selected if their content was judged to be potentially relevant to identifying neurosis. Items were phrased in question form, and test takers were instructed to answer "yes" or "no" to indicate whether each item described them accurately. Woodworth conducted a series of empirical investigations and eliminated items answered "yes" by large numbers of normal individuals. The final questionnaire consisted of 116 items. All were keyed such that a "yes" response was an indication of psychoneurosis. Although the Personal Data Sheet was never used for the purposes for which it was constructed—the war had ended by the time it was completed—both its items and Woodworth's reliance (in part) on empirical analyses for its construction served as the cornerstones for most subsequent self-report personality inventories.

With the conclusion of World War I, Woodworth abandoned his test development efforts and refocused his attention on experimental psychology. However, a number of researchers in the then-novel subdiscipline of personality psychology followed in his footsteps. Downey's (1923) Will-Temperament tests, Travis's (1925) Diagnostic Character Test, Heidbreder's (1926) Extraversion-Introversion test, Thurstone's (1930) Personality Schedule, and Allport's (1928) Ascendance-Submission measure were among the more prominent early successors to Woodworth's efforts.

Many of these efforts set the stage for contemporary personality assessment, with Hathaway and McKinley's (1943) Minnesota Multiphasic Personality Inventory (MMPI) laying the foundation for a new age of objective and empirical approaches to scale development and assessment. The MMPI assessed contemporary psychiatric syndromes, quickly became a standard for clinical personality assessment instruments, and has inspired subsequent modern developments in this field.

General Principles and Issues in Clinical Personality Assessment

Various clinical personality assessment techniques differ (to lesser and greater degrees) in terms of what they seek to assess, the sources of information they rely upon, how this information is obtained, and how it is interpreted. We discuss each of these topics in this section and end with a discussion of what constitutes evidence-based assessment.

Categorical vs Dimensional Assessment

The primary distinction in terms of what clinical personality instruments assess is between those that focus on typological versus dimensional constructs. Use of typology-based techniques is predicated on the notion that individuals may be classified into categorical types. In the area of psychopathology, most of the disorders classified with the Diagnostic and Statistical Manual of Mental Disorders, Fifth Edition (DSM-5; American Psychiatric Association, 2013), and assessed with structured interviews fall within the typological approach. For example, an individual is classified as having Schizophrenia if their symptomatic pattern is consistent with an explicit set of criteria spelled out for this condition. In some instances (e.g., Major Depression), following categorical classification, a severity rating may be applied; however, the diagnosis itself is categorical in nature.

In the domain of self-report inventories, a primary example of a typological framework is represented by the MMPI/MMPI-2 code types. As recounted by Ben-Porath and Sellbom (2023), soon after the MMPI was developed, it became clear that owing to excessive false positives, the original Clinical Scales of the inventory could not be used to differentially diagnose specific psychiatric disorders directly as the test developers, Hathaway and McKinley (1943), had intended. Instead, led by the efforts of Paul Meehl (e.g., 1956), a method for classifying test-takers into various code types based on their pattern of MMPI Clinical Scale scores was developed and became the primary interpretation method of the MMPI.

In typological assessment, once type membership (e.g., Schizophrenia, or a 27/72 MMPI code-type) is established, the individual's personality and clinical functioning can be described based on empirically identified correlates of a given type. For example, the DSM-5 includes information about a range of diagnostic features, associated features, prevalence rates, developmental course, risk and prognostic factors, suicide risk, and functional consequences related to the disorder. In the case of the MMPI/MMPI-2 code types, a broad range of personality characteristics, psychopathology symptoms, and behavioral proclivities identified through empirical research could be attributed to individuals classified as having a 27/72 code type (Graham, 2012).

Dimensional assessments emerged from the individual differences tradition or the field of differential psychology. This approach began with the work of Francis Galton, described earlier in this chapter. Trait psychologist Gordon Allport played a critical role in the development of dimensionally focused assessment. Allport (1931) posited that psychological traits, though not necessarily physical entities, are nonetheless real attributes of persons that can explain behavior rather than simply describe it. Like many subsequent dimensional models, Allport's conceptualization of traits was hierarchical. Specifically, he distinguished between *Cardinal Dispositions* (e.g., narcissism), which tend to dominate the individual's behavior; *Central Dispositions*, a relatively small number of traits that tend to be highly characteristic of the individual (e.g., conscientiousness); and *Secondary Dispositions*, which only influence behavior under certain circumstances (e.g., political attitudes).

Allport viewed traits as more than simply generalized habits. For example, repeated behaviors such as brushing one's teeth are not sufficient to qualify as traits, whereas cleanliness, which includes brushing one's teeth among other behaviors, can be viewed as a trait. Consistent with his hierarchical perspective, Allport viewed traits as only relatively independent of each other. He also viewed traits as not synonymous with moral judgments, and therefore not evaluative in nature. Finally, in an elaboration of his views on traits, Allport (1966) emphasized that specific behaviors that are inconsistent with traits are not evidence of their absence.

A significant strain of Allport's trait psychology research involved a search for the structure of personality. His work and that of others who followed in his footsteps in this area was guided by three primary assumptions: (1) That a broad range of behavioral tendencies could be reduced to a smaller number of traits that influence these behaviors; (2) that the scientific discovery of traits and the associations among them can be guided by structural examination of natural language trait descriptors (the Lexical Hypothesis); and (3) that the resulting structure will likely be hierarchical. Implications of these assumptions were that a potential source for trait descriptors is the dictionary. That is, empirical research on the structure of personality can rely on adjectives extracted from the dictionary and that the proper data analytic technique for such research was factor analysis. Implementation of this approach led Allport and Odbert (1936) to conduct a comprehensive analysis of words they extracted from an English-language dictionary, which they distilled to a set of approximately 4500 trait descriptors.

Allport and colleagues' list of trait descriptors set the framework for the dimensional and hierarchical structure of personality that has since evolved into more contemporary models. Arguably the most recognizable and accepted framework is the five-factor model (FFM) of personality or "Big 5" (Goldberg, 1990; Norman, 1963; see Tupes & Cristal, 1961 for the original work) that represents the higher order structure of personality domains reflecting neuroticism (vs. emotional stability), extraversion (vs. introversion), openness to experience (vs. rigidity), agreeableness (vs. antagonism), and conscientiousness (vs. disinhibition). The FFM, which was derived empirically via factor analyses of the aforementioned trait descriptors, has influenced subsequent theoretical accounts of personality (e.g., McCrae & Costa, 1999) as well as models of maladaptive personality and clinical psychopathology. For instance, the personality disorder trait model described in the DSM-5 Alternative Model for Personality Disorders (APA, 2013) reflects a maladaptive variant of the FFM. Further, a recent contemporary approach to organizing psychopathology dimensionally and hierarchically, the Hierarchical Taxonomy of Psychopathology (HiTOP; Kotov et al., 2017, 2021), has a structure that is similarly linked (albeit imperfectly) to the FFM (Widiger et al., 2019). The dimensional perspective is gaining more and more ground in the conception of mental disorders and mental health assessment.

Sources of Information and Interpretation

Typological and dimensional assessments rely on several information sources. As mentioned earlier, the most common among these are self-descriptions, which most often are elicited via questionnaires or interviews. The unstructured clinical interview is the primary ingredient in any psychological assessment (e.g., Lewis et al., 2021; Sommers-Flanagan et al., 2020), which serves to orient the assessment, provides for establishing a therapeutic working relationship with the person being evaluated, and allows for flexible questioning of psychosocial background and clinical symptomology. However, most evidence-based practices of assessment (see subsequent section) require multiple sources of information. Other self-reported information such as structured clinical interviews to more reliably assess various diagnostic constructs and self-report questionnaires for a more quantitative appraisal of clinical symptoms and personality traits are often preferred (e.g., Suhr & Sellbom, 2020).

Others' descriptions of the individual, obtained via the same sources, are less common, but are used to some extent. Collateral informant reports by parents and/or teachers tend to be more common for children who are less able to reliably self-report (e.g., Achenbach et al., 2020). Behavioral samples, obtained via observations that may be structured or unstructured, are also used in clinical assessment of personality and psychopathology. Performance-based assessment techniques are also used to collect important information. In cognitive assessment, various tests of maximum performance to determine neuropsychological functions, including intellectual abilities, are frequently used (Suhr & Angers, 2020). Although less commonly used in contemporary assessments, individuals' responses to ambiguous stimuli (e.g.., the ten Rorschach cards), thought to reflect various aspects of psychological functioning, are the basis of "typical" performance-based assessment techniques (Meyer & Mihura, 2020).

Two general data interpretation approaches, one clinically guided and the other empirical, are used in clinical personality assessment. Clinical interpretation tends to be impressionistic and is guided primarily by the clinician's experience, which may be grounded in theory. Clinical interpretation tends to be typological, involving impression-based typological classification and description that stems from the clinician's experience with that "type." Empirically guided interpretation, sometimes referred to as statistical, as implied by its label, is based on empirical findings of associations between test scores and relevant extra-test criteria. Its strictest form allows no role for clinical experiences or impressions in the interpretation of assessment findings. This approach can be applied to both dimensional and typological variables. Finally, clinical and empirical interpretations are not mutually exclusive. The same set of assessment data can be interpreted based both on empirical correlates and clinical experience.

Evidence-Based Principles of Assessment

Scott Lilienfeld was a champion of evidence-based practice in clinical psychology. Most of his focus on this domain was on psychological treatments (e.g., Lilienfeld et al., 2013, 2014, 2017) and a specific assessment method, the Rorschach Inkblot Method, and other performance-based (or projective) techniques (e.g., Lilienfeld et al., 2000). Although he did not contribute extensively to the literature on broader evidence-based assessment models, specifically (but see Garb et al., 2009), we believe he would have agreed that such models are critical to the practice of clinical psychology.

Numerous scholars have written about evidence-based practice in assessment (e.g., Arbisi & Beck, 2016; Bornstein, 2017; Hunsley & Mash, 2007; McFall, 2005). An evidence-based psychological assessment should be as efficient as possible, using methods with sufficient levels of reliability and validity to provide the psychologist and client with the information they need to address the referral question (Barlow, 2005). McFall (2005) indicated that to be able to conduct such evaluations, psychologists must first examine the tools at their disposal, focusing on both theory and utility. A sound theoretical model provides a solid foundation on which to base a psychological assessment and allows the psychologist to draw informative conclusions about a client. It is vital that each method or instrument adequately and accurately captures the theory or construct that it is intended to measure. For example, if the goal of a particular assessment was to determine whether an individual has a depressive disorder, the psychologist would have to know which constructs or symptoms to assess to answer this question. Measures should evidence both convergent validity (positive associations with conceptually similar constructs [e.g., hallucinations and delusions]) and discriminant validity (limited association with conceptually distinct constructs [e.g., depression and anxiety]). If a component of an assessment does not provide information relevant to the goal of answering the referral question, it is not appropriate for use in an evidence-based approach. Second, McFall (2005) emphasized the importance of evaluating the utility of psychological assessment methods and instruments. When a component of a psychological assessment adds information above and beyond what can be gained from other components, it is said to have incremental validity (Sechrest, 1963). However, the clinical utility evidence for psychological assessment continues to be understudied (e.g., Garb et al., 2009; Hunsley & Mash, 2007), though Bagby et al. (2016) reviewed the literature on how personality assessment might be useful in understanding psychotherapy outcomes.

More recently, a special series of papers in *Clinical Psychology: Science and Practice* (Arbisi & Beck, 2016) attempted to outline evidence-based practices for child (Youngstrom & Van Meter, 2016), forensic, (Archer et al. 2016), treatment (Bagby et al., 2016), and health (Butt, 2016) contexts. Sellbom and Hopwood (2016) provided generally positive comments about the progress of evidence-based assessment models in these various domains, but also opined that an underlying theme seemed to remain that these areas require further development. They concluded with the hope that "EBAs continue to develop across populations and settings that careful thought is considered with respect to (a) exactly what is being assessed, and (b) how valid innovative methods can be best integrated into psychological practice" (p. 408).

Most recently, Bornstein (2017) proposed a unified framework for evidence-based psychological assessment. More specifically, he articulated nine principles for operationalizing and implementing such, which covered the American Psychological Association's (2006) three pillars of evidence-based practice in psychology. He made the following nine points:

1. Psychologists need to have sufficient proficiency in assessment, including training in psychometrics, clinical utility, consideration of culture, and effective communication.
2. Psychologists should remain current on the theoretical and scientific advancements on the constructs they seek to assess, which should be incorporated into decisions about assessment methodology.
3. Psychologists should use empirically validated assessment instruments, and particularly those that meet design criteria for "universal tests." Such tests have been sufficiently developed and validated with consideration devoted to culture and diversity.
4. Psychologists should only interpret test scores to assess variables and outcomes with a sufficient validity base using populations to which the test-taker could be considered a member. Such evidence is important for members of cultural minority groups as well.
5. Psychologists should whenever possible use multiple methods of assessment for a given construct. They should describe the rationale for selecting each instrument and consider incremental validity evidence (i.e., empirical evidence that the methods account for unique variance in the outcome variables).
6. Psychologists should be prepared to discuss assessment method convergences and divergences carefully. Bornstein (2017) specifically commented on the fact that some methods assessing the same construct, with independent evidence for validity support, do not converge strongly (e.g., parent and teacher reports; self-report and performance-based tests). He recommended that psychologists consider divergences via the different "processes" by which information is collected (e.g., self-reported responses vs. informant reports).
7. Psychologists should self-monitor throughout the assessment process to avoid excessive reliance on heuristics (e.g., representativeness, anchoring; Tversky & Kahneman, 1974), cognitive biases (e.g., confirmation bias), and stereotypes in the evaluation of assessment data. Bornstein recommended that psychologists seek consultation as needed.
8. Psychologists should consider the "synergistic interaction" (p. 442) between clinician and client throughout the process and potential influences of these interactions on both assessment data and their interpretation.
9. Psychologists should communicate assessment results to all stakeholders using language appropriate for the person receiving the feedback. Bornstein (2017)

further argued that psychologists should communicate in a way that engages the client and facilitates growth and positive change.

From our perspective, multimethod assessment is particularly important. In many clinical contexts in which time is scarce, an unstructured clinical interview is the primary source of information. Unstructured clinical interviews do not meet the aforementioned criteria for evidence-based forms of assessment. Moreover, decades of clinical judgment research have shown subjective data sources to be inferior to objective methods and statistical approaches in the prediction of outcomes (e.g., Garb, 2005). However, as Hunsley and Mash (2007) noted, some clinical judgment is necessary to synthesize various sources of information. We argue that a good clinical assessment adheres to the general framework proposed by Bornstein and considers psychological test data, available school and medical records, collateral interviews, in addition to clinical interviews (Suhr & Sellbom, 2020). Also, whenever possible, psychologists should evaluate response bias for any self-reported data (see Ben-Porath, 2013, for a model); such assessment is critical in contexts in which an external incentive exists, such as forensic or pre-employment evaluations (Suhr & Sellbom, 2020).

Summary

Contemporary personality assessment principles typically assess psychological constructs from either typological (e.g., categorical diagnosis) or dimensional, individual differences perspectives. Numerous potential sources of information should be considered in assessment practice, including clinical interviews, psychological testing, collateral sources, and records. Evidence-based practices require multiple sources of information in addition to identifications of methods of sufficient reliability and validity, gaining and maintaining competence in the practice of psychological assessment, and good communication of assessment findings. The next major section of this chapter will consider psychological tests specifically with a focus on scale development issues and psychometric evaluation.

Development of Psychological Assessment Methods

Evidence-based scale construction is at the heart of evidence-based psychological assessment. Indeed, as noted by Clark and Watson (2019), measurement is fundamental in science as it is only with sound measurement that one can make meaningful inferences critical to clinical utility. In this section, we review two contemporary approaches to scale construction, including one deductive approach that places construct validity at the center of emphasis originally championed by Loevinger (1957) and more recently by Clark and Watson (1995, 2019), and a second more inductive approach that allows for the elaboration of theoretical constructs through scale construction. This latter approach was favored by Scott Lilienfeld in the development of the Psychopathic Personality Inventory (PPI, 1990; Lilienfeld & Andrews, 1996), which we will use as an example.

Construct Validity Approach

Central to making inferences about psychological functioning through systematic assessment is ensuring that measurement tools have strong support for validity, generally, and construct validity more specifically; validity is the most fundamental consideration in developing and evaluating assessment methods (AERA/APA/NCME, 2014; Cronbach & Meehl, 1955; Clark & Watson, 2019). Scale construction from this perspective is deductive or rational (Burisch, 1984) in that a clear a priori theoretical explication of a psychological construct guides scale development. Loevinger's (1957) monograph, published over 60 years ago, remains the sine qua non for a complete description of the foundation of evidence-based psychological measure creation. More recently, Clark and Watson (1995, 2019) have provided updated, practical guidance on how best to implement Loevinger's theoretical scheme in the context of various advancements in clinical and personality psychology assessment. Specifically, Clark and Watson (1995, 2019) emphasize three aspects of construct validity critical to the application of Loevinger's framework for evidence-based psychological assessment development: substantive, structural, and external.

Substantive validity includes ensuring that one has a clear conceptualization of the target construct(s) of interest. It is imperative that one has a comprehensive, thorough, and clear conceptual model from the onset. This conceptualization should be explicitly embedded within the existing empirical and theoretical literature, both directly relevant and more distal to the construct of interest. It is only with such a conceptualization in hand that one is best situated to move to the item-writing phase. It is important for the initial item pool to be overinclusive, ensuring that all potential aspects of the construct are captured, and that one pays careful attention to item wording.

After an exhaustive, over-inclusive item pool has been generated, one that is well-situated within the broader literature, the scale developer must next move to structural validity considerations. Such considerations begin with deciding upon a test construction strategy or item-selection strategy. Although Loevinger (1957) originally described three main conceptual models (i.e., quantitative/dimensional, class models, and more complex dynamic models), a robust literature has demonstrated that, with very rare exceptions, dimensional models fit the data best. Initial data collection must then be undertaken to begin the iterative psychometric evaluation process of scientifically grounded scale construction. This involves preliminary measure development, data collection, and psychometric evaluation, followed by additional cycles of revision of both the measure and, when appropriate, the focal construct. This process is then followed by additional data collection, psychometric evaluation, and, if needed, revision. Importantly, this necessarily implies that the validation process never formally ends resulting in the continuous elaboration of constructs and improvement of measures as the literature accumulates.

In addition to substantive and structural validity work, external validity is the third aspect of construct validity. Once strong psychometric properties of an instrument have been established, work can shift to explicit consideration of the way in which the construct of interest, as assessed by this specific scale, is situated within the immediate and broader nomological net (Cronbach & Meehl, 1955). All told, and as Clark and Watson (1995) and Clark and Watson (2019) conclude, a well-conceptualized construct, clearly situated within the theoretical and empirical literature, along with an evidence-based iterative scale construction process, is critical for scientifically rigorous scale construction. Only with assessment of constructs of interest using scales developed in this way can the science of psychology, generally, and personality psychology specifically, advance.

This construct validity approach described by Loevinger, and elaborated by Clark and Watson, is clearly evident in the development and ongoing validation efforts of the Inventory of Depression and Anxiety Symptoms (IDAS; Watson et al., 2007). Following a thorough review of the relevant literature resulting in well-conceptualized constructs clearly situated within the extant literature, the IDAS was developed to assess specific symptom dimensions of major depression and related anxiety disorders. Items were carefully written to cast a wide net, were refined through a series of internal consistency and factor analyses across multiple large samples, including both clinical and non-clinical samples, and psychometric properties of IDAS scales were confirmed in subsequently collected data from samples not included in the scale development process (Watson et al., 2007). Consistent with the iterative nature of construct validation (i.e., construct validity as an ongoing process), following the publication of the IDAS, extensive structural analyses performed on large samples resulted in the construction of the IDAS-II (Watson et al., 2012), an expanded version of the original IDAS. Overall, the IDAS is a good example of a scientifically strong instrument resulting from a rigorous scale construction process.

Exploring Psychological Constructs Through Scale Construction

A second approach to scale construction, which was favored by Scott Lilienfeld (e.g., Costello et al., 2021; Lilienfeld & Andrews, 1996), begins with an inductive process (Burisch, 1984; Cattell, 1950) as opposed to the more deductive-rational scale construction paradigm described previously. This scale construction paradigm was most prominently articulated by Auke Tellegen (e.g., Tellegen, 1982; Tellegen & Waller, 2008) in the construction of the Multidimensional Personality

Questionnaire (MPQ), which yielded a personality trait theory consisting of 11 primary traits with three higher order domains (positive emotionality, negative emotionality, and constraint). More specifically, when examining psychological constructs or sets of constructs for which the boundaries are not well articulated, the test construction process allows for the psychological constructs themselves to evolve and become better defined. In this way, the test construction process takes an exploratory approach, but one that is self-correcting, as sequential test revisions and data collections allow for a better articulated set of constructs and associated item pools. Cattell (1950) referred to this process as the *inductive-hypothetico-deductive spiral* in which the initial exploratory approach allowed for further hypothesis testing and subsequent deductive reasoning in finalizing constructs and scales.

The reader should not confuse words like *exploratory* and *inductive* with atheoretical. Tellegen and Waller (2008) make clear that the approach does not lack theoretical direction; it is merely *bi*-directional. The scale developer has psychological constructs in mind, which guide the item pool that is assembled, which casts a wide net of theoretically relevant items to capture these constructs. The initial data collection and associated analyses, however, allow for the refining of psychological constructs and scales, and perforce moves theory forward. It is important to note that this approach requires multiple sequential instances of data collection and test item revision before the process is completed.

The primary statistical technique used in this scale construction approach is exploratory factor analysis (EFA). We describe EFA in detail in the next section of this chapter. EFA allows for determining the natural structure of items within the pool through examination of their intercorrelations. A higher order structure allows for articulating specifically how these items hang together in forming constructs, preferably replicated across samples. The data may ultimately reveal a structure that is not consistent with the original target constructs, and the set of constructs are redefined accordingly.

As mentioned earlier, a good example of this approach is Lilienfeld's Psychopathic Personality Inventory (PPI; Lilienfeld, 1990; Lilienfeld & Andrews, 1996). Lilienfeld developed the PPI as part of his doctoral dissertation at the University of Minnesota. At the time, there was only one viable operationalization of the concept of psychopathic personality, the Psychopathy Checklist (PCL; Hare, 1980; later revised into PCL-R; Hare, 1991/2003), which attempted to target Hervey Cleckley's (1941) classic description. Psychopathy was not a well-defined concept at the time, with numerous theories, and the PCL-R (a clinician-rating form based on interview and institutional records) had been developed for assessment of prisoners with a substantial emphasis on antisocial and criminal behaviors, which made it unsuitable for the assessment of psychopathy in community populations. Because of the fuzzy boundaries associated with the psychopathy concept, Lilienfeld took an exploratory scale construction approach in which he identified 24 different personality constructs relevant to a host of psychopathy theories. The scale construction procedure covered three rounds of item writing and data collection using undergraduate student samples. Subsequent factor analyses of the item pools across studies ultimately revealed eight rather distinct psychopathic personality traits that were labeled

Machiavellian egocentricity, social potency, coldheartedness, carefree nonplanfulness, fearlessness, blame externalization, impulsive nonconformity, and stress immunity. Along with a PPI total score, these served as the primary scales on the PPI until further revisions of the instrument (e.g., Lilienfeld & Widows, 2005).

Evaluation of Assessment Methods

The psychometric evaluation of assessment methods is key in evidence-based assessment practice. Psychometrics is important because it allows clinical psychologists to evaluate the merits of the psychological tests they are using to measure such constructs. Empirically validated methods, including assessments (e.g., Arbisi & Beck, 2016), are critically important to clinical psychology practice. Some psychologists are involved in research. In such contexts, they must be called upon to defend their operationalizations of the psychological constructs they are studying. In this section, we will consider the evaluation of reliability, which includes various approaches to evaluating the degree of measurement error associated with test scores. We will also discuss the evaluation of internal structure, which is commonplace in psychological assessment research. Finally, we will cover various approaches to evaluating the validity of test scores as well their utility for decision-making purposes. We conclude with examples drawn from Lilienfeld's scholarship.

Reliability

All operationalizations of theoretical constructs have measurement error. No theoretical entity can be measured perfectly, at least in psychology. Therefore, test scores are always an approximation of the construct we aim to assess. The concept of reliability refers to the accuracy of construct measurement. More specifically, *classical test theory* (e.g., Nunnally & Bernstein, 1967) assumes that every observed score on a measure is composed of the "true" score and random error variance. The true score only refers to the expected value of the distribution of the repeatedly measured values and is implied to be the target property being measured (Novick, 1966); it does not refer to whether the target itself is being adequately measured, which is related to validity. Thus, there are two forms of measurement error, unsystematic and systematic. The former is random and can thus not be correlated with anything else and impacts reliability. Systematic error, on the other hand, is reliable variance that is unrelated to the target construct being measured and affects validity. In this section, we will first consider reliability.

Reliability is conceptually defined as the proportion of the total variance in test scores that is true score variance (Revelle & Condon, 2019). In reality, as typically estimated, it is actually the proportion of total variance that is systematic (i.e., non-random) and shared among test items. A higher reliability coefficient indicates that variability in the observed scores is less affected by random measurement error. Four reliability estimates are commonly used in assessment research: internal consistency reliability, test-retest reliability, alternative forms reliability, and inter-rater reliability. It is important to note that these are imperfect estimates of reliability. Because all reliability estimates come with limiting assumptions about the true score variance, the degree to which these assumptions are unmet will inform the degree to which the reliability estimate will be an underestimate of actual test score reliability.

Test-Retest Reliability This form of reliability is commonly estimated by calculating the correlation coefficient of the observed scores at two separate time points. A higher correlation between the values of the two test occasions indicates greater reliability. Test-retest reliability assumes that the true score is identical at both time points. Indeed, the relative position of an individual's score in the distribution of the population should be the same over a brief time period (Revelle & Condon, 2019). The degree to which this assumption is not met (e.g., fluctuations in actual construct levels over time; effects of re-testing), the test-retest coefficient will reflect an underestimate of reliability.

Alternate Forms Reliability Alternate forms reliability, also known as the equivalence coefficient (Geisinger, 2013), is based on two or more forms of the same test. Each form is perceived as a measure of the same construct and, additionally, the different forms are assumed to measure the same construct equally well. The error variance is contributed to by the variability among the forms. Alternate forms are generated by changing the wording of the same statement, changing the way to ask the same questions, or changing the order of questions/items (Revelle & Condon, 2017). When assessing alternate forms reliability, the two or more forms of a test are administered to the individuals on the same occasion or different occasions with a short time interval. Alternate forms reliability is estimated by computing the correlation between the measured values from the multiple forms. Similar to test-retest reliability, the application of alternate forms reliability is restricted by assumptions of having independent and identical administrations. In addition, in practice it is often challenging to generate perfectly equivalent forms. For this reason, only specialized fields, such as achievement testing in which alternate forms can be constructed at identical difficulty levels across the range of the construct being measured, tend to make use of alternate forms reliability.

Inter-rater Reliability Inter-rater reliability is estimated in contexts in which assessment approaches rely on subjective judgment. Inter-rater reliability makes use of multiple raters that review the same information (e.g., a clinical interview) and make independent ratings on a construct of interest (e.g., presence of a mental disorder). The error variance comes from the variability among the evaluations of different assessors. When two raters evaluate all targets, the easiest way is to compute the proportion of the targets that have the same categorization rated by the two assessors (e.g., presence of mental disorder). However, a better way is to account for the base rate of category assignments and consider cases where agreement among the raters is expected by chance (e.g., just guessing presence or absence results in 50% agreement) and estimate reliability based on the difference between the observed agreement and the rate of agreement by chance. Cohen's kappa (Cohen, 1960) is the commonly used approach when there are two assessors. When there are more than two assessors, Fleiss's kappa (Fleiss, 1971) can be used.

When the test scores are on an ordinal or interval scale level (e.g., scores on a Vocabulary task on an intelligence measure), inter-rater reliability does not focus on the proportion of agreement among raters (i.e., the scores provided by different assessors to be the same), but on the targets' relative positions in the distribution. A more conservative approach can take absolute score levels into account as well (i.e., in addition to rank-order agreement on individuals' Vocabulary scores are the actual magnitude of scores also in agreement). The intra-class correlation (ICC) coefficient is a common index used in these analyses. There are different forms of ICC, and their calculations are based on the analysis of different sources of variance depending on the design and assumptions (Koo & Li, 2016; Shrout & Fleiss, 1979). Their selection and use primarily depend on whether the same property is assessed by all assessors or a subset of assessors (see, e.g., Koo & Li, 2016, for a detailed discussion).

Internal Consistency Reliability The most common method of estimating reliability in personality assessment research is internal consistency, which indicates the extent to which a set of items on a scale is measuring a coherent construct. The set of items is assumed to be a random sample of all possible items for the target construct (Revelle & Condon, 2019). The items should therefore be meaningfully correlated with one another to reflect the same underlying construct. The non-shared variability among the items thus reflects the error variance among replications (Revelle & Condon, 2019). The two most well-known methods using this approach in the context of classical test theory are KR20 (Kuder & Richardson, 1937) for dichotomous item responses and coefficient alpha (Guttman, 1945; Cronbach, 1951) for continuous responses. Both methods consider the average inter-correlation among the items and are influenced by the number of items sampled, with more observations increasing the confidence in the estimate (Revelle & Condon, 2019).

These classical approaches to estimate internal consistency reliability come with important limitations. First, the reliability coefficients assume the underlying items are all measuring the same unidimensional construct, which makes them potentially problematic estimates for multidimensional constructs. Second, a scale score can have a low alpha coefficient (despite an acceptable average inter-item correlation) due to its brevity or have a high alpha coefficient by including a large number of construct-irrelevant items. As such, it is not a good estimate of either internal structure or unidimensionality (Revelle & Condon, 2019). Third, it is assumed that items are equally useful in approximating the true score across all levels of such scores and thus all provide equal information about the underlying construct (which is referred to as tau-equivalence). However, such an assumption is rarely met in clinical assessment where items do differ in their associations with an underlying latent construct (Raykov, 1997).

As a latent model-based alternative to classical test theory approaches to internal consistency, McDonald (1970) introduced the omega coefficient as a metric to evaluate scale reliability under the factor analysis approach. It captures reliability in terms of quantifying the proportion of error variance in observed item scores that is not accounted for by a latent construct. In latent factor modeling, such as confirmatory factor analysis, latent trait values are considered the "true scores" as these are estimated without random measurement error or item-specific systematic measurement error. Reliability of a test then indicates the extent to which the observed values are explained by a latent trait. Moreover, omega accounts for the item characteristics and the heterogeneity in item-to-latent trait associations. The true score variance is weighted by the factor loadings of the items on the latent factor and thus does not assume tau equivalence.

However, although the omega coefficient improves upon some of the limitations of coefficient alpha, it is not a magical solution. It assumes a well-fitting one-factor confirmatory factor analysis model, which becomes less likely as the number of items increases, especially in personality assessment research (Shou et al., 2022). In addition, the formula for calculating omega still favors longer scales, as the overall impact of measurement error attenuates as the number of items increases (see, e.g., Revelle & Condon, 2019).[1] Revelle and Condon (2019) therefore argued that relying on omega-hierarchical, which requires the estimation of the general factor variance, provides for a more accurate estimate of internal consistency reliability and unidimensionality than the original McDonald's omega, which considers the total reliable sources of variances in item scores. However, this method is less practical as it requires more complicated latent factor models.

Internal Structure

Precursors to contemporary factor analysis became available almost as soon as correlation matrices could be calculated (see, e.g., Mulaik, 2010, for a review). Scholars such as Charles Spearman used the correlation method to calculate matrices to evaluate higher-order factors for inter-related variables, and in the case of Spearman, a higher-order model of intelligence (Spearman, 1904). Subsequent scholars (e.g.,

[1] For instance, let's assume a scale with three items. Each item has a latent factor loading of 0.75, which means that the proportion of variance unaccounted for in each item is.50 ($(1-0.75)^2$). The formula for omega is the squared sum of factor loadings divided by the total variance (i.e., squared sum of factor loadings and sum of item residual variances). A three item scale would yield an omega coefficient of 0.77. A five-item scale with the same factor loadings (and thus, the same amount of measurement error associated with each item) would yield an omega coefficient of.85. See Revelle and Condon (2019) for a more sophisticated illustration.

Cattell, 1943; Thurstone, 1938) ultimately advocated for the exploratory factor analysis principles and methods that are frequently used today.

Factor analysis has been the most commonly used latent variable modeling method in psychology during the past several decades (see, e.g., Sellbom & Tellegen, 2019). In factor analysis, the observed variables are predicted by one or more latent factors, which are assumed to "cause" a person to respond in a particular way (e.g., the reason a person endorsed the item "most of the time I feel sad" is because they have high levels of depression). The latent factor explains the variance that the observed indicators (e.g., test items in assessment research) have in common. There are two main types of factor analysis, exploratory and confirmatory, both of which have different applications (Brown, 2014). In psychological assessment research, the primary purpose is either to uncover a previously unknown underlying structure of a set of test items when the construct is believed to be multidimensional (e.g., psychopathy, PTSD, neuroticism) or to test a particular hypothesis about structure (e.g., a psychopathy measure should have three underlying factors measuring affective, interpersonal, and behavioral traits). Both types of analysis inform construct validity (discussed in a subsequent section) in different ways (Shou et al., 2022).

Exploratory Factor Analysis EFA is used when there is no specific theory about the number of latent factors and the association among observed variables and latent factors.[2] EFA is often used to determine the number of latent factors among the observed variables and the item-to-factor combinations. For example, in the case of knowing how many distinct latent factors are underlying the symptoms of the Comprehensive Assessment of Psychopathic Personality-Self-Report, Sellbom et al. (2021) used EFA to determine the higher-order structure in three separate samples. They observed that the covariances among the 33 symptoms could be parsimoniously accounted for by three higher-order factors.

The two most frequently discussed processes in EFA are factor extraction and rotation, both of which are centered on the key goal of EFA—producing interpretable results (Goretzko et al., 2019). By default, factors in EFA can be extracted until no more common variance can be extracted from two or more measured properties. All observed properties are linked to, or predicted by, all extracted factors. Factors extracted in this way may not be interpretable in a straightforward manner. Various methods have been proposed for factor extraction (Goretzko et al.,

[2] Some scholars use principal components analysis (PCA) for this same purpose. PCA should not be confused with EFA, however, because it is not based on the common factor model as it does not parcel out shared and unique variances (Mulaik, 2010). Rather, PCA is a more simplistic procedure that attempts to maximize the amount of variance for which can be accounted in the indicators rather than making assumptions about causation. Some scholars nonetheless argue that PCA might be advantageous to EFA because it is more simplistic, is less prone to problematic solutions, and PCA and EFA often yield similar results. However, others (e.g., Brown., 2014; Fabrigar et al., 1999) have generally refuted these arguments as solutions are indeed dissimilar under various conditions (e.g., few indicators per factor, small communalities [i.e., amount of variance accounted for in an indicator by all factors]), and more generally, analyses should be applied based on the underlying theoretical assumptions made about associations among variables.

2019) with an objective method called parallel analysis being viewed as superior (Auerswald & Moshagen, 2019). The decision concerning the number of factors to extract should also incorporate considerations of interpretability and theory. When two or more factors can be extracted, rotation methods are usually applied to produce a simple structure to facilitate factor interpretation. A simple structure aims to make each item have a high factor loading on one single factor while having as low a loading on other factors as possible (Cai, 2013; Thurstone, 1947). The selection of rotation methods depends on whether one would assume that the latent factors are correlated (oblique) or independent (orthogonal). EFA is often used for scale development with consideration of the preceding two processes (factor extraction and rotation).

Confirmatory Factor Analysis CFA is typically used when a researcher already has a theoretically informed model on how different observed properties relate to one another and how and the degree to which they are explained by a set of latent factors. The model is specified a priori based on theory (e.g., the number of factors; how the factors and items are linked). The model is then estimated using a method that is appropriate for the underlying assumptions (e.g., maximum likelihood for continuous, normally distributed data). The model is subsequently evaluated through a series of structural equations to recreate the observed variance-covariance matrix; the degree of discrepancy between the model-implied and observed matrices informs on the plausibility of the model, and this is objectively evaluated through a series of model fit indices. If the model parameters (e.g., factor loadings, factor correlations) are consistent with theory and the model fit indices are in an acceptable range based on expert recommendations (e.g., Hu & Bentler, 1999), the model is accepted.

Item Response Theory A highly related method to CFA is item response theory (IRT; e.g., Lord & Novick, 1968). IRT is used to specifically evaluate the item parameters of categorical test items that can be fitted to a unidimensional latent construct. IRT describes how a latent trait can influence the probability of one endorsing a response category, which can be a correct response (e.g., in cognitive or achievement testing) or a keyed response (e.g., in personality testing). There are multiple IRT models available; in clinical and personality assessment, one parameter (also known as Rasch models; Rasch, 1960) and two parameter models are most common (Rouse et al., 1999). The default parameter is the difficulty parameter (b) which indicates the location on the latent trait (theta, θ) at which there is a 50% probability that an individual responds "correctly" (or, in personality, in the keyed direction) to an item. An above average b parameter means a more difficult item or one that requires a higher severity of the construct to be endorsed, and vice versa. In two-parameter models, a discrimination (a) parameter determines the sensitivity of item response in relation to the latent trait and indicates the amount of information an item may provide about the latent trait (Lord & Novick, 1968). The a parameter is also directly related to the amount of information that is provided by an item across theta levels, with the peak information occurring at the b parameter theta level.

IRT also provides for a modern test theory estimation of reliability, which is usually reflected by test information across the latent construct levels. More specifically, item information indicates the amount of information that an item could provide for each level of the latent trait (Price, 2016) and is often used as an indicator of precision of an item in assessing a particular level of latent trait. As articulated by Thomas (2019), item information is conditional on the latent trait level and can vary across the different levels. Greater levels of information mean less uncertainty in the estimated value for the target. Test information, on the other hand, is the aggregate item information at each latent trait level and is used to indicate the precision of the test in assessing a particular level of latent trait (Lord & Novick, 1968; Morizot et al., 2009). The standard error of measurement (SEM) in IRT is the inverse of the square root of information and also varies across the different latent trait levels. An examination of a test information function (with associated SEM values) can inform the test user at what latent trait levels the most reliable information is available as well as at what levels more error than reliable information is likely to be present in measurement. This is in stark contrast to classical test theory estimates of reliability, which assume equal reliability across the entire range of test scores. For instance, in the recent development of the Personality Disorder Severity scale for ICD-11 (PDS-ICD-11; Bach et al., 2021), Bach and colleagues demonstrated that, as expected in a community sample generally free of serious dysfunction, the PDS-ICD-11 scores only provided reliable information in the range of mean scores to 3 standard deviations above the mean. Classical test theory estimates would have assumed equal reliability of every single scale score.

Validity

The *Standards of Educational and Psychological Assessment* (AERA/APA/NCME, 2014) define validity as "the degree to which evidence and theory support the interpretation of test scores for proposed uses of tests" and "statements about validity should refer to particular interpretation for specified uses" (p. 11). The validation process involves accumulating evidence to support the proposed interpretation of the assessment results. Thus, the current framework of validity emphasizes sources and forms of evidence that can be used for the process of validation. A historical and theoretical analysis of the validity concept is beyond the scope of this chapter (see Cronbach & Meehl, 1955, and Messick, 1995, for more historical accounts; Borsboom & Mellenbergh, 2004, for a contemporary perspective on "causal" validity). In this chapter, we provide basic explanations of the most common forms of validation: content, criterion, construct, and incremental validity.

Content Validity Content validity refers to the degree to which the content of a measure fully represents a theoretical construct (Haynes et al., 1995). For instance, a structured clinical interview that claims to measure DSM-5 Post-traumatic Stress Disorder (PTSD) should clearly canvass information that pertains to all PTSD criteria, including exclusionary criteria. Content validity is a dynamic property, as the representativeness of items of a construct can change over time and in different environments. Definitions of psychological constructs can evolve with time as researchers develop more knowledge about the constructs. There are two common violations of content validity. First, content underrepresentativeness occurs when the full theoretical domain has not been captured. For instance, the DSM-5 criteria for Antisocial Personality Disorder are a poor representation of psychopathic personality (e.g., Sellbom & Boer, 2019) because they do not sufficiently incorporate many of the affective and interpersonal deficiencies most scholars find to be at the core of the disorder (e.g., Cooke et al., 2012). Second, construct irrelevance can also impact content validity. If a psychopathy scale contains items related to vocational interests, these would detract from the content validity of that measure.

Criterion-Related Validity Criterion-related validity indicates the degree to which test scores converge with criterion variables with which the test is supposed to converge (Cronbach & Meehl, 1955). There are definitions and applications of criterion validity in the literature that seem to depend on how "criterion variables" are defined. The term is often mixed with several other key validity terms such as convergent validity. For the purposes of the present chapter, criterion variables are defined as other measures of the same construct, directly conceptually relevant constructs, or conceptually relevant behaviors or outcomes (Shou et al., 2022). Criterion validity is concurrent when the scores of a test and criterion variables are obtained at the same time (often called *concurrent validity*), or predictive/postdictive when the criterion variables are measured after/before the current test (often called *predictive/postdictive validity*) (Grimm & Widaman, 2012; Shou et al., 2022). Criterion validity is often examined through correlations between test scores and external criterion variables, and these correlations are interpreted based on the magnitude that the researcher would expect.

Construct Validity Construct validity is synonymous with the definition of validity itself. It is the degree to which scale scores capture the theoretical construct that a scale is meant to measure. All other forms of validity inform construct validity, so they are not mutually exclusive. But construct validity is often broader in its evaluation than the other forms of validity. The pillars of evaluating construct validity concern evaluating evidence for convergent and discriminant validity. Convergent validity refers to how well the test scores converge with other variables based on theoretical expectations, whereas discriminant validity indicates how test scores diverge from other variables that assess different, non-overlapping constructs. Criterion-related validity, for instance, speaks to convergent validity, but the latter is broader, and encompasses any convergent evidence that would be expected from theory, and thus, not just specific external criteria directly related to the construct being measured. For instance, the Psychopathic Personality Inventory (PPI) scores would be expected to converge with other psychopathy measures (criterion validity) but also authoritarian attitudes and behaviors (convergent validity), but not with scores on an intelligence scale (discriminant validity).

A critical feature of construct validity, which is informed by convergent and discriminant validity evidence, is elaborating on the nomological network associated with scale scores (Cronbach & Meehl, 1955). As stated earlier, construct validation is an ongoing process that builds on a network of associations of scale scores, which, in turn, helps the field come to an improved articulation of the underlying construct actually being measured by a scale. Furthermore, construct validity can be evaluated in many different ways, including (but not limited to) examining whether conceptually expected group differences on scale scores emerge, correlations with external criterion measures, whether the internal factor structure conforms to conceptual expectations, and whether experimental manipulation that should produce change in a theoretical construct results in changes in test scores.

Incremental Validity Incremental validity concerns the extent to which test scores provide unique information about a construct relative to that which is offered by existing measures of the same construct (Hunsley & Meyer, 2003). Incremental validity is also important in deciding if an additional test is necessary in the assessment context. If the addition of a test does not provide important new information about the person being evaluated, its addition only results in cost of time and effort with no added utility. For instance, a clinician might want to determine whether the Rorschach Inkblot Method and the MMPI yield incremental useful information in the prediction of treatment outcomes. The clinician therefore reviews the literature to determine if the two tests actually increment one another in this prediction (see, e.g., Meyer, 2000, for one such example).

A common statistical method of evaluating incremental validity is the hierarchical regression model in which scores of one test is entered into the first step, and scores of a second test into the second step. If the test scores in the second step has a unique additional contribution to the model fit, such as resulting in a significant change in R^2, it has incremental validity relative to the other tests.

Examples Scott Lilienfeld contributed substantially to the personality assessment literature through scale development (as articulated earlier) and validation. Here we provide two examples to illustrate some of the points just discussed. In one of his final empirical papers, Lilienfeld and his students (Costello et al., 2021) developed and evaluated a measure of Left-Wing Authoritarianism. Because the construct was deemed insufficiently defined from a theoretical perspective, they employed Tellegen's approach to exploring psychological constructs through scale construction. They subjected their broad item pool to a series of factor analyses, settling primarily on an exploratory approach, which yielded three broad domains of Antihierarchical Aggression, Anticonventionalism, and Top-Down Censorship. Costello et al. (2021) subsequently validated their new LWA scale in a series of samples across multiple studies, including against personality questionnaires, political attitudes, behavioral tasks, and cognitive variables.

Berg et al. (2015) examined the construct validity of the PPI coldheartedness scale, which they argued had been an oft-neglected subscale of the PPI, yet possibly representative of the core features of the psychopathy construct. They used a large sample of 1158 university students who had been administered the PPI-Revised (Lilienfeld & Widows, 2005) and various other personality scales, including Big Five traits, impulsivity, depression, and anxiety. They examined convergent validity in that they hypothesized that coldheartedness would be correlated with low levels of all five Big 5 traits, but in particular low Extraversion, Agreeableness, and Neuroticism. They also expected negative correlations with depression and anxiety given that coldheartedness represents poverty in affective experiences. Finally, they expected a positive association with the sensation seeking aspects of impulsivity, but negative associations with more affect-laden aspects of impulsivity. Their findings demonstrated mixed support for convergent validity. Observed correlations were generally (albeit imperfectly) in line with expectations, though the magnitude for some was weak. As to whether the coldheartedness scale added incremental validity above and beyond other PPI-R scales, they estimated a hierarchical regression model and found that the scale incremented predictions of low agreeableness and low openness to experience, but none of the other external criteria. Berg et al. concluded that whereas the coldheartedness scale clearly overlapped with other PPI-R trait scales, it operationalizes a distinct and important psychological construct embedded within the psychopathy trait constellation.

Summary and Conclusions

This chapter was written in honor of the late Professor Scott O. Lilienfeld, who contributed substantially and impressively to the field of clinical personality assessment. We have covered a brief history of personality assessment, the general principles of such assessment, with a particular emphasis on evidence-based approaches, which was of great importance to him. We also covered contemporary scale construction approaches, including the one favored strongly by Lilienfeld himself (and developed by one of his graduate school mentors, Auke Tellegen; e.g., Tellegen & Waller, 2008), which has strong empirical grounding. We ended the chapter with a discussion of contemporary psychometric principles.

It is our hope that the reader will have attained an introductory perspective on important scientific and applied principles in clinical personality assessment. We share Professor Lilienfeld's view that reliance on evidence-based assessment practices that include multiple sources of information, with the important ingredient of well-validated psychological tests, is key to the clinical assessment process. The psychometric principles covered here provide an introductory guide for researchers who want to learn more about scale development and how to evaluate both scales they develop as well as those that operationalize the constructs they want to study. Clinicians should be mindful of these principles because not all tests are created equal and evidence-based assessment requires remaining up-to-date with the literature on the psychometric properties of tests being considered for use.

References

Achenbach, T. M., Ivanova, M. Y., & Rescorla, L. A. (2020). Multi-informant assessment of psychopathology from preschool through old age. In M. Sellbom & J. A. Suhr (Eds.), *Cambridge handbook of clinical assessment and diagnosis* (pp. 123–134). Cambridge University Press.
Allport, G. W. (1928). A test for ascendance-submission. *Journal of Abnormal and Social Psychology, 23*, 118–136.
Allport, G. W. (1931). What is a trait of personality? *Journal of Abnormal and Social Psychology, 25*, 368–372.
Allport, G. W. (1966). Traits revisited. *American Psychologist, 21*, 1–10.
Allport, G. W., & Odbert, H. S. (1936). Trait-names: A psycho-lexical study. *Psychological Monographs, 47*(1), 1–171. https://doi.org/10.1037/h0093360
American Educational Research Association, American Psychological Association, & National Council on Measurement in Education. (2014). *Standards for educational and psychological testing*. American Educational Research Association.
American Psychiatric Association. (2013). *Diagnostic and statistical manual of mental disorders* (5th ed.). Author.
American Psychological Association. (2006). Evidence-based practice in psychology. *American Psychologist, 61*(4), 271–285. https://doi.org/10.1037/0003-066X.61.4.271
Arbisi, P. A., & Beck, J. G. (2016). Introduction to the special series "empirically supported assessment". *Clinical Psychology: Science and Practice, 23*(4), 323–326. https://doi.org/10.1111/cpsp.12182
Archer, R. P., Wheeler, E. M. A., & Vauter, R. A. (2016). Empirically supported forensic assessment. *Clinical Psychology: Science and Practice, 23*(4), 348–364. https://doi.org/10.1111/cpsp.12171
Auerswald, M., & Moshagen, M. (2019). How to determine the number of factors to retain in exploratory factor analysis: A comparison of extraction methods under realistic conditions. *Psychological Methods, 24*(4), 468–491. https://doi.org/10.1037/met0000200
Bach, B., Brown, T. A., Mulder, R. T., Newton-Howes, G., Simonsen, E., & Sellbom, M. (2021). Development and initial evaluation of the ICD-11 personality disorder severity scale: PDS-ICD-11. *Personality and Mental Health, 15*(3), 223–236.
Bagby, R. M., Gralnick, T. M., Al-Dajani, N., & Uliaszek, A. A. (2016). The role of the five-factor model in personality assessment and treatment planning. *Clinical Psychology: Science and Practice, 23*(4), 365–381. https://doi.org/10.1111/cpsp.12175
Barlow, D. H. (2005). What's new about evidence-based assessment? *Psychological Assessment, 17*(3), 308–311. https://doi.org/10.1037/1040-3590.17.3.308
Ben-Porath, Y. S. (2013). Self-report inventories: Assessing personality and psychopathology. In J. R. Graham, J. A. Naglieri, & I. B. Weiner (Eds.), *Handbook of psychology: Assessment psychology* (pp. 622–644). John Wiley & Sons.
Ben-Porath, Y. S., & Butcher, J. N. (1991). The historical development of personality assessment. In C. E. Walker (Ed.), *Clinical psychology: Historical and research foundations* (pp. 121–156). Plenum Press.
Ben-Porath, Y. S., & Sellbom, M. (2023). *Interpreting the MMPI-3*. University of Minnesota Press.
Berg, J. M., Hecht, L. K., Latzman, R. D., & Lilienfeld, S. O. (2015). Examining the correlates of the coldheartedness factor of the psychopathic personality inventory–revised. *Psychological Assessment, 27*(4), 1494–1499. https://doi.org/10.1037/pas0000129
Bornstein, R. F. (2017). Evidence-based psychological assessment. *Journal of Personality Assessment, 99*(4), 435–445. https://doi.org/10.1080/00223891.2016.1236343
Borsboom, D., Mellenbergh, G. J., & van Heerden, J. (2004). The concept of validity. *Psychological Review, 111*(4), 1061–1071. https://doi.org/10.1037/0033-295X.111.4.1061
Brown, T. A. (2014). *Confirmatory factor analysis for applied research*. Guilford Press.

Burisch, M. (1984). You don't always get what you pay for: Measuring depression with short and simple versus long and sophisticated scales. *Journal of Personality, 18*(1), 81–98. https://doi.org/10.1016/0092-6566(84)90040-0

Butt, Z. (2016). In pursuit of empirically supported assessment for use in medical settings. *Clinical Psychology: Science and Practice, 23*(4), 382–402. https://doi.org/10.1111/cpsp.12176

Cai, L. (2013). Factor analysis of tests and items. APA handbook of testing and assessment in psychology, Vol. 1: Test theory and testing and assessment in industrial and organizational. *Psychology, 1*, 85–100.

Cattell, R. B. (1943). The description of personality: Basic traits resolved into clusters. *Journal of Abnormal and Social Psychology, 38*, 476–506.

Cattell, R. B. (1950). *Personality: A systematic theoretical and factual study* (1st ed.). McGraw-Hill. https://doi.org/10.1037/10773-000

Cattell, R. B. (1965). *The scientific analysis of personality*. Penguin Books.

Cattell, R. B. (1979). *Personality and learning theory* (Vol. 1). Springer.

Clark, L. A., & Watson, D. (1995). Constructing validity: Basic issues in objective scale development. *Psychological Assessment, 7*(3), 309–319. https://doi.org/10.1037/1040-3590.7.3.309

Clark, L. A., & Watson, D. (2019). Constructing validity: New developments in creating objective measuring instruments. *Psychological Assessment, 31*(12), 1412–1427. https://doi.org/10.1037/pas0000626

Cleckley, H. (1941). *The mask of sanity*. Mosby.

Cohen, J. (1960). A coefficient of agreement for nominal scales. *Educational and Psychological Measurement, 20*, 37–46.

Cooke, D. J., Hart, S. D., Logan, C., & Michie, C. (2012). Explicating the construct of psychopathy: Development and validation of a conceptual model, the comprehensive assessment of psychopathic personality (CAPP). *International Journal of Forensic Mental Health, 11*(4), 242–252.

Costello, T. H., Bowes, S. M., Stevens, S. T., Waldman, I. D., Tasimi, A., & Lilienfeld, S. O. (2021). Clarifying the structure and nature of left-wing authoritarianism. *Journal of Personality and Social Psychology*. Advance online publication. https://doi.org/10.1037/pspp0000341

Cronbach, L. J. (1951). Coefficient alpha and the internal structure of tests. *Psychometrika, 16*(3), 297–334.

Cronbach, L. J., & Meehl, P. E. (1955). Construct validity in psychological tests. *Psychological Bulletin, 52*(4), 281–302. https://doi.org/10.1037/h0040957

Downey, J. E. (1923). *The will-temperament and its testing*. World Book.

Dubois, P. L. (1970). *A history of psychological testing*. Allyn & Bacon.

Eysenck, J. J., & Eysenck, S. B. G. (1975). *Manual for the Eysenck personality questionnaire*. Educational and Industrial Testing Service.

Fabrigar, L. R., Wegener, D. T., MacCallum, R. C., & Strahan, E. J. (1999). Evaluating the use of exploratory factor analysis in psycho-logical research. *Psychological Methods, 4*(3), 272–299. https://doi.org/10.1037/1082-989X.4.3.272

Fleiss, J. L. (1971). Measuring nominal scale agreement among many raters. *Psychological Bulletin, 76*(5), 378–382.

Galton, F. (1884). Measurement of character. *Fortnightly Review, 42*, 179–185.

Garb, H. N. (2005). Clinical judgment and decision making. *Annual Review of Clinical Psychology, 1*, 67–89. https://doi.org/10.1146/annurev.clinpsy.1.102803.143810

Garb, H. N., Lilienfeld, S. O., Nezworski, M. T., Wood, J. M., & O'Donohue, W. T. (2009). Can quality improvement processes help psychological assessment meet the demands of evidence-based practice? *Scientific Review of Mental Health Practice, 7*(1), 17–25.

Geisinger, K. F. (2013). Reliability. In K. F. Geisinger (Ed.), *APA handbook of testing and assessment in psychology: Vol. 1. Test theory and testing and assessment in industrial and organizational psychology* (Vol. 1, pp. 21–41). American Psychological Association.

Goldberg, L. R. (1990). An alternative "description of personality": The big-five factor structure. *Journal of Personality and Social Psychology, 59*(6), 1216–1229. https://doi.org/10.1037/0022-3514.59.6.1216

Goretzko, D., Pham, T. T. H., & Bühner, M. (2019). Exploratory factor analysis: Current use, methodological developments and recommendations for good practice. *Current Psychology*, 1–12.

Graham, J. R. (2012). *MMPI-2: Assessing personality and psychopathology* (5th ed.). Oxford University Press.

Grimm, K. J., & Widaman, K. F. (2012). Construct validity. APA handbook of research methods in psychology, Vol 1: Foundations. *Planning, Measures, and Psychometrics, 1*, 621–642.

Guttman, L. (1945). A basis for analyzing test-retest reliability. *Psychometrika, 10*(4), 255–282.

Hare, R. D. (1980). A research scale for the assessment of psychopathy in criminal populations. *Personality and Individual Differences, 1*, 111–119.

Hare, R. D. (1991/2003). *The Hare psychopathy checklist-revised* (2nd ed.). Multi-Health Systems.

Hathaway, S. R., & McKinley, J. C. (1943). *The Minnesota multiphasic personality inventory*. University of Minnesota Press.

Haynes, S. N., Richard, D. C. S., & Kubany, E. S. (1995). Content validity in psychological assessment: A functional approach to concepts and methods. In psychological assessment, *7*(3), 238–247.

Heidbreder, E. (1926). Measuring introversion and extraversion. *Journalof Abnormal and Social Psychology, 21*, 120–134.

Heymans, G., & Wiersma, E. (1906). Beitragezurspezillenpsychologie auf grundeinermassenunterschung [Contribution of psychological specialists to personality analysis]. *Zeitschrift fur Psychologie, 43*, 81–127.

Hoch, A., & Amsden, G. S. (1913). A guide to the descriptive study of personality. *Review of Neurology and Psychiatry, 11*, 577–587.

Hu, L. T., & Bentler, P. M. (1999). Cutoff criteria for fit indexes in covariance structure analysis: Conventional criteria versus new alternatives. *Structural Equation Modeling: A Multidisciplinary Journal, 6*(1), 1–55.

Hunsley, J., & Mash, E. J. (2007). Evidence-based assessment. *Annual Review of Clinical Psychology, 3*(1), 29–51. https://doi.org/10.1146/annurev.clinpsy.3.022806.091419

Hunsley, J., & Meyer, G. J. (2003). The incremental validity of psychological testing and assessment: Conceptual, methodological, and statistical issues. *Psychological Assessment, 15*(4), 446–455. https://doi.org/10.1037/1040-3590.15.4.446

Keller, J., Hicks, B. D., & Miller, G. A. (2000). Psychophysiology in the study of psychopathology. In J. T. Cacioppo, L. G. Tassinary, & G. G. Berntson (Eds.), *Handbook of psychophysiology* (pp. 719–750). Cambridge University Press.

Koo, T. K., & Li, M. Y. (2016). A guideline of selecting and reporting intraclass correlation coefficients for reliability research. *Journal of Chiropractic Medicine, 15*(2), 155–163.

Kotov, R., Krueger, R. F., Watson, D., Achenbach, T. M., Althoff, R. R., Bagby, R. M., Brown, T. A., Carpenter, W. T., Caspi, A., Clark, L. A., Eaton, N. R., Forbes, M. K., Forbush, K. T., Goldberg, D., Hasin, D., Hyman, S. E., Ivanova, M. Y., Lynam, D. R., Markon, K., et al. (2017). The hierarchical taxonomy of psychopathology (HiTOP): A dimensional alternative to traditional nosologies. *Journal of Abnormal Psychology, 126*(4), 454–477. https://doi.org/10.1037/abn0000258

Kotov, R., Krueger, R. F., Watson, D., Cicero, D. C., Conway, C. C., DeYoung, C. G., et al. (2021). The hierarchical taxonomy of psychopathology (HiTOP): A quantitative nosology based on consensus of evidence. *Annual Reviewo Of Clinical Psychology, 17*, 83–108.

Kuder, G. F., & Richardson, M. W. (1937). The theory of the estimation of test reliability. *Psychometrika, 2*(3), 151–160.

Lewis, K. C., Spruch-Feiner, A., & Ridenour, J. M. (2021). Clinical interviewing. In G. Asmundsen (Ed.), *Comprehensive clinical psychology* (Vol. 2nd). Section 4: Assessment. Elsevier.

Lilienfeld, S. O. (1990). *Development and preliminary validation of a self-report measure of psychopathic personality* (Vol. I and II). Doctoral dissertation, University of Minnesota.

Lilienfeld, S. O., & Andrews, B. P. (1996). Development and preliminary validation of a self-report measure of psychopathic personality traits in noncriminal population. *Journal of Personality Assessment, 66*(3), 488–524.

Lilienfeld, S. O., & Widows, M. R. (2005). *Psychopathic personality inventory-revised.* Psychological Assessment Resources.

Lilienfeld, S. O., Wood, J. M., & Garb, H. N. (2000). The scientific status of projective techniques. *Psychological Science in the Public Interest, 1*(2), 27–66.

Lilienfeld, S. O., Ritschel, L. A., Lynn, S. J., Cautin, R. L., & Latzman, R. D. (2013). Why many practitioners are resistant to evidence-based practice in clinical psychology: Roo causes and constructive remedies. *Clinical Psychology Review, 33*, 883–900. http://dx.doi.org/j.cpr.2012.09.008

Lilienfeld, S. O., Lynn, S. J., Ritschel, L. A., Cautin, R. L., & Latzman, R. D. (2014). Why ineffective psychotherapies can appear to work: A taxonomy of causes of spurious therapeutic effectiveness. *Perspectives on Psychological Science, 9*, 355–387. https://doi.org/10.1177/1745691614535216

Lilienfeld, S. O., Lynn, S. J., O'Donohue, W. T., & Latzman, R. D. (2017). Epistemic humility: An overarching educational philosophy for clinical psychology programs. *The Clinical Psychologist, 70*(2), 6–14.

Loevinger, J. (1957). Objective tests as instruments of psychological theory. *Psychological Reports, 3*, 635–694. https://doi.org/10.2466/PR0.3.7.635-694

Lord, F. M., & Novick, M. R. (1968). *Statistical theories of mental test scores*. Addison-Wesley.

McCrae, R. R., & Costa, P. T. (1999). The five-factor theory of personality. In J. S. Wiggins (Ed.), *The five-factor model of personality: Theoretical perspectives* (2nd ed., pp. 51–87). Guilford Publications.

McDonald, R. P. (1970). The theoretical foundations of principal factor analysis, canonical factor analysis, and alpha factor analysis. *British Journal of Mathematical and Statistical Psychology, 23*(1), 1–21.

McFall, R. (2005). Theory and utility: Key themes in evidence-based assessment: Comment on the special section: Developing guidelines for the evidence-based assessment of adult disorders. *Psychological Assessment, 17*(3), 312–323. https://doi.org/10.1037/1040-3590.17.3.312

Meehl, P. E. (1956). Wanted—A good cook-book. *American Psychologist, 11*(6), 263–272. https://doi.org/10.1037/h0044164

Messick, S. (1995). Validation of psychological assessment. *American Psychologist, 50*(9), 741–749.

Meyer, G. J. (2000). Incremental validity of the rorschach prognostic rating scale over the MMPI ego strength scale and IQ. *Journal of Personality Assessment, 74*(3), 356–370.

Meyer, G. J., & Mihura, J. L. (2020). Performance-based techniques. In M. Sellbom & J. A. Suhr (Eds.), *Cambridge handbook of clinical assessment and diagnosis* (pp. 278–290). Cambridge University Press.

Morizot, J., Ainsworth, A. T., & Reise, S. P. (2009). Toward modern psychometrics. In R. W. Robins, R. C. Fraley, & R. F. Krueger (Eds.), *Handbook of research methods in personality psychology* (pp. 407–423). Guilford Press.

Mulaik, S. A. (2010). *Foundations of factor analysis*. CRC Press.

Norman, W. T. (1963). Toward an adequate taxonomy of personality attributes: Replicated factor structure in peer nomination personality ratings. *The Journal of Abnormal and Social Psychology, 66*(6), 574–583. https://doi.org/10.1037/h0040291

Novick, M. R. (1966). The axioms and principal results of classical test theory. *Journal of Mathematical Psychology, 3*(1), 1–18.

Nunnally, J. C., & Bernstein, I. H. (1967). *Psychometric theory*. McGraw-Hill Inc.

Price, L. R. (2016). *Psychometric methods: Theory into practice*. Guilford Publications.

Raykov, T. (1997). Scale reliability, Cronbach's coefficient alpha, and violations of essential tau-equivalence with fixed congeneric components. *Multivariate Behavioral Research, 32*(4), 329–353.

Revelle, W., & Condon, D. M. (2017). Reliability. *The Wiley Handbook of Psychometric Testing: A Multidisciplinary Reference on Survey, Scale and Test Development, 2–2*, 709–749.
Revelle, W., & Condon, D. M. (2019). Reliability from α to ω: A tutorial. *Psychological Assessment, 31*(12), 1395–1411. https://doi.org/10.1037/pas0000754
Rouse, S. V., Finger, M. S., & Butcher, J. N. (1999). Advances in clinical personality measurement: An item response theory analysis of the MMPI-2 PSY-5 scales. *Journal of Personality Assessment, 72*(2), 282–307.
Rasch, G. (1960). Probabilistic models for some intelligence and attainment tests. Copenhagen: Danish Institute for Educational Research.
Sechrest, L. (1963). Incremental validity: A recommendation. *Educational and Psychological Measurement, 23*(1), 153–158.
Sellbom, M., & Boer, D. P. (2019). Psychopathy vs antisocial personality disorder. In R. D. Morgan (Ed.), *The SAGE encyclopedia of criminal psychology* (pp. 1197–1199). Sage Publications.
Sellbom, M., & Hopwood, C. J. (2016). Evidence-based assessment in the 21st century: Comments on the special series papers. *Clinical Psychology: Science and Practice, 23*(4), 403–409. https://doi.org/10.1111/cpsp.12183
Sellbom, M., & Tellegen, A. (2019). Factor analysis in psychological assessment research: Common pitfalls and recommendations. *Psychological Assessment, 31*(12), 1428–1441. https://doi.org/10.1037/pas0000623
Sellbom, M., Liggins, C., Laurinaitytė, I., & Cooke, D. J. (2021). Factor structure of the comprehensive assessment of psychopathic personality-self-report (CAPP-SR) in community and offender samples. *Psychological Assessment, 33*(10), 927–939. https://doi.org/10.1037/pas0001029
Shou, Y., Sellbom, M., & Chen, H. F. (2022). 4.02. Fundamentals of measurement in clinical psychology. In G. J. G. Asmundsen (Ed.), *Comprehensive Clinical Psychology* 2nd edition, vol. 4 (pp. 17–35). Elsevier.
Shrout, P. E., & Fleiss, J. L. (1979). Intraclass correlations: Uses in assessing rater reliability. *Psychological Bulletin, 86*(2), 420–428.
Sommers-Flanagan, J., Johnson, V. I., & Rides At The Door, M. (2020). Clinical interviewing. In M. Sellbom & J. A. Suhr (Eds.), *Cambridge handbook of clinical assessment and diagnosis* (pp. 113–122). Cambridge University Press.
Spearman, C. (1904). "General intelligence," objectively determined and measured. *American Journal of Psychology, 15*, 201–293.
Suhr, J., & Angers, K. (2020). Neuropsychological testing and assessment. In M. Sellbom & J. A. Suhr (Eds.), *Cambridge handbook of clinical assessment and diagnosis* (pp. 191–207). Cambridge University Press.
Suhr, J. A., & Sellbom, M. (2020). Introduction to the handbook of clinical assessment and diagnosis. In M. Sellbom & J. A. Suhr (Eds.), *Cambridge handbook of clinical assessment and diagnosis* (pp. 1–6). Cambridge University Press.
Tellegen, A. (1982). *Brief manual for the multidimensional personality questionnaire*. University of Minnesota Press.
Tellegen, A., & Waller, N. G. (2008). Exploring personality through test construction: Development of the multidimensional personality questionnaire. In G. J. Boyle, G. Matthews, & D. H. Saklofske (Eds.), *The SAGE handbook of personality theory and assessment* (*Personality measurement and testing*) (Vol. 2, pp. 261–292). Sage.
Thomas, M. L. (2019). Advances in applications of item response theory to clinical assessment. *Psychological Assessment, 31*(12), 1442–1455. https://doi.org/10.1037/pas0000597
Thurstone, L. L. (1930). A neurotic inventory. *Journal of Social Psychology, 1*, 3–30.
Thurstone, L. L. (1938). *Primary mental abilities*. University of Chicago Press.
Thurstone, L. L. (1947). *Multiple factor analysis*. University of Chicago Press.
Travis, R. C. (1925). The measurement of fundamental character traits by a new diagnostic test. *Journal of Abnormal and Social Psychology, 18*, 400–425.

Tupes, E. C., & Christal, R. E. (1961). *Recurrent personality factors based on trait ratings (USAF ASD technical report no. 61–97)*. Lackland Air Force Base, Texas: U.S. Air Force.

Tversky, A., & Kahneman, D. (1974). Judgment under uncertainty: Heuristics and biases. *Science (American Association for the Advancement of Science), 185*(4157), 1124–1131. https://doi.org/10.1126/science.185.4157.1124

Watson, D., O'Hara, M. W., Simms, L. J., Kotov, R., Chmielewski, M., McDade-Montez, E. A., Gamez, W., & Stuart, S. (2007). Development and validation of the inventory of depression and anxiety symptoms (IDAS). *Psychological Assessment, 19*(3), 253–268. https://doi.org/10.1037/1040-3590.19.3.253

Watson, D., O'Hara, M. W., Naragon-Gainey, K., Koffel, E., Chmielewski, M., Kotov, R., Stasik, S. M., & Ruggero, C. J. (2012). Development and validation of new anxiety and bipolar symptom scales for an expanded version of the IDAS (the IDAS-II). *Assessment, 19*(4), 399–420. https://doi.org/10.1177/1073191112449857

Wells, F. L. (1914). The systematic observation of the personality—In its relation to the hygiene of the mind. *Psychological Review, 21*, 295–333.

Widiger, T. A., Sellbom, M., Chmielewski, M., Clark, L. A., DeYoung, C. G., Kotov, R., et al. (2019). Personality in a hierarchical model of psychopathology. *Clinical Psychological Science, 7*(1), 77–92.

Woodworth, R. S. (1920). *Personal data sheet*. Stoeling.

Youngstrom, E. A., & Van Meter, A. (2016). Empirically supported assessment of children and adolescents. *Clinical Psychology: Science and Practice, 23*(4), 327–347. https://doi.org/10.1037/h0101738

Toward a New, Improved Paradigm for Experimental Psychopathology Research … Or What We Would Talk About with Scott Over Coffee in a Dinkytown Cafe

Christopher J. Patrick and Mark F. Lenzenweger

> *Give me coffee every time...Give me coffee, coffee, coffee...And let me tell you, you have found yourself a friend...*
> *– Freedy Johnston*

It is our great privilege and pleasure to contribute a chapter to this volume in honor of our late friend and colleague, Scott Lilienfeld. Scott was a unique and powerful figure in the psychological science field. He blended a piercing critical intellect with a gracious personal style and a brilliant sense of humor. He was unfailingly brave in his willingness to challenge empirically tenuous ideas and practices—ranging from projective inkblot testing (Lilienfeld et al., 2000, 2002), to eye movement desensitization and reprocessing (Lilienfeld, 1996), to microaggressions (Lilienfeld, 2017)—and drew a lot of not-so-friendly fire for doing so. Yet, at the same time, he was also broad-minded, deeply knowledgeable on a wide range of topics, ecumenical and integrative in his thinking, and open to embracing new ideas when supported by data. He was a captivating public speaker, a superb research collaborator, a generous and effective mentor of students, and among the most talented writers in our discipline.

C. J. Patrick (✉)
Department of Psychology, Florida State University, Tallahassee, FL, USA
e-mail: cpatrick@psy.fsu.edu

M. F. Lenzenweger
Department of Psychology, State University of New York at Binghamton, Binghamton, NY, USA

Weill Cornell Medical College, New York, NY, USA
e-mail: mlenzen@binghamton.edu

C. L. Cobb et al. (eds.), *Toward a Science of Clinical Psychology*,
https://doi.org/10.1007/978-3-031-14332-8_9

Scott trained in the Psychology Department at the University of Minnesota, long renowned for its contributions in the areas of clinical and personality assessment, psychopathology research and theory, psychophysiology, and large-scale longitudinal twin research. In this chapter, we argue that key developments in these areas over the years at Minnesota and elsewhere call for fundamental shifts in how we think about and conduct experimental psychopathology (EP) research. We propose that for EP to advance, the next generation of scholars would do well to consider the viewpoints presented in this chapter. We offer these ideas and perspectives for their heuristic value, not as fixed in stone or dogmatic. Our intent is to stimulate constructive thought rather than to gripe or finger-wag.

The Classic Experimental Psychopathology Paradigm

The bases for this chapter derive from our reflections on our respective primary research programs in experimental psychopathology—psychopathic personality (psychopathy) in the case of first author Patrick, and schizophrenia and the associated latent liability construct, schizotypy, in the case of co-author Lenzenweger. We obviously acknowledge that EP covers a panoply of other pathological conditions and processes; however, our views are necessarily constrained by the substantive vantage points from which we view the field. That said, the study of psychopathy and of schizotypy and schizophrenia have encouraged many to think critically about how laboratory research on complex mental conditions might progress to best fulfill the aim of illuminating etiology and pathogenesis. For example, how and why should one experimentally study fear in psychopathy, or sustained attention (e.g., Cornblatt & Keilp, 1994; Lenzenweger et al., 1991) in schizotypy and schizophrenia—rather than relying on subjective ratings of low fear or impaired attention, respectively, for these conditions? These domains of psychopathology have served as vigorous and persistent targets for scientific investigation, owing both to their devastating impact on individual health and societal welfare as a whole and to their opaque psychological nature—as one could see from reviewing decades of issues of one of the leading journals in the field, the *Journal of Abnormal Psychology* (now *Journal of Psychopathology and Clinical Science*). Finally, by way of historical context, we note that experimental psychopathology has been in existence for over 100 years (e.g., since laboratory studies of word association performance in schizophrenia conducted by Carl Jung in the early 1900s), predating by many decades both the current *zeitgeist* of "clinical science" in psychology and the Neo-Kraepelian revolution (or, the re-emergence of the importance of descriptive phenomenology and diagnostic classification, moving away from psychoanalysis and its focus on dreams, free associations, and unconscious processes as well as its minimal regard for diagnosis) in psychiatry which began in the late 1970s.

It is helpful to begin by reflecting on a definition of experimental psychopathology. One of us proposed the following definition some years ago:

> Experimental psychopathology is the psychological science discipline that uses the methods of the experimental psychology laboratory in conjunction with quantitative analytic approaches to gain leverage on etiology and pathogenesis of psychopathology, within a brain-based (genomic, endophenotype, neurobiological) diathesis-stressor matrix (Lenzenweger, 2010, p. 19).

This definition harbors a number of important assumptions, both substantive and methodological, that provide guidance to the selection of research approaches and modes of exploration in experimental psychopathology.

Consistent with the foregoing definition, we each were taught that EP is something of a hybrid psychological science subdiscipline supported by scientific clinical psychology (or "clinical science" in today's parlance), experimental psychology, cognitive and affective (neuro)science, psychometrics and measurement, genetics/genomics, psychophysiology and neurobehavioral systems, statistical analysis, and taxonomic/classification sciences. Importantly, each of these conceptual pylons supporting EP as a subdiscipline ultimately helped to serve a common mission. That common mission has been and remains simply *the understanding of the etiology, determining underlying processes, and pathogenesis of psychopathology*. That is, the task of experimental psychopathology is to illuminate the causes and progressive unfolding of mental illness, in all its representations, and across levels of analysis. This task stands in contrast to the more typical traditional clinical psychology and clinical psychiatry approaches that have been (and remain) nearly completely focused on assessment/diagnosis and treatment of mental disorders.

As argued previously by one of us (Lenzenweger, 2020), experimental psychopathology emerged largely out of the efforts and discoveries made by psychologists that began to probe the nature of mental disorders using the methods of the experimental psychology laboratory. The relevance of the early work by pioneers of psychology (Wundt, Fechner, James, Pavlov) in setting the stage for laboratory research on psychopathology through their work on normative psychological phenomena is relatively obvious. However, EP as an active approach unto itself is seen most clearly in the case of early work that emerged in efforts to psychologically dissect and understand genuine, expressed (diagnosable) mental disorders. For example, David Shakow represents an example of an early psychologist applying the methods of the experimental psychology laboratory to the study of schizophrenia (see, e.g., Rodnick & Shakow, 1940). His work led to years of controlled laboratory assessments of cognitive processes that focused on objective performance indexes, such as reaction time and signal detection parameters, rather than subjective impressions of poor attention processing in schizophrenia patients (e.g., Nuechterlein et al., 2004). Another is David Lykken, who undertook pioneering work using multiple laboratory methods to test hypotheses regarding fear and anxiety in psychopathy. Lykken's (1957) report of his doctoral research findings served as inspiration for subsequent studies of emotional (e.g., Fowles, 1980; Hare, 1978) and cognitive processing impairments in psychopathy (e.g., Patterson & Newman, 1993) that have remained influential to this day. The work of these early pioneers was characterized by experimental rigor, conceptual clarity, and sophisticated quantification, along with careful data collection and specific hypothesis testing using laboratory methods. This collection of features exemplifies the essence of EP today, and continues to define its conceptual foundations, scientific values, and methodological ethos. As noted by Lenzenweger (2020), "experimental psychopathology is grounded in the rigorous collection and testing of empirical data in the laboratory, *not* (as Professor Brendan Maher once quipped to [one of us]) in "overstuffed leather chairs, glasses of sherry, and the world of theory devoid of data." (p. 94)

Finally, although developed primarily by psychologists, the experimental psychopathology approach came to be embraced over time by many research-oriented psychiatrists during the neo-Kraepelinian revolution of the late-1970s and 1980s. Psychiatry's adoption of EP along with other scientific-empirical approaches, as an alternative to understanding psychopathology in mentalistic (e.g., psychodynamic) terms, clearly influenced the sea change in article content during the 1970s and 1980s in what had long been treatment/clinically oriented outlets such as the *Archives of General Psychiatry* (now *JAMA Psychiatry*) and the *American Journal of Psychiatry*. The emergence of psychopharmacology in psychiatry during this time also helped to stimulate interest in the underlying nature of psychopathology among psychiatrists.

We clearly cannot touch on all aspects of the experimental psychopathology approach that warrant coverage, nor can we predict with certainty where the field will be going in the decades ahead. Nonetheless, we hope to offer some beneficial guidance and food for thought, for contemporary researchers as well as scholars to come. As inspiration for this task, the two of us imagined ourselves as co-participants in a lively conversation with our late friend Scott, enjoying a coffee together in one of the venerable Dinkytown cafes bordering the University of Minnesota's West Bank campus.

Reasons for Reconsidering How We Conduct Experimental Psychopathology Research

Clearly, the presence or absence of psychopathology in an individual is a state conferred by nature rather than one manipulated by experimental design. In Cronbach's (1957) "two disciplines" perspective, the fact that the experimenter cannot control (or randomly assign) who develops a mental illness places the study of psychopathology squarely within a correlational framework. That said, consistent with Cronbach's view, one can still probe the nature of psychological illness using experimental protocols by including psychopathology-affected persons in laboratory studies that include elements of both correlational and experimental approaches. For many decades, experimental psychopathology has done just that. There have been innumerable laboratory studies in which a target pathology group has been included for comparison against a non-pathological (healthy) group or a separate-pathology group, or in which similarly affected individuals have been assigned to different conditions of interest.

Findings from EP studies of these types have shaped how we think about understanding the nature of psychopathology in several important ways today. The many years of laboratory research focusing on cognitive, affective, and behavioral systems, and processes associated with them, have provided an organizational focus for the National Institute of Mental Health's (NIMH) program of research funding, and served as the foundation for scientific initiatives such as the NIMH Research Domain Criteria (RDoC) framework. The steady and thoughtful use of both careful clinical description and a continuous-graded perspective on psychopathological signs and symptoms, coupled with the powerful statistical approach of factor analysis, have contributed to the emergence of an influential new hierarchical system for characterizing psychopathology we discuss later (i.e., HiTOP; Kotov et al., 2017). Nonetheless, we wish to discuss, in no particular order, issues that we view as unresolved or in need of critical thought in the EP approach. Indeed, we suggest that for experimental psychopathology to continue to support the mission of understanding etiology and pathogenesis in mental disorders these issues will need to be addressed.

Diagnostic Issues: Clinical Targets for Experimental Psychopathology Research

Focus on Single Disorders and "Matched" Controls Traditionally, EP research has sought to identify differences in responding on laboratory measures between participants diagnosed with a particular disorder in comparison to "control" participants not diagnosed as such. Particular emphasis has been placed on non-report-based indicators[1] of psychological processes (e.g., brain and other physiological variables; performance measures from behavioral tasks), considered to be more objective indicators of mechanisms contributing to psychological dysfunction. In many studies, a single specific ("pure") diagnostic group (e.g., participants with major depressive disorder) is compared against a "healthy control" group, matched for characteristics such as age, sex, and race. Less commonly, the target diagnostic group is compared against a separate diagnostic ("patient control") group, either in addition to or in place of the healthy control group—allowing for matching on mental health-related variables such as treatment history, medication use, and prior substance use as well as demographics.

There are notable problems with this approach. The use of categorical diagnoses in psychopathology research has been criticized itself on a number of grounds—including unreliability of binary (present vs. absent) categorical assignments, arbitrary diagnostic thresholds, and loss of information due to dichotomization (Trull & Durrett, 2005). Comparisons of a specific ("pure") diagnostic group against a healthy control group, and/or another group exhibiting a different specific

[1] By non-report-based, we mean measures from assessment modalities other than self- or other-report.

diagnosis, are also problematic—because mental disorders frequently co-occur with one another, making studies of "pure" groups unrepresentative of individuals with mental health problems generally. Additionally, the practice of "matching" groups in EP research on selected participant characteristics is also problematic because it has long been known that matching two groups on the basis of a feature characteristic of one group likely yields mismatch on other variables of interest. For example, matching a group of normal subjects on measured intelligence (IQ) to the IQ of a sample of schizophrenia-affected patients (who on average typically show lower IQ scores) will almost certainly yield a highly atypical sample of "normal" subjects with respect to IQ and, importantly, shape correlational associations among other underlying factors (e.g., education, SES).

Relatedly, the statistical removal of the effects of what are deemed to be "nuisance" variables (e.g., sex, age, SES, education) from data based on normal and pathological samples is likely to impact the nomological (or stochastological) network for a research study (i.e., patterns of relations among hypothesized constructs and their observable manifestations in the form of measured variables) in some manner that cannot be known to the investigator (see Meehl, 1971, 1978; Miller & Chapman, 2001). Stated differently, many investigators seek to the remove the effects of what they consider a "nuisance variable" merely because two groups differ on that variable, a move guided by the assumption that removal of the influence of the nuisance variable from observed correlations makes the resulting (controlled) correlations "correct" somehow. In his classic piece on this practice, Meehl (1971) trenchantly criticized the assumptions and effects of such control approaches and he spelled out several plausible causal chains in the possible etiology of schizophrenia and how the statistical removal of the effects of social class from obtained correlations for high school social activities and later schizophrenia would likely corrupt these plausible causal chains. Clearly, nature delivers up samples of people that show considerable variation on both those variables of central theoretical interest to the experimental psychopathologist as well as variation on a host of background variables. Nonetheless, one continues to field or witness queries regarding matching of subjects and control of nuisance variables in colloquia, poster sessions, conference addresses, and NIMH study sections. Modern approaches have been developed for statistically accounting for background variables when samples need to be constructed for comparison. One such statistical approach we recommend for this purpose is propensities analysis, developed by Rubin and colleagues (e.g., Rosenbaum & Rubin, 1985).

Categorical** Versus **Dimensional Diagnosis A major trend in the study of psychopathology over the past four decades has been a shift away from a categorical (e.g., traditional psychiatric diagnostic) toward a dimensional approach to psychopathology assessment and description, involving the use of continuous-score profiles to characterize individuals along multiple symptom or maladaptive trait dimensions (Kotov et al., 2017; Widiger & Mullins-Sweatt, 2007). Notable advantages have been identified in the use of a dimensional system relative to a binary (present vs. absent) categorical system for diagnosis. These include increased reliability of measurement, enhanced ability to differentiate among individuals owing to greater sensitivity to individual differences, and ability to accommodate the occurrence of systematic comorbidity (or, minimally, covariation; see Fossati et al., 2000, or Lenzenweger & Clarkin, 2005) among different disorders as traditionally defined. The HiTOP framework, mentioned earlier, is the most comprehensive system of this kind available at this time. It organizes psychopathological features of various disorders hierarchically, from narrow symptom and trait facets at its lowest level, to intermediate-level subdimensions reflecting convergence among lower-level features, to broad spectrum dimensions at the highest (superordinate) levels.

A dimensional system such as HiTOP holds potential to address some of the above-noted problems with the traditional EP comparative groups approach. The enhanced reliability and measurement precision of a dimensional approach is expected to translate into higher and more stable relations of diagnostic scores with predictors of interest. The development of inventories for assessing disorder spectra of the HiTOP model (e.g., internalizing, externalizing) at different levels of specificity (from facet symptoms/trait to broad factors; e.g., Krueger et al., 2007; Simms et al., 2022; Watson et al., 2007) allows for feasible testing of predictive relations across different disorder dimensions, and for evaluating the contributions of specific versus common disorder elements as contributors to observed relations (Conway et al., 2019, 2022). However, we should note that while the HiTOP model has generated considerable intellectual excitement in EP and other fields, the model and methodological approach is not without its detractors (e.g., Haeffel et al., 2022).

In this context, we encourage contemporary experimental psychopathologists and those interested in the quantitative classification of psychopathology to ask probing questions as we move ahead with a more dimensional conceptualization of psychopathology. For example, does continuity in measurement at the phenotypic level correspond in a monotonic manner to the quantitative distribution of a construct at the latent level? What do we take as statistical and substantive evidence of the validity of asserting the dimensionality of a construct? To wit, does the dimensional approach represent a data-driven theoretically coherent perspective, or is it more of a methodological preference? How shall we best proceed to confirm the dimensionality of a construct? Namely, what approach should we use to establish dimensionality beyond factor analysis (which must find dimensional structure) and what alternative approaches can be used that do not assume dimensionality—as the moral equivalent to the null in testing the hypothesis of dimensionality?

There is one other key limitation of the traditional EP research strategy, irrespective of whether a categorical or dimensional approach is used to characterize participants. The limitation has to do with method and construct dissimilarity between diagnostic assignments or scores, which are report-based (most typically interview-based clinician ratings, or participant self-ratings), and lab measures that are non-report-based. For example, EP studies frequently aim to differentiate diagnostic and control groups on the basis of task performance or physiological reactivity scores. In this case, observed differences are expected to be modest at best, owing to method mismatch (different measurement modalities) as well as construct mismatch (dissimilarity in measured attributes; Campbell & Fiske, 1959; Patrick et al., 2013, 2019). In traditional EP research, the report-based diagnostic variable is treated as a fixed target—that is, as the *actual* psychological characteristic ("attribute-in-truth") onto which indicators from other measurement modalities are to be "mapped." This represents a serious handicap in efforts to relate non-report-based measures to diagnostic attributes—arguably the core aim of EP research. What is needed to enhance covariation between the two is to allow other-modality indicators to enter into the diagnostic target (i.e., group assignment or dimensional score), rather than keeping it fixed. We expand upon this point in the sections that follow.

Measurement Issues: Factors Limiting Covariation Between Diagnostic Variables and Non-report Variables

Score Reliability of Lab-Task Measures One very basic issue that did not receive adequate attention in EP research until quite recently is the reliability of scores for lab-task behavioral and physiological measures within and across test sessions (internal consistency, test-retest stability). It is well-known that reliability constrains the level of validity coefficients that can be observed for a test measure. Findings of extremely low reliability for "tried and true" laboratory measures such as emotional Stroop interference (i.e., slower color-naming of emotional vs. neutral words; Strauss et al., 2005) and neuroimaging-assessed amygdala reactivity to fearful faces (Elliott et al., 2020) have drawn serious attention to this issue in EP research. These and many other lab-task measures rely on condition-difference scores, which become less reliable to the extent that individual condition scores covary.

One wonders why such measures were not evaluated sooner and routinely for reliability. We suspect a few reasons. One is that, as noted earlier, EP researchers have traditionally viewed non-report-based lab measures as more directly indicative of mechanisms contributing to psychological dysfunction. Another is that traditional EP is based in experimental psychology and has typically relied on analysis of variance (ANOVA) statistics, which focus on task-condition effects and between-group differences, rather than on psychometric analyses, which focus on variation in scores across individuals. Related to this, task procedures selected for EP studies are typically ones that have yielded robust, replicable overall-sample effects in prior research (e.g., robust affective-neutral condition differences, on average; or, robust distraction-no distraction condition differences, on average)—presumed to be indicative of some process such as emotional activation, or attentional impairment. The assumption is that these tasks will show reliable enough *variation across subjects* to yield robust group differences in average task effects. However, variability in scores across subjects falls within the province of psychometrics, where it is well known that score reliability limits observed associations. A further assumption, considered next, is that variation in task effects across subjects can be expected to reflect *the same psychological process* as average (i.e., overall sample) task effects.

Average Task Effects *Versus* ***Inter-individual Variation in Task Effects*** Report-based scale measures are generally designed to measure psychological attributes of individuals relative to others (e.g., intelligence, anxiousness), through items chosen to index variations in the target attribute *across individuals*. By contrast, lab-experimental tasks have historically been developed to index psychological *processes* or *states* of interest (e.g., fear activation, inhibition of dominant responses), with the emphasis in task development being to maximize *average task effects* by optimizing condition-manipulations to limit variability across individuals. Moreover, while extensive effort is routinely devoted to confirming that variations in psychometric scale scores reflect individual differences in the attribute of interest (e.g., by showing that they covary with conceptually-related criterion measures but not conceptually-unrelated measures), researchers do not commonly undertake systematic validation work to confirm that variations in a neurophysiological-task measure reflect *individual differences in extent of engagement of the specific process* the task is designed to measure—as opposed to variation in some other process or processes.

As an example, a lab task procedure that has been widely used to investigate reward function in studies of psychopathology is the neuroimaging monetary incentive delay (MID) task (Knutson et al., 2000), in which brain activation is measured during anticipation and subsequent receipt of gain outcomes (i.e., monetary rewards) as compared to no-gain or loss outcomes. The use of this task in clinical studies is premised on the idea that differences in brain activation between patient and non-patient groups, or across individuals within a sample, are indicative of variations in reward sensitivity or responsiveness. However, the validity of MID-task brain activation scores for indexing individual differences in responsiveness to reward (i.e., dispositional reward sensitivity) remains to be demonstrated. Doing so would require demonstration of reliable convergent relations with previously validated measures of reward sensitivity, and consistent divergent (discriminant) associations with well-established measures of conceptually distinct attributes (e.g., threat sensitivity).

Method Variance A major challenge in seeking to identify replicable lab-task indicators of psychological characteristics or conditions, mentioned earlier, is that psychological attributes are generally operationalized in a separate measurement modality—that of self- or other-report. Owing to method variance, defined as systematic variability in scores attributable to distinct influences operating within a particular measurement modality (Campbell & Fiske, 1959), comparably reliable and valid measures of a target construct will covary more strongly with one another when operationalized in the same as compared to a different modality of assessment. For example, two validated self-report measures of fearfulness would be expected to exhibit stronger relations with one another (0.6–0.8 range) than either would with an overt behavioral or physiological measure of fear reactivity. More specifically, reliable measures of the same construct from the same modality are likely to correlate strongly (0.6–0.8 range), whereas measures of the same construct from different modalities are expected to correlate only moderately (0.3–0.5).

Correlations for measures of *only somewhat related* constructs from different modalities are expected to be even lower (i.e., 0.1–0.3).

Because lab-task measures can be expected to index constructs only somewhat related to those assessed by report-based measures of an attribute (which focus on self-ascriptions of general proclivities), correlations of task behavioral and physiological variables with report-based measures are likely to fall in the 0.1–0.3 range. Consistent with this, recent large-*N* studies of relations between brain-response variables and report-based phenotypes point to only modest effect sizes (e.g., Castellanos-Ryan et al., 2014; Hicks et al., 2007; Marek et al., 2022; Yancey et al., 2016). Specialized research strategies are needed to cope with the limiting effects of method variance on associations between measures from different assessment modalities. The final major section of this chapter discusses an example of such a strategy.

Specificity of Lab-Task Measures as Indicators of Target Attributes Apart from how reliable particular lab-task measures are, and to what extent they contain method-specific variance, a further issue is how selectively they index a specific attribute of interest (e.g., reduced sensitivity to rewarding outcomes, as related to depression) as opposed to other attributes. In short, how cleanly do they measure the attribute or construct of interest? Or, in statistical terms: How much of the reliable variance in the lab-task measure reflects the attribute of interest? This is important to consider because variation across individuals in a task effect of interest (e.g., brain reactivity to a cue for reward, relative to a non-reward cue) can reflect participant characteristics separate from the main attribute the task is designed to measure (e.g., reward sensitivity). Examples in this case might include attributes such as anxiousness or distractibility that affect neural reactivity within the task separately from reward sensitivity.

Perkins et al. (2017) illustrated this point by showing that a single neurophysiological measure can contain variance related to separate psychological attributes. The focus of this work was an electrocortical (ERP) measure of reactivity to abrupt acoustic stimuli occurring within a picture-viewing task—the noise-probe P3. This ERP component is a variant of the well-known P3 response that occurs to rarely occurring ("oddball") stimuli within a target detection task, as evidenced by an *r* of ~0.3 between the two in this study. However, the noise-probe P3 is distinct from the oddball P3 in that it occurs to an unexpected, intense stimulus (i.e., noise burst) that is perceived as aversive by most subjects. Perkins et al. reported opposing associations of two questionnaire-assessed traits, threat sensitivity and disinhibition, with amplitude of noise-probe P3 in a picture-viewing task. The two traits, which were uncorrelated with each other, accounted for separate portions of variance in noise-probe P3. In addition, analyses revealed that probe-P3's association with disinhibition was attributable to variance in common with the oddball-P3 response, whereas its relation with threat sensitivity was not. The authors' interpretation was that the P3 response to noise-probe stimuli contains a component of variance reflecting a disinhibition-related process indexed by other variants of P3 (e.g., a general impairment in elaborative post-processing of stimulus events; Foell et al., 2016; Patrick et al., 2016), along with a separate component of variance reflecting a fear-related process not represented in other variants of P3 (e.g., heightened vigilance following the occurrence of an unexpected aversive event; see Drislane et al., 2013).

A different scenario pertaining to specificity of measurement is one in which a neurophysiological measure taps variation in a distinct process across individuals that relates to different psychological attributes. An example of this might be a neurophysiological measure of arousability, such as change in alpha-frequency EEG activity during performance of a cognitive task (Ray & Cole, 1985), that relates to different psychological attributes which include a common element of arousability (e.g., sociability and sensation seeking). In this case, the two attributes would be expected to overlap in their associations with this neurophysiological measure (i.e., if variations in a common brain process account for observed associations of each). Conceptually, this would indicate an element of similarity between the two attributes that is not evident in the modality of self-report.

These two scenarios highlight potential discontinuity between how attributes are represented in modalities of person-report and lab-task response. In the first, correlations of separate portions of variance in a single neurophysiological measure with two distinct trait variables indicate that different attribute-related processes are tapped by the same neural reactivity index. In turn, this encourages a shift toward viewing the neural measure as multidimensional rather than unitary—and considering methods by which differing portions of variance in the measure might be parsed to index different attributes (e.g., quantitative methods such as structural equation modeling or multidimensional item-response modeling; Balsis et al., 2018). In the second scenario, relations of a common component of variance in a single neurophysiological measure with two putatively distinct traits suggests a role for some shared brain process in each. This could serve as an impetus for reconfiguring the two traits into three individual difference dimensions—one reflecting their mutual association with neurophysiological arousability and the other two reflecting separate (and perhaps more psychological-experiential) aspects of each.

Score Aggregation Report-based assessments of psychological attributes typically involve aggregation of scores across different items of an inventory or scale. Aggregating across items operates to harmonize responses to thematically related but non-identical indicators around a common dimension of variation representing the target attribute. For example, self-report items such as "I frequently attend parties" and "I seek out positions of leadership" are less clearly indicative of extraversion when considered alone than when combined together with other items pertaining to outgoingness, friendliness, assertiveness, and activity level. Combining across multiple item-indicators results in lesser weighting of portions of variance in individual item responses that are unrelated to the target attribute, whether systematic (e.g., indicative of other attributes) or unsystematic in nature (e.g., related to carelessness or misreading).

Target-attribute related variance in lab-task measures will invariably be entangled with non-relevant components of variance, thereby necessitating some means of isolating the variance of interest. One approach to achieving this is to aggregate across different attribute-related lab-task measures. Aggregation results in lesser weighting of portions of variance in individual indicators that are unrelated to the target attribute, to the extent the indicators covary mainly due to their mutual relations with the attribute of interest (i.e., they are "locally independent", in latent-variable modeling terms). Aggregation is particularly useful for distilling attribute-related variance when lab-task measures are of different types or come from separate task procedures—because in these cases less of the covariance among indicators will reflect non-attribute related influences they share.

An example of this comes from work on reduced P3 amplitude as an indicator of externalizing proneness (disinhibition). This association has been demonstrated most frequently for P3 response to rare target stimuli in visual oddball tasks; consistent with expectation, the magnitude of this association is modest (~0.2; e.g., Hicks et al., 2007; Yancey et al., 2013), indicating that about 4.4% of the portion of variance in oddball-target P3 response that is reliable (i.e., ~ 0.9, based on split-half estimation; Perkins et al., 2017) relates to externalizing proneness. However, other variants of P3 covary with externalizing proneness at similar levels, including ones derived from separate tasks as well as ones measured in the same oddball task (Nelson et al., 2011; Patrick et al., 2013). Variants of P3 from different tasks correlate less highly with one another (0.2–0.4) than variants measured in the same task (0.6 or higher; Nelson et al., 2011; Venables et al., 2018), indicating that a greater proportion of the covariance among different-task P3s reflects variance related to externalizing proneness (e.g., Burwell et al., 2016).

As a demonstration of this, Nelson et al. (2011) showed that the externalizing-related variance in P3 measures from three separate tasks (oddball, flanker, and choice-feedback) could be effectively distilled using factor analysis. Whereas the three individual P3 measures correlated only modestly with one another (median $r = 0.26$) and with a criterion measure of externalizing proneness, scores on a factor reflecting their shared variance correlated above 0.4 with scores on the externalizing criterion. Moreover, a factor analysis incorporating scores on the externalizing criterion together with the P3 brain measures yielded a single common factor on which all variables loaded to similar marked degrees (0.44–0.60). The latter result highlighted the possibility of quantifying externalizing proneness (disinhibition) as an individual difference dimension residing between self-report and neurophysiological assessment modalities.

In the next section, we describe a methodological strategy by which EP research could seek to address the measurement issues enumerated in this section and thereby amplify relations between diagnostic variables (phenotypes) of interest and lab-task behavioral and physiological measures. We describe how this methodological strategy can serve the aim of identifying biobehavioral processes associated with, and perhaps contributing to, psychological dysfunction.

A Methodological Strategy for Amplifying Relations Between Diagnostic Phenotypes and Lab-Task Variables in EP Research

In the approach described here, clinically relevant traits assessed via self- or other-report are viewed as nodes within the empirical subspace of a conceptual-empirical ("nomological"; Cronbach & Meehl, 1955; see also Meehl, 1978) network, which connect more closely to nodes reflecting report-based diagnostic phenotypes, and more distally to behaviorally- and biologically-defined characteristics. In turn, nodes of each type within the empirical subspace of the network connect to hypothetical constructs in the theoretical subspace of the network. From this standpoint, trait constructs can be operationalized in terms of nodes reflecting different modalities of measurement in the empirical subspace, or on the other hand, deduced from regions of the empirical space at the intersection of different-modality measures. More specific to the current context, operationalizations of clinically relevant traits can be systematically revised to incorporate biological and behavioral measures, and thereby serve as effective interfaces between diagnostic phenotypes and biobehavioral measures.

Description of the Strategy The methodological strategy we describe provides a means to quantify diagnostic constructs through combined use of report-based measures and lab-task measures. This approach focuses on biobehavioral trait constructs such as threat sensitivity, reward sensitivity, inhibitory control, and affiliative capacity, which can be conceptualized in both psychological and biological-behavioral terms (Depue & Iacono, 1989; Depue & Lenzenweger, 2001; Lenzenweger & Depue, 2020; Patrick et al., 2019); these hypothetical trait constructs serve as anchors for integrating measures from different modalities into trait assessments with power to predict criterion measures across different measurement modalities (e.g., self- and other-rated symptoms; behavioral performance measures; brain-response variables).

This measurement-based strategy focuses on trait-dispositional constructs because traits are by definition trans-situational and show broad predictive power for clinical-psychological and performance outcomes when assessed using report-based measures (e.g., Kotov et al., 2017; Krueger & Tackett, 2003; Samuel & Widiger, 2008; Widiger, 2013). However, our proposed strategy focuses on trait constructs of a particular type—that is, *biobehavioral traits*, reflecting classes of behavior theorized to relate to distinct evolved-adaptive systems of the brain (Lang, 1994, 1995; Miller & Cohen, 2001). As an example, the biobehavioral construct of threat sensitivity can be conceptualized as proneness to react more or less strongly to acute aversive stimuli (Yancey et al., 2016), as a function of constitutional and environmental influences that affect detection and processing of such stimuli and the degree to which they prompt activation of the brain's defensive motivational system (e.g., Fanselow, 1994; Lang, 1995). Defined this way, variations in this trait can be expected to contribute, on average and across people, to self-perceptions of fearfulness in relation to threats of various types encountered in everyday life, brain and bodily reactivity within different situations involving threat, and inclination to enter versus avoid threat contexts and overt-measurable behavior within such contexts. This conception of biobehavioral dispositions reflects a realist position (e.g., Borsboom et al., 2004; Tellegen, 1991), in which traits are viewed as psychobiological networks or structures (Allport, 1937; Eysenck, 1967) encompassing internal representations of percepts, actions/reactions, and semantics (e.g., connotations, interpretations, perspectives, beliefs) that can affect measured variables in different modalities (Lang, 1979, 1994). Such traits are also arguably driven by basic neurobehavioral systems that are well conserved and manifest themselves not only in humans, but also in the behavior of other mammals mutatis mutandis (Depue & Lenzenweger, 2001; Lenzenweger & Depue, 2020).

The approach proceeds in a series of iterative steps that lead to progressive modification of the initial conceptualization of the target trait. First, efforts are made to identify *reliable behavioral and physiological indicators*, from psychologically relevant tasks, of a target attribute assessed through self- or other-report. Psychometrically sound scale measures of attributes conceptualized in biobehavioral terms are recommended as initial referents for this "mapping" process because they are coherent and reliable as well as efficient and inexpensive. However, to be considered a viable index of a biobehavioral construct, the scale measure should be composed of conceptually relevant items or item-sets that have been shown to relate to one or more established biobehavioral indicators of the attribute. Examples include scale measures of trait disinhibition that relate to cognitive-task performance (e.g., Brennan & Baskin-Sommers, 2018; Young et al., 2009) and P3 brain response (e.g., Brislin et al., 2019; Yancey et al., 2013; see next subsection), and scale measures of dispositional fear/fearlessness that relate to effective performance under threat (e.g., Yancey et al., 2019, in press) and aversive startle potentiation (e.g., López et al., 2013; Yancey et al., 2016; see also Kramer et al., 2012). Using the trait scale as a provisional referent, further research is undertaken to identify new, replicable indicators of the trait from these other modalities.

Once additional indicators have been identified, analyses can be undertaken to evaluate their covariance *structure*, in part to refine neurophysiological quantification of the target attribute, and also to clarify the functional meaning of the neural indicators themselves (e.g., by considering common vs. unique processing demands of lab-tasks they derive from). This is followed by efforts to (a) update conceptualization of the target attribute to incorporate insights gained from the structural analysis of neurophysiological indicators, (b) modify the psychometric scale measure of the target construct to reflect the neurally informed conceptualization, and (c) apply understanding of relevant neural processes to create new lab tasks expected to yield more robust brain indicators of the target attribute. This process continues iteratively to the point where an optimal set of physiological tasks/measures exists for operationalizing the targeted biobehavioral construct in a precise and reliable manner.

Empirical Illustration: Multi-Modal Quantification of Inhibitory Control Capacity Relying on research demonstrating associations for multiple variants of P3 brain response and performance on different cognitive-control tasks with general proneness to externalizing problems (e.g., Nelson et al., 2011; Patrick et al., 2013; Young et al., 2009), Venables et al. (2018) worked to develop a multi-modal approach to quantifying the biobehavioral trait construct of inhibitory control (inhibition-disinhibition), conceptualized as externalizing proneness. These authors collected multiple indicators of inhibitory control from three different modalities of measurement (self-report, behavioral performance, neurophysiology) and characterized their interrelations within and across modalities through use of structural modeling. The self-report indicators were four scale measures of trait disinhibition reflecting general externalizing proneness (cf. Drislane & Patrick, 2017), the behavioral performance indicators were measures of performance from four different inhibitory control tasks (cf. Young et al., 2009), and the neurophysiological indicators were four variants of P3 brain response from three separate visual-motor tasks (cf. Nelson et al., 2011).

Relations among these various indicators were characterized in terms of a higher-order model in which indicators from each modality (self-report, behavioral response, neurophysiology) defined lower-order modality factors, which loaded in turn onto a general, higher-order factor representing covariance across the three measurement modalities. This structural model accounted for covariance among the 12 indicators quite well, as indicated by good fit according to statistical indices. The demonstration of a coherent broad factor accounting for covariation among these different sets of indicators accords with the view of inhibitory control as a latent disposition that influences measurable responses in different modalities.

Certain aspects of the model warrant specific mention. First, within the fully unconstrained model, in which loading parameters were freely estimated (both for individual indicators on modality factors and for modality factors on the higher-order factor), the behavioral-response and neurophysiological modality factors loaded more strongly onto the general factor (−0.60 and − 0.77, respectively) than did the self-report modality factor (0.40). The implication is that the general factor of the unconstrained model reflected variation across participants in brain reactivity and behavioral performance more so than variation in self-perceived proclivities. Owing to this, scores on the general factor correlated more highly with criterion measures from the modality of behavioral response (i.e., other task-performance variables) and neurophysiology (i.e., a separate variant of P3) than with self-report criterion measures of externalizing problems (i.e., scales assessing antisocial conduct, alcohol/drug abuse, and impulsive-erratic personality disorder symptoms). The authors' interpretation was that the general factor of this model had "shifted away" from the modality of psychological self-description toward the modalities of lab-task behavioral and neurophysiological response. An interesting corollary finding was that scores on the general model factor of the model were uncorrelated with a scale measure of socially desirable responding, whereas scores on the self-report modality factor showed a significant negative correlation. The implication is that multi-domain assessments of clinically relevant attributes may be less susceptible to well-known response biases.

Another notable aspect of the Venables et al. (2018) study pertains to an alternative version of the structural model in which the loadings of the three lower-order modality factors onto the higher-order general factor were constrained to be equal, rather than being allowed to freely vary. This model accounted comparably well for covariance patterns as the unconstrained model, as evidenced by similar statistical fit. However, the general factor of this alternative model correlated more strongly with criterion measures of externalizing problems than the general factor of the unconstrained model—owing to greater representation of disinhibition-scale variance in the general factor of the former. The implication is that different versions of the general inhibition-disinhibition factor can be specified (by constraining loadings of modality factors, or by including other types of indicators in the model and/or modeling the data differently) to fulfill different assessment aims. For example, the general factor of the unconstrained model would likely be more effective for quantifying levels of inhibitory control in studies of neurophysiological processes/mechanisms. By contrast, the general factor of the constrained model would likely be more effective for clinical diagnosis and decision-making.

An additional point regarding the Venables et al. (2018) model is that it focused on the trait of inhibition-disinhibition conceptualized in a highly specific manner—as resistance versus susceptibility to impulse-control problems (externalizing proneness). Externalizing proneness differs from other ostensibly related concepts such as impulsivity, (dys)constraint (lack of self-control), and (un)conscientiousness in the personality literature (e.g., Berg et al., 2015; Costa Jr & McCrae, 1992; Tellegen & Waller, 2008; Whiteside & Lynam, 2001) in that it derives not just from report-based data. It is grounded as well in behavioral genetic research on the externalizing spectrum of problems and traits (e.g., Krueger et al., 2002; Young et al., 2000) and in work identifying brain and task-performance measures related to externalizing problems and characterizing the etiological basis of their relations (e.g., Hicks et al., 2007; Yancey et al., 2013; Young et al., 2009). Studies that have evaluated relations of purely self-report-based measures of impulsivity with behavioral task measures of inhibitory control or dysconstraint have found weak or negligible associations (Friedman et al., 2020; Sharma et al., 2014). Similarly, Bowyer et al. (2020) found that maladaptive personality traits converged effectively with brain response indicators when configured to reflect externalizing proneness, but not when configured to reflect self-report defined dimensions. These differences in findings highlight the importance of utilizing scale measures with direct empirical links to biobehavioral data in working to establish multi-modal operationalizations of clinically relevant biobehavioral traits.

Concluding Thoughts in Our Imagined Conversation with Scott

As we ponder our imagined Dinkytown cafe conversation with Scott, we can easily picture him wanting to continue batting around ideas for many more hours. The following are just a few of the additional topics we could imagine turning to: (1) reductionism in experimental psychopathology; (2) the challenge of establishing causal relations based on observational/correlational data (e.g., the weakness of causal inference in traditional structural equation modeling versus newer approaches such as Rubin's (2005) causal model); (3) the difficulty of building empirical bridges from the genomic level of analysis to experimental psychopathology laboratory studies; (4) the utility of blind empirical approaches to understanding data versus theory-guided approaches (e.g., structure arising from machine learning algorithms as compared to substantive considerations and construct development/refinement); (5) how best to elucidate the personality and psychopathology interface (i.e., should we work from the neurobehavioral systems level of analysis out to phenotypic manifestations, or begin with phenotypic manifestations and follow them down to underlying systems); (6) embracing the importance of *emergence* and emergent phenomena in understanding psychopathology, given the abundance of emergent phenomena in the world (e.g., birds flocking, ant colonies, the game of chess) and the critical importance of emergent conceptualizations in fields as divergent as condensed matter and material physics, to animal behavior, to meteorology, to contemporary cognitive neuroscience (Depue & Lenzenweger, 2001; Lenzenweger & Depue, 2020), a view that Scott also adopted over time (e.g., Lilienfeld et al., 2019); (7) how best to analyze our data (e.g., the critical importance of principled exploratory data analysis, judicious post hoc discovery, the context of discovery vs. the context of justification, the limits of administrative solutions to scientific problems [e.g., pre-registration of studies]); (8) the critical importance of using time passage as a lever to understand the etiology and unfolding of psychopathology when no experimental protocol will do (e.g., the value of data that is yielded by prospective longitudinal research in psychopathology; cf. Lenzenweger, 2006, 2021) versus the appeal of cross-sectional studies; and (9) last, but not least, the importance of the perennial admonition from the late Professor Brendan Maher (1966, 2003) to the field of experimental psychopathology, namely, to "count, don't rate"--that is, to do all we can to steer away from self- and other-rating measures in the study of psychopathology, and instead rely on measures that reflect enumerating or tallying up discrete quantitative indicators of the phenomenon of interest (or, by way of analogy, consider that we don't simply look at a stack of groceries on the checkout conveyer belt at the supermarket and subjectively rate their cost, rather we add up the prices using the method of counting).

As a final word, we encourage readers of this chapter to discover what Scott himself had to say about many of these topics by delving into his rich and voluminous writings, which will carry forward as continuing sources of scholarly insight and inspiration—including Lilienfeld (1994, 1995, 2007), Lilienfeld et al. (2008,

2010), Lilienfeld and Widows (2005), and Morgan and Lilienfeld (2000), to name but a few. Our hope is that through exposure to Scott's written works, and recordings of his lectures available online, others will also imagine the wide range of topics they would choose to discuss over coffee with Scott.

References

Allport, G. W. (1937). *Personality: A psychological interpretation*. Holt.

Balsis, S., Choudhury, B. S., Geraci, L., & Patrick, C. J. (2018). Alzheimer's disease assessment: A review and illustrations focusing on item response theory techniques. *Assessment, 25*, 360–373.

Berg, J. M., Latzman, R. D., Bliwise, N. G., & Lilienfeld, S. O. (2015). Parsing the heterogeneity of impulsivity: A metaanalytic review of the behavioral implications of the UPPS for psychopathology. *Psychological Assessment, 27*, 1129–1146.

Borsboom, D., Mellenbergh, G. J., & van Heerden, J. (2004). The concept of validity. *Psychological Review, 111*(4), 1061–1071.

Bowyer, C. B., Joyner, K. J., Latzman, R. D., Venables, N. C., Foell, J., & Patrick, C. J. (2020). A model-based strategy for interfacing trait domains of the DSM-5 AMPD with neurobiology. *Journal of Personality Disorders, 34*, 586–608.

Brennan, G. M., & Baskin-Sommers, A. R. (2018). Brain-behavior relationships in externalizing: P3 amplitude reduction reflects deficient inhibitory control. *Behavioral Brain Research, 337*, 70–79.

Brislin, S. J., Patrick, C. J., Flor, H., Nees, F., Heinrich, A., Drislane, L. E., Yancey, J. R., et al. (2019). Extending the construct network of trait disinhibition to the neuroimaging domain: Validation of a bridging scale for use in the European IMAGEN project. *Assessment, 26*(4), 567–581.

Burwell, S. J., Malone, S. M., & Iacono, W. G. (2016). One-year developmental stability and covariance among oddball, novelty, go/no-go, and flanker event-related potentials in adolescence: A monozygotic twin study. *Psychophysiology, 53*, 991–1007.

Campbell, D. T., & Fiske, D. W. (1959). Convergent and discriminant validation by the multitrait-multimethod matrix. *Psycholological Bulletin, 56*(2), 81–105.

Castellanos-Ryan, N., Struve, M., Whelan, R., Banaschewski, T., Barker, G. J., Bokde, A. L., et al. (2014). Neural and cognitive correlates of the common and specific variance across externalizing problems in young adolescence. *American Journal of Psychiatry, 171*(12), 1310–1319.

Conway, C. C., Forbes, M. K., Forbush, K. T., Fried, E. I., Hallquist, M. N., Kotov, R., Patrick, C. J., et al. (2019). A hierarchical taxonomy of psychopathology can transform mental health research. *Perspectives on Psychological Science, 14*(3), 419–436.

Conway, C. C., South, S. C., Forbes, M. K., & the HiTOP Consortium. (2022). A hierarchical taxonomy of psychopathology (HiTOP) primer for mental health researchers. *Clinical Psychological Science, 10*(2), 236–258.

Cornblatt, B. A., & Keilp, J. G. (1994). Impaired attention, genetics, and the pathophysiology of schizophrenia. *Schizophrenia Bulletin, 20*, 31–46.

Costa, P. T., Jr., & McCrae, R. R. (1992). *Revised NEO personality inventory (NEO PI-R) and NEO five-factor inventory (NEOFFI) professional manual*. PAR.

Cronbach, L. J. (1957). The two disciplines of scientific psychology. *American Psychologist, 12*, 671–684.

Cronbach, L. J., & Meehl, P. E. (1955). Construct validity in psychological tests. *Psychological Bulletin, 52*, 281–302.

Depue, R. A., & Iacono, W. G. (1989). Neurobehavioral aspects of affective disorders. *Annual Review of Psychology, 40*, 457–492.

Depue, R. A., & Lenzenweger, M. F. (2001). A neurobehavioral dimensional model of personality disorders. In W. J. Livesley (Ed.), *The handbook of personality disorders* (pp. 136–176). Guilford.

Drislane, L. E., & Patrick, C. J. (2017). Integrating alternative conceptions of psychopathic personality: A latent variable model of triarchic psychopathy constructs. *Journal of Personality Disorders, 31*(1), 110–132.

Drislane, L. E., Vaidyanathan, U., & Patrick, C. J. (2013). Reduced cortical call to arms differentiates psychopathy from antisocial personality disorder. *Psychological Medicine, 43*, 825–836.

Elliott, M. L., Knodt, A. R., Ireland, D., Morris, M. L., Poulton, R., Ramrakha, S., et al. (2020). What is the test-retest reliability of common task-functional MRI measures? New empirical evidence and a meta-analysis. *Psychological Science, 31*(7), 792–806.

Eysenck, H. J. (1967). *The biological basis of personality*. Charles C. Thomas.

Fanselow, M. S. (1994). Neural organization of the defensive behavior system responsible for fear. *Psychonomic Bulletin and Review, 1*, 429–438.

Foell, J., Brislin, S. J., Palumbo, I., Perkins, E. R., & Patrick, C. J. (2016). Brain mechanisms of externalizing proneness: Results from functional MRI studies in adolescents and adults. *Psychophysiology, 53*, S15.

Fossati, A., Maffei, C., Bagnato, M., Battaglia, M., Donati, D., Donini, M., et al. (2000). Patterns of covariation of DSM-IV personality disorders in a mixed psychiatric sample. *Comprehensive Psychiatry, 41*, 206–215.

Fowles, D. C. (1980). The three arousal model: Implications of Gray's two-factor learning theory for heart rate, electrodermal activity, and psychopathy. *Psychophysiology, 17*, 87–104.

Friedman, N. P., Hatoum, A. S., Gustavson, D. E., Corley, R. P., Hewitt, J. K., & Young, S. E. (2020). Executive functions and impulsivity are genetically distinct and independently predict psychopathology: Results from two adult twin studies. *Clinical Psychological Science, 8*(3), 519–538.

Haeffel, G. J., Jeronimus, B. F., Kaiser, B. N., Weaver, L. J., Soyster, P. D., Fisher, A. J., et al. (2022). Folk classification and factor rotations: Whales, sharks, and the problems with the hierarchical taxonomy of psychopathology (HiTOP). *Clinical Psychological Science, 10*(2), 259–278.

Hare, R. D. (1978). Electrodermal and cardiovascular correlates of psychopathy. In R. D. Hare & D. Schalling (Eds.), *Psychopathic behavior: Approaches to research* (pp. 107–143). Wiley.

Hicks, B. M., Bernat, E. M., Malone, S. M., Iacono, W. G., Patrick, C. J., Krueger, R. F., & McGue, M. (2007). Genes mediate the association between P3 amplitude and externalizing disorders. *Psychophysiology, 44*, 98–105.

Knutson, B., Westdorp, A., Kaiser, E., & Hommer, D. (2000). FMRI visualization of brain activity during a monetary incentive delay task. *NeuroImage, 12*, 20–27.

Kotov, R., Krueger, R. F., Watson, D., Achenbach, T. M., Althoff, R. R., et al. (2017). The hierarchical taxonomy of psychopathology (HiTOP): A dimensional alternative to traditional nosologies. *Journal of Abnormal Psychology, 126*, 454–477.

Kramer, M. D., Patrick, C. J., Krueger, R. F., & Gasperi, M. (2012). Delineating physiological defensive reactivity in the domain of self-report: Phenotypic and etiologic structure of dispositional fear. *Psychological Medicine, 42*, 1305–1320.

Krueger, R. F., & Tackett, J. L. (2003). Personality and psychopathology: Working toward the bigger picture. *Journal of Personality Disorders, 17*(2), 109–128.

Krueger, R. F., Hicks, B. M., Patrick, C. J., Carlson, S. R., Iacono, W. G., & McGue, M. (2002). Etiologic connections among substance dependence, antisocial behavior and personality: Modeling the externalizing spectrum. *Journal of Abnormal Psychology, 111*, 411–424.

Krueger, R. F., Markon, K. E., Patrick, C. J., Benning, S. D., & Kramer, M. D. (2007). Linking antisocial behavior, substance use, and personality: An integrative quantitative model of the adult externalizing spectrum. *Journal of Abnormal Psychology, 116*(4), 645–666.

Lang, P. (1979). A bioinformational theory of emotional imagery. *Psychophysiology, 16*, 495–512.

Lang, P. J. (1994). The motivational organization of emotion: Affect-reflex connections. In S. Van Goozen, N. E. Van de Poll, & J. A. Sergeant (Eds.), *The emotions: Essays on emotion theory* (pp. 61–93). Erlbaum.

Lang, P. J. (1995). The emotion probe: Studies of motivation and attention. *American Psychologist, 50*, 372–385.

Lenzenweger, M. F. (2006). The longitudinal study of personality disorders: History, design, and initial findings. (*special essay*). *Journal of Personality Disorders, 6*, 645–670.

Lenzenweger, M. F. (2010). *Schizotypy and schizophrenia: The view from experimental psychopathology*. Guilford Press.

Lenzenweger, M. F. (2020). Conceptual foundations of experimental psychopathology: Historical context, scientific posture, and reflections on substantive and method matters. In A. G. C. Wright & M. N. Hallquist (Eds.), *The Cambridge handbook of research methods in clinical psychology* (pp. 93–104). Cambridge University Press.

Lenzenweger, M. F. (2021). Schizotypy 17 years on: Dimensions of psychosis. *Journal of Abnormal Psychology, 130*, 399–412.

Lenzenweger, M. F., & Clarkin, J. F. (2005). The personality disorders: History, development, and research issues. In M. F. Lenzenweger & J. F. Clarkin (Eds.), *Major theories of personality disorder* (2nd ed., pp. 1–42). Guilford.

Lenzenweger, M. F., & Depue, R. A. (2020). Personality disturbances as emergent phenomena reflective of underlying neurobehavioral systems: Beyond dimensional measurement, phenotypic trait descriptors, and factor analysis. *Psychopathology, 53*, 213–220.

Lenzenweger, M. F., Cornblatt, B. A., & Putnick, M. E. (1991). Schizotypy and sustained attention. *Journal of Abnormal Psychology, 100*, 84–89.

Lilienfeld, S. O. (1994). Conceptual problems in the assessment of psychopathy. *Clinical Psychology Review, 14*, 17–38.

Lilienfeld, S. O. (1995). *Seeing both sides: Classic controversies in abnormal psychology*. Brooks/Cole.

Lilienfeld, S. O. (1996). Eye movement desensitization and reprocessing (EMDR) for anxiety: Less than meets the eye? *Skeptical Inquirer, 20*, 25–31.

Lilienfeld, S. O. (2007). Psychological treatments that cause harm. *Perspectives on Psychological Science, 2*, 53–70.

Lilienfeld, S. O. (2017). Microaggressions: Strong claims, inadequate evidence. *Perspectives on Psychological Science, 12*, 138–169.

Lilienfeld, S. O., Wood, J. M., & Garb, H. N. (2000). The scientific status of projective techniques. *Psychological Science in the Public Interest, 1*, 27–66.

Lilienfeld, S. O., Wood, J. M., & Garb, H. N. (2002). The Rorschach test is scientifically questionable. *Harvard Mental Health Letter, 10*, 4–5.

Lilienfeld, S. O., Ruscio, J., & Lynn, S. J. (2008). *Navigating the mindfield: A guide to separating science from pseudoscience in mental health*. Prometheus.

Lilienfeld, S. O., Lynn, S. J., Ruscio, J., & Beyerstein, B. J. (2010). *50 great myths of popular psychology: Shattering widespread misconceptions about human behavior*. Wiley-Blackwell.

Lilienfeld, S. O., Watts, A. L., Murphy, B., Costello, T. H., Bowes, S. M., Smith, S. F., et al. (2019). Personality disorders as emergent interpersonal syndromes: Psychopathic personality as a case example. *Journal of Personality Disorders, 33*, 577–622.

Lilienfeld, S. O., & Widows, M. R. (2005). *Psychopathic Personality Inventory—Revised (PPI-R) professional manual*. Odessa, FL: Psychological Assessment Resources.

López, R., Poy, R., Patrick, C. J., & Moltó, J. (2013). Deficient fear conditioning and self-reported psychopathy: The role of fearless dominance. *Psychophysiology, 50*, 210–218.

Lykken, D. T. (1957). A study of anxiety in the sociopathic personality. *Journal of Abnormal and Social Psychology, 55*(1), 6–10.

Maher, B. A. (1966). *Principles of psychopathology: An experimental approach*. McGraw-Hill.

Maher, B. A. (2003). Psychopathology and delusions: Reflections on methods and models. In M. F. Lenzenweger & J. M. Hooley (Eds.), *Principles of experimental psychopathology: Essays in honor of Brendan A. Maher* (pp. 9–28). American Psychological Association.

Marek, S., Tervo-Clemmens, B., Calabro, F. J., Montez, D. F., Kay, B. P., Hatoum, A. S., et al. (2022). Reproducible brain-wide association studies require thousands of individuals. *Nature, 603*(7902), 654–660.

Meehl, P. E. (1971). High school yearbooks: A reply to Schwarz. *Journal of Abnormal Psychology, 77*(2), 143–148.

Meehl, P. E. (1978). Theoretical risks and tabular asterisks: Sir Karl, sir Ronald, and the slow progress of soft psychology. *Journal of Consulting and Clinical Psychology, 46*(4), 806–834.

Miller, G. A., & Chapman, J. P. (2001). Misunderstanding analysis of covariance. *Journal of Abnormal Psychology, 110*(1), 40–48.

Miller, E. K., & Cohen, J. D. (2001). An integrative theory of prefrontal cortex function. *Annual Review of Neuroscience, 24*, 167–202.

Morgan, A. B., & Lilienfeld, S. O. (2000). A meta-analytic review of the relation between antisocial behavior and neuropsychological measures of executive function. *Clinical Psychology Review, 20*, 113–136.

Nelson, L. D., Patrick, C. J., & Bernat, E. M. (2011). Operationalizing proneness to externalizing psychopathology as a multivariate psychophysiological phenotype. *Psychophysiology, 48*, 64–72.

Nuechterlein, K. H., Barch, D. M., Gold, J. M., Goldberg, T. E., Green, M. F., & Heaton, R. K. (2004). Identification of separable cognitive factors in schizophrenia. *Schizophrenia Research, 72*(1), 29–39.

Patrick, C. J., Venables, N. C., Yancey, J. R., Hicks, B. M., Nelson, L. D., & Kramer, M. D. (2013). A construct-network approach to bridging diagnostic and physiological domains: Application to assessment of externalizing psychopathology. *Journal of Abnormal Psychology, 122*(3), 902–916.

Patrick, C. J., Foell, J., Venables, N. C., & Worthy, D. A. (2016). Substance use disorders as externalizing outcomes. In T. P. Beauchaine & S. P. Hinshaw (Eds.), *Oxford handbook of externalizing spectrum disorders* (pp. 38–60). Oxford University Press.

Patrick, C. J., Iacono, W. G., & Venables, N. C. (2019). Incorporating neurophysiological measures into clinical assessments: Fundamental challenges and a strategy for addressing them. *Psychological Assessment, 31*(12), 1512–1529.

Patterson, C. M., & Newman, J. P. (1993). Reflectivity and learning from aversive events: Toward a psychological mechanism for the syndromes of disinhibition. *Psychological Review, 100*, 716–736.

Perkins, E. R., Yancey, J. R., Drislane, L. D., Venables, N. C., Balsis, S., & Patrick, C. J. (2017). Methodological issues in the use of individual brain meaures to index trait liabilities: The example of noise-probe P3. *International Journal of Psychophysiology, 111*, 245–255.

Ray, W. J., & Cole, H. W. (1985). EEG alpha activity reflects attentional demands, and beta activity reflects emotional and cognitive processes. *Science, 228*, 750–752.

Rodnick, E. H., & Shakow, D. (1940). Set in the schizophrenic as measured by a composite reaction time index. *American Journal of Psychiatry, 97*(1), 214–225.

Rosenbaum, P. R., & Rubin, D. B. (1985). Constructing a control group using multivariate matched sampling methods that incorporate the propensity score. *The American Statistician, 39*(1), 33–38.

Rubin, D. B. (2005). Causal inference using potential outcomes: Design, modeling, decisions. *Journal of the American Statistical Association, 100*(469), 322–331.

Samuel, D. B., & Widiger, T. A. (2008). A meta-analytic review of the relationships between the five-factor model and DSM-IV-TR personality disorders: A facet level analysis. *Clinical Psychology Review, 28*(8), 1326–1342.

Sharma, L., Markon, K. E., & Clark, L. A. (2014). Toward a theory of distinct types of "impulsive" behaviors: A meta-analysis of self-report and behavioral measures. *Psychological Bulletin, 140*(2), 374–408.

Simms, L. J., Wright, A. G. C., Cicero, D., Kotov, R., Mullins-Sweatt, S. N., Sellbom, M., et al. (2022). Development of measures for the hierarchical taxonomy of psychopathology (HiTOP): A collaborative scale development project. *Assessment, 29*(1), 3–16.

Strauss, G. P., Allen, D. N., Jorgensen, M. L., & Cramer, S. L. (2005). Test-retest reliability of standard and emotional Stroop tasks: An investigation of color-word and picture-word versions. *Assessment, 12*(3), 330–337.

Tellegen, A. (1991). Personality traits: Issues of definition, evidence, and assessment. In D. Cicchetti & W. M. Grove (Eds.), *Thinking clearly about psychology: Essays in honor of Paul E. Meehl, Vol. 1. Matters of public interest; Vol. 2. Personality and psychopathology* (pp. 10–35). University of Minnesota Press.

Tellegen, A., & Waller, N. (2008). Exploring personality through test construction: Development of the multidimensional personality questionnaire. In G. J. Boyle, G. Matthews, & D. H. Saklofske (Eds.), *Handbook of personality theory and testing: Personality measurement and assessment* (Vol. 2, pp. 261–292). Sage.

Trull, T. J., & Durrett, C. A. (2005). Categorical and dimensional models of personality disorder. *Annual Review of Clinical Psychology, 1*, 355–380.

Venables, N. C., Foell, J., Yancey, J. R., Kane, M. J., Engle, R. W., & Patrick, C. J. (2018). Quantifying inhibitory control as externalizing proneness: A cross-domain model. *Clinical Psychological Science, 6*, 561–580.

Watson, D., O'Hara, M. W., Simms, L. J., Kotov, R., Chmielewski, M., McDade-Montez, E. A., & Stuart, S. (2007). Development and validation of the inventory of depression and anxiety symptoms (IDAS). *Psychological Assessment, 19*(3), 253–268.

Whiteside, S. P., & Lynam, D. R. (2001). The five factor model and impulsivity: Using a structural model of personality to understand impulsivity. *Personality and Individual Differences, 30*, 669–689.

Widiger, T. A. (2013). Personality and psychopathology. *World Psychiatry, 10*(2), 103–106.

Widiger, T. A., & Mullins-Sweatt, S. (2007). Mental disorders as discrete clinical conditions: Dimensional versus categorical classification. In M. Hersen, S. M. Turner, & D. C. Beidel (Eds.), *Adult psychopathology and diagnosis* (pp. 3–33). Wiley.

Yancey, J., Venables, N., Hicks, B., & Patrick, C. J. (2013). Evidence for a heritable brain basis to deviance-promoting deficits in self-control. *Journal of Criminal Justice, 41*, 309–317.

Yancey, J. R., Venables, N. C., & Patrick, C. J. (2016). Psychoneurometric operationalization of threat sensitivity: Relations with clinical symptom and physiological response criteria. *Psychophysiology, 53*(3), 393–405.

Yancey, J. R., Bowyer, C. B., Foell, J., Boot, W. R., & Patrick, C. J. (2019). Boldness moderates the effects of external threat on performance within a task switching paradigm. *Journal of Experimental Psychology: Human Perception and Performance, 45*, 758–770.

Yancey, J. R., Bowyer, C. B., Roberts, K. E., Jones, D., Foell, J., McGlade, E. C., Yurgelun-Todd, W. R., & Patrick, C. J. (in press). Boldness moderates cognitive performance under acute threat: Evidence from a task-switching paradigm involving cueing for shock. *Journal of Experimental Psychology: Human Perception and Performance*.

Young, S. E., Stallings, M. C., Corley, R. P., Krauter, K. S., & Hewitt, J. K. (2000). Genetic and environmental influences on behavioral disinhibition. *American Journal of Medical Genetics: Neuropsychiatric Genetics, 96*, 684–695.

Young, S. E., Friedman, N. P., Miyake, A., Willcutt, E. G., Corley, R. P., Haberstick, B. C., & Hewitt, J. K. (2009). Behavioral disinhibition: Liability for externalizing spectrum disorders and its genetic and environmental relation to response inhibition across adolescence. *Journal of Abnormal Psychology, 118*, 117–130.

The Role of Temperament in the Classification and Treatment of Emotional Disorders: A Transdiagnostic Approach

Erin F. Ward-Ciesielski, Andrew J. Curreri, Brittany Woods, and David H. Barlow

Introduction

Debates about the most accurate and efficient methods to understand and classify psychopathology have been ongoing since the beginnings of such efforts. While categorical and prototypical approaches such as the Diagnostic and Statistical Manual of Mental Disorders (DSM) and International Classification of Diseases (ICD) comprise the most widely used systems at this time (American Psychiatric Association [APA], 2013; World Health Organization [WHO], 2016), one central aspect of the debate centers on the shared characteristics that present across such categories. These characteristics suggest the existence of underlying commonalities, or transdiagnostic typologies that could maximize the validity and utility of classification and highlight a more limited number of targets for treatment. Although hardly a new idea, recognition and acknowledgment of commonalities across disorders have reemerged in recent years (e.g., Bullis et al., 2019; East-Richard et al., 2020; Garland & Howard, 2014). In part, this is likely in response to the seemingly continuous proliferation of specific disorders and disorder-specific treatments driven by our categorical nosology. In this chapter, we provide a historical overview of the proliferation of categorical disorders and subsequent return to diagnostic commonalities. Further, we highlight one such commonality, temperament—in particular, neuroticism—and associated transdiagnostic approaches that target neuroticism in psychological treatments. We then highlight several avenues for continued research in the area of targeted transdiagnostic treatment.

E. F. Ward-Ciesielski (✉)
Center for Anxiety and Related Disorders, Boston University, Boston, MA, USA

A. J. Curreri · B. Woods · D. H. Barlow
Boston University, Boston, MA, USA

C. L. Cobb et al. (eds.), *Toward a Science of Clinical Psychology*,
https://doi.org/10.1007/978-3-031-14332-8_10

Brief History of the Classification of Psychological Disorders

Upon recognition of the need for a consistent, uniform classification system that could be applied internationally to organize causes of morbidity and mortality, the first version of the ICD originated in the 1850s and was ultimately the basis for the International List of Causes of Death in 1900 (Clark et al., 2017). Concurrently, organizations across the United States were engaged in efforts to specifically classify cases of mental disorders, ultimately culminating in the first edition of the DSM (APA, 1952).

The first modern edition of the ICD (ICD-6; World Health Organization [WHO], 1949), which was also the first edition to include classification of mental disorders, listed 26 categories, grouped into three broad clusters: psychoses, psychoneurotic disorders, and disorders of character, behavior, and intelligence. DSM-I (APA, 1952) was also organized into three groups: disorders with an organic basis, disorders without an identified organic basis, and "mental retardation." While the ICD and DSM were overlapping and generally similar classification systems in their early editions, with DSM-III published in 1980, the systems began to diverge (Clark et al., 2017). With this third edition, additional information regarding operationally defined, observable indicators, such as patient behaviors and patient-reported symptoms, were elaborated, and thresholds (e.g., number of criteria), duration criteria, and exclusions (e.g., due to a general medical conditions) were specified. This led to a substantial proliferation of new diagnoses, as well as additional diagnostic categories and subtypes (Kawa & Giordano, 2012). In fact, while DSM-I included about 100 disorders, in DSM-III, 265 categories of disorders were delineated. This number grew to 292 diagnoses in DSM-III-R, 297 in DSM-IV, and 298 in DSM-5 (Suris et al., 2016). These additional diagnoses are intended to provide greater specificity and reliability to inform treatments; however, criticism for this system has been pervasive for decades.

Limitations to the Proliferation of a Categorical Diagnostic Approach

A full discussion of the critiques of diagnostic classification systems over more than a century is beyond the scope of this chapter (for reviews see, for example, Brown & Barlow, 2002; Jablensky, 2016; Lilienfeld et al., 2013; Suris et al., 2016); however, three common limitations of extant diagnostic systems are relevant here. These include pervasive comorbidity, questions about whether disorders are truly discrete categories, and overlooking the multiple etiologies of psychological disorders (see Clark et al., 2017 for a comprehensive review). First, comorbidity (i.e., exhibiting characteristics that yield multiple concurrent diagnoses) is the rule rather than the exception (e.g., Hasin & Grant, 2015). For example, in a seminal paper reporting on data from more than 9000 adults from the US National Comorbidity Survey

Replication, Kessler et al. (2005) found that 45% of individuals who met criteria for any diagnosis actually met criteria for two or more. Furthermore, current and lifetime comorbidity rates among anxiety, depressive, and related disorders are high, at around 55% and 76%, respectively (Brown et al., 2001).

While it is likely that some individuals are genuinely impacted by multiple disorders simultaneously, given the use of symptoms to indicate the presence of a psychological condition, an inherent limitation involves the variable presentation of symptoms and the ways in which similar symptoms are considered diagnostic of multiple different disorders (e.g., sleep disturbance in generalized anxiety disorder and major depressive disorder). The obvious result of this limitation is the propensity for multiple diagnoses being applied with little understanding or recognition of the potential underlying processes which may better account for areas of distress or impairment than diagnostic labels. That is, it is unclear how often an individual meets criteria for multiple diagnoses relative to how often different providers label or conceptualize symptoms as indicative of separate disorders. Given poor diagnostic interrater reliability (e.g., Regier et al., 2013; Spitzer et al., 1979), at least some comorbid diagnoses are likely erroneous. In fact, field trials for the DSM-5 yielded "questionable" reliability estimates for common diagnoses like major depressive disorder and generalized anxiety disorder (Regier et al., 2013). Furthermore, even when attempting to apply broad categorical designations (e.g., internalizing vs. externalizing), research supporting these designations is inconsistent (e.g., Hasin & Grant, 2015). For example, a disorder may load onto multiple factors (e.g., borderline personality disorder; Eaton, Krueger, Keyes, et al., 2011; Eaton, Krueger, & Oltmanns, 2011). Similarly, one study found that alcohol dependence—unlike other substance use disorders—was more strongly associated with the internalizing latent factor (Kushner et al., 2012), possibly because of its frequent co-occurrence with anxiety and/or depression.

A second common critique of current diagnostic systems is that they perpetuate the notion that psychological disorders are discrete categorical constructs. That is, a person either meets a certain number of diagnostic criteria, and therefore evidences the disorder, or does not meet sufficient criteria and may end up described as "not elsewhere classified" or "unspecified." This categorical assumption has been routinely challenged and arguments for the greater accuracy of a dimensional or continuum-based approach are common (e.g., Brown & Barlow, 2009; Coghill & Sonuga-Barke, 2012; Köhne, 2020; Lilienfeld, 2014a; Luyten & Blatt, 2011); however, the continued reliance on categorical diagnostic systems further perpetuates the belief that these categories are true representations of mental illness (Hyman, 2010). In fact, this categorical assumption essentially dichotomizes what may actually be a continuum of variability and, therefore, limits the value and information provided by a diagnostic label. This categorical approach may also affect reliability of diagnostic assessment. For instance, providers may differ widely in their estimation of whether a specific diagnostic criterion has been met (e.g., a patient has *sufficient* irritability to fulfill this criterion for generalized anxiety disorder), which then affects overall diagnostic reliability.

Finally, it is well-established and widely accepted that psychological disorders develop because of varied etiological factors. The potential lure, and corresponding weakness, of a categorical diagnostic system is the idea that each disorder can be boiled down to a limited list of factors. In fact, as Clark et al. (2017) argue, understanding the myriad factors that cause disorders and the ways in which these factors interact is foundational to understanding psychopathology more comprehensively.

Shared Processes and a Transdiagnostic Approach to Psychopathology

Recognition that psychological diagnoses are imperfect and potentially obfuscate underlying processes, which therefore leads to additional inefficiencies in research and treatment efforts, is not new. In fact, the original work to revise and increase the scientific rigor of the first edition of the DSM began with the revisions for DSM-III (Clark et al., 2017). Since that time, the number of diagnoses has expanded, but our understanding of them—and particularly their underlying commonalities and etiology—has progressed less substantially. In recent years, wide-reaching efforts to challenge the extant and entrenched categorical diagnostic system have taken form (e.g., Conway et al., 2019; Cuthbert & Insel, 2013; Harkness et al., 2014). Two examples are the Research Domain Criteria initiative and the Hierarchical Taxonomy of Psychopathology.

The Research Domain Criteria (RDoC) Initiative The RDoC initiative from the National Institute of Mental Health (NIMH) is a formal and systemic example of the recognition that diagnostic categories are limited in their utility to meaningfully differentiate individuals and that an explicit focus on dimensional similarities and commonalities may be more appropriate (NIMH, n.d.). The RDoC initiative has highlighted that its intention is not to replace diagnostic systems, but instead to direct attention to the "varying degrees of dysfunction in general psychological/biological systems" (NIMH, n.d.). That is, it is intended as a research framework to encourage inquiry into shared processes, as measured in multiple ways (e.g., genetic, self-report, behavioral indices).

In brief, the RDoC framework provides a model for researchers to study psychopathology by delineating several broad domains of functioning, which are then subdivided into constructs for empirical study and can be examined across a range of indices (i.e., genes, molecules, cells, circuits, physiology, behavior, self-report). Domains are further divided into specific constructs that vary along hypothesized continuums from normal to abnormal functioning. For example, within the "negative valence systems" domain, constructs include acute threat (i.e., fear), potential threat (i.e., anxiety), sustained threat (e.g., trauma, avoidance), loss (e.g., sadness, withdrawal), and frustrative nonreward (e.g., aggression). These constructs can then be measured across indices and across the normal-to-abnormal continuum to elucidate their unique and integrated role within psychopathology. This framework provides an example of several aspects that are relevant for our larger discussion of transdiagnostic conceptualizations of psychopathology, including providing an alternative to diagnostic systems that result in considerable within-category heterogeneity, explicit targeting of the issues posed by significant comorbidity and diagnostic symptom overlap, and a focus on broad domains that underlie normal and abnormal functioning.

The first aspect relevant to a transdiagnostic conceptualization is the attempt to provide an alternative to current diagnostic systems that result in within-category heterogeneity whereby, for example, two different individuals may share only one symptom in common, yet both receive the same diagnosis of major depressive disorder. As mentioned above, the RDoC framework was intended to provide more flexibility and encouragement for research to take a noncategorical approach to understanding the continuum of functioning. By not limiting researchers to confine their investigations to heterogeneous diagnostic categories, RDoC provides a way to attempt to better understand pathological processes that may represent a more unifying understanding of the depressive presentation, for example. The second aspect relevant to a transdiagnostic conceptualization is the explicit recognition and attempt to overcome the reality of substantial diagnostic comorbidity within the current DSM or ICD nosology. In particular, the RDoC framework circumvents the requirement for researchers to differentiate between generalized anxiety disorder and social anxiety disorder, for example, by instead encouraging a definition of psychopathology based on areas of dysfunction and impairment. Whereas the DSM would distinguish these disorders based on the nature of the specific threat stimulus, RDoC provides a framework for researchers to study underlying processes that may give rise to symptoms irrespective of contextual triggers (e.g., elevated cortisol levels or anxiety sensitivity within the potential threat construct under negative valence systems). This ability to operationalize constructs of interest and forego diagnostic categories to define participant samples or populations of interest further enables more generalizable research findings and addresses previous research that has limited its scope to a single diagnostic category or a "pure" presentation, which rarely fits client presentations in practice (e.g., Hasin & Grant, 2015). And finally, the third aspect relevant to a transdiagnostic conceptualization is an emphasis on broad domains of human functioning (e.g., negative/positive valence systems, cognitive systems, arousal/regulatory systems). The RDoC's framework incorporating a multiple continuum approach addresses limitations of the categorical diagnostic approach of the DSM, which will ideally result in increased knowledge of key determinants and processes involved in psychopathology.

The RDoC initiative is not without its critics, and challenges that the initiative must address have been discussed extensively (e.g., Lilienfeld & Treadway, 2016). For example, authors have argued against the top-down approach to dictating research directions (e.g., Ross & Margolis, 2019) and have criticized the overemphasis on biological systems and measurement at the expense of behavioral indices (e.g., Lilienfeld, 2014b). Despite these criticisms, RDoC has led to a wave of research that generally incorporates a transdiagnostic approach. For instance, in a recent systematic review of 6 years of RDoC-based research, Carcone and Ruocco (2017) found that many studies examined selected constructs across more than one diagnostic category.

The Hierarchical Taxonomy of Psychopathology (HiTOP) Another recent example of a novel approach to psychological disorders is the HiTOP (Conway et al., 2019). Seeking to address the limitations of diagnostic systems based on patients meeting a certain number of criteria—which imply that even one fewer endorsed criterion is meaningfully distinct, indicative of insignificant distress or impairment, and/or overall does not warrant a diagnosis and the associated research and treatment attention—the HiTOP takes a data-driven (or quantitative nosological) approach to organizing psychopathology (Kotov et al., 2017). Where DSM and ICD base their nosology on clinical presentations that are *subsequently* studied in field trials and retroactively supported or refuted, the HiTOP approach relies on *already existing* evidence to create an improved organizational framework intended to reflect psychopathology more reliably.

Like RDoC, HiTOP provides a valuable alternative to categorical diagnostic approaches and addresses limitations of within-category heterogeneity, comorbidity and diagnostic symptom overlap, and arbitrary boundaries for "threshold" and "subthreshold" psychopathology (Kotov et al., 2018). It is an even newer system than RDoC and, as such, the broad implications and potential limitations of this framework are yet to be fully realized and are already generating meaningful criticism (Haeffel et al., 2022); however, the promise of an empirically derived organizational framework for transdiagnostic progress is noteworthy.

Summary RDoC and the HiTOP are two examples of attempts to change the way the field has come to think about psychological diagnoses. Recognizing the limitations of categorical systems with considerable commonalities that result in limited reliability and substantial comorbidity, these efforts underscore the need to continue reviewing and improving our conceptualization of psychopathology. A return to focusing on commonalities and underlying characteristics and psychological processes may be the most accurate reflection of the nature of psychopathology and the most effective way to improve our understanding of and ability to treat psychological suffering.

Brief History of Neuroticism

Neuroticism is defined as a trait-like tendency to experience frequent and intense negative emotions as well as a perception of uncontrollability of and incapability to cope with stressful experiences including intense emotional experience itself (Barlow et al., 2014; Sauer-Zavala & Barlow, 2021). This term has a rich history in clinical psychology, yet its conceptualization and application to the understanding of psychological disorders is relatively recent. Indeed, to understand the terms "neurotic," "neurosis," and "neuroticism" and their relevance to psychopathology today, it is best to examine how and why the term as it is currently used emerged.

Until 1980 and the publication of DSM-III, disorders involving the dysregulation of emotion—such as anxiety, depression, and related disorders (e.g., obsessive-compulsive or dissociative disorders)—fell into a large category, "neurotic disorders," with individuals said to have been suffering from "neurosis." However, these broad categories were largely based on theories of etiology, rather than empirical evidence. It was not until DSM-III that this balance shifted, with a trend toward a descriptive, empirically focused understanding of psychopathology. The result was an expansion of the number of categories into more narrowly defined entities and subsumed disorders. Subsequently, a wave of research on specific disorders and disorder-specific, empirically supported treatments emerged and multiplied, with greater understanding of disorders came more "splitting" of diagnostic categories to highlight their unique symptoms or course.

Alongside the disorder "splitting" research, other researchers began to realize that many of the disorders within and across diagnostic categories shared similar features and were often comorbid with one another (Brown et al., 2001). For instance, individuals with emotional disorders—anxiety, depression, and other disorders marked by emotional difficulties and dysregulation (e.g., borderline personality disorder)—compared with healthy individuals have higher levels of negative affect (e.g., Brown & Barlow, 2009) and report experiencing more frequent and intense negative emotions (Campbell-Sills et al., 2006; Mennin et al., 2005). It was becoming apparent that a hierarchical structure of anxiety, depressive, and other negative emotion-related disorders was emerging. Although this resembled a return to earlier diagnostic categories like "neurotic disorders," the significant difference was that this development was based on empirical support for the existence of broader categories, which earlier versions of the DSM lacked.

Neuroticism as an empirically derived construct existed well before the "splitting" of diagnoses in the 1980s. Eysenck (1947) first used the term in his research of personality, and it is encompassed—alongside extraversion (or positive emotionality)—in well-known personality theories such as the Big Three and Big Five (Eysenck & Eysenck, 1975). Findings from latent factor research suggested that the hierarchical structure of these emotional disorders involved two core dimensions: neuroticism/negative affect and extraversion/positive affect (Brown et al., 1998; Brown & Naragon-Gainey, 2013).

Neuroticism and the Development of Psychopathology

Clark and Watson (1991) proposed the tripartite structural theory of anxiety and depression based on these two core dimensions (neuroticism and extraversion). The theory states that anxiety and depressive disorders share a common, nonspecific component (i.e., "general affective distress") and are distinguished by psychological hyperarousal (specific to anxiety) and lack of positive affect (specific to depression). Research supporting this model followed (e.g., Brown et al., 1998; Zinbarg & Barlow, 1996); for example, Zinbarg and Barlow (1996) found a higher-order general factor that differentiated each group of participants with principal anxiety disorders (e.g., social phobia, generalized anxiety disorder) from a "no disorder" group.

In addition to structural descriptive models of anxiety and depression, earlier we had developed a theory of the etiology of emotional disorders more generally called "triple vulnerability theory" (i.e., Barlow, 1988, 2000; Barlow et al., 2014; Sauer-Zavala & Barlow, 2021). Triple vulnerability theory proposes three separate and interacting vulnerabilities: a general biological vulnerability (genetic), a general psychological vulnerability (early experiences instilling a sense of un- controllability-unpredictability), and a more specific psychological vulnerability involving learning experiences that associate negative emotion with specific foci (i.e., certain stimuli or experiences that are interpreted as threatening, such as physiological sensations in panic disorder). Notably, this theory explains how distinct disorders may emerge from shared vulnerabilities (Barlow et al., 2021; Sauer-Zavala & Barlow, 2021).

The *general biological vulnerability* is mostly defined by genetic and neurobiological contributions to temperament (Barlow, 2000). Studies suggest that the neuroticism is heritable, with poly-genetic contribution explaining 40–60% of variance in its expression (e.g., Bouchard & Loehlin, 2001; Clark et al., 1994; Hettema et al., 2001; Kendler et al., 2003; Skre et al., 1993). Like other genetic traits and dimensions of personality, neuroticism is thought to be relatively stable over the lifespan. Although exerting its greatest effect in childhood (Laceulle et al., 2013), neuroticism remains relatively stable before gradual age-related decreases later in life (Eaton, Krueger, Keyes, et al., 2011, Eaton, Krueger, & Oltmanns, 2011; Roberts & Mroczek, 2008; Roberts et al., 2006). Additionally, neurobiological indicators of neuroticism indicate heightened activity in emotion-generating structures—particularly the amygdala—and underactivation or reduced inhibition in prefrontal regions (Keightley et al., 2003; Stein et al., 2007; Westlye et al., 2011). This translates to characteristic symptoms of emotional disorders: stronger reactions to emotion-provoking stimuli and more difficulty regulating responses to them. However, a genetic predisposition for neuroticism alone will not develop into an emotional disorder (Barlow et al., 2014; Sauer-Zavala & Barlow, 2021). Rather, in isolation from the other vulnerabilities, a person with this profile may have a heightened responsiveness to stress and seem irritable or driven, but that response would not be pathological. Instead, it is the repeated early developmental learning experiences of stress—reinforcing a sense of uncontrollability and incapability to cope—that interacts with heritable predispositions to produce psychopathology.

The *general psychological vulnerability* largely refers to these early learning experiences that contribute to aversive reactivity to emotional experiences, or a sense that one cannot predict, control, or cope with stressful life experiences and associated emotions. From a theoretical perspective, research on perceived control as it relates to anxiety and depression has a considerable history. For example, the well-known models of locus of control theory (Rotter, 1954) and learned helplessness (Seligman, 1975) rely on attributions of perceived loss of control. Additionally, basic animal and human research has repeatedly established that fears and anxiety can be experimentally created, and these studies consistently do so when the research paradigm involves chronic early exposure to unpredictability and uncontrollability (Barlow et al., 2014; Sauer-Zavala & Barlow, 2021). From these fields of research, it is understood that early adverse experiences, as well as parenting styles that foster a sense of inability to cope, can interact with a genetic predisposition for neuroticism to create psychopathology (Barlow et al., 2014; Sauer-Zavala & Barlow, 2021).

These first two vulnerabilities are robustly related to anxiety and depression generally, but manifest most clearly in generalized anxiety disorder and depressive disorders (e.g., Brown, 2007; Brown et al., 1998; Mineka et al., 1998; Watson et al., 2005). The development of more specific anxiety and depressive disorders likely results from classical conditioning, instructional learning, or observation of anxiety related to specific stimuli or conditions, which constitute the third (specific psychological) vulnerability that is most proximally associated with the development of specific disorders as noted above (Barlow et al., 2014, 2021; Sauer-Zavala & Barlow, 2021).

Based on the triple vulnerability theory, we can view neuroticism as being comprised of the first two general vulnerabilities: a genetically based tendency to experience emotions strongly and frequently (stemming from the general biological vulnerability) and aversive reactivity to emotional experiences (stemming from the general psychological vulnerability). Functionally related to aversive reactivity to emotional experiences is a rigid reliance on avoidant coping strategies such as suppression, rumination, and avoidance when encountering stress related intense emotion.

Redefining Disorder Classifications

As evidenced by the previously reviewed research, there is a strong theoretical and empirical basis for the existence of a hierarchical structure of emotional disorders, with neuroticism as one higher-order latent factor. This organization warrants a more dimensional approach to diagnosis and assessment (e.g., Brown & Barlow, 2005). For example, Brown and Barlow's (2009) dimensional model proposes creating a symptom profile for each patient that consists of several constructs, central to which are the temperaments of neuroticism and extraversion, along with some more specific factors that also exist dimensionally across emotional disorders (e.g., somatic anxiety, intrusive cognitions). Extensive evaluation of the reliability and validity of this dimensional model is needed; however, initial examination of its validity has been promising (Rosellini et al., 2015; Rosellini & Brown, 2014).

Despite growing popularity of more dimensional approaches that consider personality features (e.g., HiTOP), personality and affective disorders have long been considered separate entities. Personality traits are considered stable and enduring

(American Psychiatric Association, 2013; Roberts & DelVecchio, 2000) and personality disorders have historically been perceived as more resistant to treatment (e.g., Stone, 1993), whereas emotional disorders have been seen as more transient and, therefore, treatable. As such, it can be difficult to grasp how personality traits can account for the vulnerability of emotional disorders—with or without personality psychopathology—and that targeting personality or temperamental traits is feasible in the treatment of emotional disorders. This leads to some hesitancy in considering personality traits as higher-order latent factors for emotional disorders. However, focusing on features of personality may allow for a more parsimonious approach to treatment. Transdiagnostic constructs—including anxiety sensitivity, experiential avoidance, distress intolerance, and intolerance of uncertainty—each refer to the tendency to find emotional experiences aversive, and research supports that these constructs relate to neuroticism (Barlow et al., 2014, 2021; Sauer-Zavala & Barlow, 2021). Therefore, rather than designing multiple treatments that are each intended to address the multitude of transdiagnostic constructs, targeting a higher-order factor encompassing all of them (i.e., neuroticism) may be more efficient.

Focusing on the transdiagnostic constructs (i.e., aversive reactivity to emotions) that connect personality vulnerabilities and symptoms may shed light on treatment targets that are naturally amenable to change (Barlow et al., 2021). This malleability may ultimately increase acceptability of classification based on temperamental characteristics (Sauer-Zavala & Barlow, 2021). Indeed, over the last several decades, transdiagnostic treatments have emerged, with some having a theoretical basis in temperamental features. As with disorder-specific treatments developed previously, establishing whether a transdiagnostic treatment approach constitutes evidence-based treatment will ultimately require the evaluation of not only treatment outcomes but support for the theoretical base upon which the treatment rests (e.g., David & Montgomery, 2011; Lilienfeld, 2011; Rosen & Davison, 2003). That is, evaluating the theory that (1) targeting a transdiagnostic construct is possible, (2) effective targeting impacts the construct in expected ways, and (3) this impact leads to improved treatment outcomes is essential.

Distinctions Among Transdiagnostic Approaches to Treatment

Given the limitations of diagnostic classification, and of the disorder-specific treatments that were derived from this system, treatment researchers have shifted attention to developing protocols that can be used effectively across diagnostic presentations, that is, *transdiagnostic treatments* (e.g., Dalgleish et al., 2020). As the name implies, transdiagnostic treatments are treatments that have been found efficacious in reducing symptoms of multiple disorders concurrently. Approaches to developing such treatments differ in meaningful ways, including the theoretical rationale underlying selected treatment targets, with temperament figuring prominently in the development of a subset of transdiagnostic approaches.

In a recent review of transdiagnostic approaches, Dalgleish et al. (2020) distinguish between two classes of transdiagnostic treatments: *universal interventions* and *modular interventions*. Universal interventions, such as the Unified Protocol for Transdiagnostic Treatment of Emotional Disorders (UP; Barlow et al., 2018), utilize the same broadly applicable therapeutic elements for all patients regardless of presenting diagnosis. In contrast, modular interventions, such as Shaping Healthy Minds (Black et al., 2018), consist of various self-contained treatment elements that can be selected and ordered based on each individual patient's presentation. However, the authors argue that many of the transdiagnostic treatments in existence are not rooted in a clear theoretical framework, posing a challenge for the field moving forward (see also Lilienfeld, 2014c).

The authors describe a treatment model whereby some proportion of patients may remit simply based on nonspecific treatment factors (e.g., alliance, expectancy), some based on common processes (e.g., shared treatment elements across treatments drawn from the same theoretical framework, such as challenging distorted cognitions in cognitive behavioral therapy), and some based on diagnosis-specific processes (e.g., treatment elements meant to target specific diagnostic features, such as behavioral activation in depression). One implication of this model is that for treatments to be most efficacious, they may require both common *and* diagnosis-specific elements. This suggests that, at least when it comes to treating someone's primary diagnosis, transdiagnostic protocols may actually be *less* effective than diagnosis-specific protocols if they fail to include diagnosis-specific elements.

Sauer-Zavala et al. (2017b) offer a slightly contrasting framework for understanding distinctions among transdiagnostic approaches to treatment. Within this framework, treatments are classified based on the nature of the processes they target. Treatments that target several constructs using several independent treatment elements are *modular treatments*, defined in the same way as in Dalgleish et al. (2020). Another class, *universally applied therapeutic principles*, refers to interventions that broadly apply a guiding therapeutic strategy regardless of diagnostic presentation (e.g., resolving psychic conflict in psychodynamic psychotherapy, correcting distorted thinking in cognitive therapy). Finally, some transdiagnostic treatments may be considered *shared mechanisms treatments*, meaning they target specific empirically identified mechanisms underlying classes of disorders. Whereas universally applied therapeutic principles approaches are informed by broad theories of approaches to treatment, shared mechanisms treatments are informed by models of psychopathology that are drawn from basic science research into the core processes that maintain certain classes of disorders.

In the context of the hypothetical treatment model described by Dalgleish et al. (2020), any transdiagnostic treatment—really any well-delivered treatment at all—has the potential to activate nonspecific factors, regardless of how the treatment is constructed or the theory from which it is drawn. Beyond these common factors, universally applied therapeutic principles are likely to target common processes without specifically addressing disorder-specific processes, whereas modular treatments could contain components that target both common and diagnosis-specific processes based on a patient's need. Shared mechanisms treatments assume that there is a causal relationship between common and specific processes; in other words, common processes are responsible for diagnosis-specific processes. This implies that addressing common processes can lead to relief from diagnosis-specific processes without needing to address the diagnosis-specific processes directly.

Consider the example of behavioral avoidance, an emotion regulation strategy that is nearly ubiquitous across emotional disorders, involving refraining from engaging in activities that are predicted to involve uncomfortable emotions (Helbig-Lang & Petermann, 2010). In depression, people may avoid activities with potential for positive reinforcement due to an assumption that these activities will not produce an appropriate level of enjoyment. For patients with this presenting problem, a clinician is likely to recommend behavioral activation (BA), which is framed as increasing contact with valued activities that are reinforced by a sense of pleasure or accomplishment (Jacobson et al., 2001). However, in the anxiety disorders, behavioral avoidance often presents as refraining from engaging in activities that are typically associated with anxiety (e.g., giving a speech in social anxiety disorder, riding a crowded train in panic disorder; Helbig-Lang & Petermann, 2010). For patients with this presenting problem, a clinician may recommend exposure therapy (Foa & Kozak, 1986). In both cases (BA for depression and exposure for anxiety), the underlying principle is that adaptive functioning can begin to be restored by making contact with uncomfortable affect and processing these experiences. Thus, in practice, a transdiagnostic treatment based on shared mechanisms may include treatment strategies that look, on the surface, like traditional BA and exposure. However, framing these strategies transdiagnostically and connecting new therapeutic learning to a broader overarching theory can promote adaptive functioning across emotions and contexts (i.e., targeting the common process of behavioral avoidance to yield improvements in diagnosis-specific processes across depression and anxiety).

Temperamental Features as Shared Mechanisms

To be maximally effective, treatments taking the shared mechanisms approach must effectively target core mechanistic processes that are responsible for disorder-specific symptom expression. At least as it relates to the emotional disorders, neuroticism has been identified as a primary latent factor underlying disorder expression across several theoretical and empirical models of psychopathology classification (e.g., Brown & Barlow, 2009; Clark, 2005; Clark & Watson, 1991). As described above, temperamental characteristics are generally considered nonspecific vulnerabilities for psychopathology that interact with lower-level vulnerabilities and specific stressors to contribute to the etiology of specific disorders. Thus, a key takeaway for transdiagnostic treatment development for emotional disorders is that temperamental features are linked to disorder-specific symptom expression and, thus, may be an efficient target for treating the disorders to which they give rise. Of course, it is important to note that the present discussion is limited to emotional disorders which, as described above, share underlying temperamental vulnerabilities. It does not apply to other symptom presentations (e.g., psychosis) that are thought to have distinct etiological bases.

Below, we review several transdiagnostic treatment protocols that were developed to treat the emotional disorders. All of these protocols were designed to target transdiagnostic processes theorized to underlie these disorders, including neurotic temperament; as described above, the focus on these common processes is meant to foster change in disorder-specific processes across disorders simultaneously. In considering the merit of this approach, it is important to examine different types of evidence. As scientists have previously noted (e.g., David & Montgomery, 2011; Lilienfeld, 2011; Rosen & Davison, 2003), establishing empirical support for a psychological treatment requires not just evidence of change in symptoms over time, but also evidence of change in theoretically derived mechanisms. Thus, for each protocol, we will briefly describe its transdiagnostic components, review evidence of its efficacy on primary outcomes such as symptoms and functioning, and review evidence of change in transdiagnostic constructs that are plausible mechanisms of treatment effects.

The Unified Protocol

The emerging literature supporting the link between temperament and psychopathology, as well as the increasingly evident limitations of the single-diagnosis treatment paradigm, led to the development of the Unified Protocol (UP; Barlow et al., 2018; Wilamowska et al., 2010). The UP offers a model of transdiagnostic treatment aimed at neuroticism as the primary higher-order factor in the maintenance of the full spectrum of emotional disorders. Treatment strategies include cultivating non-judgmental and present-focused awareness and attention toward emotions, developing flexibility in cognitive appraisals, and acting opposite to emotion-driven urges. These skills are practiced independently within distinct modules but are then practiced simultaneously during the final phase of treatment, which involves exposure to internal (e.g., physical sensations) and external (i.e., situational) emotional cues. These so-called "emotion exposures" utilize common exposure techniques (interoceptive, imaginal, and in vivo exposures) to increase patients' contact with emotions perceived as dangerous or intolerable. Emotion exposures, in conjunction with skills learned in previous modules, facilitate emotional processing and inhibitory learning to promote effective goal-oriented behavior. Although preliminary research shows that some of its modules exert independent effects on relevant processes (Sauer-Zavala et al., 2017a)—consistent with modular models of transdiagnostic treatment—the UP is fundamentally a shared mechanisms treatment because its range of treatment strategies are meant to reduce disorder-specific symptom expressions through their effect on the underlying neuroticism.

In a large randomized controlled trial (RCT), the UP was compared to gold-standard single-diagnosis protocols (SDPs) for generalized anxiety disorder, panic disorder, social anxiety disorder, and obsessive-compulsive disorder. Results showed the UP produced equivalent reductions in principal disorder severity (Barlow et al., 2017) and severity of comorbid conditions (Jarvi Steele et al., 2018) compared to SDPs, and did so with less attrition (Barlow et al., 2017). Furthermore, with regard to the primary higher-order treatment target of neuroticism, the UP was associated with greater change in neuroticism as measured by the self-report Eysenck Personality Questionnaire (Eysenck & Eysenck, 1975) than the SDPs, controlling for symptoms of anxiety and depression (Sauer-Zavala et al., 2021). Taken together, these findings suggest that a transdiagnostic treatment can effectively and simultaneously produce change in temperamental characteristics and symptoms. Preliminary data from several smaller studies also support the efficacy of the UP in improving symptoms of depression (Sauer-Zavala et al., 2020), borderline personality disorder (Lopez et al., 2015; Sauer-Zavala et al., 2016), post-traumatic stress disorder, (Varkovitzky et al., 2018), and alcohol use disorder (Ciraulo et al., 2013), with effect sizes comparable to traditional CBT (for reviews, see Cassiello-Robbins et al., 2020; Sakiris & Berle, 2019).

Transdiagnostic Cognitive Behavioral Therapy

Another protocol that has garnered considerable empirical support is Transdiagnostic Cognitive Behavioral Therapy (tCBT; Norton, 2012). Although guided by transdiagnostic theory supporting negative affectivity (i.e., neuroticism) as a core temperamental feature across the full range of emotional disorders, tCBT was originally developed for and tested in people with primary anxiety disorders. The protocol was later slightly adapted to broaden its applicability to individuals diagnosed with primary depression. tCBT utilizes common CBT strategies to reduce negative affectivity, including restructuring automatic thoughts, a variety of exposure techniques (e.g., situational, interoceptive), and identifying and challenging core beliefs and schemas (Norton, 2012). Thus, tCBT is quite similar to the UP in its underlying theory as well as the range of strategies it uses to target negative affectivity.

tCBT has demonstrated efficacy across multiple research trials for individuals diagnosed with primary anxiety disorders (Norton & Barrera, 2012; Harris & Norton, 2019) or primary depression (Harris & Norton, 2019), and has been shown to reduce symptoms of comorbid disorders to a greater degree than diagnosis-specific manuals (Norton et al., 2013). In an evaluation of four potential treatment mechanisms (i.e., anxiety, negative affectivity, anxiety sensitivity, and intolerance of uncertainty), all four constructs decreased over treatment; however, only change in negative affectivity significantly predicted change in symptoms, supporting negative affectivity, a construct often equated with neuroticism (Brown & Barlow, 2009), as a potential mechanism of anxiety reduction (Talkovsky & Norton, 2014). The protocol's exclusive application in group settings remains unique among shared mechanisms transdiagnostic protocols, which have typically been developed as individual treatments and later adapted for group delivery (e.g., Bullis et al., 2015), or vice versa (e.g., Riccardi et al., 2017).

Emotion Regulation Therapy

The UP and tCBT share a focus on temperament, specifically neuroticism or negative affectivity, which underlies the full range of emotional disorders. Basic and translational findings in affective science suggest that a subset of emotional disorders (e.g., GAD and depression, sometimes referred to as the "distress disorders") may involve particular sensitivity to emotional cues and reliance on especially elaborative self-referential processing in coping with distress. Although negative self-referential processing (i.e., repetitive negative thinking, such as worry or rumination) is elevated across the emotional disorders (Ehring & Watkins, 2008), this process is particularly salient in treatment refractory distress disorders and poses a barrier to effective therapeutic learning (Mennin & Fresco, 2013). Drawing from these findings, Emotion Regulation Therapy (ERT; Mennin & Fresco, 2014; Renna et al., 2017) represents a mechanism-informed, emotion-focused transdiagnostic protocol for the treatment of distress disorders. Emotions are conceptualized as motivational signals that prompt behavior that is aligned with one's values and appropriate to the circumstances; thus, in ERT, the goal is to develop emotional awareness, increase behavioral flexibility, and ultimately reduce maladaptive threat appraisals. ERT includes three core elements: awareness skills training (including components such as psychoeducation and motivational cue detection), regulation skills training (e.g., mindfulness, cognitive reappraisal), and experiential exposure (e.g., valued action, experiential imagery).

An initial open trial provided support for ERT in the treatment of GAD with or without co-occurring depression (Mennin et al., 2015). A subsequent RCT replicated these findings, demonstrating that ERT produced greater improvements in anxiety and depression symptoms, functioning, and quality of life compared to a modified attention control group (Mennin et al., 2018). The latter study identified emotion regulation, mindfulness, reappraisal, and decentering (or the ability to observe one's thoughts and feelings with a sense of distance; Fresco et al., 2007) as significant mediators of all outcomes; a follow-up analysis demonstrated that changes in reappraisal and decentering temporally precede and predict changes in anxiety symptoms, suggesting that these processes may be primary mechanisms through which ERT reduces symptoms (O'Toole et al., 2019). Furthermore, neuroimaging findings have demonstrated treatment-linked changes in connectivity of neural systems implicated in emotional sensitivity and self-referential processes (Scult et al., 2019). Given that ERT was developed to improve outcomes for treatment refractory distress disorders, it has not yet been tested as a treatment for other emotional disorders (e.g., fear disorders such as panic disorder or social anxiety disorder). However, distress and fear disorders are considered emotional disorders

(Bullis et al., 2019), and are frequently comorbid (Watson, 2005), suggesting ERT may be an effective treatment across the broader range of emotional disorders.

False Safety Behavior Elimination Therapy

Whereas ERT teaches a range of emotion regulation skills to facilitate contextual learning, other approaches target specific emotion regulation strategies. For example, research has shown that individuals with anxiety disorders often rely on safety aids, which are behavioral or cognitive strategies that function to reduce anxiety in the short term (Salkovskis et al., 1999; Riccardi et al., 2017). Despite their short-term protective function, safety aids prevent individuals from fully experiencing negative affect, which impairs emotional processing and prevents corrective learning (Foa & Kozak, 1986; Craske et al., 2008). False Safety Behavior Elimination Therapy (F-SET) was designed, as the name implies, to eliminate safety aids that are used maladaptively to reduce or prevent anxiety. F-SET consists of psychoeducation, identification of safety aids, and "antiphobic activities," which refers to encouraging participants to engage with anxiety-provoking situations while behaving the opposite to their safety behavior. For example, an individual with social anxiety may be instructed to walk around in public with clothing that may attract negative attention instead of attempting to "blend in." Notably, F-SET does not involve teaching any other common cognitive or behavioral skills (e.g., cognitive restructuring), nor are patients specifically trained in traditional in vivo exposures during sessions, although antiphobic activities may involve interoceptive or situational exposures. This contrasts with most CBT protocols (transdiagnostic or otherwise) that tend to involve dedicated session time for cognitive restructuring and formal exposure exercises.

To date, F-SET has been tested in two randomized control trials for individuals with GAD, social anxiety, and/or panic disorder. A 10-session version of F-SET delivered in group format was associated with significant anxiety and depression symptom reduction compared to a waitlist control (Schmidt et al., 2012). An individually administered, brief (5-session) version of the protocol also produced significant reductions in anxiety and depression symptoms (Riccardi et al., 2017). In the latter study, mediational analysis demonstrated that reductions in avoidance mediated symptom outcomes, suggesting that eliminating safety behaviors promotes engagement with anxiety-provoking situations.

Transdiagnostic Behavior Therapy

As mechanistically transdiagnostic protocols were beginning to be developed and tested, gaps in the emerging research literature grew evident. For example, these protocols were being tested with civilian participants, failing to capture unique aspects of the military veteran identity (e.g., greater illness burden associated with psychiatric conditions, greater incidence of post-traumatic stress disorder and major depressive disorder; see Gros, 2014). To address these limitations, Gros (2014) developed Transdiagnostic Behavior Therapy (TBT), a 12- to 16-session protocol for military veterans that emphasizes various exposure techniques (e.g., situational, interoceptive, imaginal, and positive emotional/behavioral activation). Exposure forms the backbone of the protocol, as avoidance is considered the primary treatment target. TBT also includes various optional modules (e.g., response prevention, cognitive therapy, anger management) that are taught explicitly as skills to be incorporated into exposure exercises as needed. This contrasts with other transdiagnostic protocols (e.g., UP, tCBT) that view various treatment components as relatively independent yet synergistic in creating change with the target mechanism, neuroticism, or negative affectivity.

Initial evaluations of TBT for veterans with emotional disorders have shown promise as indicated by improvements on self-reported and clinician-rated indices of change in symptoms and functioning (Gros, 2014; Gros et al., 2017). Although designed for veterans, the effectiveness of TBT has also been studied in civilian samples. For example, one study compared TBT to disorder-specific protocols in participants diagnosed with panic disorder, social anxiety disorder, or OCD. Participants who underwent TBT demonstrated a similar degree of symptom reduction as those who underwent a disorder-specific protocol, although TBT evidenced greater improvement in overall impairment as measured on a self-report measure of symptom interference in daily life (Gros et al., 2019). In terms of treatment targets, studies have yet to evaluate the purported mechanism of change, avoidance reduction, as a mediator of symptom outcomes in TBT. However, TBT has been shown to effectively reduce several facets of avoidance within a transdiagnostic sample of veterans (Gros et al., 2020).

Emotion Regulation and Temperamental Change

Taken together, results from various treatment trials reviewed above support the effectiveness of shared mechanisms transdiagnostic approaches to the treatment of emotional disorders; we are aware of no published instance of a shared mechanisms transdiagnostic treatment underperforming relative to a diagnosis-specific treatment protocol. Given that the UP and tCBT were explicitly designed to target neuroticism or negative affectivity, with empirical evidence confirming treatment effects on these constructs (Sauer-Zavala et al., 2020; Sauer-Zavala et al., 2021; Talkovsky & Norton, 2014), temperamental features appear to have clinical relevance and warrant attention in treatment for emotional disorders. Other similar treatments—including ERT, F-SET, and TBT—show promise in improving emotional disorders through an explicit focus on emotion regulation strategies, including negative self-referential processing, safety-seeking behavior, and avoidance, as summarized above; however, the effect of these treatments on temperament has yet to be explored.

Of course, whether purportedly targeting neuroticism or emotion regulation, these treatments are ultimately very similar in that they draw from learning theory and research and utilize exposure-based techniques to facilitate changes in emotional processing and behavioral flexibility. For exposure to be maximally effective, individuals must necessarily eliminate avoidant emotion regulation strategies (Craske et al., 2008); thus, change in neuroticism and change in emotion regulation are both likely to occur as a function of effective emotion exposure, no matter which process is the purported target.

John and Gross (2007) have outlined a model that suggests that emotion regulation strategy use differs based on personality features; in particular, neuroticism is associated with maladaptive emotion regulation strategy use (e.g., greater rumination, less reappraisal). Currently, there is no broad consensus as to whether emotion dysregulation is considered a facet of neuroticism or whether these are truly distinct, independent constructs. For example, some neuroimaging research suggests that neuroticism is related to hyperactivation of the amygdala, which is viewed as a proxy for emotion generation (e.g., Everaerd et al., 2015; Haas et al., 2007; Stein et al., 2007). However, a meta-analysis of neuroimaging studies examining neural activity in individuals high in neuroticism failed to find a consistent relationship between neuroticism and amygdala activation (Servaas et al., 2013). Instead, neuroticism is more robustly associated with reduced connectivity between the amygdala and the ventromedial prefrontal cortex (a pathway implicated in emotional inhibition and a proxy for emotion regulation; Servaas et al., 2013; Silverman et al., 2019).

In other words, dysfunction in the ability to successfully downregulate negative emotions appears central to the definition of neuroticism above and beyond simply the frequent activation of negative emotional states. Furthermore, a structural equation modeling study in a large treatment-seeking sample of adults with emotional disorders found that the associations between various emotion regulation strategies and psychopathology were largely accounted for by neuroticism (Anderson et al., 2021). Thus, the constructs of neuroticism and emotion regulation appear to be deeply intertwined. Continued development and refinement of transdiagnostic interventions should be guided by theory that identifies both common and specific processes involved in psychopathology and links them to therapeutic processes of change (e.g., David & Montgomery, 2011; Lilienfeld, 2011; Rosen & Davison, 2003); modifying maladaptive emotion regulation strategies appears to be one "pathway to neuroticism" through which treatment can facilitate temperamental change.

Conclusions and Future Directions

Recent efforts to shift the focus of research on psychopathology to common processes and underlying features (e.g., RDoC, HiTOP) require critical examination and continued refinement; however, these approaches highlight a broader recognition and appreciation for transdiagnostic conceptualizations and have clear implications for interventions. This return to highlighting commonalities across patient presentations as an alternative to categorical diagnostic distinctions based on differential symptom presentation has led to a renewed emphasis on identifying and targeting shared transdiagnostic mechanisms, such as neuroticism. Although many treatments exist that may be described as "transdiagnostic," in that they reduce symptoms or foster improvements across diagnostic presentations, only a subset are considered *shared mechanisms* treatments that target the specific psychological processes that underlie a broad range of symptom expressions within a class of disorders such as emotional disorders. Notably, these treatments engage similar processes (e.g., aversive reactivity to emotional experience; emotion-motivated avoidant coping) to reduce levels of neuroticism (Barlow et al., 2021). This emphasis on shared mechanisms is certainly beneficial from a research standpoint, but more importantly, transdiagnostic conceptualization and treatment approaches offer possibilities to increase the reach of evidence-based psychological treatments. That is, by enabling providers to learn fewer treatments without sacrificing competency in affecting change, transdiagnostic treatments increase our potential to reach a broader population of individuals in need of treatment.

As awareness of the value of targeting underlying transdiagnostic processes across clinical presentations has grown, greater efforts to capitalize on this targeting are underway. But it would be antithetical to the value of transdiagnostic approaches for the field to move toward a proliferation of varied transdiagnostic treatments, possibly differing in only small details, much as happened with disorder-specific psychological treatments. One way to mitigate that potential pitfall is to continue to evaluate and ensure transdiagnostic treatments are grounded in theory, effectively establish and target shared mechanisms (such as temperament), and demonstrate that changes in those mechanisms account for changes in important outcomes. This continued focus on psychopathological mechanisms, and a closer targeting of these mechanisms with transdiagnostic treatments, should advance public behavioral health efforts in the most effective manner.

References

American Psychiatric Association. (1952). *Diagnostic and statistical manual of mental disorders.*

American Psychiatric Association. (2013). *Diagnostic and statistical manual of mental disorders* (5th ed.).

Anderson, G. N., Tung, E. S., Brown, T. A., & Rosellini, A. J. (2021). Facets of emotion regulation and emotional disorder symptom dimensions: Differential associations and incremental validity in a large clinical sample. *Behavior Therapy, 52*(4), 917–931. https://doi.org/10.1016/j.beth.2020.11.003

Barlow, D. H. (1988). *Anxiety and its disorders: The nature and treatment of anxiety and panic.* Guilford Press.

Barlow, D. H. (2000). Unraveling the mysteries of anxiety and its disorders from the perspective of emotion theory. *American Psychologist, 55*, 1247–1263. https://doi.org/10.1037/0003-066X.55.11.1247

Barlow, D. H., Ellard, K. K., Sauer-Zavala, S., Bullis, J. R., & Carl, J. R. (2014). The origins of neuroticism. *Perspectives on Psychological Science, 9*(5), 481–496. https://doi.org/10.1177/1745691614544528

Barlow, D. H., Farchione, T. J., Bullis, J. R., Gallagher, M. W., Murray-Latin, H., Sauer-Zavala, S., et al. (2017). The unified protocol for transdiagnostic treatment of emotional disorders compared with diagnosis-specific protocols for anxiety disorders: A randomized clinical trial. *JAMA Psychiatry, 74*(9), 875–884.

Barlow, D. H., Farchione, T. J., Sauer-Zavala, S., Murray Latin, H., Ellard, K. K., Bullis, J. R., et al. (2018). *Unified protocol for the transdiagnostic treatment of emotional disorders: Therapist guide* (2nd ed.). Oxford University Press.

Barlow, D. H., Curreri, A. J., & Woodard, L. S. (2021). Neuroticism and disorders of emotion: A new synthesis. *Current Directions in Psychological Science, 30*(5), 410–417.

Black, M., Hitchcock, C., Bevan, A. O Leary, C., Clarke, J., Elliot, R., Watson, P., ..., & Dalgleish, T. (2018). The HARMONIC trial: study protocol for a randomized controlled feasibility trial of Shaping Healthy Minds-a modular transdiagnostic intervention for mood, stressor-related and anxiety disorders in adults. *BMJ Open, 8, e024546.* https://doi.org/10.1136/bmjopen-2018-024546

Bouchard, T. J., Jr., & Loehlin, J. C. (2001). Genes, evolution, and personality. *Behavior Genetics, 31*, 243–273. https://doi.org/10.1023/A:1012294324713

Brown, T. A. (2007). Temporal course and structural relationships among dimensions of temperament and DSM-IV anxiety and mood disorder constructs. *Journal of Abnormal Psychology, 116*(2), 313–328. https://doi.org/10.1037/0021-843X.116.2.313

Brown, T. A., & Barlow, D. H. (2002). Classification of anxiety and mood disorders. In D. H. Barlow (Ed.), *Anxiety and its disorders: The nature and treatment of anxiety and panic (2nd ed., pp. 292–327). New York: Guilford Press.*

Brown, T. A., & Barlow, D. H. (2005). Dimensional versus categorical classification of mental disorders in the fifth edition of the diagnostic and statistical manual of mental disorders and beyond: Comment on the special section. *Journal of Abnormal Psychology, 114*(4), 551–556. https://doi.org/10.1037/0021-843X.114.4.551

Brown, T. A., & Barlow, D. H. (2009). A proposal for a dimensional classification system based on the shared features of the DSM-IV anxiety and mood disorders: Implications for assessment and treatment. *Psychological Assessment, 21*(3), 256.

Brown, T. A., & Naragon-Gainey, K. (2013). Evaluation of the unique and specific contributions of dimensions of the triple vulnerability model to the prediction of DSM-IV anxiety and mood disorder constructs. *Behavior Therapy, 44*(2), 277–292. https://doi.org/10.1016/j.beth.2012.11.002

Brown, T. A., Chorpita, B. F., & Barlow, D. H. (1998). Structural relationships among dimensions of the DSM-IV anxiety and mood disorders and dimensions of negative affect, positive affect, and autonomic arousal. *Journal of Abnormal Psychology, 107*(2), 179–192. https://doi.org/10.1037/0021-843X.107.2.179

Brown, T. A., Campbell, L. A., Lehman, C. L., Grisham, J. R., & Mancill, R. B. (2001). Current and lifetime comorbidity of the DSM-IV anxiety and mood disorders in a large clinical sample. *Journal of Abnormal Psychology, 110*(4), 585–599. https://doi.org/10.1037/0021-843X.110.4.585

Bullis, J. R., Sauer-Zavala, S., Bentley, K. H., Thompson-Hollands, J., Carl, J. R., & Barlow, D. H. (2015). The unified protocol for transdiagnostic treatment of emotional disorders: Preliminary exploration of effectiveness for group delivery. *Behavior Modification, 39*(2), 295–321.

Bullis, J. R., Boettcher, H., Sauer-Zavala, S., Farchione, T. J., & Barlow, D. H. (2019). What is an emotional disorder? A transdiagnostic mechanistic definition with implications for assessment, treatment, and prevention. *Clinical Psychology: Science and Practice, 26*(2), e12278.

Campbell-Sills, L., Barlow, D. H., Brown, T. A., & Hofmann, S. G. (2006). Acceptability and suppression of negative emotion in anxiety and mood disorders. *Emotion, 6*(4), 587–595. https://doi.org/10.1037/1528-3542.6.4.587

Carcone, D., & Ruocco, A. C. (2017). Six years of research on the National Institute of Mental Health's Research Domain Criteria (RDoC) Initiative: A systematic review. *Frontiers in Cellular Neuroscience, 11*, 46. https://doi.org/10.3389/fncel.2017.00046

Cassiello-Robbins, C., Southward, M. W., Wilner Tirpak, J., & Sauer-Zavala, S. (2020). A systematic review of Unified Protocol applications with adult populations: Facilitating widespread dissemination via adaptability. *Clinical Psychological Review, 78, 101852.* https://doi.org/10.1016/j.cpr.2020.101852

Ciraulo, D. A., Barlow, D. H., Gulliver, S. B., Farchione, T., Morissette, S. B., Kamholz, B. W., et al. (2013). The effects of venlafaxine and cognitive behavioral therapy alone and combined in the treatment of co-morbid alcohol use-anxiety disorders. *Behaviour Research and Therapy, 51*(11), 729–735.

Clark, L. A. (2005). Temperament as a unifying basis for personality and psychopathology. *Journal of Abnormal Psychology, 114*(4), 505–521. https://doi.org/10.1037/0021-843X.114.4.505

Clark, L. A., & Watson, D. (1991). Tripartite model of anxiety and depression: Psychometric evidence and taxonomic implications. *Journal of Abnormal Psychology, 100*(3), 316–336.

Clark, L. A., Watson, D., & Mineka, S. (1994). Temperament, personality, and the mood and anxiety disorders. *Journal of Abnormal Psychology, 103*, 103–116. https://doi.org/10.1037/0021-843X.103.1.103

Clark, L. A., Cuthbert, B., Lewis-Fernández, R., Narrow, W. E., & Reed, G. M. (2017). Three approaches to understanding and classifying mental disorder: ICD-11, DSM-5, and the National Institute of Mental Health's Research Domain Criteria (RDoC). *Psychological Science in the Public Interest, 18*(2), 72–145. https://doi.org/10.1177/1529100617727266

Coghill, D., & Sonuga-Barke, E. J. S. (2012). Annual research review: Categories versus dimensions in the classification and conceptualization of child and adolescent mental disorders—Implications of recent empirical study. *Journal of Child Psychology and Psychiatry, 53*(3), 469–489.

Conway, C. C., Forbes, M. K., Forbush, K. T., Fried, E. I., Hallquist, M. N., Kotov, R., et al. (2019). A hierarchical taxonomy of psychopathology can transform mental health research. *Perspectives on Psychological Science, 14*(3), 419–436.

Craske, M. G., Kircanski, K., Zelikowsky, M., Mystkowski, J., Chowdhury, N., & Baker, A. (2008). Optimizing inhibitory learning during exposure therapy. *Behaviour Research and Therapy, 46*(1), 5–27.

Cuthbert, B. N., & Insel, T. R. (2013). Toward the future of psychiatric diagnosis: The seven pillars of RDoC. *BMC Medicine, 11*, 126.

Dalgleish, T., Black, M., Johnston, D., & Bevan, A. (2020). Transdiagnostic approaches to mental health problems: Current status and future directions. *Journal of Consulting and Clinical Psychology, 88*(3), 179.

David, D., & Montgomery, G. H. (2011). The scientific status of psychotherapies: A new evaluative framework for evidence-based psychosocial interventions. *Clinical Psychology: Science and Practice, 18*(2), 89–99.

East-Richard, C., Mercier, A. R., Nadeau, D., & Cellard, C. (2020). Transdiagnostic neurocognitive deficits in psychiatry: A review of meta-analyses. *Canadian Psychology/Psychologie Canadienne, 61*(3), 190–214.

Eaton, N. R., Krueger, R. F., Keyes, K. M., Skodol, A. E., Markon, K. E., Grant, B. F., & Hasin, D. S. (2011). Borderline personality disorder co-morbidity: Relationship to the internalizing-externalizing structure of common mental disorders. *Psychological Medicine, 41*(5), 1041–1050.

Eaton, N., Krueger, R., & Oltmanns, T. (2011). Aging and the long-term stability of the internalizing spectrum of personality and psychopathology. *Psychology and Aging, 26*, 987–993.

Ehring, T., & Watkins, E. R. (2008). Repetitive negative thinking as a transdiagnostic process. *International Journal of Cognitive Therapy, 1*(3), 192–205.
Everaerd, D., Klumpers, F., van Wingen, G., Tendolkar, I., & Fernández, G. (2015). Association between neuroticism and amygdala responsivity emerges under stressful conditions. *NeuroImage, 112*, 218–224.
Eysenck, J. J. (1947). *Dimensions of personality*. Kegan Paul.
Eysenck, H. J., & Eysenck, S. B. G. (1975). *Manual of the Eysenck personality questionnaire*. Hodder and Stoughton.
Foa, E. B., & Kozak, M. J. (1986). Emotional processing of fear: Exposure to corrective information. *Psychological Bulletin, 99*(1), 20.
Fresco, D. M., Moore, M. T., van Dulmen, M. H., Segal, Z. V., Ma, S. H., Teasdale, J. D., & Williams, J. M. (2007). Initial psychometric properties of the experiences questionnaire: validation of a self-report measure of decentering. *Behavior Therapy, 38, 234–246.* https://doi.org/10.1016/j.beth.2006.08.003
Garland, E. L., & Howard, M. O. (2014). A transdiagnostic perspective on cognitive, affective, and neurobiological processes underlying human suffering. *Research on Social Work Practice, 24*(1), 142–151.
Gros, D. F. (2014). Development and initial evaluation of Transdiagnostic Behavior Therapy (TBT) for veterans with affective disorders. *Psychiatry Research, 220*(1–2), 275–282.
Gros, D. F., Szafranski, D. D., & Shead, S. D. (2017). A real world dissemination and implementation of Transdiagnostic Behavior Therapy (TBT) for veterans with affective disorders. *Journal of Anxiety Disorders, 46*, 72–77.
Gros, D. F., Merrifield, C., Rowa, K., Szafranski, D. D., Young, L., & McCabe, R. E. (2019). A naturalistic comparison of group Transdiagnostic Behaviour Therapy (TBT) and disorder-specific cognitive behavioural therapy groups for the affective disorders. *Behavioural and Cognitive Psychotherapy, 47*(1), 39–51.
Gros, D. F., Shapiro, M. O., & Allan, N. P. (2020). Efficacy of transdiagnostic behavior therapy on transdiagnostic avoidance in veterans with emotional disorders. *Journal of Clinical Psychology, 76*(1), 31–39.
Haas, B. W., Omura, K., Constable, R. T., & Canli, T. (2007). Emotional conflict and neuroticism: Personality-dependent activation in the amygdala and subgenual anterior cingulate. *Behavioral Neuroscience, 121*(2), 249.
Haeffel, G. J., Jeronimus, B. F., Fisher, A. J., Kaiser, B. N., Weaver, L. J., Vargas, I., et al. (2022). The Hierarchical Taxonomy of Psychopathology (HiTOP) is not an improvement over the DSM. *Clinical Psychological Science, 10*(2), 285–290. https://doi.org/10.1177/21677026211068873
Harkness, A. R., Reynolds, S. M., & Lilienfeld, S. O. (2014). A review of systems for psychology and psychiatry: Adaptive systems, personality psychopathology five (PSY-5), and the DSM-5. *Journal of Personality Assessment, 96*(2), 121–139.
Harris, K. R., & Norton, P. J. (2019). Transdiagnostic cognitive behavioral therapy for the treatment of emotional disorders: A preliminary open trial. *Journal of Behavior Therapy and Experimental Psychiatry, 65*, 101487.
Hasin, D. S., & Grant, B. F. (2015). The National Epidemiological Survey on Alcohol and Related Conditions (NESARC) Waves 1 and 2: Review and summary of findings. *Social Psychiatry and Psychiatric Epidemiology, 50*(11), 1609–1640. https://doi.org/10.1007/s00127-015-1088-0
Helbig-Lang, S., & Petermann, F. (2010). Tolerate or eliminate? A systematic review on the effects of safety behavior across anxiety disorders. *Clinical Psychology: Science and Practice, 17(3), 218–233.* https://doi.org/10.1111/j.1468-2850.2010.01213.x
Hettema, J. M., Neale, M. C., & Kendler, K. S. (2001). A review and meta-analysis of the genetic epidemiology of anxiety disorders. *American Journal of Psychiatry, 158*(10), 1568–1578. https://doi.org/10.1176/appi.ajp.158.10.1568
Hyman, S. H. (2010). The diagnosis of mental disorders: The problem of reification. *Annual Review of Clinical Psychology, 6*, 155–179.

Jablensky, A. (2016). Psychiatric classifications: Validity and utility. *World Psychiatry, 15*(1), 26–31. https://doi.org/10.1002/wps.20284

Jacobson, N. S., Martell, C. R., & Dimidjian, S. (2001). Behavioral activation treatment for depression: Returning to contextual roots. *Clinical Psychology: Science and Practice, 8(3), 255–270.* https://doi.org/10.1093/clipsy.8.3.255

Jarvi Steele, S., Farchione, T. J., Cassiello-Robbins, C., Ametaj, A., Sbi, S., Sauer-Zavala, S., & Barlow, D. H. (2018). Efficacy of the Unified Protocol for transdiagnostic treatment of comorbid psychopathology accompanying emotional disorders compared to treatments targeting single disorders. *Journal of Psychiatric Research, 104*, 211–216.

John, O. P., & Gross, J. J. (2007). Individual differences in emotion regulation. In J. Gross (Ed.), *Handbook of emotion regulation*. The Guilford Press.

Kawa, S., & Giordano, J. (2012). A brief historicity of the Diagnostic and Statistical Manual of Mental Disorders: Issues and implications for the future of psychiatric canon and practice. *Philosophy, Ethics, and Humanities in Medicine, 7*, 2. https://doi.org/10.1186/1747-5341-7-2

Keightley, M. L., Seminowicz, D. A., Bagby, R. M., Costa, P. T., Fossati, P., & Mayberg, H. S. (2003). Personality influences limbic-cortical interactions during sad mood induction. *NeuroImage, 20*, 2031–2039. https://doi.org/10.1016/j.neuroimage.2003.08.022

Kendler, K. S., Prescott, C. A., Myers, J., & Neale, M. C. (2003). The structure of genetic and environmental risk factors for common psychiatric and substance use disorders in men and women. *Archives of General Psychiatry, 60*, 929–937. https://doi.org/10.1001/archpsyc.60.9.929

Kessler, R. C., Chiu, W. T., Demler, O., & Walters, E. E. (2005). Prevalence, severity, and comorbidity of twelve-month DSM-IV disorders in the National Comorbidity Survey Replication (NCS-R). *Archives of General Psychiatry, 62*(6), 617–627.

Köhne, A. C. J. (2020). The relationalist turn in understanding mental disorders: From essentialism to embracing dynamic and complex relations. *Philosophy, Psychiatry, & Psychology, 27*(2), 119–140.

Kotov, R., Krueger, R. F., Watson, D., Achenbach, T. M., Althoff, R. R., Bagby, R. M., et al. (2017). The Hierarchical Taxonomy of Psychopathology (HiTOP): A dimensional alternative to traditional nosologies. *Journal of Abnormal Psychology, 126*(4), 454–477.

Kotov, R., Krueger, R. F., & Watson, D. (2018). A paradigm shift in psychiatric classification: The Hierarchical Taxonomy of Psychopathology (HiTOP). *World Psychiatry, 17*(1), 24–25.

Kushner, M. G., Wall, M. M., Krueger, R. F., Sher, K. J., Maurer, E., Thuras, P., & Lee, S. (2012). Alcohol dependence is related to overall internalizing psychopathology load rather than to particular internalizing disorders: Evidence from a national sample. *Alcoholism: Clinical and Experimental Research, 36*(2), 325–331.

Laceulle, O., Ormel, J., Aggen, S., Neale, M., & Kendler, K. (2013). Genetic and environmental influences on the longitudinal structure of neuroticism: A trait-state approach. *Psychological Science, 24*, 1780–1790. https://doi.org/10.1177/0956797613481356

Lilienfeld, S. O. (2011). Distinguishing scientific from pseudoscientific psychotherapies: Evaluating the role of theoretical plausibility, with a little help from Reverend Bayes. *Clinical Psychology: Science and Practice, 18*(2), 105–112.

Lilienfeld, S. O. (2014a). DSM-5: Centripetal scientific and centrifugal antiscientific forces. *Clinical Psychology: Science and Practice, 21*, 269–279.

Lilienfeld, S. O. (2014b). The Research Domain Criteria (RDoC): An analysis of methodological and conceptual challenges. *Behavior Research and Therapy, 62*, 129–139.

Lilienfeld, S. O. (2014c). Why ineffective psychotherapies appear to work: A taxonomy of causes of spurious therapeutic effectiveness. *Perspectives on Psychological Science, 9*(4), 355–387.

Lilienfeld, S. O., & Treadway, M. T. (2016). Clashing diagnostic approaches: DSM-ICD versus RDoC. *Annual Review of Clinical Psychology, 12*, 435–463.

Lilienfeld, S. O., Smith, S. F., & Watts, A. L. (2013). Issues in diagnosis: Conceptual issues and controversies. In W. E. Craighead, D. J. Mikllowitz, & L. W. Craighead (Eds.), *Psychopathology: History, diagnosis, and empirical foundations* (2nd ed., pp. 1–35). Wiley.

Lopez, M. E., Stoddard, J. A., Noorollah, A., Zerbi, G., Payne, L. A., Hitchcock, C. A., et al. (2015). Examining the efficacy of the unified protocol for transdiagnostic treatment of emotional disorders in the treatment of individuals with borderline personality disorder. *Cognitive and Behavioral Practice, 22*(4), 522–533.

Luyten, P., & Blatt, S. J. (2011). Integrating theory-driven and empirically-derived models of personality development and psychopathology: A proposal for DSM V. *Clinical Psychology Review, 31*(1), 52–68.

Mennin, D. S., & Fresco, D. M. (2013). What, me worry and ruminate about DSM-5 and RDoC? The importance of targeting negative self-referential processing. *Clinical Psychology: Science and Practice, 20*(3), 258–267.

Mennin, D. S., & Fresco, D. M. (2014). Emotion regulation therapy. In J. J. Gross (Ed.), *Handbook of emotion regulation* (2nd ed.). The Guilford Press.

Mennin, D. S., Heimberg, R. G., Turk, C. L., & Fresco, D. M. (2005). Preliminary evidence for an emotion dysregulation model of generalized anxiety disorder. *Behaviour Research and Therapy, 43*(10), 1281–1310. https://doi.org/10.1016/j.brat.2004.08.008

Mennin, D. S., Fresco, D. M., Ritter, M., & Heimberg, R. G. (2015). An open trial of emotion regulation therapy for generalized anxiety disorder and cooccurring depression. *Depression and Anxiety, 32*(8), 614–623.

Mennin, D. S., Fresco, D. M., O'Toole, M. S., & Heimberg, R. G. (2018). A randomized controlled trial of emotion regulation therapy for generalized anxiety disorder with and without co-occurring depression. *Journal of Consulting and Clinical Psychology, 86*(3), 268.

Mineka, S., Watson, D., & Clark, L. A. (1998). Comorbidity of anxiety and unipolar mood disorders. *Annual Review of Psychology, 49*, 377–412. https://doi.org/10.1146/annurev.psych.49.1.377

National Institute of Mental Health. (n.d.). *About RDoC*. Retrieved April 28, 2021, from https://www.nimh.nih.gov/research/research-funded-by-nimh/rdoc/about-rdoc.shtml

Norton, P. J. (2012). *Group cognitive-behavioral therapy of anxiety: A transdiagnostic treatment manual*. The Guilford Press.

Norton, P. J., & Barrera, T. L. (2012). Transdiagnostic versus diagnosis-specific CBT for anxiety disorders: A preliminary randomized controlled noninferiority trial. *Depression and Anxiety, 29*(10), 874–882.

Norton, P. J., Barrera, T. L., Mathew, A. R., Chamberlain, L. D., Szafranski, D. D., Reddy, R., & Smith, A. H. (2013). Effect of transdiagnostic CBT for anxiety disorders on comorbid diagnoses. *Depression and Anxiety, 30*(2), 168–173.

O'Toole, M. S., Renna, M. E., Mennin, D. S., & Fresco, D. M. (2019). Changes in decentering and reappraisal temporally precede symptom reduction during Emotion Regulation Therapy for generalized anxiety disorder with and without co-occurring depression. *Behavior Therapy, 50*(6), 1042–1052.

Regier, D. A., Narrow, W. E., Clarke, D. E., Kraemer, H. C., Kuramoto, J., Kuhl, E. A., & Kupfer, D. J. (2013). DSM-5 field trials in the United States and Canada, part II: Test-retest reliability of selected categorical diagnoses. *The American Journal of Psychiatry, 170*(1), 59–70. https://doi.org/10.1176/appi.ajp.2012.12070999

Renna, M. E., Quintero, J. M., Fresco, D. M., & Mennin, D. S. (2017). Emotion regulation therapy: A mechanism-targeted treatment for disorders of distress. *Frontiers in Psychology, 8*, 98.

Riccardi, C. J., Korte, K. J., & Schmidt, N. B. (2017). False safety behavior elimination therapy: A randomized study of a brief individual transdiagnostic treatment for anxiety disorders. *Journal of Anxiety Disorders, 46*, 35–45.

Roberts, B. W., & DelVecchio, W. F. (2000). The rank-order consistency of personality traits from childhood to old age: A quantitative review of longitudinal studies. *Psychological Bulletin, 126*(1), 3–25. https://doi.org/10.1037/0033-2909.126.1.3

Roberts, B. W., & Mroczek, D. (2008). Personality trait change in adulthood. *Current Directions in Psychological Science, 17*(1), 31–35. https://doi.org/10.1111/j.1467-8721.2008.00543.x

Roberts, B., Walton, K., & Viechtbauer, W. (2006). Patterns of mean-level change in personality traits across the life course: A meta-analysis of longitudinal studies. *Psychological Bulletin, 132*, 1–25. https://doi.org/10.1037/0033-2909.132.1.1

Rosellini, A. J., & Brown, T. A. (2014). Initial interpretation and evaluation of a profile-based classification system for the anxiety and mood disorders: Incremental validity compared to DSM-IV categories. *Psychological Assessment, 26*(4), 1212–1224. https://doi.org/10.1037/pas0000023

Rosellini, A. J., Boettcher, H., Brown, T. A., & Barlow, D. H. (2015). A transdiagnostic temperament-phenotype profile approach to emotional disorder classification: An update. *Psychopathology Review, 2*(1), 110–128. https://doi.org/10.5127/pr.00

Rosen, G. M., & Davison, G. C. (2003). Psychology should list empirically supported principles of change (ESPs) and not credential trademarked therapies or other treatment packages. *Behavior Modification, 27*(3), 300–312. https://doi.org/10.1177/0145445503253829

Ross, C. A., & Margolis, R. L. (2019). Research Domain Criteria: Strengths, weaknesses, and potential alternatives for future psychiatric research. *Molecular Neuropsychiatry, 5*, 218–235.

Rotter, J. B. (1954). *Social learning and clinical psychology*. Prentice-Hall.

Sakiris, N., & Berle, D. (2019). A systematic review and meta-analysis of the Unified Protocol as a transdiagnostic emotion regulation based intervention. *Clinical Psychological Review, 72, 101751*. https://doi.org/10.1016/j.cpr.2019.101751

Salkovskis, P. M., Clark, D. M., Hackmann, A., Wells, A., & Gelder, M. G. (1999). An experimental investigation of the role of safety-seeking behaviours in the maintenance of panic disorder with agoraphobia. *Behaviour Research and Therapy, 37*(6), 559–574.

Sauer-Zavala, S., & Barlow, D. H. (2021). *Neuroticism: A new framework for emotional disorders and their treatment*. Guilford Press.

Sauer-Zavala, S., Bentley, K. H., & Wilner, J. G. (2016). Transdiagnostic treatment of borderline personality disorder and comorbid disorders: A clinical replication series. *Journal of Personality Disorders, 30*(1), 35–51.

Sauer-Zavala, S., Cassiello-Robbins, C., Conklin, L. R., Bullis, J. R., Thompson-Hollands, J., & Kennedy, K. A. (2017a). Isolating the unique effects of the unified protocol treatment modules using single case experimental design. *Behavior Modification, 41*(2), 286–307.

Sauer-Zavala, S., Gutner, C. A., Farchione, T. J., Boettcher, H. T., Bullis, J. R., & Barlow, D. H. (2017b). Current definitions of "transdiagnostic" in treatment development: A search for consensus. *Behavior Therapy, 48*(1), 128–138.

Sauer-Zavala, S., Bentley, K. H., Steele, S. J., Tirpak, J. W., Ametaj, A. A., Nauphal, M., et al. (2020a). Treating depressive disorders with the Unified Protocol: A preliminary randomized evaluation. *Journal of Affective Disorders, 264*, 438–445.

Sauer-Zavala, S., Fournier, J. C., Steele, S. J., Woods, B. K., Wang, M., Farchione, T. J., & Barlow, D. H. (2021). Does the unified protocol really change neuroticism? Results from a randomized trial. *Psychological Medicine, 51*(14), 2378–2387. https://doi.org/10.1017/S0033291720000975

Schmidt, N. B., Buckner, J. D., Pusser, A., Woolaway-Bickel, K., Preston, J. L., & Norr, A. (2012). Randomized controlled trial of false safety behavior elimination therapy: A unified cognitive behavioral treatment for anxiety psychopathology. *Behavior Therapy, 43*(3), 518–532.

Scult, M. A., Fresco, D. M., Gunning, F. M., Liston, C., Seeley, S. H., García, E., & Mennin, D. S. (2019). Changes in functional connectivity following treatment with emotion regulation therapy. *Frontiers in Behavioral Neuroscience, 13*, 10.

Seligman, M. E. P. (1975). *Helplessness: On depression, development and death*. Freeman Press.

Servaas, M. N., Van Der Velde, J., Costafreda, S. G., Horton, P., Ormel, J., Riese, H., & Aleman, A. (2013). Neuroticism and the brain: A quantitative meta-analysis of neuroimaging studies investigating emotion processing. *Neuroscience & Biobehavioral Reviews, 37*(8), 1518–1529.

Silverman, M. H., Wilson, S., Ramsay, I. S., Hunt, R. H., Thomas, K. M., Krueger, R. F., & Iacono, W. G. (2019). Trait neuroticism and emotion neurocircuitry: Functional magnetic resonance imaging evidence for a failure in emotion regulation. *Development and Psychopathology, 31*(3), 1085–1099.

Skre, I., Onstad, S., Torgersen, S., Lygren, S., & Kringlen, E. (1993). A twin study of DSM–III–R anxiety disorders. *Acta Psychiatrica Scandinavica, 88*, 85–92. https://doi.org/10.1111/j.1600-0447.1993.tb03419.x

Spitzer, R. L., Forman, J. B., & Nee, J. (1979). DSM-III field trials, I: Initial interrater diagnostic reliability. *American Journal of Psychiatry, 136*, 815–817. https://doi.org/10.1176/ajp.136.6.815

Stone, M. H. (1993). *Abnormalities of personality: Within and beyond the realm of treatment. W W Norton & Co.*

Stein, M. B., Simmons, A. N., Feinstein, J. S., & Paulus, M. P. (2007). Increased amygdala and insula activation during emotion processing in anxiety-prone subjects. *American Journal of Psychiatry, 164*(2), 318–327.

Suris, A., Holliday, R., & North, C. S. (2016). The evolution of the classification of psychiatric disorders. *Behavioral Sciences, 6*(1), 5. https://doi.org/10.3390/bs6010005

Talkovsky, A. M., & Norton, P. J. (2014). Mediators of transdiagnostic group cognitive behavior therapy. *Journal of Anxiety Disorders, 28*(8), 919–924.

Varkovitzky, R. L., Sherrill, A. M., & Reger, G. M. (2018). Effectiveness of the unified protocol for transdiagnostic treatment of emotional disorders among veterans with posttraumatic stress disorder: A pilot study. *Behavior Modification, 42*(2), 210–230.

Watson, D. (2005). Rethinking the mood and anxiety disorders: A quantitative hierarchical model for DSM-V. *Journal of Abnormal Psychology, 114(4), 522–536.* https://doi.org/10.1037/0021-843X.114.4.522

Watson, D., Gamez, W., & Simms, L. J. (2005). Basic dimensions of temperament and their relation to anxiety and depression: A symptom-based perspective. *Journal of Research in Personality, 39*(1), 46–66. https://doi.org/10.1016/j.jrp.2004.09.006

Westlye, L. T., Bjørnebekk, A., Grydeland, H., Fjell, A. M., & Walhovd, K. B. (2011). Linking an anxiety-related personality trait to brain white matter microstructure: Diffusion tensor imaging and harm avoidance. *Archives of General Psychiatry, 68*, 369–377. https://doi.org/10.1001/archgenpsychiatry.2011.24

Wilamowska, Z. A., Thompson-Hollands, J., Fairholme, C. P., Ellard, K. K., Farchione, T. J., & Barlow, D. H. (2010). Conceptual background, development, and preliminary data from the unified protocol for transdiagnostic treatment of emotional disorders. *Depression and Anxiety, 27*(10), 882–890.

World Health Organization. (1949). *International statistical classification of diseases, injuries, and causes of death, 6th revision*. Author.

World Health Organization. (2016). *International statistical classification of diseases and related health problems (10th ed.).*

Zinbarg, R. E., & Barlow, D. H. (1996). Structure of anxiety and anxiety disorders: A hierarchical model. *Journal of Abnormal Psychology, 105*, 181–193.

Challenges and Opportunities for Experimental Psychopathology and Translational Research

Michael T. Treadway

Introduction

A primary goal of translational research is to leverage the explanatory power of well-controlled, experimentally rigorous studies to develop mechanistic hypotheses that may help unravel the mysterious psychological and biological sequela that give rise to psychiatric conditions. Because well-controlled experiments for relevant variables are often not possible in clinical populations (e.g., controlling a prenatal environment, or random assignment to manipulation likely to produce severe depression), translational research fills an important gap in understanding potential causes. The term "translational research" is loosely defined, and can be applied to animal or human studies performed with a specific clinical condition or application in mind, or to clinical intervention studies that have been critically informed by basic science. While not a strict requirement, a common goal among studies in this area has been to transverse multiple levels of analysis, most often measures of systems neuroscience (functional brain signals, brain morphology, or hormone levels) with some aspect of individual symptomatology such as depressed mood or avoidance due to anxiety. In practice, this endeavor has largely revolved around the tools of experimental psychopathology (i.e., "tasks"), with which researchers attempt to develop measures that can link behavior observed in animal models (and the associated knowledge regarding their underlying neural mechanisms) with clinical signs and symptoms observed in patients. Examples of such tasks include the use of simple Pavlovian or instrumental conditioning paradigms that have widely been used to identify the roles of the mesolimbic dopamine system (Pessiglione et al., 2006) and fronto-amygdala circuitry in mediating reinforcement learning and fear conditioning (Phelps et al., 2004; Phelps & LeDoux, 2005), respectively; the use of

M. T. Treadway (✉)
Emory University, Atlanta, GA, USA
e-mail: mtreadway@emory.edu

C. L. Cobb et al. (eds.), *Toward a Science of Clinical Psychology*,
https://doi.org/10.1007/978-3-031-14332-8_11

effort-based decision-making paradigms to assess dopamine-linked motivational circuitry (Soder et al., 2021; Treadway et al., 2012b; Wardle et al., 2011); or the use of reaction-time tasks to probe mechanisms of attention (Disner et al., 2011; Gotlib et al., 2004), among many others.

Once behavioral and biological convergence between animals and humans has been established (e.g., the same behavioral effect occurs in response to a common pharmacological manipulation), these tasks are then applied as functional assays for relevant symptom domains or cognitive processes in clinical populations. In the case of mood disorders commonly characterized by anhedonia, fatigue, and low energy, reinforcement learning and effort based decision-making tasks have been used to test a conceptual link to alterations in mesolimbic DA function (Admon et al., 2016; Huys et al., 2013; Treadway et al., 2012a). Similarly, fear-conditioning experiments have been used in patients with post-traumatic stress disorder (PTSD) to isolate a possible role for an over-active amygdala (Milad et al., 2007, 2009).

These are but a small number of examples meant to illustrate a broader point, which is that translational research is critically dependent on the presumed fidelity of identified behavioral tasks as measures of *both* the hypothesized neural system and the symptomatic construct of interest. In this way, the requirements for translational measures in experimental psychopathology are both broader and more specific than the traditional desiderata of psychological assessment, such as construct validity (Cronbach & Meehl, 1955). Broader in that they seek to capture multiple levels of analysis, and narrower in that they seek to constrain the psychological construct of interest (e.g., "fear") to a particular circuitry (e.g., "fear-resulting-from-amygdala-over-reactivity-due-to-enhanced-noradrenergic-innervation") so as to distinguish it from other potential biological mechanisms that may give rise to similar subjective experiences.

Successes and Failures

In the area of psychopathology, translational research has undoubtedly been very successful for certain types of questions. Perhaps most prominently, the core prerequisite of translational research has largely been validated; that is, it is indeed possible to translate task-based measures from animals to humans, and to "back-translate" human behaviors into animal paradigms with a high degree of fidelity, as illustrated by the examples of reinforcement learning, fear condition, and effort-based decision-making cited above. Further, many of these behavioral paradigms have revealed phylogenetically conserved functions (i.e., effects of catecholamines on attention and vigor) for key brain areas and neurotransmitters. In this way, translational research appears to be built on a solid foundation.

The next consideration is whether and how translational research has informed our understanding of mental illness. Here, the track record is more mixed. On the one hand, translational research has undeniably helped to answer the question of *where* in the body and the brain the biological mechanisms of particular symptoms are likely to occur. Put more colloquially, it has helped us to identify the "key players": brain areas, cell types, genes, and signaling proteins that may confer risk and dictate treatment responses to various conditions. However, the diagnostic and prognostic utility of this information has been limited. For example, just knowing that the amygdala contributes to anxiety or that dopamine can modulate motivation does not do much to address the question of *how* illness is caused in any meaningful sense. Moreover, the complex nature of this circuitry means that at the biological level, there are exponentially greater potential causes for the same behavior, as any disruption along underlying pathways may give rise to disruption. In other words, knowing that the amygdala may be hyper-active *on average* in a given clinical population does not offer actionable intelligence for treating a given patient. To paraphrase the opening lines of Tolstoy's *Anna Karenina*, healthy biological systems largely function the same way, but each system failure is unique. Indeed, after decades of small effect sizes and poor replication for many candidate genes or neuroimaging studies seeking to isolate causal biomarkers for psychiatric conditions, some have speculated that perhaps every diagnosed patient must be considered as "an exemplar or a rare disease model" (Paulus & Thompson, 2019).

I would suggest this view is overly pessimistic. In reality, we are likely to find that certain types of system failures (i.e., pathophysiology) are more frequent than others, giving hope to the notion of precision medicine—interventions that are targeted to the individual on the basis of a detailed understanding of that individual's pathophysiology—that has been helpful in other forms of behavioral health. Nevertheless, current practices in translational research may need substantial revision to unlock its potential. In the following sections, I outline some of these issues and suggest some possible steps towards remediation.

Current Challenges for Translational Research

The question as to why translational research has yet to produce a clear etiological and pathophysiological basis for clinical diagnoses has remained at the forefront of reviews, commentaries, and criticisms of field. Many answers have been proposed, including low statistical power, (Button et al., 2013), insufficiently precise hypotheses and definitions (Huys et al., 2016), small effect sizes (Paulus & Thompson, 2019), and so-called "shallow-phenotyping" (i.e., reliance on brief or imprecise measurements for a single construct; Phillips & Kendler, 2021). In this section, I try to identify several less frequently invoked issues that I believe pose additional challenges for translational research as it is commonly practiced. In particular, I focus on common assumptions that guide the practice of experimental psychopathology and how they might be modified to improve both ecological validity and identification of contributing biological causes.

Temporal Stability of Target Symptoms An often-unspoken assumption of experimental psychopathology is that the objects of our study—the signs and symptoms of psychopathology—are relatively stable through time. That is, a person diagnosed with major depressive disorder on a Monday can be counted upon to report anhedonia, fatigue, guilt, dysphoric mood, and poor sleep on a Thursday. This was a critical assumption for experimental psychopathology researchers, as it provided license for individuals to assume that target deficits would be easily measurable once a diagnosis had been established. For example, if seeking to test the possibility that a negative information processing bias as a neurocognitive mechanism in major depressive disorder (MDD), a researcher might expect that the administration of task at any point within 1-month of the clinical interview would be appropriate for detecting the deficit if this hypothesis is true.

There is now fairly consistent evidence, however, that this assumption is invalid. Indeed, while early, small-sample ambulatory assessment (AA) suggested a high degree of stability (e.g., consistent low mood in patients), much larger, more comprehensive studies have found otherwise. In one analysis of prior ambulatory assessment studies, it was found that patients with anxiety or mood disorders showed greater variability (as determined by mean sum of successive differences, MSSD) as compared to matched controls (Treadway & Leonard, 2016). In a more recent large sample study of "mood homeostasis" in >25,000 participants, it was found that mood stability was a hallmark of psychological health, rather than distress. Indeed, it was suggested that individuals with psychological disorders often lack the full complement of necessary coping tools to maintain a positive mood in the face of daily challenges and stressors. In contrast, individuals without current disorders are more adept at flexibility regulating their mood through adjusting their activities and commitments or reaching out for social support (Taquet et al., 2020). It is also worth noting that the general conclusion from these more recent AA methodologies and sophisticated computational modeling paradigms would not be surprising to a clinician working today or 50 years ago. Even the most severe forms of mental illness, such as delusions or dissociation, show variability in their symptoms and have been known to experience moments of "lucidity" (Marder & Freedman, 2014; Peterson et al., 2021).

Taken together, clinical case studies and rigorous experimental evidence all challenge the common practice of treating depression diagnosis and severity as a "steady-state," even over relatively short periods of time. This issue has been raised many times before, but is worth revisiting in light of the new evidence. Further, when seeking to measure neuro-cognitive mechanisms, this raises two additional concerns discussed below.

Mismatched Sampling Frequency If we accept that most symptoms show dynamic oscillations over time (be they periodic, stochastic, or context-dependent), then the timing of biological and experimental assessments becomes critical. When seeking to identify a neurocognitive mechanism for such symptoms, it is therefore critical to consider the proposed relationship between the mechanism and symptomatic expression. Certain classes of biological causes may reflect an individual's "average level" of a symptom and be relatively unrelated to fluctuations (Treadway & Leonard, 2016). For example, individuals with various prefrontal lesions can be expected to show a decremented performance on various neurocognitive tasks. However, they will also have "good days and bad days" during which their performance varies somewhat around their mean due to unknown factors. In such cases, however, it is highly unlikely that the causes of such performance variation would be attributable to structural variation in their prefrontal lesion. Rather, it makes much more sense to consider the lesion as a cause for the lowered "average level" of performance.

In contrast, for a highly variable phenomenon such as an epileptic seizure, temporal lobe activity during periods of quiescence will be wholly uninformative, while the explanatory power of measured activity *during* seizure is sufficient for neurosurgical intervention. As such, it is standard practice in the treatment of severe epilepsy cases to monitor implanted recording electrodes in epileptic patients for one or more weeks to determine the proper location. Unlike lesions, it is the precise temporal coupling between the variance of regional synchronous neural activity and the "symptoms" of seizures that defines the causation. Trying to infer the location of cortical areas that contribute to a patient's epilepsy by sampling neural activity occurring in between seizures would be meaningless.

Accessibility of Symptom Experiences Of all the challenges listed above, perhaps the most daunting and least discussed is the issue of accessing symptom experience during the process of measurement. All organisms are generally motivated to avoid unpleasant mental states, and patients suffering from psychological disorders are no exception. For experimental psychopathologists, this presents a particularly thorny challenge; whereas the history of clinical assessment has largely depended on the ability of patients to *report* on symptoms that may have recently occurred (which has its own caveats and pitfalls), the premise of experimental psychopathology paradigms is to transiently invoke the requisite conditions and contexts such that patients *experience* their symptoms in-the-moment. While it may be the case that a tearful patient enters a moment of profound sadness, guilt, or shame when answering probing questions during a clinical interview, that is no guarantee that such emotions are present and actively shaping behavior when they are completing a computer task an hour later.

The assumption of patient access to their symptomatic states has of course been embedded within the prior assumptions relating to their temporal stability, where it has been assumed that clinical symptoms are so intransigent and inescapable, that there is little need to consider the issue further. To illustrate this point with a few examples, this assumption requires that the patient doesn't just report that they seem to be "jumpy" and frequently over-react, he or she experiences that same manifestation of anxiety when learning to differentiate abstract cues from a mild electric shock or a white noise blast; or it requires that the patient access a sense of hopelessness, pessimism, and being overwhelmed when deciding whether to rapidly push a button or squeeze a handgrip for money. The challenge is even more pronounced when dealing with more acutely painful symptoms such as self-loathing, loneliness, shame, or intense fear. Most of us have pronounced psychological defenses that are engaged to suppress or alter these intense emotions, which may manifest as other symptoms, such as dissociation, flattened affect, fatigue, or distraction. Thus, even when a task is successful in creating the necessary conditions for symptom access, the temporal window will likely be brief, resulting in high rates intra- and inter-individual variability.

It is also worth noting that this phenomenon is not restricted to intense emotional or affective symptoms. If a researcher is seeking to understand behavioral or neural mechanisms of a putative cognitive distortion such as "black-and-white thinking" or "personalization," (Beck & Beck, 1995) they may be frustrated to find that their target subjects fail to exhibit such cognitive styles during a simple learning task, despite reporting them as frequent problems in their daily lives. Such would be an example of a task design that implicitly assumes an excessive degree of temporal stability and context-independence to the expression such thought distortions.

There are of course clear exceptions to this concern, and was with most aspects of psychopathology, they are clearer to identify in the extremes. Individuals with severe, vegetive depression will likely show more reliable impairments in reinforcement learning, and individuals with addiction in the acute phases of substance abstinence will likely experience frequent, intense cravings that can be readily measured experimentally. Nevertheless, the majority of targeted constructs in psychopathology research are likely difficult to access due to their inherent variability, context-specific nature, and reflexive suppression in response to the sheer anguish they induce.

Recommendations for Future Research

Given the challenges listed above, how can we improve experimental psychopathology methods in service of translational research? First and foremost, careful consideration of the timing and nature of clinical assessments and their hypothesized relationship to the timing and temporal stability of biological assessments will go a long way to addressing several of these concerns. In short, the assumption of symptom stability should be re-examined. By extension, short-term longitudinal sampling with ambulatory assessment or other "wearables" methods should be employed wherever possible to as to gain some purchase on intra-individual variability. These data will enhance the sensitivity of the experiment regardless of whether the proposed biological substrate is hypothesized to relate to "average level" of a symptom (as in a lesion) or to the variability of a symptom (as in a seizure).

The broader use of ambulatory assessment protocols also provides a mean of capturing the experience of symptomatic states as they can provide data over a much longer time frame than a typical laboratory visit. One may further be tempted to leverage ambulatory data as a means of deciding when a particular task should be performed, so as to capture task data during an optimal window of experience. This approach may be fruitful, though it runs the risk that act of performing a task may meaningfully shift attention away from the symptomatic state that the task attempts to measure (a variation of the "observer effect" in physics, which states that the act of measuring a physical system inexorably alters the quantity being measured).

An additional approach, now widely advocated, is the use of computational methods that can be used to extract more precise signals with less information loss from behavioral data. For example, behavioral performance during a preference may occasionally reflect lapses in attention, distraction, or gradual fatigue over the course of the task that are not captured by conventional summary statistics (e.g., mean of choice A over choice B). Modeling approaches can thereby help reduce noise as well as incorporate more sophisticated hypotheses related to task dynamics. Often subsumed within the general label of "computational psychiatry," this approach can also be used to inform task design and to identify latent forms of information processing (e.g., prediction errors or state-transition probabilities) that have no direct behavioral correlate but may meaningfully relate to neural signals. Finally, there is a nascent, yet exciting field of more immersive paradigms using virtual reality and other platforms to create complex, ecologically valid environments. These have long been used in the context of PTSD treatment, but are not being employed in service of psychopathology research for a diverse array of conditions, from specific phobia to suicide (Franklin et al., 2019; Reggente et al., 2018).

Conclusions

Translational research—abetted by careful experimental work at multiple levels—has made great progress in helping us uncover the gross anatomy of psychological distress and suffering. And yet, clear application to clinical practice has largely remained elusive. Much emphasis has been placed on the need for well-powered studies, more sensitive biological measurement techniques, and more sophisticated analytical pipelines. While this is all true, there remains a central role for psychological measurements with excellent validity. Fulfilling the promise of translational research will therefore require special attention to the methods and practices of experimental psychopathology.

References

Admon, R., Kaiser, R. H., Dillon, D. G., Beltzer, M., Goer, F., Olson, D. P., et al. (2016). Dopaminergic enhancement of striatal response to reward in major depression. *American Journal of Psychiatry, 174*(4), 378–386.

American Psychiatric, A. (2013). *Diagnostic and statistical manual of mental disorders (DSM-5®)*. American Psychiatric Publishing.

Beck, J. S., & Beck, A. T. (1995). *Cognitive therapy: Basics and beyond*. Guilford Press.

Button, K. S., Ioannidis, J. P., Mokrysz, C., Nosek, B. A., Flint, J., Robinson, E. S., & Munafò, M. R. (2013). Power failure: Why small sample size undermines the reliability of neuroscience. *Nature Reviews Neuroscience, 14*(5), 365–376.

Cronbach, L. J., & Meehl, P. E. (1955). Construct validity in psychological tests. *Psychological Bulletin, 52*(4), 281.
Disner, S. G., Beevers, C. G., Haigh, E. A., & Beck, A. T. (2011). Neural mechanisms of the cognitive model of depression. *Nature Reviews Neuroscience, 12*(8), 467–477.
Franklin, J. C., Huang, X., & Bastidas, D. (2019). Virtual reality suicide: Development of a translational approach for studying suicide causes. *Behaviour Research and Therapy, 120*, 103360.
Gotlib, I. H., Krasnoperova, E., Yue, D. N., & Joormann, J. (2004). Attentional biases for negative interpersonal stimuli in clinical depression. *Journal of Abnormal Psychology, 113*(1), 121–135. https://doi.org/10.1037/0021-843X.113.1.1212004-11098-014[pii]
Huys, Q. J., Pizzagalli, D. A., Bogdan, R., & Dayan, P. (2013). Mapping anhedonia onto reinforcement learning: A behavioural meta-analysis. *Biology of Mood & Anxiety Disorders, 3*(1), 12.
Huys, Q. J. M., Maia, T. V., & Frank, M. J. (2016). Computational psychiatry as a bridge from neuroscience to clinical applications. *Nature Neuroscience, 19*(3), 404–413.
Insel, T., Cuthbert, B., Garvey, M., Heinssen, R., Pine, D. S., Quinn, K., et al. (2010). Research domain criteria (RDoC): Toward a new classification framework for research on mental disorders. *American Journal of Psychiatry, 167*(7), 748–751. https://167/7/748[pii]10.1176/appi.ajp.2010.09091379
Lilienfeld, S. O., Lynn, S. J., Ruscio, J., & Beyerstein, B. L. (2011). *Great myths of popular psychology: Shattering widespread misconceptions about human behavior* (Vol. 50). Wiley.
Marder, S. R., & Freedman, R. (2014). *Learning from people with schizophrenia*. Oxford University Press.
Milad, M. R., Wright, C. I., Orr, S. P., Pitman, R. K., Quirk, G. J., & Rauch, S. L. (2007). Recall of fear extinction in humans activates the ventromedial prefrontal cortex and hippocampus in concert. *Biological Psychiatry, 62*(5), 446–454.
Milad, M. R., Pitman, R. K., Ellis, C. B., Gold, A. L., Shin, L. M., Lasko, N. B., et al. (2009). Neurobiological basis of failure to recall extinction memory in posttraumatic stress disorder. *Biological Psychiatry, 66*(12), 1075–1082.
Onitsuka, T., Hirano, Y., Nemoto, K., Hashimoto, N., Kushima, I., Koshiyama, D., et al. (2022). Trends in big data analyses by multicenter collaborative translational research in psychiatry. *Psychiatry and Clinical Neurosciences, 76*(1), 1–14.
Paulus, M. P., & Thompson, W. K. (2019). The challenges and opportunities of small effects: The new normal in academic psychiatry. *JAMA Psychiatry, 76*(4), 353–354.
Pessiglione, M., Seymour, B., Flandin, G., Dolan, R. J., & Frith, C. D. (2006). Dopamine-dependent prediction errors underpin reward-seeking behaviour in humans. *Nature, 442*(7106), 1042–1045. https://doi.org/10.1038/nature05051
Peterson, A., Clapp, J., Largent, E. A., Harkins, K., Stites, S. D., & Karlawish, J. (2021). What is paradoxical lucidity? The answer begins with its definition. *Alzheimer's & Dementia 18*(3).
Phelps, E. A., & LeDoux, J. E. (2005). Contributions of the amygdala to emotion processing: From animal models to human behavior. *Neuron, 48*(2), 175–187. https://doi.org/10.1016/j.neuron.2005.09.025
Phelps, E. A., Delgado, M. R., Nearing, K. I., & LeDoux, J. E. (2004). Extinction learning in humans: Role of the amygdala and vmPFC. *Neuron, 43*(6), 897–905.
Phillips, M. L., & Kendler, K. S. (2021). Three important considerations for studies examining pathophysiological pathways in psychiatric illness: In-depth phenotyping, biological assessment, and causal inferences. *JAMA Psychiatry, 78*(7), 697–698.
Reggente, N., Essoe, J. K.-Y., Aghajan, Z. M., Tavakoli, A. V., McGuire, J. F., Suthana, N. A., & Rissman, J. (2018). Enhancing the ecological validity of fMRI memory research using virtual reality. *Frontiers in Neuroscience, 12*, 408.
Satel, S., & Lilienfeld, S. O. (2013). *Brainwashed: The seductive appeal of mindless neuroscience*. Basic Civitas Books.
Soder, H. E., Cooper, J. A., Lopez-Gamundi, P., Hoots, J. K., Nunez, C., Lawlor, V. M., et al. (2021). Dose-response effects of d-amphetamine on effort-based decision-making and reinforcement learning. *Neuropsychopharmacology, 46*(6), 1078–1085.

Taquet, M., Quoidbach, J., Gross, J. J., Saunders, K. E., & Goodwin, G. M. (2020). Mood homeostasis, low mood, and history of depression in 2 large population samples. *JAMA Psychiatry, 77*, 944.

Treadway, M. T., & Leonard, C. V. (2016). Isolating biomarkers for symptomatic states: Considering symptom–substrate chronometry. *Molecular Psychiatry, 21*, 1180–1187.

Treadway, M. T., Bossaller, N. A., Shelton, R. C., & Zald, D. H. (2012a). Effort-based decision-making in major depressive disorder: A translational model of motivational anhedonia. *Journal of Abnormal Psychology, 121*(3), 553–558. https://doi.org/10.1037/a0028813

Treadway, M. T., Buckholtz, J. W., Cowan, R. L., Woodward, N. D., Li, R., Ansari, M. S., et al. (2012b). Dopaminergic mechanisms of individual differences in human effort-based decision-making. *Journal of Neuroscience, 32*(18), 6170–6176. https://doi.org/10.1523/jneurosci.6459-11.2012

Wardle, M. C., Treadway, M. T., Mayo, L. M., Zald, D. H., & de Wit, H. (2011). Amping up effort: Effects of d-amphetamine on human effort-based decision-making. *Journal of Neuroscience, 31*(46), 16597–16602. https://doi.org/10.1523/jneurosci.4387-11.2011

Wood, J. M., Teresa, P. M., Garb, H. N., & Lilienfeld, S. O. (2001). The misperception of psychopathology: Problems with the norms of the Comprehensive System for the Rorschach. *Clinical Psychology: Science and Practice, 8*(3), 350–373.

The Nomological Net of Scott Lilienfeld's Psychopathic Personality Inventory Scales

Lee Anna Clark, Lilian Dindo, Elizabeth McDade-Montez, Krista Kohl, Alex Casillas, Rob Latzman, and David Watson

The Nomological Net of the Psychopathic Personality Inventory Scales

Scott Lilienfeld was not one to shy away from controversy. At the same time, he always sought to reconcile conflicting views, to find their similarities and to explain their differences from a scientific perspective. This was the spirit that he brought to his work in the highly contentious field of psychopathy. In Lilienfeld et al. (2015), he and colleagues examined the major points of debate in the field and concluded that they reflect two broad conceptualizations of psychopathy. To oversimplify, one conceptualization views psychopathy as a distinct entity in nature, whereas the other conceptualizes it as a combination of characteristics that reflect a diverse array

Supplementary Information The online version contains supplementary material available at [https://doi.org/10.1007/978-3-031-14332-8_12].

L. A. Clark (✉)
Department of Psychology, University of Notre Dame, Notre Dame, IN, USA
e-mail: la.clark@nd.edu

L. Dindo
University of Houston, Houston, TX, USA

E. McDade-Montez
Capitola, CA, USA

K. Kohl · A. Casillas
University of Iowa, Iowa City, IA, USA

R. Latzman
Georgia State University, Atlanta, GA, USA

D. Watson
University of Notre Dame, Notre Dame, IN, USA

C. L. Cobb et al. (eds.), *Toward a Science of Clinical Psychology*,
https://doi.org/10.1007/978-3-031-14332-8_12

of higher and lower order personality dimensions each of which is continuous across an adaptive–maladaptive spectrum. Lilienfeld et al. (2015) hypothesized that this bifurcation of views reflected the historic split between basic personality research and psychopathology research, which widened in the mid-1960s when the *Journal of Abnormal and Social Psychology* split into the *Journal of Abnormal Psychology* and a new *Journal of Personality and Social Psychology* (see Watson & Clark, 1994, for a fuller description of these changes in the field). In the mid-1990s, however, both Lilienfeld (e.g., Lilienfeld & Andrews, 1996) and we (e.g., Watson et al., 1994) sought to close this gap by demonstrating the close connections between basic dimensions of personality and various forms of psychopathology and, over the past few decades, relations between personality and psychopathology increasingly have been the focus of research.

This research has indicated that personality disorders (PD), as defined by the *Diagnostic and Statistical Manual of Mental Disorders* (*DSM-5*, Section II [*DSM-5*-II]; APA, 2013), as well as personality pathology not explicitly defined by *DSM*, such as psychopathy, may be understood to a large extent as extreme variants of common personality traits (e.g., Clark, 2007; Livesley & Jang, 2000; Widiger & Simonsen, 2005). As such, as stated earlier, Lilienfeld, Lynam, Widiger, and others have proposed that psychopathy is best viewed as a constellation of maladaptive personality characteristics rather than as a qualitatively distinct disorder (e.g., Krueger, 2006; Lilienfeld et al., 2015; Lynam & Derefinko, 2006; Marcus et al., 2013; Miller & Lynam, 2012; Widiger, 1998).

Psychopathy was described originally in extensive detail by Cleckley in *The Mask of Sanity* and, although the criminal consequences of this form of pathology are often the most visible, personality features are at the core of this classic definition (Cleckley, 1941/1976). Cleckley's criteria for identifying psychopathy included descriptions of deficient emotional reactivity (e.g., absence of nervousness, poverty of affect) and interpersonal functioning (e.g., pathological egocentricity and incapacity for love, unresponsiveness in interpersonal situations, superficial charm; impersonal sexuality), as well as the disinhibited/antisocial tendencies (e.g., unreliability, poorly motivated antisocial behaviors) that are characteristic of the disorder. He attributed these problems to a congenital peculiarity or deficit that contributes strongly to the etiology of psychopathy. Hare's Psychopathy Checklist (PCL; Hare, 1991), now revised (PCL-R; Hare, 2003), was developed to assess Cleckley's psychopathy (although it does not follow Cleckley's conceptualization in every respect), and quickly became the gold standard for diagnosing psychopathy. However, it was designed to assess psychopathy in forensic samples and involves a lengthy procedure including an interview and data from prison files, so numerous self-report measures of psychopathy were subsequently developed, both to simplify assessment and to be more appropriate for use with non-incarcerated as well as forensic samples.

The focus of this chapter, the Psychopathic Personality Inventory (PPI; Lilienfeld & Andrews, 1996), was one such measure. It consists of eight basic scales, but not long after its publication, factor analyses of its scales were found to yield two dominant factors: One, labeled Fearless Dominance (FD), was marked by the Stress Immunity, Fearlessness, and Social Influence scales, and the other, self-centered impulsivity (SCI), by the Rebellious Nonconformity, Alienation, Blame Externalization, and Carefree Nonplanfulness scales.[1] The Coldheartedness scale did not load on either factor (Benning et al., 2003, 2005; Patrick et al., 2006). Although most of the ensuing PPI research focused on its higher order factors, some researchers questioned whether they accurately reflect the PPI's structure, especially their replicability across sample type. For example, Neumann et al. (2008) criticized use of the factors based on the low-to-moderate intercorrelations of their component scales, reporting an average of .36 for the FD scales and .22 for the SCI scales in a large offender sample. Lilienfeld and Andrews (1996) had reported similar values of .30 and .25, respectively, in their seminal article. Together with the moderate percentage of the PPI's common variance accounted for by the two factors (e.g., Benning et al., 2003 reported a value just over 50%, and Neumann et al., 2008, 43%), these data indicate that there is a great deal of specificity in the basic scales that may be valuable to consider in terms of the nomological net of psychopathic personality traits, beyond what can be gleaned from use of higher order factors. Elucidating that network is a primary purpose of the current chapter.

Relations Between Higher Order Factors of Psychopathy and Personality

Notably, early factor analyses of the PCL-R also yielded two factors (e.g., Hare, 1991, 1998; Harpur et al., 1989). Factor 1 reflects psychopathy's core interpersonal and affective features (e.g., lack of remorse or guilt, manipulativeness), whereas Factor 2 taps an impulsive, antisocial lifestyle (e.g., lack of realistic, long-term goals; irresponsibility). Whether the PCL-R and PPI factors reflect the same construct has been the subject of much debate. Some researchers (e.g., Edens et al., 2008; Miller & Lynam, 2012) have noted that the PCL-R factors are moderately strongly correlated (e.g., around .50; Hare, 1991), whereas the PPI factors are essentially orthogonal (e.g., $r = .12$ per Marcus et al.'s, 2013 meta-analysis). Moreover, correlations between the two measures' respective factors tend to be rather low (e.g., Marcus et al., 2013, reported meta-analytic correlations of .21 and .15 for the two sets of factors, respectively).

However, other researchers (e.g., Benning et al., 2003) linked the PPI FD and SCI with PCL-R Factors 1 and 2, respectively, on the basis of their patterns of correlations with external validators. There are now two meta-analyses of both the PCL-R and PPI factors' correlations with the higher order factors of personality, so considerable data are available to adjudicate this debate. Examining first the PCL-R, Lynam and Derefinko (2006) and Lilienfeld et al. (2015) both reported meta-analytic

[1] The scale names of the PPI and its revision, the PPI-R, are slightly different. We use the latter's scale names throughout this chapter, given their now more common use and very high degree of similarity between the two scale sets.

results between psychopathy and personality, focused primarily on Hare's (1991) Psychopathy Check List-Revised (PCL-R) and the Big-Five of personality. They found that Factor 1—psychopathy's core interpersonal and affective features—and Factor 2—an impulsive, antisocial lifestyle—both relate to low A. They also found that Factor 2 related to low C and to N, although in both cases, Lynam and Derefinko (2006) found stronger relations (−.45 vs. −.27 for C and .34 vs. 18 for N). Neither PCL-R factor related to Extraversion in either analysis. Finally, only Lynam and Derefinko (2006) found that Factor 1 related mildly to low C ($r = -.22$).

Turning to the PPI, Miller and Lynam (2012) conducted meta-analyses of relations between the PPI factors and higher order scales of both the Big-Five and Big-Three (e.g., Eysenck & Eysenck, 1975; Tellegen & Waller, 2008) models of personality. They found that FD was primarily related to low N ($rs = -.50$) and high E (mean $r = .48$) of the Big-Five and Big-Three models, whereas SCI was related to low A ($r = -.49$) and low C ($r = .51$) of the Big Five, low Constraint ($r = -.54$) of the Big Three, and also moderately to N in both models (mean $r = .33$).[2] The meta-analysis of Marcus et al. (2013), examining the PPI with Big-Three-model traits, yielded similar—but generally weaker—results, perhaps because they co-analyzed psychopathology and personality measures (e.g., they considered anxiety and depression measures both to assess N, along with more purely personality trait measures).

Comparing across the two pairs of analyses (i.e., PCL-R and PPI, respectively, with personality), there were three "universals," all involving Factor 2 and SCI: Both correlated moderately strongly with low A and low C (rs for A = −.35 to −.49; $M = -.43$; rs for C = −.27 to −.51; $M = -.42$) and moderately with N (rs = .15 to .34; $M = .27$). These results provide strong support for the contention that PCL-R Factor 2 and PPI SCI reflect highly similar constructs, whereas PCL-R Factor 1 and PPI FD are quite distinct. The purpose of our study was thus twofold: First, we sought to probe the nature of the higher order PPI factors in relation to not only higher order, but also lower order personality traits, as well as measures of "real world behavior." Second, as mentioned previously, we aimed to elucidate the nomological net of the lower order psychopathic personality traits themselves, outside of the context of these higher order factors.

[2] Currently, the usual terms for the first two Big-Three dimensions are Negative Emotionality (NEM) and Positive Emotionality (PEM), but for simplicity, we use the Big-Five terms Neuroticism and Extraversion.

Method

Procedures

We conducted three studies, all with undergraduates enrolled in introductory psychology classes at a large midwestern public university. Participants in all three samples completed the PPI and one or more other personality and/or behavioral paper-and-pencil questionnaires in a large group setting after giving written informed consent. All study procedures were approved the University's Institutional Review Board.

Participants

The first sample included 578 students (70% reported being female, 94% white), of whom 547 (71% female, 95% white) completed the PPI. Mean age was 19.4 years in both the total sample and PPI completers. The second sample included 399 students (63% of whom reported being female), of whom 388 (63% female) completed the PPI. Other demographic data were not collected in this sample, but the population from which they were drawn was primarily White and ranged in age between 18 and 23 years.[3] The third sample included 332 male (92% white) students, collected explicitly to correct the gender imbalance of the other two samples, all of whom completed the PPI. We report here only on the subsets of participants who completed the PPI.

Measures[4]

Psychopathic Personality Inventory (PPI; Lilienfeld & Andrews, 1996) The PPI is a 187-item self-report measure designed to assess psychopathic personality characteristics in a non-incarcerated population. Responders use a 4-point Likert-type scale: false, mostly false, mostly true, true. The measure has eight factor analytically derived scales that assess various traits relevant to the broad construct of psychopathy: Machiavellian Egocentricity, Blame Externalization, Carefree Nonplanfulness, Rebellious Nonconformity, Fearlessness, Social Influence, Stress Immunity, and Coldheartedness. Internal consistency reliabilities (Cronbach's

[3] Participants' exact age and ethnicity was not recorded. However, age and ethnicity estimates are based from the enrollment statistics of the Elementary Psychology course from which participants were drawn.

[4] Descriptive statistics for all measures are provided in Supplemental Table 1.

alpha) in the current study ranged from .77 to .87; average interitem correlations (AICs) from .14 to .87 (see Table 1).

DIS-I (Dindo et al., 2009) The DIS-I is a 65-item, factor analytically derived measure of five correlated, content-distinct traits related to disinhibition that measure both high and low levels of the dimension: Manipulativeness (e.g., "It is easy for me to take advantage of others"), Prosociality (which has two subscales, Considerateness and Goal Orientation; e.g., "I am attentive to other people's feelings," and "I have high standards of achievement for myself," respectively), Distractibility (e.g., "I have a hard time staying focused for long periods of time"), Risk Taking (e.g., "I enjoy taking risks"), and Orderliness (e.g., "I am bothered by messiness and clutter"). Respondents rate each item on a 5-point Likert scale ranging from "strongly disagree" to "strongly agree." All scales had strong internal consistency reliabilities in the current sample (coefficient alpha range = .80–.88; AICs = .29–.38). The DIS-I was collected in Sample 1.

Revised NEO Personality Inventory (NEO PI-R; Costa & McCrae, 1992) The NEO PI-R is a 240-item measure that assesses the domains of the Big-Five of personality—Neuroticism (N), Extraversion (E), Openness (O), Agreeableness (A), and Conscientiousness (C)—each of which is composed of six lower order facets.

Table 1 Intercorrelations of the psychopathic personality inventory scales

Scales (Number of items)	1	2	3	4	5	6	7	8
1. Machiavellian Egocentrism (30)	*.86 (.17)*							
2. Blame Externalization (18)	.53	*.85 (.24)*						
3. Carefree Nonplanfulness (20)	.41	.35	*.82 (.19)*					
4. Rebellious Nonconformity (17)	.46	.35	.42	*.80 (.19)*				
5. Fearlessness (19)	.41	**.14**	**.19**	.56	*.86 (.24)*			
6. Social Influence (24)	**.20**	**-.08**	**-.05**	**.26**	.39	*.87 (.22)*		
7. Stress Immunity (11)	**-.04**	**-.34**	**-.09**	**.16**	.38	.44	*.79 (.23)*	
8. Coldheartedness (21)	**.32**	**.06**	**.32**	**.10**	**.10**	**.01**	**.21**	*.77 (.14)*
Average Interscale Correlations	.34	.17	.16	.32	.34	.16	.23	.11
Fearless Dominance	.25	-.11	.03	.43	**.78**	**.76**	**.79**	.14
Self-centered Impulsivity	**.79**	**.76**	**.71**	**.75**	.44	.11	-.11	.25

Note: $N = 1267$. Correlations ≤ **.35** are in **bold** (61%; 17 of 28) for the scales. For the factors, the stronger of each scale's two correlations is in bold. Correlations in red denote the correlation between two scales each of which correlates most strongly with the other. Alpha coefficients (average interitem correlations; AIC) are shown in italics in the diagonal. If considered as an eight-item scale, the alpha coefficient (AIC) of the PPI would be .70 (.23). Average interscale correlation for scales 1 through 5 (typically termed "Self-Centered Impulsivity") was .42 (alpha = .73); that for scales 5 through 7 (Fearless Dominance) was .40 (alpha = .63). The average discriminant correlation was .12 without and .13 with Coldheartedness.

Respondents rated each item on a 5-point Likert scale ranging from "strongly disagree" to "strongly agree." In the current sample, the scales' internal consistency reliabilities (alphas) were very high for the domain scales (alpha range = .86–.91; AICs = .17–.25) and moderate to high for the facet scales (alpha range = .49–.82; median = .71; AICs = .11–.36; median = .23). The NEO PI-R was collected in Sample 1.

Schedule for Nonadaptive and Adaptive Personality (SNAP; Clark, 1993) and General Temperament Survey (GTS; Clark & Watson, 1990) The SNAP is a 375-item, true-false format, self-report questionnaire designed to assess personality characteristics relevant to both the normal and abnormal range. The SNAP yields scores on three scales—Negative Temperament (NT), Positive Temperament (PT), and Disinhibition (DIS)—that are largely unrelated to one another ($|r|$s =.07–.27) and that measure the core of the Big Three dimensions of personality, plus 12 more specific trait scales each primarily associated with one of the Big Three core scales. For example, mistrust and self-harm are associated with NT, exhibitionism and entitlement with PT, and impulsivity and (low) workaholism with DIS (see Table 2 for a complete scale list). In addition, DIS has two subscales—Antisocial Behavior and Carefree Orientation—that correlate .40–.50 with each other and that are strongly negatively related to Big-Five Agreeableness and Conscientiousness, respectively. The SNAP was collected in Sample 2; a subset of Sample 3 participants (n = 182) also completed the SNAP.[5]

The GTS is a 90-item derivative of the SNAP that includes only NT, PT, and DIS (and their subscales). It was collected in Sample 1 and its scales were merged with the parallel SNAP scales in the other two samples in all relevant analyses. Across all three samples, internal consistency reliabilities (Cronbach's alpha) for the Big Three core scales were high (.83–.89); those for the DIS subscales were .71. Alphas for the other scales (collected in Samples 2 and 3) ranged from .77 to .85; median = .81.

Personal Lifestyles Questionnaire (PLQ; Muhlenkamp & Brown, 1983; cited in Mahon et al., 2002) The PLQ is a 24-item questionnaire designed to assess health-related behaviors. Participants are asked to indicate the extent to which they engage in various behaviors. Items are endorsed on a 4-point Likert-type scale from "almost always" to "never." We used factor analysis to group the items into three scales: A 7-item Healthful Habits scale (e.g., getting adequate sleep, exercising regularly, limiting caffeine; alpha = .68, AIC = .23); a 7-item Hazardous Behaviors scale (e.g., not wearing a seatbelt, driving after drinking, heavy smoking; alpha = .66, AIC = .22); and a 6-item Self-Care scale (e.g., getting together with friends, confiding concerns, reserving time for relaxation, annual health-care appointments; alpha = .60, AIC = .20).[6] The PLQ was collected in Sample 1.

---

[5] The SNAP is now in its 2nd edition (SNAP-2; Clark et al., 2014), but the scales completed by our participants are identical to those in the SNAP-2.

[6] The factor loading matrix for the three-factor solution is available in Supplemental Table 2.

Table 2 Correlations of the two higher order psychopathic personality inventory scales with personality traits and related behavior

Scale	Sample size	Fearless Dominance	Self-Centered Impulsivity
Five Factor Model Domains – SNAP scales, All Samples; NEO scales, Sample 1[a]			
Miller and Lynam (2012) *N*	*2561*	**−.50**	*.30*
Marcus et al. (2013) *NEM*	*8571*	*−.35*	*.30*
NEO PI-R Neuroticism	538	**−.57***	.23
SNAP Negative Temperament	1112	−.49	.24
Miller and Lynam (2012) *E*	*2561*	*.48*	*−.11*
Marcus et al. (2013) *PEM*	*5715*	*.39*	*−.02*
NEO PI-R Extraversion	538	.37	−.20
SNAP Positive Temperament	1112	.37	−.22
Miller and Lynam (2012) *A*	*2561*	*−.10*	*−.49*
NEO PI-R Agreeableness	538	−.12	**−.58**
Marcus et al. *(2013) SS*	*1441*	***.51***	***.50***
SNAP Disinhibition	1112	.37	**.71***
SNAP Antisocial Behavior	1112	.33	**.61**
Miller and Lynam (2012) *C*	*2561*	*−.25*	***−.51***
Miller and Lynam (2012) *CON*	*2561*	*−.25*	***−.51***
Marcus et al. *(2013) CON*	*5280*	*−.04*	***−.44***
NEO PI-R Conscientiousness	538	.02	**−.56**
SNAP Carefree Behavior	1112	.22	**.57**
Miller and Lynam (2012) *O*	*2298*	*−.25*	*.04*
NEO PI-R Openness	538	.18	−.14
Disinhibition Inventory – Sample 1			
Manipulativeness	536	.11	**.66***
Prosociality	536	.08	**−.54**
Goal Orientation	536	.13	−.49
Considerateness	536	.01	−.46
Risk-taking	536	**.61***	.27
Distractibility	536	−.18	.38
Orderliness	536	−.14	−.20
SNAP-2 Lower Order Traits – Samples 2 and 3			
Manipulativeness	570	.24	**.68***
Mistrust	570	−.09	.47
Aggression	570	.18	.49
Self-harm	570	−.15	.37
Impulsivity	570	.40	**.61**
Propriety	570	−.25	−.34
Workaholism	570	.01	−.17
Exhibitionism	570	.44	.13
Energy	1112	.31	−.13
Positive Affect	1112	.41	−.11
Detachment	570	−.24	.22

(continued)

Table 2 (continued)

Scale	Sample size	Fearless Dominance	Self-Centered Impulsivity
Entitlement	570	.25	.11
Dependency	570	−.42	.05
Eccentric Perceptions	570	.09	.41
Five Factor Model Facets – Sample 1			
N Anxiety	538	**−.55***	−.03
N Depression	538	−.43	.17
N Hostility	538	−.20	.37
N Self-consciousness	538	**−.55***	.02
N Vulnerability	538	**−.54***	.23
E Gregariousness	538	.22	−.14
E Assertiveness	538	.46	−.03
E Trust	538	.16	−.39
E Straightforwardness	538	−.21	**−.53***
A Altruism	538	.04	−.45
A Compliance	538	−.15	−.41
A Modesty	538	−.24	−.33
A Tender-Mindedness	538	−.16	−.28
C Competence	538	.15	−.42
C Dutifulness	538	.06	−.47
C Achievement Striving	538	.07	−.41
C Self-Discipline	538	.09	−.48
C Deliberation	538	−.18	−.46
O Aesthetics	538	.07	−.13
O Feelings	538	−.01	−.28
Personal Lifestyle Questionnaire – Sample 1			
Hazardous Behaviors	539	.18	.47*
Healthful Habits	539	−.22	.22
Self-Care	539	−.16	.15
Behaviors Questionnaire – Sample 2			
Antisocial Behaviors	389	.14	**.52***
Irresponsible Behaviors	389	.21	.44

Note. *N* Neuroticism, *NEM* Negative Emotionality, *NEO PI-R* NEO Personality Inventory Revised, *SNAP* Schedule for Nonadaptive and Adaptive Personality, *E* Extraversion, *A* Agreeableness, *SS* Sensation Seeking, *C* Conscientiousness, *O* Openness. Each scale's stronger correlation, regardless of sign, is noted as follows: those ≥ .35 and < .50 are underlined; those ≥ .50 are bolded.
*The strongest correlation of each factor (within ± .01) in each section.
[a]Plus Miller and Lynam's (2012) and Marcus et al. (2013)'s meta-analyses for comparison; these are shown in italics.

Behaviors Questionnaire (BQ) The BQ is a 50-item questionnaire developed for this study to assess the frequency with which an individual has engaged in a range of externalizing behaviors during the previous week, month, or year. Participants respond using a 1 (zero times) to 4 (more than five times) Likert-type scale. We used factor analysis to develop two scales: A 21-item Antisocial Behaviors scale (e.g., vandalism, ticketed for public intoxication, leaving a restaurant without paying, starting physical fights; alpha = .83; AIC = .19) and a 15-item Irresponsible Behaviors scale (e.g., multiple one-night stands; unplanned/unprotected sex; frequent drug and alcohol use, regularly skipping class, going out the night before an important test; alpha = .81, AIC = .22).[7] The BQ was collected in Sample 2.

Results

Two-Factor Structure of the Psychopathic Personality Inventory

We first assessed whether the typical two-factor structure (i.e., that of Benning et al., 2003) was seen in our data, and found that it was.[8] Fearless Dominance was marked by Stress Immunity, Social Influence, and Fearlessness (loadings .55–.73), and SCI was marked by Machiavellian Egocentrism, Blame Externalization, Rebellious Nonconformity and Carefree Nonplanfulness (loadings .60–.74). Blame Externalization and Rebellious Nonconformity cross-loaded −.31 and .30, respectively, on FD, and Fearlessness cross-loaded .39 on SCI; all other cross-loadings were <.30. The two factors correlated negligibly (r = .15), and accounted for 38% (24% and 14%, respectively) of the common variance. We created unit-weighted factor-based scales using each factor's primary markers after standardizing the scales to weight them equally within factor. The interscale correlations within factors were somewhat higher than those typically found in the literature—means were .40 and .42 among the FD and SCI scales, respectively—but still low enough to indicate there is potentially valuable information in the nomological net of the basic scales. Nonetheless, given that considerable research has examined the correlates of the PPI factors (indeed, more than those of its basic scales), we first present our findings involving FD and SCI.

Relations with Higher Order Personality Traits As shown in the top portion of Table 2, our results largely replicated Miller and Lynam's stronger findings (vs. the weaker ones of Marcus et al., 2013). Further, in our data, FD related more moderately to SNAP DIS (the opposite pole of Big-Three Constraint) and its Antisocial Behavior subscale (rs = .37 and .33, respectively) compared to the .51 found by Marcus et al. (2013). In addition, we found a stronger relation between SCI and SNAP DIS (r = .71) than was found in either meta-analysis between SCI and low

[7] The factor loading matrix for the two-factor solution is available in Supplemental Table 3.

[8] The factor loading matrix for the two-factor solution is available in Supplemental Table 4.

Constraint (−.52 and −.44, respectively), most likely because DIS focuses more on the maladaptive end of the dimension, as does SCI, than do measures of Constraint in other Big-Three instruments.

Relations with Lower Order Personality Traits Given the distinctiveness of FD (compared to PCL-R Factor 1) and that the PPI's higher order factors mask a great deal of scale-level specificity, we also examined the factors' nomological net in relation to lower order personality traits (see Table 2). In relation to the DIS-I (Dindo et al., 2009), the strongest correlates were between FD and Risk-taking ($r = .61$) and between SCI and Manipulativeness ($r = .66$) and Prosociality ($r = -.54$), including both its subscales (*r*s = −.49 and −.46 for Goal Orientation and Considerateness, respectively). Distractibility also correlated .38 with SCI, but Orderliness correlated only weakly with both factors ($|rs| \leq .20$).

The strongest correlations of the PPI factors with the lower order SNAP scales involved SCI: .68 with Manipulativeness, and .61 with Impulsivity. Both factors also had several correlations in the .40s: SCI correlated with Mistrust, Aggression, and Eccentric Perceptions (*r*s = .47, .49, and .41, respectively), whereas FD correlated with Impulsivity, Exhibitionism, Positive Affect, and (low) Dependency (*r*s = .40, .44, .41, and −.42, respectively).

With the NEO PI-R facets, FD had the stronger set of relations: Of the N facets, Anxiety, Depression, Self-consciousness and Vulnerability all had strong negative relations (*r*s = −.55, −.43, −.55, and −.54, respectively), plus E Assertiveness correlated .46. On the other hand, only A Straightforwardness correlated >.50 ($r = .53$) with SCI, whereas a large number of scales correlated between .35 and .49. Other than N Hostility ($r = .37$), all of these such correlations were with facets of A (three additional facets) and C (five of the six—all but Orderliness).

Relations with Health and Externalizing Behaviors Table 2 also displays correlations between the PPI factors and indices of behaviors assessed with the PLQ and BQ. The only PLQ correlation ≥ .35 was between SCI and Hazardous Behaviors ($r = .47$). However, Healthful Habits did correlate modestly with both factors: $r = -.22$ with FD and $r = .22$ with SCI. Similarly, SCI correlated with both scales of the Behaviors Questionnaire, which assesses only externalizing behaviors: $r = .52$ with Antisocial Behaviors and $r = .44$ with Irresponsible Behaviors, which also correlated .21 with FD.

PPI Scale-level Correlations

In sum, our PPI results at the higher order factor level largely replicate those found in the literature, so we turn now to the heart of the chapter—explicating the nature of the basic personality traits that the PPI assesses, proceeding in the same order as before: Higher order personality traits, then lower order traits, and finally health and externalizing behaviors.

Relations with Higher Order Personality Traits In Table 3, we see that Stress Immunity is strongly negatively correlated with N/NT, and Blame Externalization has a moderate positive relation with N/NT, whereas Social Influence correlated −.37 with NEO PI-R N, but only −.29 with SNAP NT. However, Social Influence was moderately strongly correlated with both E and PT (*r*s = .50 and .48, respectively); Carefree Nonplanfulness also correlated moderately (*r* = −.38) with E, but < .20 with SNAP PT. Thus, the correlation of the higher order factor FD with N and E reflects the largely separate contributions of Stress Immunity and Social Influence, respectively.

Not surprisingly, most of the strong correlations between the PPI basic scales and higher order personality traits were in the domains of Agreeableness and Conscientiousness. Both Machiavellian Egocentrism and Carefree Nonplanfulness correlated ≥ .35 with all scales in these domains. NEO PI-R A correlated negatively more strongly with Machiavellian Egocentrism (*r* = −.64) and NEO PI-R C with Carefree Nonplanfulness (*r* = −.67), with cross correlations of −.35 and −.37, respectively, whereas SNAP DIS correlated strongly (*r*s > .60) with both PPI scales, as well as correlating in the .50s with both Rebellious Nonconformity and Fearlessness. All other correlations of Blame Externalization and Rebellious Nonconformity were between −.35 and −.48. Thus, two of the four scales that constitute SCI are primarily responsible for that factor's correlations with A and C. It also should be noted that Coldheartedness correlated −.43 with NEO PI-R A and −.40 with NEO PI-R O.

Relations with Lower Order Personality Traits Turning to lower order personality dimensions, shown in Table 4, the value of these examinations becomes particularly clear. First, concerning the DIS-I, there were four pairs of PPI—DISI-I scales in which each was most strongly correlated with the other: PPI Machiavellian Egocentrism with DIS-I Manipulativeness (*r* = .72), Carefree Nonplanfulness with Goal Orientation (*r* = −.60), Fearlessness with Risk-taking (*r* = .65) and Coldheartedness with Considerateness (*r* = −.49). Of the other four PPI scales, Blame Externalization correlated strongly with DIS-I Manipulativeness (*r* = .52), as well as correlating around −.40 with Prosociality and both its subscales, and Rebellious Nonconformity correlated .42 with both Manipulativeness and Risk-taking. However, Social Influence correlated moderately only with Risk-taking (*r* = .43) and Stress Immunity only with Distractibility (*r* = −.36), underscoring (as seen in Table 2) that, except for Risk-taking, the DIS-I scales are associated primarily with PPI SCI.

Similarly, there were four sets of PPI—SNAP scales in which each correlated most strongly with the other: PPI Machiavellian Egocentrism with SNAP Manipulativeness (*r* = .70) and Antisocial Behavior (*r* = .68), Blame Externalization with Mistrust (*r* = .64), Carefree Nonplanfulness with Carefree Behavior (*r* = .65) and Impulsivity (*r* = .62), and Social Influence with Exhibitionism (*r* = .66). The only other correlations ≥ |.50| were Rebellious Nonconformity with Impulsivity (*r* = .57) and Propriety (*r* = −.50) and Machiavellian Egocentrism with Aggression

Table 3 Correlations of the Psychopathic Personality Inventory scales with domain-level personality traits

Scales	Machvlln Egoctrsm	Blame Extrnlzn	Carefree Nonplnflns	Rebellious Noncmfrm	Fearless-ness	Social Influence	Stress Immunity	Cold-hrtdnss
				Neuroticism/ Negative Temperament				
NEO PI-R Neuroticism	.11	.38	.23	-.02	-.25	-.37	**-.68*†**	-.22
SNAP Negative Temperament	.17	<u>.44</u>	.09	.01	-.19	-.29	**-.67*†**	-.25
				Extraversion/ Positive Temperament				
NEO PI-R Extraversion	-.08	-.28	-.19	-.07	.17	**.50†**	.20	-.21
SNAP Positive Temperament	-.07	-.17	-.38	-.06	.19	<u>.48†</u>	.21	-.20
				Agreeableness/Conscientiousness vs. Disinhibition				
SNAP Disinhibition	**.64*†**	.35	**.61**	**.58†**	**.51†**	.25	.07	.17
NEO PI-R Agreeableness	**-.64*†**	<u>-.48†</u>	-.35	-.35	-.19	-.17	.07	<u>-.43†</u>
SNAP Antisocial Behavior	**.67*†**	.37	.36	<u>.46</u>	<u>.45</u>	.25	.07	.17
NEO PI-R Conscientiousness	-.37	-.35	**-.67*†**	-.36	-.18	.07	.18	-.17
SNAP Carefree Behavior	<u>.42</u>	.24	**.65*†**	<u>.45</u>	.34	.14	.02	.11
				Openness to Experience				
NEO PI-R Openness	-.20	-.18	-.19	.13	.10	.18	.14	<u>-.40†</u>

Note: Sample size is 538 for NEO PI-R scales, Sample size is 1112 for SNAP scales, *NEO PI-R* Revised NEO Personality Inventory, *GTS* General Temperament Survey, *DIS-I* Disinhibition Inventory, *SNAP* Schedule for Nonadaptive and Adaptive Personality, *Machvlln Egoctrsm* Machiavellian Egocentrism, *Extrnlzn* Externalization, *Nonplnflns* Nonplanfulness, *Noncmfrm* Nonconformity, *Cold-hrtdnss* Cold-heartedness. Correlations (absolute values) ≥ .50 are **bolded**; |*r*s| ≤ .50 and ≥ .40 are <u>underlined</u>
*Highest correlation in row within ±.03; †highest correlation in column within ±.03; in red when these converge

($r = .56$). Workaholism correlated only with Carefree Nonplanfulness ($r = -.46$), and Dependency only with Stress Immunity ($r = -.46$). Positive Affect, Energy, Entitlement, and Detachment all correlated moderately with Social Influence (*r*s = .50, .48, .36, and −.43), again indicating that Social Influence is an Extraversion-domain scale. Coldheartedness' strongest SNAP correlate was Dependency; *r* was only −.22.

Among the NEO PI-R facet scales, there were six pairs of direct correspondences with the PPI scales: PPI Machiavellian Egocentrism and A Straightforwardness correlated most strongly with each other ($r = -.62$); Blame Externalization and A Trust $r = -.50$; Carefree Nonplanfulness correlated −.58 and −.56 with, respectively, C Achievement Striving and Self-Discipline; Social Influence and E Assertiveness $r = .62$; Stress Immunity and N Vulnerability $r = -.63$; and Coldheartedness −.44 correlated with both A Tender-Mindedness and O Feelings. Both Machiavellian Egocentrism and Blame Externalization also correlated in the .40–.55 range with other A and C facets, respectively and, in addition, Blame Externalization, Social Influence, and Stress Immunity each had several other moderate correlations, mostly negative, with A for the first and with N for the latter two scales. However, Rebellious Nonconformity correlated only with A Straightforwardness and C Deliberation

(rs = −.36) and Fearlessness' strongest facet correlation was −.34 with C Deliberation.[9]

Relations with Health and Externalizing Behaviors Finally, at the bottom of Table 4 are correlations with participants' self-reported behaviors. Once again, Machiavellian Egocentrism and Carefree Nonplanfulness dominated the relations, with the former correlating .46 with Antisocial Behaviors and .38 with Hazardous Behaviors, and the latter correlating .44 with both Antisocial Behaviors and Irresponsible Behaviors. Only one other correlation reached the .40 level—Rebellious Nonconformity with Hazardous Behaviors, although there was a smattering of other correlations between .35 and .40 for the four SCI component scales. Fearlessness, Social Influence, Stress Immunity, and Coldheartedness, however, had no correlates ≥.30. Nonetheless, Healthful Habits and Self-Care had some low positive relations (.21–.28) with Social Influence and Stress Immunity, indicating that some individuals high in these psychopathic personality traits engage in positive health behaviors.

Summary of Strong Correlations of the PPI Basic Scales

We have reported a large number of correlations between the PPI scales and many other personality and behavioral measures, so it is useful to summarize the consistent patterns that have emerged from these analyses. We present these data in Table 5, arranged—to the extent possible—by the strongest correlations for each PPI scale. Machiavellian Egocentrism is clearly a marker of low A; more specifically, however, it taps manipulativeness and deceitfulness versus being truthful and straightforward. Blame Externalization is also a low-A facet that quite specifically reflects Mistrustfulness. Carefree Nonplanfulness marks low C and specifically taps whimsically impulsive behavior versus deliberate, disciplined behavior that is directed towards achieving one's goals. In fact, it might be considered a reverse-keyed marker of C, given that 80% of its items are reverse keyed (e.g., I think about long-term goals; strive to be the best). Rebellious Nonconformity is a less focused trait—it taps the same characteristics as Machiavellian Egocentrism and particularly Carefree Nonplanfulness but in a more diffuse way, at least in the array of scales that we collected.

Fearlessness is specifically focused on Risk-taking in our analyses. As such, it is not surprising that it correlated from .78 to .84 with the Boldness scale (Sellbom & Phillips, 2013) of Patrick's (2010) Triarchic Psychopathy Measure. Interestingly, it correlated with SNAP DIS, especially its Antisocial Behavior facet (rs = .51 and

[9]Given correlations of these magnitudes, the question of content overlap naturally arises, so we compared the items of several of the more highly correlated scale pairs. We found that they often had key terms in common (e.g., fear and worry in Stress Immunity, Neuroticism, and Negative Temperament) but the item similarities did not go beyond that level of overlap.

Table 4 Correlations of the psychopathic personality inventory with lower order personality traits and related behaviors

Scales	Machvlln Egoctrsm	Blame Extrnlzn	Carefree Nonplnflns	Rebellious Noncmfrm	Fearless-ness	Social Influence	Stress Immunity	Cold-hrtdnss
			Disinhibition inventory – Sample 1 (*N* = 536)					
Manipulativeness	**.72*†**	**.52†**	.41	.42†	.25	.15	-.14	.32
Prosociality	-.39	-.45	**-.56***	-.29	-.06	.10	.15	-.42
Goal Orientation	-.27	-.40	**-.60*†**	-.28	-.01	.13	.20	-.26
Considerateness	-.42	-.39	-.39	-.23	-.08	.06	.07	**-.49*†**
Risk-taking	.24	-.02	.21	.42†	**.65*†**	.43†	.30	.02
Distractibility	.24	.31	.44*	.19	.04	-.08	-.36†	-.08
			SNAP Lower Order Traits – Samples 2 and 3 (*N* = 581)					
Manipulativeness	**.70*†**	.43	.42	.47	.36	.17	.02	.14
Antisocial Behavior	**.67*†**	.37	.36	.46	.45	.25	.07	.17
Mistrust	.34	**.64*†**	.17	.21	.08	-.09	-.22	-.06
Aggression	**.56***	.42	.24	.26	.32	.17	-.08	.19
Carefree Behavior	.42	.24	**.65*†**	.45	.34	.14	.02	.11
Impulsivity	.41	.23	**.62*†**	**.57**	.46†	.27	.18	.10
Propriety	-.11	.03	-.44	**-.50***	-.25	-.09	-.23	-.16
Workaholism	-.01	.12	-.46*	-.19	-.02	.11	-.06	-.09
Exhibitionism	.24	.01	.04	.12	.26	**.66*†**	.15	-.05
Energy	-.01	-.05	-.37	-.05	.18	.40*	.13	-.16
Positive Affect	-.05	-.20	-.26	.00	.20	.48*	.25	-.17
Detachment	.13	.24	.11	.15	-.07	-.43*	-.10	.11
Entitlement	.31	.08	-.12	.07	.16	.36*	.08	-.04
Dependency	.02	.20	.08	-.15	-.22	-.31	-.46*	-.22
			Five Factor Model Facets – Sample 1 (*N* = 536)					
A Straightforwardness	**-.62*†**	-.39	-.30	-.36†	-.25	-.24	.00	-.29
A Modesty	**-.51**	-.17	-.12	-.23	-.15	-.33	-.08	-.29
A Altruism	-.42	-.38	-.32	-.25	-.09	.06	.12	-.35
A Compilance	-.43	-.31	-.26	-.29	-.21	-.20	.07	-.24
A Trust	-.31	**-.50*†**	-.22	-.16	.02	.09	.25	-.21
N Hostility	.34	.41	.27	.14	-.03	-.06	-.36	.07
C Achievement Striving	-.24	-.24	**-.58*†**	-.24	-.08	.10	.14	-.15
C Self-Discipline	-.32	-.34	**-.56*†**	-.29	-.10	.09	.22	-.11
C Deliberation	-.34	-.22	**-.52**	-.36†	-.34	-.10	.03	-.08
C Competence	-.23	-.33	**-.51**	-.23	-.06	.16	.26	-.13
C Dutifulness	-.39	-.32	**-.53**	-.26	-.11	.06	.20	-.23
E Assertiveness	.08	-.09	-.15	.06	.18	**.62*†**	.28	.00
N Vulnerability	.09	.33	.29	-.01	-.24	-.36	**-.63*†**	-.11
N Depression	.00	.33	.15	.03	-.14	-.37	-.48*	-.22
N Self-consciousness	-.05	.21	-.02	-.11	-.30	-.49*	-.48*	-.24
E Gregariousness	-.02	-.22	-.05	-.13	.08	.39	.07	-.09
A Tender-Mindedness	-.33	-.18	-.21	-.14	-.15	-.11	-.09	-.44*†
O Feelings	-.25	-.26	-.23	-.14	-.09	.12	-.03	-.44*†
O Aesthetics	-.20	-.09	-.21	.07	.02	.14	.03	-.38
			Personal Lifestyles Questionnaire – Sample 1 (*N* = 510)					
Hazardous Behaviors	.38*†	.36†	.32†	**.40†**	.28†	.10	.02	.14†
Healthful Habits	-.11	-.27*	-.21	-.08	.08	.21	.21†	-.06
Self-Care	-.07	-.20	-.09	-.10	.02	.28†*	.10	-.11
			Behaviors Questionnaire – Sample 2 (*N* = 388)					
Antisocial Behaviors	.46*†	.37†	.44*†	.34	.20	.10	.01	.19†
Irresponsible Behaviors	.37	.19	.44*†	.39†	.29†	.15†	.04	.11

Note: *Machvlln Egoctrsm* Machiavellian Egocentrism, *Extrnlzn* Externalization, *Nonplnflns* Nonplanfulness, *Noncmfrm* Nonconformity, *Cold-hrtdnss* Cold-heartedness, *SNAP* Schedule for Nonadaptive and Adaptive Personality correlations (absolute values) $\geq$ .50 are **bolded**; $|rs| \leq$ .50 and $\geq$ .35 are underlined

*For each measure, highest correlation in row within ±.03; †highest correlation in column within ±.03, for each measure; in red when these converge.

.45, respectively), but not with either A or C, even though DIS correlated −.57 with C and −.40 with A. Social Influence acts like a facet of Extraversion, and specifically reflects Exhibitionism and Assertiveness; it also taps low N to a certain extent, but is largely unrelated to either A or C. Stress Immunity, in turn, is clearly a marker of low N as it correlates most highly with higher order measures of N (vs. specific facets) and, again, does not correlate with either A or C. Thus, it might be considered a reverse-keyed measure of N, given that 73% (8 of 11) of its items are reverse-keyed (e.g., "easily flustered under pressure" is a Stress Immunity item, reverse-keyed). The correlational patterns of the scales that are components of the FD factor has led to a debate in the literature regarding whether the factor and its components can be considered aspects of psychopathy (e.g., see Lilienfeld et al., 2012; Miller & Lynam, 2012; Lynam & Miller, 2012). We discuss later how we might understand this pattern. Finally, Coldheartedness appears to be a facet of low A, correlating most strongly with the A facet Tender-Mindedness and DIS-I Considerateness. Once again, one might say it actually measures Tender Considerateness, as 95% of its items are keyed in that direction.

It is important to take note of those scales that are named for their reverse-keyed end and to consider (1) whether they should be renamed to reflect their primary keying direction and (2) the extent to which they actually measure the construct for which they are currently named. That is, lacking or being low on a construct is not necessarily equivalent to being high on its opposite end. For example, not being sad is not the same as being happy; not being mean is not the same as being nice. It seems that there may be relatively few constructs that are truly bipolar, such that when two unipolar scales are created to replace a bipolar scale, they are often only weakly correlated. However, this statement is based more on years of experience with measure development than on established research results, because a literature search reveals that there has been little substantive work into this important question, representing a critical lacuna that should be addressed in the future.

Turning to the behavioral questionnaires, it is noteworthy that only the component scales of SCI (i.e., and not those of FD) correlated with these measures, and they correlated only with the scales tapping hazardous health behaviors and not the two scales that assess positive health habits (thus, apropos the above paragraph on bipolarity, it appears that positive and negative health habits also are not clear opposites). Machiavellian Egocentrism was the most strongly correlated scale with PLQ Hazardous Behaviors and with BQ Antisocial Behaviors, whereas Carefree Nonplanfulness was the strongest correlate of BQ Irresponsible Behaviors. Blame Externalization and Rebellious Nonconformity also had several correlations in the .35–.40 range with these scales.

For comparison, we also include in Table 5 the correlations of the various scales with the two PPI higher order factors. As can been seen, in the vast majority (83%) of cases, a specific PPI scale correlates with at least one of the various scales more strongly than either of the factors, ranging from trivial differences of .01 to as large a difference as .22 (SNAP Exhibitionism correlates .66 with Social Influence but only .44 with FD), with an overall mean difference of .10. In contrast, in the six

Table 5 Summary of strong correlations between the psychopathic personality inventory scales and other measures

Scales	Machvlln Egoctrsm	Blame Extrnlzn	Carefree Nonplnfl	Rebellious Noncmfrm	Fearless-ness	Social Influence	Stress Immunity	Cold-hrtdnss	FD	SCI
Personality Traits										
DISI Manipulativeness	**.72*†**	**.52**	.41	.42	.25	.15	-.14	.32	.11	**.66**
SNAP Manipulativeness	**.70*†**	.43	.42	.47	.36	.17	.02	.14	.24	**.68**
SNAP Disinhibition	**.64**	.35	**.61**	**.58†**	**.51**	.25	.07	.17	.37	**.71*†**
SNAP Antisocial Behavior	**.67***	.37	.36	.46	.45	.25	.07	.17	.33	**.61**
NEO E Straightforwardness	**-.62***	-.39	-.30	-.36	-.25	-.24	.00	-.29	-.21	**-.53**
NEO PI-R Agreeableness	**-.64***	-.48	-.35	-.35	-.19	-.17	.07	-.43	-.12	**-.58**
SNAP Mistrust	.34	**.64*†**	.17	.21	.08	-.09	-.22	-.06	-.09	.47
NEO E Trust	-.31	**-.50***	-.22	-.16	.02	.09	.25	-.21	.16	-.39
NEO PI-R Conscientiousness	-.37	-.35	**-.67*†**	-.36	-.18	.07	.18	-.17	.02	**-.56**
SNAP Carefree Behavior	.42	.24	**.65*†**	.45	.34	.14	.02	.11	.22	**.57**
DISI Goal Orientation	-.27	-.40	**-.60***	-.28	-.01	.13	.20	-.26	.13	-.49
SNAP Impulsivity	.41	.23	**.62***	**.57†**	.46	.27	.18	.10	.40	**.61**
NEO C Achievement Striving	-.24	-.24	**-.58***	-.24	-.08	.10	.14	-.15	.07	-.41
NEO C Self-Discipline	-.32	-.34	**-.56***	-.29	-.10	.09	.22	-.11	.09	-.48
NEO C Competence	-.23	-.33	**-.51***	-.23	-.06	.16	.26	-.13	.15	-.42
NEO C Dutifulness	-.39	-.32	**-.53***	-.26	-.11	.06	.20	-.23	.06	-.47
NEO C Deliberation	-.34	-.22	**-.52***	-.36	-.34	-.10	.03	-.08	-.18	-.46
DISI Risk-taking	.24	-.02	.21	.42	**.65*†**	.43	.30	.02	**.61†**	.27
SNAP Exhibitionism	.24	.01	.04	.12	.26	**.66*†**	.15	-.05	.44	.13
NEO E Assertiveness	.08	-.09	-.15	.06	.18	**.62***	.28	.00	.46	-.03
NEO PI-R Extraversion	-.08	-.28	-.19	-.07	.17	**.50***	.20	-.21	.37	-.20
SNAP Positive Temperament	-.07	-.17	-.38	-.06	.19	.48*	.21	-.20	.37	-.22
NEO PI-R Neuroticism	.11	.38	.23	-.02	-.25	-.37	**-.68*†**	-.22	**-.57*†**	.23
SNAP Negative Temperament	.17	.44	.09	.01	-.19	-.29	**-.67*†**	-.25	-.49	.24
NEO N Vulnerability	.09	.33	.29	-.01	-.24	-.36	**-.63***	-.11	**-.54*†**	.23
NEO N Anxiety	-.08	.14	.01	-.18	-.36	-.29	**-.59***	-.28	**-.55*†**	-.03
NEO N Depression	.00	.33	.15	.03	-.14	-.37	-.48*	-.22	-.43	.17
NEO N Hostility	.34	.41	.27	.14	-.03	-.06	-.36	.07	-.20	.37
NEO N Self-consciousness	-.05	.21	-.02	-.11	-.30	-.49	-.48	-.24	**-.55*†**	.02
DISI Considerateness	-.42	-.39	-.39	-.23	-.08	.06	.07	-.49*†	.01	-.46
NEO A Tender-Mindedness	-.33	-.18	-.21	-.14	-.15	-.11	-.09	-.44*	-.16	-.28
NEO O Feelings	-.25	-.26	-.23	-.14	-.09	.12	-.03	-.44*	-.01	-.28
Behavioral Questionnaires										
PLQ Hazardous Behaviors	.41	.37	.34	.40	.28	.12	.01	.13	.18	.47*
BQ Antisocial Behaviors	.46	.37	.44	.34	.20	.10	.01	.19	.14	.52*
BQ Irresponsible Behaviors	.37	.19	.44*	.39	.29	.15	.04	.11	.21	.44*

Note: Machvlln Egoctrsm Machiavellian Egocentrism, *Extrnlzn* Externalization, *Nonplnfl* Nonplanfulness, *Rebellious Noncmfrm* Rebellious Nonconformity, *Cold-hrtdnss* Cold-heartedness, *DISI* Disinhibition Inventory, *SNAP* Schedule for Nonadaptive and Adaptive Personality, *PI-R* Personality Inventory-Revised, *PLQ* Personal Lifestyles Questionnaire, *BQ* Behaviors Questionnaire, *N* Neuroticism, *A* Agreeableness, *O* Openness, *PLQ* Personal Lifestyle Questionnaire, *BQ* Behaviors Questionnaire. Correlations (absolute values) ≥ .50 are **bolded**; |*rs*| ≤ .50 and ≥ .40 are underlined

*Highest correlation in row within ±.03; †highest correlation in column within ±.03; in red when these converge

cases in which the association with a factor scale is stronger, the range of differences from the lower orders scales' correlations is from .01 to .07, with a mean difference of .05.

Further, a specific PPI scales has a direct correspondence with one of the various scales (i.e., each is the other's strongest correlate) in 10 cases, whereas there are only two such relations with the PPI factor scales: SNAP Disinhibition and SCI (both higher order scales) are each other's strongest correlates ($r = .71$), and NEO Self-consciousness and Fearless Dominance correlate most strongly with each other ($r = -.55$).

Discussion

We have presented data documenting that the four component scales of PPI higher order SCI factor reflect various aspects of low A and C, with each having a particular focus. Specifically, Machiavellian Egocentrism correlated with Manipulativeness (*r*s = .70–.72), Blame Externalization with Mistrust (*r* = .64), and Carefree Nonplanning with the interrelated scales of Carefree Behavior (*r* = .65), Impulsivity (*r* = .62), and low Achievement Striving (*r* = .60). Rebellious Nonconformity also related to Impulsivity (*r* = .57), but related to low Propriety (.50) and five other scales in the .40–.49 range, as well, so its content was a bit more diffuse. The SCI scales also relate to various externalizing behaviors.

In contrast, the three component scales of FD by-and-large do not relate to either A or C (although FD does correlate strongly with SNAP DIS, which, turn, *is* strongly related to both A and C), nor do they correlate with externalizing behaviors. Instead, Fearlessness reflects the specific trait of Risk-taking (*r* = .65); Social Influence reflects Exhibitionism (*r* = .66) and Assertiveness (*r* = .62), both facets of E; and Stress Immunity taps low Anxiety (*r* = .63) and Vulnerability (*r* = 59), facets of N. Coldheartedness, which forms its own factor, reflects low Considerateness (*r* = .49) and the Tender-Mindedness (*r* = .44), facet of A. Thus, whether researchers should focus on the higher order factors or the lower order scales depends on the aims of their investigation, whether they are interested in discerning broad patterns, for which the simplicity of using the factor scales may be preferred, or are probing a phenomenon to understand it in greater specificity, for which the individual scales confer the clear advantage of providing more information. That said, those who choose to investigate at the factor level should be aware of the specificity that these factors mask, whereas those choosing to investigate phenomena at the scale level should be aware that their results may implicate broader patterns.

Broadening the Focus to All of Personality Pathology

In terms of the issue with which we began this chapter—namely, whether psychopathy is a unique and qualitatively distinct disorder or best viewed as a constellation of maladaptive personality characteristics—we clearly join Scott Lilienfeld in interpreting the data as more strongly supportive of latter view. Importantly, however, we do not view this debate in isolation, but rather place it in the context of the broader debate of whether personality pathology as a whole domain is best characterized (1) categorically, as it has been traditionally in the DSM and the International Classification of Diseases, Versions 6 through 10 (ICD; World Health Organization, 1949, 1992), and still is in Section II of *DSM-5*; (2) fully dimensionally as it is in the International Classification of Diseases, 11th Edition; or (3) in a hybrid dimensional-categorical fashion, as exemplified in the Alternative Model of Personality Disorder (AMPD) in Section III of *DSM-5*.

The advantage of considering psychopathy within this larger context is that the perspective of dimensional (or hybrid) models (e.g., ICD-11 and AMPD, respectively) is useful to consider in the debate about whether (1) the PPI traits that do not tap aspects of low A and C (i.e., the three component scales of the FD factor) should nonetheless be considered psychopathic traits, as Lilienfeld et al. (2012) contend, or (2) instead reflect psychologically healthful characteristics, including aspects of both low N and high E, particularly social assertiveness, which Miller and Lynam (2012) summarized as stable extraversion (Eysenck & Rachman, 1965) and argue are not central to psychopathy. The primary element that both the AMPD and ICD-11 bring to the table is that personality traits are the second of their two main criteria, the first being maladaptive personality functioning.

The theoretical basis for requiring impairment in personality functioning, as well as personality traits in the maladaptive range, to diagnose personality pathology was first introduced into the personality-disorder research literature by Livesley et al. (1994), subsequently developed by Livesley and Jang (2000, 2005), and finally adapted for inclusion in the AMPD. However, the concepts they introduced into this literature had earlier origins, including in the work of Allport (1937), who wrote that "…personality is something and personality does something…" (p. 48), and who later elaborated that personality is "the dynamic organization within the individual of those psychophysical systems that determine… characteristic behavior and thought" (1961, p. 28). Livesley and Jang also drew on work in evolutionary psychology, specifically that of Plutchik (1980), who described universal life tasks that all individuals need to achieve to function successfully in society.[10] Finally, they incorporated concepts from cognitive psychology, for example, "how individuals *interpret* life tasks of work, play, intimacy, power, and health … envisaging alternative future selves, and devising cognitive strategies to guide behavior in relevant situations" (Cantor, 1990, p. 735, emphasis added).

Livesley and Jang (2005) integrated these varied perspectives with the clinical literature on personality dysfunction and proposed that PD reflects "the failure to achieve one or more of the following: (1) stable and integrated representations of self and others; (2) the capacity for intimacy, to function adaptively as an attachment figure, and/or to establish affiliative relationships; and (3) adaptive functioning in the social group [including] prosocial behavior and/or cooperative relationships" (p. 264).

This work's influence on the AMPD can be seen in its first criterion and, subsequently, also that of ICD-11 PD model. Specifically, in the AMPD, Criterion A is "Moderate or greater impairment in personality (self/interpersonal) functioning, manifested by difficulties in two or more of the following four areas: Identity, self-direction, empathy, and intimacy" (APA, 2013, p. 770). Each of the four areas is further defined and five levels of functioning are delineated from (0) Little or no impairment to (4) Extreme impairment, with Level 2, Moderate impairment, required for diagnosis (see APA, 2013, pp. 775–778). The ICD-11 criterion is highly

---

[10] More recent work in this general area has been done by the Organisation for Economic Co-operation and Development (e.g., see https://www.oecd.org/officialdocuments/publicdisplaydocumentpdf/?cote=EDU/WKP(2018)9&docLanguage=En)

similar and, importantly, this personality-functioning severity rating (Mild, Moderate, or Severe) is the only required PD diagnostic criterion (https://icd.who.int/browse11/l-m/en#/http%3a%2f%2fid.who.int%2ficd%2fentity%2f941859884). Thus, a major difference between the two systems is that the AMPD requires at least one pathological trait—its Criterion B (APA, 2013, p. 761), whereas the ICD-11 model's trait and pattern specifiers (https://icd.who.int/browse11/lm/en#/http%3a%2f%2fid.who.int%2ficd%2fentity%2f1128733473) are optional, although clinicians are strongly encouraged to use them.

A second difference between the two models is that the AMPD's Criterion B is a specific list of 25 personality trait facets organized into five domains (APA, 2013, pp. 779–781), which essentially are the five-factor model domains, with Psychoticism substituted for Openness. In contrast, the ICD-11 PD model describes five trait domains—the five-factor model domains minus Openness plus Anankastia—a trait domain reflecting perfectionism and a high need for control—plus a specific Borderline pattern based directly on the *DSM-IV* PD criteria.

Finally, as mentioned earlier, the AMPD is a hybrid model, providing criteria for six specific personality disorder diagnoses, using combinations of aspects of both Criterion A and Criterion B. "Individuals who have a pattern of impairment in personality functioning and maladaptive traits that matches one of the six defined personality disorders should be diagnosed with that personality disorder. … Individuals whose personality functioning or trait pattern is substantially different from that of any of the six specific personality disorders should be diagnosed with Personality Disorder-Trait Specified (PD-TS)" (APA, 2013, p. 771). However, a diagnosis of PD-TS can be based on *any* specific trait facet that fits within the five domains, even if it is not in the list of 25, which brings the discussion back around to psychopathy, (or psychopathic personality disorder, if you will), because it could be diagnosed using the AMPD model.[11] For example, it would not be difficult to argue that a PD-TS diagnosis should be given to individuals who (a) meet the AMPD's personality impairment criterion (e.g., have few to no clear life goals, have low empathy and generally poor interpersonal relationships), (b) do not evidence pathological levels of at least six of the seven traits that define Antisocial Personality Disorder in the AMPD (viz., manipulativeness, deceitfulness, callousness, hostility, risk taking, impulsivity, and irresponsibility), and (c) have a pathologically high level of risk taking (i.e., Fearlessness) and/or dominance (i.e., Social Influence), and/or a pathologically low level of N (i.e., Stress Immunity, such that, for example, they do not become concerned even in emergency situations when circumstances warrant concern); in other words, if they were high on FD, but not SCI.

In brief, individuals with personality impairment who have one or more prominent PPI traits that are typically, but not perhaps exclusively, associated with healthy adaptivity might be diagnosed with psychopathy per either the *DSM-5* Section II or III model. This is essentially the argument that Lilienfeld et al. (2012) made when they likened such an individual to Lykken's primary psychopath. On the other hand,

[11] Of course, it also could be diagnosed in *DSM-5*, Section II, using "Other Specified Personality Disorder" (APA, 2013, p. 684), but that is often deemed a "wastebasket category," whereas PD-TS is meant to be an important alternative to the other six specific PDs.

Miller and Lynam (2012) opined that one should be "cautious in concluding that individuals with high scores on PPI FD alone are psychopathic" (p. 321). Taking this statement literally, then, from the perspective of the AMPD or ICD-11, we agree entirely, because personality disorder cannot be diagnosed in these systems on the basis of "statistically abnormal" traits alone, that is, without evidence of personality impairment. This, in fact, is perhaps the primary reason that Livesley has argued throughout his career that (a) a clear definition of personality disorder is imperative and (b) the *DSM* system of diagnosing personality disorders on the basis of meeting a limited set of descriptors, many (but not all) of which are specific manifestations of personality traits, is quite inadequate (see Livesley et al., 1994, for a particularly cogent critique).

If, conversely, personality impairment is present, then a diagnosis should be considered. However, we think that the debate about relations of psychopathy with the component traits of FD goes even deeper and, at its core, is back to the more fundamental question of whether distinct entities within the broad domain of personality pathology to which one can give specific diagnostic labels actually exist at all. If there is no such entity that can be labeled psychopathy, then arguments about its core characteristics can be considered scientifically irrelevant or, perhaps to overstate the point a bit, at least are no more scientific than arguments about whether unicorns have horns or Santa Claus has a beard that is as white as snow.

We acknowledge that it is extremely easy to get pulled into debates about specific types of personality pathology. One need only glance at a few issues of the *Journal of Personality Disorders* or *Personality Disorders: Theory, Research, and Treatment* to see that belief in an entity called "Borderline Personality Disorder" is alive and well. Note that we use the term "belief" deliberately, because there is virtually no scientific evidence to support the view that Borderline Personality Disorder, or any other specific type of personality pathology, including psychopathy, exists as a discrete entity in nature.

To sum up our view, we will know that the field has matured when the use of diagnostic labels, other than as convenient heuristics, disappears entirely and is replaced with deeper understanding of how personality traits—which are themselves useful constructs rather than discrete entities in nature—and personality processes arise, and how they are maintained, disrupted, or developed over the course of individuals' lives.

We recognize that this chapter is a somewhat unusual contribution to a Festschrift in that it reads more like an empirical-research journal publication than a "traditional" chapter, but we would like to think that Scott would be pleased to see it included in volume intended to honor him, because it demonstrates how his work fits into—and can be influential in—the broader field of scientific psychology which was a particularly noteworthy hallmark of his research.

References

Allport, G. W. (1937). *Personality: A psychological interpretation*. Holt.

Allport, G. W. (1961). *Pattern and growth in personality*. Holt, Rhineholt, & Winston.

American Psychiatric Association. (2013). *Diagnostic and statistical manual of mental disorders* (5th ed.). Author.

Benning, S. D., Patrick, C. J., Hicks, B. M., Blonigen, D. M., & Krueger, R. F. (2003). Factor structure of the psychopathic personality inventory: Validity and implications for clinical assessment. *Psychological Assessment, 15*(3), 340–350.

Benning, S. D., Patrick, C. J., Blonigen, D. M., Hicks, B. M., & Iacono, W. G. (2005). Estimating facets of psychopathy from normal personality traits: A step toward community epidemiological investigations. *Assessment, 12*(1), 3–18.

Cantor, N. (1990). From thought to behavior: "Having" and "doing" in the study of personality and cognition. *American Psychologist, 45*, 735–750.

Clark, L. A. (1993). *Schedule for nonadaptive and adaptive personality*. University of Minnesota Press.

Clark, L. A. (2007). Assessment and diagnosis of personality disorder: Perennial issues and emerging conceptualization. *Annual Review of Psychology, 58*, 227–258.

Clark, L. A., & Watson, D. (1990). *General temperament survey* [Unpublished manuscript]. University of Iowa.

Clark, L. A., Simms, L. J., Wu, K. D., & Casillas, A. (Eds.). (2014). *Schedule for nonadaptive and adaptive personality-2nd edition: Manual for administration, scoring, and interpretation*. University of Minnesota Press.

Cleckley, H. (1941/1976). *The mask of sanity* (6th ed.). C.V. Mosby.

Costa, P. T., & McCrae, R. R. (1992). *NEO personality inventory – revised*. Sigma Assessment Systems.

Dindo, L., McDade-Montez, E., Sharma, L., Watson, D., & Clark, L. A. (2009). Development and initial validation of the Disinhibition Inventory (DIS-I): A multifaceted measure of disinhibition. *Assessment, 16*, 274–291.

Edens, J. F., Poythress, N. G., Lilienfeld, S. O., Patrick, C. J., & Test, A. (2008). Further evidence of the divergent correlates of the Psychopathic Personality Inventory factors: Prediction of institutional misconduct among male prisoners. *Psychological Assessment, 20*, 86–91.

Eysenck, H. J., & Eysenck, S. B. G. (1975). *Manual of the Eysenck personality questionnaire*. Hodder & Stoughton.

Eysenck, H. J., & Rachman, S. (1965). *The causes and cures of neurosis: An introduction to modern behaviour therapy based on learning theory and the principles of conditioning*. RR Knapp.

Hare, R. D. (1991). *Manual for the revised psychopathy checklist*. Multi-Health Systems.

Hare, R. D. (1998). Psychopathy, affect, and behavior. In D. J. Cooke, A. E. Forth, & R. D. Hare (Eds.), *Psychopathy: Theory, research, and implications for society* (pp. 105–137). Kluwer Academic Publishers.

Hare, R. D. (2003). *The Hare psychopathy checklist-revised*. Multi-Health Systems.

Harpur, T. J., Hare, R. D., & Hakstian, A. R. (1989). Two-factor conceptualization of psychopathy: Construct validity and assessment implications. *Psychological Assessment, 1*, 6–17.

Krueger, R. F. (2006). Perspectives on psychopathy: Toward an integration. In C. J. Patrick (Ed.), *Handbook of psychopathy* (pp. 193–204). Guilford.

Lilienfeld, S. O., & Andrews, B. P. (1996). Development and preliminary validation of a self-report measure of psychopathic personality traits in noncriminal populations. *Journal of Personality Assessment, 66*(3), 488–524.

Lilienfeld, S. O., Patrick, C. J., Benning, S. D., Berg, J., Sellbom, M., & Edens, J. F. (2012). The role of fearless dominance in psychopathy: Confusions, controversies, and clarifications. *Personality Disorders, Theory, Research, and Treatment, 3*(3), 327–340.

Lilienfeld, S. O., Watts, A. L., Francis Smith, S., Berg, J. M., & Latzman, R. D. (2015). Psychopathy deconstructed and reconstructed: Identifying and assembling the personality building blocks of Cleckley's chimera. *Journal of Personality, 83*(6), 593–610.

Livesley, W. J., & Jang, K. L. (2000). Toward an empirically based classification of personality disorder. *Journal of Personality Disorder, 14*, 137–151.

Livesley, W. J., & Jang, K. L. (2005). Differentiating normal, abnormal, and disordered personality. *European Journal of Personality, 19*, 257–268.

Livesley, W. J., Schroeder, M. L., Jackson, D. N., & Jang, K. L. (1994). Categorical distinctions in the study of personality disorder: Implications for classification. *Journal of Abnormal Psychology, 103*, 6–17.
Lynam, D. R., & Derefinko, K. J. (2006). Psychopathy and personality. In C. J. Patrick (Ed.), *Handbook of psychopathy* (pp. 133–155). Guilford.
Lynam, D. R., & Miller, J. D. (2012). Fearless dominance and psychopathy: A response to Lilienfeld et al. *Personality Disorders, Theory, Research, and Treatment, 3*, 341–353.
Mahon, N. E., Yarcheski, T. J., & Yarcheski, A. (2002). The revised Personal Lifestyle Questionnaire for early adolescents. *Western Journal of Nursing Research, 25*, 533–547.
Marcus, D. K., Fulton, J. J., & Edens, J. F. (2013). The two-factor model of psychopathic personality: Evidence from the Psychopathic Personality Inventory. *Personality Disorders, Theory, Research, and Treatment, 4*, 67–76.
Miller, J. D., & Lynam, D. R. (2012). An examination of the Psychopathic Personality Inventory's nomological network: A meta-analytic review. *Personality Disorders, Theory, Research, and Treatment, 3*, 305–326.
Muhlenkamp, A. F., & Brown, N. J. (1983). *The development of an instrument to measure health practices*. Paper presented at the American Nurses Association Council of Nurse Researchers Conference.
Neumann, C. S., Malterer, M. B., & Newman, J. P. (2008). Factor structure of the Psychopathic Personality Inventory (PPI): Findings from a large incarcerated sample. *Psychological Assessment, 20*, 169–174.
Patrick, C. J. (2010). Conceptualizing the psychopathic personality: Disinhibited, bold,… Or just plain mean? In R. T. Salekin & D. R. Lynam (Eds.), *Handbook of child adolescent psychopathy* (pp. 15–48). Guilford Press.
Patrick, C. J., Edens, J. F., Poythress, N. G., Lilienfeld, S. O., & Benning, S. D. (2006). Construct validity of the psychopathic personality inventory two-factor model with offenders. *Psychological Assessment, 18*(2), 204–208.
Plutchik, R. (1980). A general psychoevolutionary theory of emotion. In R. Plutchik & H. Kellerman (Eds.), *Emotion: Theory, research and experience* (pp. 3–33). Academic Press.
Sellbom, M., & Phillips, T. R. (2013). An examination of the triarchic conceptualization of psychopathy in incarcerated and nonincarcerated samples. *Journal of Abnormal Psychology, 122*, 208–214.
Tellegen, A., & Waller, N. G. (2008). Exploring personality through test construction: Development of the Multidimensional Personality Questionnaire. In G. J. Boyle, G. Matthews, & D. H. Saklofske (Eds.), *The SAGE handbook of personality theory and assessment, vol 2: Personality measurement and testing* (pp. 261–292). Sage.
Watson, D., & Clark, L. A. (1994). Introduction to the Special Issue on personality and psychopathology. *Journal of Abnormal Psychology, 103*(1), 3.
Watson, D., Clark, L. A., & Harkness, A. R. (1994). Structures of personality and their relevance to psychopathology. *Journal of Abnormal Psychology, 103*, 18–31.
Widiger, T. A. (1998). Psychopathy and normal personality. In D. J. Cooke, A. E. Forth, & R. D. Hare (Eds.), *Psychopathy: Theory, research, and implications for society* (pp. 47–68). Kluwer Academic Publishers.
Widiger, T. A., & Simonsen, E. (2005). Alternative dimensional models of personality disorder: Finding a common ground. *Journal of Personality Disorders, 19*(2), 110–130.
World Health Organization. (1949). *International statistical classification of diseases, injuries, and causes of death, 6th revision*. Author.
World Health Organization. (1992). *International statistical classification of diseases and related health problems, 10th revision*. Author.

Part IV
Psychotherapy: Critical Issues and New Directions

Clinical Practice Guidelines: When Efficacy Is Not Enough: An Essay in the Honor of Scott O. Lilienfeld

Steven D. Hollon

Introduction

I first met Scott Lilienfeld when he was a graduate student at the University of Minnesota back in the Fall of 1980. Scott had a strong interest in understanding psychopathy and pseudoscience and came to Minnesota to work with David Lykken who was the leading expert with respect to each. I had my own history with Lykken, who had resigned from the department when I was hired. It was nothing personal; he resigned because the department refused to interview his advisee Bill Iacono (a far superior candidate) so as to not become too "inbred"—a very strange position for a faculty to take that was comprised of Lykken, Meehl, Tellegen, Gottesman, and Berscheid, all trained at Minnesota. I had an open hour on my schedule and, unaware that he had resigned in protest over my being invited, I crossed campus to drop in uninvited at his office in psychiatry research. We had a lovely chat about the uses and abuses of the polygraph (I was doing a physiological dissertation in which I was trying to deconfound prediction and control—which cannot be done) and eight years later when I left for Vanderbilt, Lykken and Auke Tellegen took me out for a farewell lunch.

Scott was one of the brightest people that I have ever met and one of the most iconoclastic. He was a perfect match to Lykken, both in interests and intellect, and one of the most interesting students I have ever taught (I did the course on behavior therapy in those days, and Scott wanted to know not just how things were done and if they worked but how they worked and how we knew). Minnesota was the home of "dust bowl" empiricism and perhaps the premier individual differences program of its day. The graduate students had the benefit of taking courses on philosophy of science with Meehl and personality with Tellegen, among other superb and

S. D. Hollon (✉)
Department of Psychology, Vanderbilt University, Nashville, TN, USA
e-mail: steven.d.hollon@vanderbilt.edu

C. L. Cobb et al. (eds.), *Toward a Science of Clinical Psychology*,
https://doi.org/10.1007/978-3-031-14332-8_13

thought-evoking offerings. Scott soaked up the wisdom of the faculty like a sponge, but he was never an easy "sell." He challenged conventional wisdom and could "smell" opinions not wholly based on fact. Like the best students, he pushed the faculty as hard as they pushed him, and it was clear that he was destined for greater things.

Clinical Practice Guidelines and Empirically Supported Treatments

I lost track of Scott after we left Minnesota in 1985 for Vanderbilt (my partner Judy Garber finished her doctorate with Paul Meehl, and it was time for her to go on the academic job market), but he resurfaced again in my professional life about a quarter century later when I served as the Chair of the steering committee advising the American Psychological Association (APA) on the generation of clinical practice guidelines (CPGs). I want to pick the story up from the point Scott and I intersected once again to illustrate what a profound effect he had on both me and the larger field, but first there is some needed background.

Empirically Supported Treatments

In the late 1990s my long-time friend and colleague Dianne Chambless invited me to join her on the lead article in a special issue in the *Journal of Consulting and Clinical Psychology* (*JCCP*) defining empirically supported therapies (ESTs; Chambless & Hollon, 1998). Dianne and I had gotten to know each other when we were doing internships at different institutions in Philadelphia. Don Klein, the pharmacological theorist who first separated panic from the other anxiety disorders (since it showed a specific response to antidepressant medications and an episodic course), would come to town periodically to visit Aaron (Tim) Beck, and Tim would invite Dianne and me to join for lunch and extended conversations. Dianne had done one of the original theoretical conceptualizations of agoraphobia and panic disorder (what she considered to be a "fear of fear"; Goldstein & Chambless, 1978). She and Klein carried on a spirited debate as to whether panic was psychological or biological in nature, and I did the same with respect to depression. Tim smiled on as he moderated.

Dianne and I went our separate ways (she to the University of Georgia and then American University and me to the University of Minnesota and then Vanderbilt) before we reconnected on the National Institute of Mental Health (NIMH) Psychosocial and Biobehavioral Treatments Subcommittee of the Treatment Development and Assessment Research Review Committee. In those days, serving on a NIMH review committee was like taking part in a high-powered seminar.

Grants were fewer in number, and each got at least an hour's discussion. I learned a lot from Dianne and other committee members like Ellen Frank, Marsha Linehan, and Jan Fawcett. Virtually all the grants that we reviewed focused on randomized controlled trials that tested the efficacy of different psychosocial interventions and debates over the methods involved were intense.

The 1990s saw an effort by Division 12 of APA to identify a set of empirically supported treatments (ESTs) that could be said to be efficacious in the treatment of a variety of psychological disorders, and Dianne was tapped to lead the effort (Task Force on Promotion and Dissemination of Psychological Procedures, 1995; Chambless et al., 1996). The criterion the Task Force adopted paralleled those used by the Food and Drug Administration (FDA) to determine whether a medication could go to market; all that was required was two or more positive trials (significant differences relative to some other treatment or control condition). These seemed to me to be a reasonable (and if somewhat minimal) criteria but listing of treatments that met that standard created quite a firestorm, since most of the treatments that did were cognitive or behavioral in nature. Advocates of more traditional dynamic and humanistic psychotherapies were unnerved at the prospect that their interventions would have to be subjected to empirical disconfirmation to prove their worth, even though it was Rogers and his humanistic colleagues who did some of the first randomized controlled trials to test the efficacy of psychotherapy (Rogers & Dymond, 1954). When Dianne was invited to chair the special issue for *JCCP*, she invited me to join her on a lead article that would lay out the criteria for the specific reviews to follow, along with a justification for what we chose and why we did.

The Empire Strikes Back

It was about that time that I started serving on APA committees that addressed issues relevant to how treatments were evaluated. The first should have been a non-controversial effort to develop criteria for evaluating treatment guidelines developed by third-party payers for the purpose of denying legitimate claims for service; what the companies did was to sell one set of guidelines to their corporate payers and use a second covert set to deny promised coverage [American Psychological Association (APA), 2002]. That project should not have been controversial since we were protecting the public and the profession from what could only be considered fraud on the part of the insurance industry, but even the notion of going to the experimental literature raised the hackles of advocates of the more traditional therapies. It took us less than two years to generate a template and more than eight years to get it passed by APA Council.

My second involvement with APA was on a presidential task force ostensibly empaneled to broaden the criteria by which treatments were evaluated to address the concerns of advocates of the more traditional psychotherapies but was intended instead to undercut the reliance on outcome data from randomized controlled trials [APA Presidential Task Force on Evidence Based Practice (EBP), 2006]. After much debate and considerable verbal fireworks, we adopted a tripartite model in which the best empirical data would be leavened with clinical expertise and patient preferences to identify the optimal treatment for a given individual. While I very much believe that patients have a right to the treatment of their choice, I do think that at least there should be an informed choice with the clinician obligated to lay out the pros and cons of the available alternatives for the patient to choose among. We have a "doors" problem in this country such that patients often get the treatment preferred by the therapist they happen to see, not the treatment that might be best for them or the one they would prefer. If a patient comes to me who would do better with a treatment I cannot provide, I think it is my obligation to inform the patient and offer the optimal referral. Clinical expertise (my preference) should not be allowed to trump the empirical literature in terms of what I recommend. Some types of information are just more valuable than others (there is a hierarchy of informative designs with randomized controlled trials at the top), and we were able to hold the line against those who wanted to give equal weight to clinical expertise.

Clinical Practice Guidelines

In 2010, I was invited to chair the Advisory Steering Committee (ASC) that the APA commissioned to come up with a plan for generating clinical practice guidelines (CPGs). The move to generate guidelines was not without controversy; a large segment of the governing Council viewed it as a "backdoor" attempt to put imprimatur of the organization on the mostly cognitive and behavioral ESTs and opposed any efforts to rely on anything other than clinical judgment to evaluate the efficacy of treatments. However, the proportion of nonpsychotic patients (most people treated for mental health issues) treated with psychotherapy had declined sharply in the two decades since the introduction of the selective serotonin reuptake inhibitors (SSRIs) largely because they were safe enough for primary care physicians to prescribe (Marcus & Olfson, 2007). The leadership of APA (successive elected presidents and some of the more prescient members of Council) recognized that this was neither good for the public nor the profession and pressed ahead with a plan for APA to develop its own CPGs as a counter.

The original ASC was comprised of nine members drawn from a range of different theoretical orientations and employments including research academicians and practicing clinicians. Internal divisions were not so great as in my earlier APA committee experiences, and we became a harmonious group that moved in a relatively rapid fashion to formulate a plan for generating CPGs. We were aided greatly by two outside influences. I had gotten to know Steve Pilling at the University of London who oversaw the psychotherapy side of the National Institute of Clinical and Health Evaluation (NICE) for the National Health Service (NHS) in the United Kingdom (UK) and had the opportunity to sit in as an observer at one of the meetings of their guideline panel on depression. The experience was truly revelatory to me as I watched a multidisciplinary group of scientists and practitioners (including nonprofessional with "lived experience") evaluate the existing empirical evidence in a manner that was leavened with clinical judgment and patient preference. At my request we invited Professor Pilling to fly to Washington to meet with the ASC to lay out what they did in NICE and why they did it in that fashion, which he did much to our edification.

The other seminal event that helped us move our process along was the publication of a pair of "how to" manuals by the Institute of Medicine (IOM), now the National Academy of Medicine, that provided guidelines for conducting systematic reviews (IOM, 2011a) and processing the resultant information through a multidisciplinary panel balanced with respect to theoretical orientation and profession (IOM, 2011b). What the IOM summarized were emerging "best practices" with respect to generating CPGs, largely consistent with practices already adopted by NICE, that held across the entirety of medicine and mental health.

The ASC largely bought into these recommendations although with some misgivings on the part of some members. One concern was that we were "buying into" the medical model since practicing clinicians often equate controlled research with pharmacotherapy. Most of the practices employed in pharmacological research were developed by research psychologists in response to the need to evaluate the effectiveness of educational programs (Fiske et al., 1970). Little new effort gets expended without a reason, and it was Eysenck's critique of the effectiveness of psychotherapy that got the process started with respect to treatment research (Eysenck, 1953). In brief, what Eysenck did was to take existing third-party payer records and compared outcomes for those "on the dole" for mental health issues who did versus did not pursue psychotherapy and found no difference between the groups. The article set off a firestorm of responses in the form of randomized controlled trials (RCTs), with some of the leading humanistic psychotherapists in the lead (Rogers & Dymond, 1954). These early trials were somewhat primitive by modern standards, but they did involve true experiments in which patients were randomized to conditions and outcomes compared at some future time. It would be nearly a decade before psychiatry caught up methodologically with the use of placebo-controlled trials and then only in response to pressure from the FDA to generate evidence of efficacy and safety to bring a novel medication to market. The subsequent quarter century of research clearly showed that psychotherapy works better than its absence, albeit for reasons still open to debate (Luborsky et al., 1975). I am always bemused when I hear my colleagues rail against adopting a "medical model" in evaluating treatment efficacy since the methods essentially came from us.

Another concern was that randomized controlled trials tended to "cherry pick" easy patients who were not representative of the complexities often encountered in clinical practice. This is one of the core issues raised with respect to the distinction between efficacy trials (done under carefully controlled conditions with diagnostically "clean" patients) versus effectiveness trials (done under real-world conditions with the kinds of diagnostically "messy" seen in actual clinical practice). Although that may have been the case in the early days of outcome research, it is clearly not the case any longer, and the kinds of patients treated in RCTs are representative of the kinds of patients treated in everyday applied clinical settings (Stirman et al., 2005).

What the ASC came up with was a tripartite definition of clinical outcomes based on the nature of the comparison in the trial (Hollon et al., 2014). In brief, a treatment can be *efficacious* if it works better than its absence, *specific* if it exceeds the generic benefits of simply going into treatment (expectation of change and contact with a therapist), and *superior* if it exceeds another specific intervention (Mohr et al., 2009). Different types of control conditions are required for each: (1) some type of no or minimal treatment condition is sufficient to establish efficacy (although these are surprisingly difficult to implement in an ethical fashion); (2) some type of non-specific control like a pill-placebo (PLA) or generic supportive psychotherapy is necessary to establish specificity; and (3) some other specific intervention is required to establish superiority. The three types of outcomes are like Russian-nesting dolls; if you establish superiority, you perforce establish specificity; and if you establish specificity, you perforce establish efficacy, unless the comparator has a negative nocebo effect as can be the case for some "wait list" controls (Furukawa et al., 2014).

No one nowadays would generate a CPG without first conducting a systematic review summarized via meta-analyses, but no one generating a CPG would simply add text to the summary indices generated by those meta-analyses. Instead, they would bring together a multidisciplinary guideline panel comprised of members with different theoretical perspectives to review the results, as the IOM recommends and NICE implements. CPGs bring judgment back into the process and use the principle of adversarial collaboration from cognitive psychology in which biases are not so much eliminated (since they often cannot be) as balanced to be offsetting (Mellers et al., 2001). It is important to remember that meta-analyses are simply summaries of the empirical data in a literature and not necessarily directly interpretable in and of themselves. The quality of treatment implementation varies across studies as does the rigor of the controls and most quantitative analyses do not adequately capture that variation across trials. In any literature, there are often *"silver bullet" studies* in which internal validity is preserved, the comparison condition(s) stringent, and the samples wholly representative. If, for example, a particular type of psychotherapy can hold its own with antidepressant medications in a trial in which both are superior to PLA in a clinical sample, that speaks to the efficacy and specificity of both interventions (see for example DeRubeis et al., 2005 or Dimidjian et al., 2006, for placebo-controlled comparisons of cognitive therapy and behavioral activation respectively to antidepressant medications). The data are critical and something that we always want to see, but the data do not interpret themselves, and this is where experience and judgment rule the day.

Theoretical Plausibility Enters Consideration

This is where Scott reenters the tale. Scott was not a treatment researcher per se, but he is widely considered the foremost authority on pseudoscience in psychology (see for example Lilienfeld, 2011 or Lilienfeld et al., 2003). Scott defined pseudoscientific practices as those that "possess the superficial appearance of science but lack its substance" (Lilienfeld & Landfield, 2008, p. 1216; see also Lilienfeld, 1998). Pseudoscientific practices lack adequate empirical support to back up their extravagant claims, and their claims are frequently extravagant. He went on to note that pseudoscientific practices are neither necessarily entirely invalid or ineffective nor that those who promote them are necessarily charlatans (many believe if the efficacy of their interventions), but the assertions associated with these practices greatly outstrip the quality of the available scientific evidence (Lilienfeld et al., 2012).

What Scott argued most persuasively (I think) is that it is not sufficient for a treatment to be efficacious (better than its absence) to be recommended in a CPG, it also is necessary that its underlying theoretical rationale be plausible. In essence, he argued for the *theoretical plausibility* of the model on which the treatment was based. Numerous examples abound in psychology (and in medicine) of instances in which an intervention worked for largely nonspecific reasons (hope and expectation) that was based on a theory that was not supported by the best available science of the day and often so clearly wrong as to be implausible. Mesmer had a treatment that worked but that posited the existence of invisible force fields (animal magnetism) that could be manipulated by the laying on of hands. No such invisible force fields exist (although we did not know that at the time), and the success of his approach was better explained by the notion of suggestion that in later decades formed the basis for hypnosis and even later still psychoanalysis. If we do not know enough to know that an explanatory theory is clearly inconsistent with the known principles of science, then it is simply prescientific; but if we know that the theory underlying a particular intervention could not possibly be true, then we are dealing with pseudoscience. A century ago, Harry Houdini (the great magician) and Sir Arthur Conan Doyle (the creator of Sherlock Holmes) set out find the truth behind spiritualism, Houdini to expose charlatans (and naive "true believers") in their midst and Conan Doyle to prove that the supernatural did in fact exist. Scott was the modern-day descendant of Houdini exposing pseudoscience in psychology from assessment to treatment.

The various energy field therapies for trauma represent perhaps the most egregious example of pseudoscience in the current psychotherapy literature. These interventions work (they are better than their absence) but likely for largely nonspecific reasons. They also are popular with the practicing professionals and the public, in large part because they promise quick relief in an almost "magical" fashion (flirting with the supernatural is endemic). The theory on which they are based is clearly specious; there are no "auras" emanating from people who have been the victims of trauma (or anyone else) and the "laying on of hands" or other presumptive manipulations of these purported fields cannot possibly be the reason why these treatments "work." Scott quite reasonably took me to task for allowing pseudoscience in through the "back door" by not including theoretical plausibility as a criterion that must be met, and I appreciate the correction that he offered. The ASC has learned from my failing and now incorporates *theoretical plausibility* as a necessary criterion that a treatment must meet to be recommended in a guideline. This is a change for the better and attributable to Scott.

Scott believed that it is not only important to consider theoretical plausibility, but it is also important to identify scientifically supported mechanisms that mediate or moderate treatment effects, as others have pointed out (Rosen & Davison, 2003; David et al., 2018; David & Montgomery, 2011). Scott had interesting things to say about this in relation to plausibility and harmful interventions (Lilienfeld, 2011).

Treatments That Cause Harm

I reconnected with Scott in the early years of this century when Sona Dimidjian and I were asked to do an article for the *American Psychologist* that picked up on his classic treatise on treatments that do harm (Lilienfeld, 2007). The first question that we had for the editors who contacted us was why they had not simply approached Scott to update his earlier article and, although we never got a clear answer, it was apparent to us that they considered his views too radical for a mainstream psychological audience. We called Scott in Atlanta discuss the matter with him, and he was not surprised and a little bit bemused. He well understood that he was considered something of a "gadfly" by mainstream psychology and that he was unlikely to be approached by APA to do an update for their flagship journal. We talked it over with him at some length and decided to go forward only when he encouraged us to do so (Dimidjian & Hollon, 2010). We are proud of the article we produced but consider it more scholarly and temperate than the excesses and abuses that Scott described (who knew that people had suffocated going through "rebirthing therapy" before Scott did his expose).

Not everyone responds to treatment and some patients do get worse, but deterioration is mercifully minimal in most mainstream therapies. For example, only 5–7% of patients deteriorated in treatment (end of treatment scores higher than when they started), and only 1% showed reliable deterioration (end-point scores a standard deviation higher than when they started) in a large individual patient meta-analysis of over 1700 patients randomized to either cognitive behavior therapy or medication treatment for depression (Vittengl et al., 2016). Such findings with respect to mainstream treatments are somewhat reassuring but may give a false sense of security. Psychotherapy treatment studies often fail to report negative outcomes at the level of the individual patient level (industry-funded trials are required to do so by the FDA), but the ASC has learned to scour the published literature for such events and to track them down with personal communications to the authors when no such reporting can be found. We have long done a better job of reporting severe adverse effects in trials comparing psychotherapy to medication (because it is standard practice in the latter), but it is only now becoming standard in psychotherapy trials in large part because of the advent of the CPGs. This too reflects Scott's impact on the field, and the field is much the better for it.

Pseudoscience in Continuing Education

Scott was twice elected president of the Society for the Science of Clinical Psychology (SSCP), the only person to serve two terms. In 2016, I joined Scott (as incoming president for his second term) and Mitch Prinstein (the outgoing president) in meeting with Cynthia Belar, Ph.D, the chief executive officer of the APA at the time, and Antoinette (Toni) Minniti, who oversees the Office of CE Sponsor Approval (CESA), to discuss the issue of credits being given for pseudoscience offerings. What we found was that Drs. Belar and Minniti shared our concerns about the things that were being offered (in addition to numerous pseudoscience offerings on treatments like "energy field" therapy, there was even one offering on how to conduct exorcisms) and were as committed as we were to actively promoting science and maintaining the scientific integrity of the courses that were offered for CE credits (Hollon, 2016).

What they lacked at that time were the resources to screen the large number of potential programs offered with the degree of scientific rigor in the over 800 proposals that they receive a year. Moreover, APA does not accredit specific programs. Rather they accredit sponsors who propose multiple programs in any given year, not all intended for psychologists. Some egregious courses could well slip through, especially if they are ectoplasmic. Toni reminded us that there is a formal complaint process and encouraged members of SSCP to get active in reporting specific programs that seemed to fall outside the bounds or settled science (Minniti, 2016). We have followed up on her suggestion and filed complaints against some of the more egregious offerings. That and an increment in staffing has also helped to some extent.

The greater problem is that some advocates of pseudoscience offerings are litigious. If their offerings are disallowed, they are ready and able to bring suit against the APA to force their inclusion. CESA can disallow the more egregious offerings (exorcism is out) but not those interventions that have some empirical base. Dozens of RCTs attest to the efficacy of energy field therapy (mostly comparisons against its absence that should yield positive results for largely nonspecific reasons) and even a journal to publish such outlandish pseudoscientific claims. If APA tries to prevent such workshops from being presented it likely will be sued and, in a society that believes that the position of the stars at the time of birth predicts personality, the outcomes of such lawsuits could be dire.

There is a potential solution and that lies with the CPGs. Lyn Bufka, the APA staffer who has been the prime mover behind the guideline process for over two decades, brought a lawyer from APA's legal department to meet with members of SSCP and interested parties at the annual convention in San Francisco in 2018. What the lawyer told us (my apologies but I cannot remember her name) was that APA could not single out specific interventions for exclusion without risk of lawsuit unless they had been evaluated along with other more reasonable interventions and found wanting by a duly impaneled group. In effect, if the clinical guideline process adopted *theoretical plausibility* as a criterion that must be met to recommend a treatment and ruled that the pseudoscience offerings did not, then APA could justify excluding such offerings from CE credits. What we could not do was to rule them out in an arbitrary fashion, but we could subject them to the same criteria that other treatments had to meet, and if they were found wanting (as they certainly would), then we could exclude them.

The ASC has subsequently adopted *theoretical plausibility* as a necessary criterion that any intervention must meet in order to be recommended in a guideline. I had initially resisted his entreaties because of my ambivalence about Eye Movement Desensitization and Reprocessing (EMDR). The theory was clearly specious but not implausible and, from my perspective, anything that increased the likelihood that traditional clinicians would be comfortable enough to encourage their patients to relive their trauma represented an advance. That said, Scott brought me around and the others who have taken my place on the ASC and we now consider theoretical plausibility as a necessary criterion.

Summary and Conclusions

Scott Lilienfeld was an iconoclast who did more to rid the field of pseudoscientific thinking than anyone else of his generation. Other chapters in this text attest to his impact on psychopathology and assessment, but he also had a profound effect on treatment and what we are willing to accept as a field. He elevated the notion of *theoretical plausibility* to a status comparable to efficacy when evaluating the suitability of treatments. It is not enough that a treatment can be shown to work (relative to its absence), but it also must be based on a theory that is plausible give current scientific standards. Charlatans and hucksters (and their often well-intended fellow travelers) offer treatments that often appear too good to true and all too often that is the case. Scott was not a treatment researcher, but no one in his generation had a greater impact on how we evaluate treatments. Lykken and Meehl would be proud.

References

American Psychological Association (APA). (2002). Criteria for evaluating treatment guidelines. *American Psychologist, 57*, 1052–1059.

APA Presidential Task Force on Evidence Based Practice (EBP). (2006). Evidence-based practice in psychology. *American Psychologist, 61(4)*, 271–285.

Chambless, D. L., & Hollon, S. D. (1998). Defining empirically supported therapies. *Journal of Consulting and Clinical Psychology, 66*, 7–18.

Chambless, D. L., Sanderson, W. C., Shoham, V., Bennett Johnson, S., Pope, K. S., Crits-Christoph, P., Baker, M., Johnson, B., Woody, S. R., Sue, S., Beutler, L., Williams, D. A., & McCurry, S. (1996). An updated on empirically validated therapies. *Clinical Psychologist, 49*, 5–18.

David, D., & Montgomery, G. H. (2011). The scientific status of psychotherapies: A new evaluative framework for evidence-based psychosocial interventions. *Clinical Psychology: Science and Practice, 18*, 89–98.

David, D., Lynn, S. J., & Montgomery, G. (2018). *Evidence based psychotherapy: The state of the science and practice*. Wiley.
Dimidjian, S., & Hollon, S. D. (2010). How would you know if psychotherapy was harmful? *American Psychologist, 65*, 21–33.
DeRubeis, R. J., Hollon, S. D., Amsterdam, J. D., Shelton, R. C., Young, P. R., Salomon, R. M., O'Reardon, J. P., Lovett, M. L., Gladis, M. M., Brown, L. L., & Gallop, R. (2005). Cognitive therapy vs. medications in the treatment of moderate to severe depression. *Archives of General Psychiatry, 62*, 409–416. https://doi.org/10.1001/archpsyc.62.4.409
Dimidjian, S., Hollon, S. D., Dobson, K. S., Schmaling, K. B., Kohlenberg, R. J., Addis, M. E., Gallop, R., McGlinchey, J. B., Markley, D. K., Gollan, J. K., Atkins, D. C., Dunner, D. L., & Jacobson, N. S. (2006). Behavioral activation, cognitive therapy, and antidepressant medication in the acute treatment of major depression. *Journal of Consulting and Clinical Psychology, 74*, 658–670. https://doi.org/10.1037/0022-006X.74.4.658
Eysenck, H. J. (1953). The effects of psychotherapy. *Journal of Counselling Psychology, 16*, 319–324.
Fiske, D. W., Hunt, H., Luborsky, L., Orne, M. T., Parloff, M. G., Reiser, M. F., & Tuma, A. H. (1970). The planning of research on effectiveness of psychotherapy. *Archives of General Psychiatry, 22*, 22–32.
Furukawa, T. A., Noma, H., Caldwell, D. M., Honyashiki, M., Shinohara, K., Imai, H., Chen, P., Hunot, V., & Churchill, R. (2014). Waiting list may be a nocebo condition in psychotherapy trials: A contribution from network meta-analysis. *Acta Psychiatrica Scandinavia, 130*, 181–192. https://doi.org/10.1111/acps.12275
Goldstein, A. J., & Chambless, D. L. (1978). A reanalysis of agoraphobia. *Behavior Therapy, 9*, 47–59.
Hollon, S. D. (2016). Exorcizing the demons that plague continuing education (CE). *Clinical Science, 19(3)*, 2–4.
Hollon, S. D., Areán, P. A., Craske, M. G., Crawford, K. A., Kivlahan, D. R., Magnavita, J. J., Ollendick, T. H., Sexton, T. L., Spring, B., Bufka, L. F., Galper, D. G., & Kurtzman, H. (2014). Development of clinical practice guidelines. *Annual Review of Clinical Psychology, 10*, 213–241.
Institute of Medicine (IOM). (2011a). *Finding what works in health care: Standards for systematic reviews*. National Academy Press.
Institute of Medicine (IOM). (2011b). *Clinical practice guidelines we can trust*. National Academy Press.
Lilienfeld, S. O. (1998). Pseudoscience in contemporary clinical psychology: What it is and what we can do about it. *The Clinical Psychologist, 51*, 3–9.
Lilienfeld, S. O. (2007). Psychological treatments that cause harm. *Perspectives on Psychological Science, 2*, 53–70.
Lilienfeld, S. O. (2011). Distinguishing scientific from pseudoscientific psychotherapies: Evaluating the role of theoretical plausibility, with a little help from Reverend Bayes. *Clinical Psychology: Science and Practice, 18*, 105–112. https://doi.org/10.1111/j.1468.2850.2011.01241.x
Lilienfeld, S. O., & Landfield, K. (2008). Science and pseudoscience in law enforcement: A user-friendly primer. *Criminal Justice and Behavior, 35*, 1215–1230.
Lilienfeld, S. O., Lynn, S. J., & Lohr, J. M. (Eds.). (2003). *Science and pseudoscience in clinical psychology*. Guilford Press.
Lilienfeld, S. O., Ammirati, R., & David, M. (2012). Distinguishing science from pseudoscience in school psychology: Science and scientific thinking as safeguards against human error. *Journal of School Psychology, 50*, 7–36. https://doi.org/10.1016/j.jsp.2011.09.006
Luborsky, L., Singer, B., & Luborsky, L. (1975). Comparative studies of psychotherapies: Is it true that "Everyone has won and all must have prizes". *Archives of General Psychiatry, 32*, 995–1008.

Marcus, S. C., & Olfson, M. (2007). National trends in the treatment for depression from 1998 to 2007. *Archives of General Psychiatry, 67(12)*, 1265–1273. https://doi.org/10.1001/archgenpsychiatry.2010.151
Mellers, B., Hertwig, R., & Kahneman, D. (2001). Do frequency representations eliminate conjunction effects? An exercise in adversarial collaboration. *Psychological Science, 12(4)*, 269–275.
Minniti, A. (2016). Comment on quality continuing education. *Clinical Science, 19(3)*, 2–4.
Mohr, D. C., Spring, B., Freedland, K. E., Beckner, V., Areán, P., Hollon, S. D., Ockene, J., & Kaplan, R. (2009). The selection and design of control conditions for randomized controlled trial of psychological interventions. *Psychotherapy and Psychosomatics, 78*, 275–284.
Rogers, C. R., & Dymond, R. (1954). *Psychotherapy and personality change.* University of Chicago Press.
Rosen, G. M., & Davison, G. C. (2003). Psychology should list empirically supported principles of change (ESPs) and not credential trademark therapies or other treatment packages. *Behavior Modification, 27*(3), 300–312. https://doi.org/10.1177/0145445503027003003
Stirman, S. W., DeRubeis, R. J., Crits-Christoph, P., & Rothman, A. (2005). Can the randomized controlled trial literature generalize to non-randomized patients? *Journal of Consulting and Clinical Psychology, 73*, 127–135.
Task Force on Promotion and Dissemination of Psychological Procedures. (1995). Training in and dissemination of empirically-validated psychological treatments: Report and recommendations. *Clinical Psychologist, 48*, 3–23.
Vittengl, J. R., Jarrett, R. B., Weitz, E., Hollon, S. D., Twisk, J., Cristea, I., David, D., DeRubeis, R. J., Dimidjian, S., Dunlop, B. W., Faramarzi, M., Hegerl, U., Kennedy, S. H., Kheirkhah, F., Mergl, R., Miranda, J., Mohr, D. C., Rush, A. J., Segal, Z. V., Siddique, J., Simons, A. D., & Cuijpers, P. (2016). Divergent outcomes in cognitive behavioral therapy and pharmacotherapy for adult depression. *American Journal of Psychiatry, 173(5)*, 481–490.

New Perspectives in Cognitive Theory and Therapy

Aaron T. Beck, Molly R. Finkel, Aaron P. Brinen, and Scott H. Waltman

Case Example: P.J.

P.J. is a third-year graduate student at a large research university where he plans to obtain his Ph.D. in Chemistry. P.J. could be described as a mild-mannered man who is ordinarily calm, peaceful, and passive. For the most part, P.J. seems eager to please his friends, family members, and professors; however, when he is provoked, his personality changes rapidly and drastically. In this altered personality state, he can become angry, verbally abusive, and is motivated to use physical force to express his aggression. On one occasion when P.J. "lost his cool," he began to shout at his neighbor who accidentally tossed a baseball in his driveway. On another occasion, he pushed his girlfriend during an argument. P.J. has described that he is a totally different person when he is in the angry state. We have found that individuals like P.J. experience a change of schematic activation (i.e., increased funneling of information through certain belief systems), which leads to a specific modal activation (i.e., increased prevalence of specific cognitions, affect, physiology, motivations, and compensatory behaviors) that accounts for his seemingly holistic change in personality. In contrast to his earlier mode, in which he wants to succeed and

A. T. Beck
Department of Psychiatry, Perelman School of Medicine, University of Pennsylvania, Philadelphia, PA, USA

M. R. Finkel (✉)
Ferkauf Graduate School of Psychology, Yeshiva University, New York, NY, USA
e-mail: mfinkel2@mail.yu.edu

A. P. Brinen
Department of Psychiatry and Behavioral Sciences, Vanderbilt University Medical Center, Nashville, TN, USA

S. H. Waltman
Pacific University, Forest Grove, Oregon, USA

C. L. Cobb et al. (eds.), *Toward a Science of Clinical Psychology*,
https://doi.org/10.1007/978-3-031-14332-8_14

affiliate closely with people, he changes in the second mode to perceiving the opposing individual as an adversary, an enemy, and somebody who he must defend himself against—which explains his change in presentation.

While analyzing this short example, an important question to consider is, "What model of personality and psychopathology could be applied to best understand P.J. as a whole person?"

From the perspective of the medical model, one might conceptualize P.J.'s angry states as being caused by irregularities in the biological processes related to impulse control, emotion regulation, etc. From a strictly psychosocial perspective, one might delve into environmental stressors, social and cultural factors, and individual cognitive-affective experiences that have led to his states of anger. While both models may be relevant and useful, we also note that a there are many other important theoretical components to flesh out (particularly to be included within the psychosocial model). Through discussing some of these components including adaptation/maladaptation (Beck & Haigh, 2014), levels of cognitive processing (Waltman & Sokol, 2017), the theory modes (Beck et al., 2020b), and evolutionarily based drives (Beck & Bredemeier, 2016), we can more comprehensively analyze the case of P.J., the transient behaviors of everyday life, and more holistically describe the formation of psychopathology.

The Cognitive Model and the Theory of Modes

The basic tenet of the Generic Cognitive Model is that the perception of a situation directly influences emotion, physiology, and behavior (Beck, 1963, 1964). The Generic Cognitive Model holds that situation-specific thoughts or automatic thoughts (i.e., "He always messes with me in the morning") are often brief and fleeting, take the form of a thought or image, and are regarded as true without reflection or evaluation. These automatic thoughts stem from an underlying belief system and influence how we feel and what we do. As cognitive therapy holds a robust tradition of research and scientific inquiry, cognitive theory and therapy have evolved over the years (Beck, 1963, 1964, 1979, 1996; Beck & Bredemeier, 2016; Beck et al., 2020a; Beck & Haigh, 2014; Clark & Beck, 1999; Waltman & Sokol, 2017). Consistent with the notion of Darwinian evolution, adaptations to the model have often resulted from new challenges or opportunities. An advance in the cognitive model is the inclusion of something called *modes* (Beck et al., 2020b; Beck, 1999; Beck & Haigh, 2014; Clark & Beck, 1999).

Modes were initially understood to be the activation of schema (a pattern of thought) and the associated coping/compensatory strategies. Modal activation describes a person's current emotional-cognitive-behavioral state (see Fassbinder et al., 2016). A few examples of modes are anger mode, depressed mode, and anxious mode. The concept of modes was first introduced in the schema therapy literature to account for rapid changes in the presentation of clients with borderline personality disorder. Schema therapists noted that when these individuals would become dysregulated, they would have extreme thinking patterns, high emotional activation, and engage in impulsive behaviors (see Fassbinder et al., 2016; Young, 1999). Alternatively, when these people were regulated, their thinking would not be extreme, their emotions were not elevated, and their behavior was not impulsive; these different presentations representing different modal states (Fassbinder et al., 2016). As the Generic Cognitive Model has been revised over the years, other modes have been identified (e.g., depressive mode; Beck & Haigh, 2014).

In previous writings on the Theory of Modes (Beck et al., 2020b), we defined a mode as either adaptive or maladaptive based on the relative fit between internal and external demands. Additionally, we stated that continued activation of particular maladaptive modes over a prolonged duration often denotes psychopathology. For example, the prolonged duration of needing certainty (internal demand) about the future (external demand) leading to persistent and immense worry and functional impairment may be defined as generalized anxiety. In our current discussion, we are extending this theory to consider adaptation, maladaptation, and psychopathology as existing on a continuum with evolutionary aspects in mind, this being consistent with the Generic Cognitive Model (see Beck & Haigh, 2014; Waltman & Sokol, 2017). Specifically, we suggest that due to changes in our internal and external environments, changes in our societal and cultural norms, shifts in how humans allocate internal cognitive resources, etc., functions that may have been adaptive in earlier phases of human evolution may now be labeled maladaptive, and even psychopathological (Nesse, 2019). More recently, our understanding of modes has expanded (see Beck et al., 2020b), as will be illustrated in the current chapter.

As described in the case example above, individuals' personalities can shift drastically and holistically depending on their fit with their environment at any given moment. These different personality states that become temporarily activated are labeled as modes. Examples of personality states that are modes include being angry, depressed, and paranoid. These modes are reflexive and when activated, become expressed even though the individual[1] may prefer not to express them. The operation of the mode follows a trajectory of processes as follows: activation of the relevant beliefs leads to cognitive conceptualization of the situation which leads to a combination of affect and motivation. If the mode is uninhibited (see Craske et al., 2014), it leads directly to behavior. These specific modes represent the state of personality at a given time.[2] As modes serve an evolutionary function of meeting situational demands, there is likely a biodiversity of modes (Beck & Haigh, 2014). We will review a sampling of these modes below with a method for categorization.

[1] The word "individual" is used throughout the chapter in most cases to refer to persons seeking or receiving mental health services.

[2] In the extreme form, for example in Dissociative Identity Disorder, the mode takes on a life of its own, detached from the rest of the personality (Lynn et al., 2006).

Personality as an Agent of Adaptation

Fundamental to our current theory of personality is the concept that the personality is the agent of adaptation. Ordinarily, individuals have the capacity to switch from one mode to another in order to attempt to find a fit between their endogenous internal components (demands, drives, goals, values, and desires, such as being connected to one's family or seeking employment) and the external situational factors (Beck & Bredemeier, 2016). The function of personality, therefore, is to provide the intangible aspects of the individual (thoughts, feelings, motivations, etc.) that allow the person to connect and adapt to the outside world. Optimally, there is a good fit between an individual's internal circumstance, drives, and desires (including cognitive, affective, motivational, and behavioral components) and the external situational demands. We would label this proper fit as *adaptation*. However, when this fit between the internal and external demands is poor, one could label this as *maladaptation*. An example of this type of maladaptation is P.J. becoming intensely angry at his neighbor who has thrown a ball onto his driveway. Here, P.J. has angry cognitions and a desire to be respected and a motivation to retaliate through verbal aggressiveness, and yet, the external situational factors would not necessarily warrant this level of reaction. Thus, there is a mis-fit between the internal and external demands. While this example is more interpersonal in nature, this dynamic of poor fit between internal and external demands is also evidenced in various forms of psychopathology.

Determining what is adaptive also might require a multidimensional, or intersectional lens. The adaptivity of a specific modal activation is dependent on context, and on an individual level there is a diversity of considerations including group and individual identities pertaining to age, gender identity, sexual orientation, ethnic and racial identity, acculturation, ability, religious identity, and other demographic factors, which can be dimensional considerations (see Hays & Iwamasa, 2006; Waltman, 2013). Further, an individual's modal response might vary in adaptiveness throughout the day as the concordance between modal expression and environmental demands might shift depending on setting and cultural contexts, this necessitating cross-cultural code-switching (see Molinsky, 2007). For example, a discussion about coworker with a spouse versus business partner may require a switch in delivery (e.g., tone, content, affective expression) based on a number of cultural factors (e.g., common vs. different identities, power differentials). Thus, psychological flexibility is broadly a marker for mental health and wellness (see Levin et al., 2012).

The presence of anxiety or some other signal of distress is not necessarily a sign of maladaptation. An adaptive response to an external or internal danger (e.g., a pain in the chest) may involve anxiety which is a signal of a threat (in this case, a threat of an organic disease causing the chest pain). Another example of an adaptive yet negative affective response would be the experience of grief and sadness after a breakup of a romantic relationship or death of a loved one. In both examples, we would call the responses adaptive because they are realistic and concordant to the stimulus situation. In cases of maladaptation, often symptoms of distress are present in a way that is discordant, disproportionate, or unrealistic (see Gellatly & Beck, 2016). As discussed below, a common goal of psychotherapy is to foster adaptation through the process of cognitive modification which can be achieved through a plurality of methods (Lorenzo-Luaces et al., 2015) including recovery-oriented processes (Beck et al., 2020a, b), interpersonal learning in a group setting (Yalom, 1995), corrective emotional experiences (Silberschatz, 2013), and the use of Socratic Dialogue (Waltman et al., 2020).

Cognition: Levels of Cognitive Processing and Cognitive Content Within a Mode

If we examine the case of P.J. once more, we can note that he is aware of the fact that he often exaggerates and/or misinterprets the degree of the offense. He does not take any time to step back from the situation to assess other perspectives than his own and does not employ coping strategies that could reduce his urge to become angry. In this angry mode, P.J.'s personality, which includes his cognitive, affective, motivational, and behavioral faculties, is largely being driven by an automatic, rapid, and reflexive stream of cognitive processing that uses minimal cognitive resources. This rapid processing stream may have originated early in human evolution due to its necessity in upholding the evolutionary drives (e.g., safety, reproduction). Individuals can change a maladaptive response to an adaptive response through the reflective apparatus (i.e., *superordinate processing domain*) which brings about cognitive modification resulting in changes to beliefs, affect, motivation, and behavior (see Lorenzo-Luaces et al., 2015). This apparatus is comprised of metacognitive processing such as problem solving, perspective taking, and adaptive coping. This critical reflective, superordinate stream of processing is consistently underutilized by P.J. in this angry state, thus, leading to a maladaptive fit with his environment. Importantly, the use of reflective oversight processing requires significant utilization of cognitive resources, which often individuals do not have access to in more extreme states of maladaptation (i.e., overactivation of the limbic system and corresponding emotional dysregulation).[3]

The cognitive content of the mode is largely determined by cognitive schemas, underlying sets of thoughts, expectancies, or generalizations categorized together based on prior experiences, social relationships, cultural norms, etc. (e.g., "others are threatening" is a schema). The cognitive schemas are relatively stable structures which serve to help guide and shape individuals' perceptions of events and to categorize these perceptions and pre-existing notions of the self, others, and the outside world (i.e., the cognitive triad); When activated, cognitive schemas generate

[3] The reflexive and reflective domains of processing are similar to the concept of fast and slow thinking coined by Daniel Kahneman (2011) (although the levels of cognitive processing described in the current formulation were inspired by earlier work by Beck on cognitive theory and therapy (Beck, 1964, 1979, etc.).

automatic thoughts (Beck, 1952) and automatic commands, that is, engaging in violent behavior or "acting out" (Beck & Haigh, 2014).

As stated above, maladaptive responses may occur when there is a poor fit between the mode and the total situation. The most common course of a poor fit is the presence of bias in the cognitive processing of the total situation (Beck, 1963, 1964). Individuals are "programmed" with certain biases embedded in the cognitive schemas (Beck & Haigh, 2014). Cognitive biases can be the answer to the question of what is involved when two individuals have different responses to the identical situation. Despite the same external stimulus, the individuals will draw on information from their previous experiences, present needs, drives, aspirations, and expectations in forming their unique reaction. Examples of cognitive biases include personalization, confirmatory bias, externalizing bias, among others. Here, one person's cognitive schema may create a more smooth, adaptive fit with the external stimulus and the corresponding mode that becomes activated would be labeled as adaptive.

These biases in processing are common in interpersonal situations, particularly in those situations involving close relationships. Generally, cognitive biases lead to well-known distortions such as selective abstraction, overgeneralization, and exaggeration (e.g., catastrophizing) and minimizing. Examples of the use of these biases include individuals who are particularly sensitive to any behavior that resembles a put down, such as seeing overprotective behavior as patronizing. Individuals also may exaggerate the significance of a sarcastic comment by a partner with the thought (emanating from a cognitive schema), "She doesn't respect me." Another common distortion, particularly among individuals who are medically orientated, would be, "My pain in the chest means I'm having a heart attack." Because cognition is the first personality domain to be activated in a given mode, cognitive biases often lead to the activation of entire maladaptive modes based on this biased framework.

In addition to the types of cognitive biases being determined by cognitive schemas, the schemas also impact two other aspects of the modes: the *degree of charge* and the *density* (see Beck et al., 2020b). The degree of charge depends to a large extent on the cognitive processing. When the cognitive processing is hyper-charged, then the mode is hyper-charged which carries over to the impulse, affect, and behavior. For example, cognitive schemas, which shape the automatic reflexive cognitive processing, can become overactivated in response to a stimulus danger, disadvantage, or defeat. This highly charged processing can then determine the corresponding emotional, motivational, and behavioral response. Similarly, when a schema has been drawn on consistently, it becomes structuralized and can reflect a "habitual" personality trait. This may lead to activation of modes with greater density. Modal density can impact the likelihood of the mood becoming activated, the period in which a mode is activated, as well as the difficulty in shifting from one mode to another.

All of psychopathology can be conceived of as the paradigm of the four building blocks: perception of gain, loss, threat, and offense. This paradigm is fitted into the

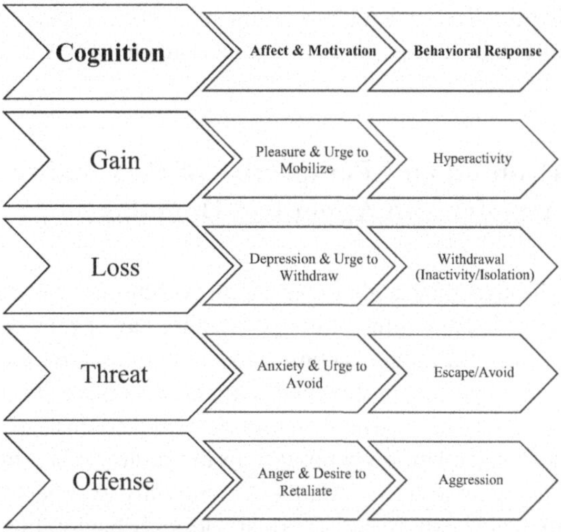

Fig. 1 Sequence of activation of the mode (The primary pathway that is discussed throughout the chapter is illustrated in Fig. 1. The authors acknowledge that the sequence of modal activation leads to not only behavior, but consequences based on the behaviors, which can lead back in a cyclical manner to cognition, affect, motivation, and future behaviors)

temporal sequence of perception (cognition or belief), affect and motivation, and then behavior (see Fig. 1). In the case of psychopathology, it is well established that individuals have strong negative cognitive schemas which maintain the negative automatic thoughts and impact feelings, motivations, and behaviors (symptomatology) greatly (Beck & Haigh, 2014). Generally, when these cognitive biases become more extreme, the mental health condition moves along this same trajectory and becomes more severe. Relatedly, the flexibility of cognitive bias or the ability to reverse this belief system becomes more difficult in more severe cases. These negative cognitive schemas (and associated biased cognitive processing) lead to biased perception of events, a negative self-identity (i.e., inferior, inadequate, unlovable, inefficacious), and a negative image of the outside world (i.e., rejecting, hostile, dangerous).

These negative schemas tend to form in part due to individuals' experience of adverse formative life events (Beck, 2020). The meanings derived from the experiences, repeated failures, rejections, and vulnerabilities remain salient and often overlay a biased negative interpretation on to current events which are inherently neutral or even positive. For example, P.J.'s school years involved children bullying him and he learned, "People hurt you." When the ball is thrown into his yard, he interprets the neutral stimulus (poorly thrown ball) through the lens and interprets the event, "he is always messing with me." In these situations, the individual is likely to ignore the more realistic explanation (e.g., "he's a bad ball thrower") and instead, selects the more negative, less likely explanation (Beck & Haigh, 2014). The individual not only discounts or ignores the data that are contradictory to the positive interpretation, but if the event is in the least bit negative, the individual exaggerates it. Just as these negative perceptions and expectancies are enhanced in cases of psychopathology, the positive sector of personality becomes minimized or dormant. Therefore, it is common to see individuals experience a lack of positive expectation and interpretation of events, a lack of gratification, blunted positive affect, lack of productive motivation, etc. (Beck & Haigh, 2014).

Evolutionary Perspective of Personality and Psychopathology: Aversive and Appetitive Domains

Through thousands of years of evolutionary processes such as natural selection, specific paradigms of the personality have persisted over time. In a hunter gatherer society, the hunter is confronted by both aversive and appetitive stimuli. When hunters are successful (experiencing an appetitive stimulus), they experience pleasure, satisfaction, or gain. A natural response to this satisfaction would be to continue to seek satisfaction via hunting in the future. When hunters are unsuccessful (experiencing an aversive stimulus), commonly experiencing danger, challenge, or defeat, they may experience a corresponding behavioral response (e.g., withdrawal, avoidance, aggression) as well as an affective response (e.g., anxiety, dysphoria or anger). The adaptive functions that are promoted by the protection against aversive/negative stimuli and promotion of the positive/appetitive stimuli include survival, sociality, sexuality, reproduction, achievement, competition, and independence.

Despite the evolutionary progress of humans over time, the aversive and appetitive domains still provide an overarching framework for conceptualizing psychopathology in modern times. Under the umbrella of the two domains, there are clusters of specific modes which include the cognitions/affects/motivations and behavior with a similar theme (e.g., an anxious mode or depressed mode would fall under the aversive sector of personality). When the mode is increased in intensity, dominance, and duration, it is labeled a disorder and the specific affect and behaviors are labeled as symptoms (according to the Diagnostic and Statistical Manual (DSM-5) (American Psychiatric Association, 2013). In terms of mode activation, psychopathological modes remain activated for a prolonged period and/or may have an extreme cognitive content or meaning.

For example, the dysthymic/aversive disorders, namely depression, anxiety, and violence, represent maladaptive exaggerations of everyday aversive cognitive interpretations of loss, threat, and offense, and corresponding affective reactions of sadness, anxiety, and anger. In anxiety for example, the cognitive content is provided by the cognitive schemas which may have the meaning of threat. For example, in social anxiety the cognition might be, "I am vulnerable in social situations and will be rejected if I stick my neck out." The individual responds with anxiety and uses avoidance techniques to withdraw from the situation (i.e., flight reaction), and avoidance serves to temporarily inhibit the incorporation of any new data from the environment.

In depression, the pre-existing cognitive schema provides a meaning attached to the situation that pertains to loss, disappointment, self-criticism, etc. The person overgeneralizes and makes a value judgment about the self, for example, "I am stupid, worthless, no good, etc." Therefore, there is a self-attribution of the loss and associated affects of sadness and hopelessness. In disorders that contain violence, anger, and aggression, the individual attaches the meaning of loss here as well, but attributes the cause of the loss to another individual who has criticized or let the individual down, and thus responds with anger and a sense of devaluation, which may or may not be expressed.

While anxiety, depression, and anger can become globalized, these presentations are qualitatively different from that of individuals with severe mental illness (SMI; Garety et al., 2001). Neurobiological dysfunctions are involved in the active psychotic process (Morrison et al., 2000); however, psychosis is not an individual's personality (see Beck et al., 2020b). External and internal adversities can drive a number of maladaptive schemas. Importantly, there is generally a difference in the cognitive content of individuals with SMI, compared to the non-psychotic individuals. Given that the SMI individuals face challenges in so many areas of functioning related to positive, negative and disorganized symptomatology, as well as intense self-stigmatization and stigma from the outside world, these individuals maintain robust negative attitudes with much broader content (Beck et al., 2020b). Indeed, their sense of helplessness, lack of confidence, and limited motivation are permeated with judgments regarding their personal self as useless, a bad person, etc. (Grant & Beck, 2009). This broadly encompassing negative cognitive content in SMI populations includes negative views (of the self and others) regarding sociality, ability, pleasure, communication, trust, control, and many other facets.

The key element in the disorders (as opposed to the transient modal activation and reactions to everyday life) is the element of bias. Thus, in anxiety disorders, the individual bias is one of magnification (i.e., catastrophizing; Gellatly & Beck, 2016; Waltman & Palermo, 2019) and overgeneralization. A similar bias can be observed in the extreme activation in depression, anger, and aggressive disorders. Thus, the difference between the adaptive response (and modal activation) and the pathological response is the introduction of situation-incongruent bias based on previously stored cognitive schemas and cognitive processing aspects of the modal activation.

When the modes are in the aversive state (e.g., depression, anxiety, or aggression, schizophrenia), the therapeutic strategy is to diffuse these modes. This is done through various cognitive and behavioral methods (Beck & Haigh, 2014). A hallmark of the cognitive and behavioral therapies is the use of collaborative empiricism, a scientifically driven testing of the ideas as a team of equals (see Waltman et al., 2020), which results in cognitive modification (see Lorenzo-Luaces et al., 2015). This process diffuses maladaptive modal activation. While the emphasis is on diffusing the aversive modes, we also have the option of activating the appetitive modes (these modes have to do with safety, self-confidence, scopophilia, optimism, etc.). In recent years, there has been an increased emphasis on fostering change through reinforcing strengths and recovery-oriented methods (Beck et al., 2020a, b; Padesky & Mooney, 2012).

The appetitive and aversive modes are diametrically situated and function similar to a seesaw. Activation of the appetitive mode causes deactivation of the aversive mode (and vice versa). Thus, a savvy therapist has two routes to bringing about change in modal activation. Traditional cognitive and behavioral methodology would be to target a reduction in the aversive mode through restructuring unhelpful cognitions and modifying behaviors that are incongruent with adaptation. Strengths-based and recovery-oriented methods would be more focused on directly cultivating appetitive modal activation and increasing those experiences serving as evidence to modify existing schema.

Modal Activation: A Continuum from Transient Reactions to Psychopathology

In everyday life, the various transient cognitions serve the purpose of alerting the individual to a problem or new stimulus. After these cognitions are activated, individuals then experience a variety of affects, which also serve an alerting function, and tend to be more propelling compared to cognitions. In psychopathology, the cognitions and affects also provide an alert to the individual. However, the activated psychopathological mode contains biased cognitions (interpretation) based on stored cognitive schemas, exaggerated affective responses that are disproportionate to the circumstance, and prolonged activation of the entire maladaptive mode. Below we will describe numerous modes that can represent non-psychotic disorders if in exaggerated form.

In the case of anxiety, for example, the individual's reaction to stimuli with the meaning of threat/danger leads to an activation of the "anxious mode." Chronic activation of the anxious mode leads to a modal response that is easily triggered and often hyper-charged. Thus, in anxiety disorders, there is either a bias that exaggerates the perceived risk and/or an exaggerated or prolonged anxious reaction which cannot be handled by avoidance.

Loss of self-esteem or loss of empowerment leads to depression or sadness. If an individual feels insecure or inferior, then the perception of loss of value or power can also lead to depression. The difference between an episode of sadness versus clinical depression is based on an exaggeration and prolongation of negative beliefs (i.e., negatively biased evaluations of the aspects of one's life, and perceptions of oneself as a failure or helpless). The same stimulus can lead to anger when the individual perceives the devaluation of another as an offense and feels relatively safe in attacking the offender. Continued expression of this angry affect and behavior can lead to turmoil in social and interpersonal relationships.

In each of these presentations, one critical similarity is the exaggerated maladaptive cognitive and emotional responses to stimulus situations (often labeled as catastrophizing in the field of cognitive therapy (Ellis, 1962). Catastrophizing has been found to be a transdiagnostic process, present across psychopathology (Gellatly & Beck, 2016; Waltman & Palermo, 2019). Catastrophizing is central to anxiety in that the catastrophic beliefs lead to an ineffective coping strategy of avoidance, whereas in depression and suicide the catastrophic thinking patterns lead to an ineffective coping strategy of withdrawal paired with hopelessness. Both of these being examples of the aversive modes in action.

Within the appetitive domain, individuals naturally try to increase the frequency and intensity of experienced satisfaction, pleasure, euphoria, etc. If pleasure seeking extends beyond being transient and fitting to the individual's external environment, we may describe this as an "addiction mode." Therefore, an exaggeration of the positive benefits of the addictive behaviors or in other words a maladaptive engagement (which leads to physiological and psychological dependence and later withdrawal symptoms upon attempting to eliminate an addiction), would be labeled an addictive disorder, including both substance abuse and behavioral addiction (i.e., sex, virtual gaming, gambling, shopping, and possibly work-related activity).

In both domains, a major theme or problem is the perceived (or real) lack of control. With anxiety one defends oneself or controls the situation through the impulse to avoid or through actual behavioral avoidance. In depression, one already feels defeated and so withdraws (the attempt at control) in order to avoid further defeat, loss, etc. In the case of anger, one expresses the anger in order to control another person and prevent the other person from insulting or controlling them to a greater extent. In substance use disorders and other addictions, the main mechanism is seeking gratification/pleasure and controlling either one's interface with their surroundings, their outward identity in the presence of others, their affective expression, or motivation via the use of the addictive substance or behavior. In the case of addiction, the search for control often times leads to a self-image of being out of control and/or been controlled by the psychological and physiological dependence.

The extension of the mode to a disorder depends on the duration and degree of disability, represented by components of the mode. are diagnosed as "symptoms" such as generalized anxiety disorder are simply exaggerations of the adaptive affect and cognitions of the modes. A central portion of the theory represents the excessive pathological state as being on a continuum with the adaptive state. This is well demonstrated with research on the relationship between anxiety and performance. Low levels of anxiety can increase focus, motivation, and effective behavioral strategies; however, as anxiety becomes excessive performance suffers (Eysenck & Calvo, 1992).

From this perspective, psychopathology represents an extension and magnification of an adaptive, transient reactions. The syndromes may also occasionally arise from the continual repetition of the transient reactions. Thus, the major difference between a transiently activated mode (either adaptive or maladaptive) and a psychopathological mode is not the primary emotion that is activated. In fact, as we noted above, the cognitive content and primary emotions seem to remain the same regardless of the intensity of the stimulus event. Instead, the difference is in the intensity, exaggeration, and prolonged nature of the mode (including cognitive schema or meaning of the event). For example, it has previously been demonstrated that personality disorders represent normative personality traits in extreme or overly rigid presentations (Trull & Durrett, 2005; Wiggins & Pincus, 1989). With this framework, mental health professionals can begin to better understand why individuals given mental health diagnoses often find themselves "stuck" in one mode. Thus, the therapeutic goal becomes activating adaptive modes that can offset the durable and exaggerated maladaptive psychopathological modes. Below we will discuss an iteration of cognitive therapy developed specifically for helping individuals shift into adaptive modes, work towards aspirations, and foster recovery

Psychotherapy

When individuals first appear for psychotherapy, they are apprehensive regarding the therapist's reaction to them and may feel vulnerable when they reveal their "innermost secrets." Additionally, new clients may hesitate to talk about subjects that embarrass them and make them feel vulnerable, such as their anger, narcissism, and independent needs. The skillful, flexible therapist responds initially with unconditional acceptance (see Rogers, 1995) and then fortifies the individual's strengths by expressing appreciation for the individual's courage in sharing the self-revelations. The therapy from then on progresses to build on the individual's positive assets, accomplishments, goals, strengths, etc.

There are two complimentary cognitive approaches to treatment that can follow the above description of the trajectory of treatment and the therapeutic relationship. These two approaches share a basis in the cognitive model but have fundamental differences in the demeanor of the therapist. In one approach, the therapist uses logic and reasoning to correct the aversive evaluations of the self and the task. This could include reviewing past experiences which contradict the aversive interpretations (examining the evidence) or using cognitive reframing to consider a stimulus situation from a different, more adaptive perspective. Across the span of psychopathology, this approach has been directed towards the "symptoms" and specifically, a reduction in various cognitive patterns, negative affect, and maladaptive behavior patterns. This is the standard cognitive therapy approach.

As we previously mentioned, the factor of control is critical across many forms of psychopathology. From the perspective of the standard cognitive therapy approach, the therapist may guide the individual in session towards recognizing maladaptive thought patterns about control, restructure and reframe their perspective on feeling out of control or what it may take to gain control back in their lives, and in series of focused interventions, gain skills to un-learn some of their negative cognitive biases regarding control. For example, in the case of anger, the individual must learn that the act of striking the partner does not lead to the partner becoming more compliant but leads to a destruction of the relationship. In substance use disorders, it is important to re-establish control over the falsity of assumptions such as "the only way to enjoy oneself is through accomplishment or drug taking" and engage in new learning that enhances the self-image and creates new thinking patterns. In the case of anxiety, we try to switch to the mode in which the object is perceived in terms of its realistic threat and the individual is perceived more realistically in terms of ability to handle the threat, thereby reinstating a greater sense of control.

The other approach maintains a more positive, strengths-based, and recovery focus. In recent years, the attention of many psychotherapists has shifted from looking at the specific symptomatology in an isolative fashion or working towards the overt correction of various misinterpretations, to a broader, more trans-diagnostic approach that aims to view individuals holistically and activate the total personality. For example, for those with serious mental health conditions, the therapeutic program entitled Recovery Oriented Cognitive Therapy (CT-R) aims to activate these broad aspects of personality, such as being efficient, valuable, a good person, independent. (Beck et al., 2020b) and focuses on underlying adaptive meanings behind surface level maladaptive modes. It is important to note that both traditional cognitive therapy and CT-R are directed at cognitive modification. However, the critical difference in CT-R is the importance of activating positive cognitions and reinforcing the affirmative meanings from positive experiences, rather than deactivating negative cognitions.[4]

The CT-R approach aims to foster the appetitive aspect of the personality. The therapist attempts to activate past and present positive evaluations of the self through a number of positive experiences. This learning (or re-learning) is experiential in that it relies on action as a therapeutic modality. Importantly, the CT-R therapist designs experiences in an individualistic manner and works with the individual to provide opportunity for meeting the individual's aspirations. In collaboratively setting an individual's aspirations, the clinical staff member might ask the individual "What would you like your life to be like when you get out of the hospital?" Once the individual has set their aspirations, the therapy focuses on skills building, problem solving, mastery, control, etc. Symptoms are targeted as they impede progress towards these aspirations. For example, one individual was fixed on the idea of becoming a famous playwright. He understood multiple important meanings underling this aspiration. These included his ability to be a valuable member of a team, his ability to entertain people through his writing, and providing pleasure to audience members who would enjoy the plays. When he thought about these different meanings with his clinical care team, he found that he could maintain these desired meanings while pursuing the aspiration and understanding that becoming a famous playwright is a process and not guaranteed. These critical discussions about the meanings behind individuals' grander aspirations or the meaning of a successful experience were fulfilled by being an usher and can be strengthened throughout the course of treatment. While the previous example describes an individual with a specific career aspiration, often CT-R trained staff have observed that when institutionalized individuals became engaged in daily activities of their own choosing (such as washing the dishes or folding the laundry) that they became animated and their overall functioning, sense of self-worth and altruism improved among other factors.

[4] This more holistic approach was also supported by considerable research summarized by Wood and Tarrier (2010).

Another more specific intervention is particularly effective in tapping into individual's positive and adaptive personality attributes. During the therapy session, the therapist reverses roles and encourages the individual to educate the therapist about topics that the individual is particularly knowledgeable and the therapist deficient about. In this way, the therapist builds up the individual's self-confidence, equalizes the therapeutic relationship, and makes it more natural, while also undercutting the individual's regressive tendencies. There are also additional CT-R strategies that are used to indirectly offset positive symptoms. In the application of CT-R to the positive symptoms of schizophrenia, we have found that by inferring the perceived deficiency of a particular asset and strengthening that perceived deficiency or desired trait through targeted, personalized activities, we are able to indirectly reduce the positive symptom. This experience is used as an experiment to test the individual's beliefs about controllability of the positive symptoms. For example, with individuals experiencing grandiose delusions, we found that the following was effective in eliminating the delusion from the individual's discussion with clinical staff and themselves. One individual experienced the grandiose delusion that he was God. Clinical staff understood this delusion as a perceived deficiency in his experienced altruism and lack of access and ability to help others in need while in the hospital. Therefore, staff designed activities for him to become engaged with other members of the unit in leading a volunteer group that would help the community through food donations, neighborhood clean-ups, etc. In doing so, he reinforced beliefs about his abilities to be socially connected and helpful to others. This intervention gets at the heart of what CT-R represents, namely by understanding the whole person, not just symptoms in isolation, staff can help to provide opportunities for a surge of positive, adaptive experiences that can offset symptoms by focusing on the individuals desires, assets, and aspirations.

Through a process of engagement, clinical providers can act as catalysts for these processes that foster the appetitive domains, and classic cognitive strategies can be used to facilitate adaptive schematic processing to help with generalization of new learning. It is critical that clinical staff not only help to promote meaningful action and interventions but also collaboratively draw conclusions about the meanings and feelings associated with successful experiences and the individual's strengths, assets, opportunities, and capabilities. For example, even after small success experience, members of an individual's care team would assist in drawing conclusions what a successful experience says about the individual, what the experience denotes about how the individual can relate to others, and even discussing whether the individual may be willing to try a similar activity again. Some specific examples include a therapist saying, "You showed courage in going to group therapy today and discussing sensitive topics" or asking, "What did the fact that you enjoyed interreacting with other people today say about you?" These positive interactions with the clinical staff also help to reverse the stigmatization imposed by the clinical staff onto individuals.

Thus, the overarching treatment target across psychopathology is not put in terms of "changing of the person" but rather in terms of transformation of the individual from durable, prolonged maladaptive modes, to a stable and fortified adaptive mode. This adaptive mode includes an openness to take in multiple perspectives and obtain new learning, a problem-solving component, and heighted access to metacognitive or superordinate processing. It is also important to note that this adaptive mode can be fleeting or momentary if individuals maintain strong negative biases and thus, the mode needs to be continually invigorated with new learning experiences which provide positive meanings such as control, mastery, and a greater degree of hope. These meanings and found purpose in individuals' lives can also have a more generalized positive impact on the broader views of the self-identity. For example, someone with alcohol dependence might a shift away from perceiving oneself as an "addict" or "drunk," particularly if other more adaptive components of their personality have been activated or strengthened. It also should be noted that the focus is not on relief of symptoms, but rather, personal development and attainment of purpose and meaning in life. Thus, in this approach, the developing individuals' aspirations and the concordant plan to attain these aspirations and move towards recovery comes naturally and serves as a learning opportunity to correct maladaptive schema.

Summary and Future Directions

We have presented a unified theory of personality, adaptation, psychopathology, and psychotherapy. We attempted to demonstrate how the individual responds to danger, defeat, disempowerment, and devaluation respectively with anxiety, sadness, and anger. We also spell out how each motivation is expressed: flight, withdrawal, and craving. We also show how the excessive craving for satisfaction can lead to addiction (even appetitive modes can become maladaptive if out of balance).

In our thinking about a productive model of psychopathology and psychotherapy, we have stuck to the cognitive model, but have paid more attention to the positive aspects of personality, and, in so doing, created a more holistic model. In this model, we perceive the disorders as encompassing a maladaptive formation of the standard adaptive features of personality: the disorders represent an exaggeration of the adaptive modes and are generally labeled according to which aspect of the mode is most salient (neuroses representing an exaggeration of the automatic thoughts/cognitions, the affective disorders such as anxiety and depression representing the exaggerating or distorted affects, and the behavioral disorders such as suicide, self-mutilation, violent behavior, addictions and obsessive compulsive disorder (OCD) representing salience of maladaptive actions). It is to be noted that for each disorder, the cognitive model (Cognition > Affect > Motivation) remains intact. The differences between each disorder can be located in the belief system, which consists of formulas and algorithms. In addition, the disorders may be divided into the aversive domain (which includes anxiety, depression) and its counter appetitive domain (which encompasses addictive disorders). Experienced clinicians generally use an integrative approach with their outpatients, applying logic and reason to the beliefs and automatic thoughts, but also setting up goals, and keeping track of positive experience as tools in their armamentarium. This integrative approach coordinates well with the cognitive model of personality and psychopathology.

The efficacy of recovery oriented cognitive therapy (CT-R) is ripe for validation. A series of randomized control trials is crucially indicated. Best practices would suggest that any positive results are replicated at new sites by independent researchers (Chambless & Hollon, 1998). If this intervention is found to be successful for individuals with severe and persistent mental illness, then it should also be determined whether the therapy is effective for individuals with less severe presentations. As promising results are found, researchers should look to test the efficacy of CT-R across a range of diagnoses and presentations. As the appetitive and aversive domains are thought to be diametrically opposed and inversely related, researchers should examine the treatment effects of CT-R on both traditional treatment targets (i.e., symptom reduction) and recovery-oriented treatment targets (e.g., Sociality Scale; Beck et al., 2020b; Temporal Experience of Pleasure Scale; Gard et al., 2006, 2007). Moreover, as CT-R and more traditional forms of cognitive therapy are viewed here as compatible, researchers may benefit from assessing both the comparative effects of these treatments and the potential additive effects of combined forms of therapy. Importantly, it might be that new measures need to be constructed and validated as this innovation represents a paradigm shift. For example, outcome measures such as purpose, meaning, compassion, fulfillment of aspirations, connectedness to community, amongst others, could be explored as outcome measures on newly developed scales for professionals utilizing CT-R in both clinical and research capacities. Further, as cognitive modification is thought to be the mechanism of change, researchers should include measures of underlying beliefs (e.g., Dysfunctional Attitude Scale; Beck et al., 1991). Finally, researchers should consider using sophisticated designs that gather data at various points of time to allow for predictive models to be made to clarify and validate the model. In closing, curiosity and an empirical mindset are core values of the practice of cognitive behavioral therapy (CBT) and of the namesake of this edited textbook; the future of CBT will be guided by the science.

References

American Psychiatric Association. (2013). *Diagnostic and statistical manual of mental disorders* (5th ed.). Author.

Beck, A. T. (1952). Successful outpatient psychotherapy of a chronic schizophrenic with a delusion based on borrowed guilt. *Psychiatry, 15*(3), 305–312.

Beck, A. T. (1963). Thinking and depression I. Idiosyncratic content and cognitive distortions. *Archives of General Psychiatry, 9*, 324–333. https://doi.org/10.1001/archpsyc.1963.01720160014002

Beck, A. T. (1964). Thinking and depression II. Theory and therapy. *Archives of General Psychiatry, 10*(6), 561–571. https://doi.org/10.1001/archpsyc.1964.01720240015003

Beck, A. T. (1979). *Cognitive therapy and the emotional disorders*. Meridian.

Beck, A. T. (1996). *Beyond belief: A theory of modes, personality, and psychopathology*.

Beck, A. T. (1999). *Prisoners of hate: The cognitive basis of anger, hostility, and violence*. HarperCollins.

Beck, J. S. (2020). *Cognitive behavior therapy, third edition: Basics and beyond.* Guilford Publications.
Beck, A. T., & Bredemeier, K. (2016). A unified model of depression: Integrating clinical, cognitive, biological, and evolutionary perspectives. *Clinical Psychological Science, 4*(4), 596–619.
Beck, A. T., & Haigh, E. A. P. (2014). Advances in cognitive theory and therapy: The Generic Cognitive Model. *Annual Review of Clinical Psychology, 10*, 1–24. https://doi.org/10.1146/annurev-clinpsy-032813-153734
Beck, A. T., Brown, G., Steer, R. A., & Weissman, A. N. (1991). Factor analysis of the Dysfunctional Attitude Scale in a clinical population. *Psychological Assessment: A Journal of Consulting and Clinical Psychology, 3*(3), 478–483.
Beck, A. T., Finkel, M. R., & Beck, J. S. (2020a). The theory of modes: Applications to schizophrenia and other psychological conditions. *Cognitive Therapy and Research.* https://doi.org/10.1007/s10608-020-10098-0
Beck, A. T., Grant, P. M., Inverso, E., Brinen, A., & Perivoliotis. (2020b). *Recovery oriented cognitive therapy for serious mental health conditions*. The Guilford Press.
Chambless, D. L., & Hollon, S. D. (1998). Defining empirically supported therapies. *Journal of Consulting and Clinical Psychology, 66*(1), 7–18.
Clark, D. A., & Beck, A. T. (1999). *Scientific foundations of cognitive theory and therapy of depression*. Wiley.
Craske, M. G., Treanor, M., Conway, C. C., Zbozinek, T., & Vervliet, B. (2014). Maximizing exposure therapy: An inhibitory learning approach. *Behaviour Research and Therapy, 58*, 10–23.
Ellis, A. (1962). *Reason and emotion in psychotherapy*. Lyle Stuart.
Eysenck, M. W., & Calvo, M. G. (1992). Anxiety and performance: The processing efficiency theory. *Cognition & Emotion, 6*(6), 409–434.
Fassbinder, E., Schweiger, U., Martius, D., Brand-de Wilde, O., & Arntz, A. (2016). Emotion regulation in schema therapy and dialectical behavior therapy. *Frontiers in Psychology, 7*, 1–19.
Gard, D. E., Gard, M. G., Kring, A. M., & John, O. P. (2006). Anticipatory and consummatory components of the experience of pleasure: A scale development study. *Journal of Research in Personality, 40*(6), 1086–1102.
Gard, D. E., Kring, A. M., Gard, M. G., Horan, W. P., & Green, M. F. (2007). Anhedonia in schizophrenia: Distinctions between anticipatory and consummatory pleasure. *Schizophrenia Research, 93*(1-3), 253–260.
Garety, P. A., Kuipers, E., Fowler, D., Freeman, D., & Bebbington, P. E. (2001). A cognitive model of the positive symptoms of psychosis. *Psychological Medicine, 31*(2), 189–195.
Gellatly, R., & Beck, A. T. (2016). Catastrophic thinking: A transdiagnostic process across psychiatric disorders. *Cognitive Therapy and Research, 40*(4), 441–452.
Grant, P. M., & Beck, A. T. (2009). Defeatist beliefs as a mediator of cognitive impairment, negative symptoms, and functioning in schizophrenia. *Schizophrenia Bulletin, 35*(4), 798–806.
Hays, P. A., & Iwamasa, G. Y. (2006). *Culturally responsive cognitive-behavioral therapy.* American Psychological Association.
Kahneman, D. (2011). *Thinking, fast and slow*. Macmillan.
Levin, M. E., Hildebrandt, M. J., Lillis, J., & Hayes, S. C. (2012). The impact of treatment components suggested by the psychological flexibility model: A meta-analysis of laboratory-based component studies. *Behavior Therapy, 43*(4), 741–756.
Lorenzo-Luaces, L., German, R. E., & DeRubeis, R. J. (2015). It's complicated: The relation between cognitive change procedures, cognitive change, and symptom change in cognitive therapy for depression. *Clinical Psychology Review, 41*, 3–15.
Lynn, S. J., Fassler, O., Knox, J. A., & Lilienfeld, S. O. (2006). Dissociation and dissociative identity disorder: Treatment guidelines and cautions. In *Practitioner's guide to evidence-based psychotherapy* (pp. 248–257). Springer.
Molinsky, A. (2007). Cross-cultural code-switching: The psychological challenges of adapting behavior in foreign cultural interactions. *Academy of Management Review, 32*(2), 622–640.

Morrison, A. P., Wells, A., & Nothard, S. (2000). Cognitive factors in predisposition to auditory and visual hallucinations. *British Journal of Clinical Psychology, 39*(1), 67–78.

Nesse, R. M. (2019). *Good reasons for bad feelings: Insights from the frontier of evolutionary psychiatry*. Penguin.

Padesky, C. A., & Mooney, K. A. (2012). Strengths-based cognitive–behavioural therapy: A four-step model to build resilience. *Clinical Psychology & Psychotherapy, 19*(4), 283–290.

Rogers, C. R. (1995). *On becoming a person: A therapist's view of psychotherapy*. Houghton Mifflin Harcourt.

Silberschatz, G. (2013). *Transformative relationships: The control mastery theory of psychotherapy*. Routledge.

Trull, T. J., & Durrett, C. A. (2005). Categorical and dimensional models of personality disorder. *Annual Reviews Clinical Psychology, 1*, 355–380.

Waltman, S. H. (2013). Cross-cultural considerations for differentiating between religiosity and psychosis. *Health and Interprofessional Practice, 1*(4), eP1041.

Waltman, S. H., & Palermo, A. (2019). Theoretical overlap and distinction between rational emotive behavior therapy's awfulizing and cognitive therapy's catastrophizing. *Mental Health Review Journal, 24*(1), 44–50.

Waltman, S., & Sokol, L. (2017). the generic cognitive model of cognitive behavioral therapy: A case conceptualization-driven approach. In S. Hofmann & G. Asmundson (Eds.), *The science of cognitive behavioral therapy* (pp. 3–18). Academic.

Waltman, S. H., Codd, R. T., McFarr, L. M., & Moore, B. A. (2020). *Socratic questioning for therapists and counselors: Learn how to think and intervene like a cognitive behavior therapist*. Routledge.

Wiggins, J. S., & Pincus, A. L. (1989). Conceptions of personality disorders and dimensions of personality. *Psychological Assessment: A Journal of Consulting and Clinical Psychology, 1*(4), 305.

Wood, A. M., & Tarrier, N. (2010). Positive clinical psychology: A new vision and strategy for integrated research and practice. *Clinical Psychology Review, 30*(7), 819–829.

Yalom, I. D. (1995). *The theory and practice of group psychotherapy*. Basic Books.

Young, J. E. (1999). *Cognitive therapy for personality disorders: A schema-focused approach*. Professional Resource Press.

The Future of Cognitive Therapy

Dean McKay and Jonathan Abramowitz

A volume honoring the memory of Scott Lilienfeld by necessity would critically consider the future of cognitive therapy. It is not because one emphasis of his work was on the benefits and limitations of cognitive therapy, but because Scott focused on errors in thinking that might lead clinicians to apply methods unsupported by science, regardless of how well-meaning they may be. The scope of work on these biases in clinical practices ranges from influential volumes covering the entire corpus of clinical practice (i.e., Lilienfeld et al., 2015) to highly specific appraisals of methods with dubious scientific merit (i.e., dolphin-assisted therapy for autism; Marino & Lilienfeld, 1998).

While Scott was generally favorable toward cognitive therapy (or, more broadly, cognitive-behavioral therapy), he noted that clinical psychology, like all health sciences, should be attentive to the potential that any treatment may have adverse effects, and thus would be suitable for critical scrutiny (i.e., Lilienfeld, 2007). One of us (DM) had the opportunity to co-author works with Scott, and the experience had a profound professional impact. One central feature to our collaboration was identification of cognitive errors and logical fallacies. And it is this central theme that is the core of the present chapter. Specifically, the aim of this chapter is to honor Scott's legacy by discussing how cognitive therapy must include an explicit role for logical fallacies, and methods for clinicians to avoid them, in delivering treatment. This includes an expanded role for examining the connection between language and human cognition. This connection is well known in other sciences (i.e., linguistics) but generally de-emphasized or ignored altogether in the training of cognitive therapists.

D. McKay (✉)
Department of Psychology, Fordham University, The Bronx, NY, USA
e-mail: mckay@fordham.edu

J. Abramowitz
University of North Carolina-Chapel Hill, Chapel Hill, NC, USA

C. L. Cobb et al. (eds.), *Toward a Science of Clinical Psychology*,
https://doi.org/10.1007/978-3-031-14332-8_15

Cognitive Therapy: A Brief Overview

Cognitive therapy in its current form is built on two complementary frameworks. One emphasizes the identification of thinking errors that individuals make in reaction to everyday situations. The dominant conceptual work underpinning cognitive therapy comes from Beck et al. (1979), Ellis (1962), and Meichenbaum (1977). While there are distinctions among the three conceptualizations from Beck, Ellis, and Meichenbaum, the core feature is identification of specific spontaneously occurring (i.e., "automatic") maladaptive patterns of thinking, and guiding clients to alter these patterns. The underlying premise is that the spontaneously occurring thoughts and interpretations are influenced by more deeply held (i.e., "core") dysfunctional beliefs and ideas, and that when a given situation (e.g., a poor grade) is interpreted in light of such cognitions (e.g., "I will never amount to anything"), it spurs distress (e.g., depression). Accordingly, distress is alleviated through therapeutic challenges to the veracity of these patterns of thinking. Collectively, the advent of this approach heralded the "cognitive revolution" that swept through the broader field of psychology in the 1960s and 1970s and even turned some behavior therapists into cognitive-behavior therapists. Detractors suggested that the arrival of the cognitive revolution was simply a reification of hypothetical constructs (i.e., Greenwood, 1999), whereas others modified their laboratory theories to account for the causal role ascribed to thoughts (such as the learned helplessness theory of depression; Alloy et al., 1984).

A central feature in cognitive therapy, as described by Beck, Ellis, and Meichenbaum, is to identify and isolate words and phrases that may emerge from daily events. These words and phrases in turn lead to emotional reactions. To facilitate treatment, these words and phrases are targeted by the clinician, and clients are instructed to challenge these in their daily lives through direct disputation from evidence. Thus, if a client engages in "black or white thinking," they would be trained to identify a *range* of options rather than focus exclusively on the polar extremes. Clients who might "discount the positive/amplify the negative" would be taught to understand that the negative side of an argument comes with possible benefits that have been overlooked (discounted). For "overimportance of thoughts," a client would be guided to illustrate how thoughts need not be heeded or may not be indicative of anything about the client's personal characteristics. These are just a few of many ways that cognitive therapists might aid clients in challenging and correcting cognitive errors.

Cognitive therapy, in the form described by Beck, Ellis, and Meichenbaum, came to be fully integrated into behavior therapy when experimental and treatment research showed that it was difficult to separate cognition from behavior. On the one hand, cognitive interventions, such as behavioral experiments (to test the validity of old and new ways of thinking), often include features that resemble exposure therapy, a behavioral technique (i.e., Bennett-Levy et al., 2004). On the other hand, direct behavioral interventions have been shown to lead to changes in cognitive distortions (i.e., in OCD; Abramowitz et al., 2005). In its current form, cognitive therapy has been extensively applied, although presently empirical support emphasizes the combination of cognitive therapy with behavioral therapy (Newman et al., 2021). On closer inspection in the research literature, there is not as much evidence to support the sole use of cognitive therapy as its supporters might assert. For example, in a recent patient-level meta-analysis, Furukawa et al. (2021) found that Internet-delivered cognitive therapy had an effect size no different from other non-specific therapies. Further, the clinical practice guidelines for depression published by the American Psychological Association concluded there was insufficient evidence to recommend cognitive therapy (McQuaid et al., 2019). This is significant considering that depression was the first condition for which cognitive therapy was systematically evaluated, in comparisons against medication (discussed in Hollon & Beck, 2013).

As research into cognitive distortions grew, it was increasingly recognized that not only were there spontaneously occurring thoughts, which may give rise to emotional reactions, but also environmental factors prompted a bias toward (or away) from accurate information. This in turn leads to biases in how information is encoded, processed, and recalled, which in turn impact judgments. Clinical scientists drew on basic cognitive experimental work to adapt laboratory methods in assessing biases in attention, memory, and judgment in relation to different emotional states (i.e., MacLeod et al., 1999). The careful accumulation of principles of cognitive biases that distort memory processes and associated downstream behaviors influenced some practitioners of cognitive therapy as described by Beck, Ellis, and Meichenbaum by highlighting ways to educate and target anticipated cognitive errors that could in turn be targeted in treatment. More recently, computer-based interventions to target these automatic processes (i.e., attention retraining, Cisler & Koster, 2010; Knowles et al., 2016; Price et al., 2016) have been developed with some beneficial effects on anxiety and depression (Hallion & Ruscio, 2011).

Training in Cognitive Therapy

As with any psychotherapeutic method, training in proper implementation is crucial for it to benefit the client. Many clinicians report that they practice cognitive therapy in some form. For example, in a survey of over 2000 therapists, approximately 69% reported using cognitive therapy (discussed in Brown, 2013). As noted earlier, cognitive therapy has increasingly been subsumed under the more general cognitive-behavioral therapy heading, and as a result it is more difficult to determine proportions of clinicians who administer cognitive therapy alone. Indeed, the merging of cognitive therapy with behavior therapy was viewed as a natural outcome given the methods of cognitive therapy involve at least some behavioral targets (such as via behavioral experiments; i.e., Bennett-Levy et al., 2004), and since behavioral interventions often include some cognitive interventions to address reticence for engagement (such as in exposure therapy; Richard & Lauterbach, 2006). However, it is reasonable to assume that cognitive therapy may be practiced more frequently than behavior therapy among self-described CBT practitioners. One reason for this assumption is that, at least in the case of anxiety alleviation, clinicians often express reservations due to typically unfounded concerns about risks to clients (Farrell et al., 2016).

Aside from the aforementioned behavioral experiments, cognitive therapy includes several therapeutic strategies that require considerable training in proper implementation. At its core, the approach involves cognitive disputation and restructuring. Cognitive disputation involves identifying dysfunctional beliefs held by the client, and challenging these beliefs for their accuracy. For some clinicians early in their training or who are new to this approach, cognitive disputation could be simply interpreted as identifying ways the client is wrong in their beliefs. This would be one central clinical error, and has been identified as a factor in client dropout (Kim et al., 2016). The clearest way to avoid clinical errors of this sort is through careful training. In order to properly apply cognitive therapy, it would be maximally effective to begin early in graduate training, through coursework, and follow with clinical applications at each level of training. As there is increasing recognition that many therapists did not have the opportunity to receive formal training in cognitive therapy, post-graduate training has begun to be offered, in some highly specialized areas. For example, the International Obsessive Compulsive Disorder Foundation has a behavior therapy training institute, and a corresponding expert consultation program, to ensure more clinicians can deliver specialized care for the disorder. There has been a recognition that structured training, and not just attending a few workshops, is essential for the health of the broader cognitive-behavioral therapy movement (McKay, 2014).

Looking to the Future

Language and Thought in Cognitive Therapy—Client Targets

Considering the fundamental unit of intervention in cognitive therapy is the adjustment of words and propositions, it is natural to expect that cognitive theorists would stress the linguistic models of how language itself shapes thought (such as the Sapir-Whorf hypothesis; discussed in Joseph, 1996). Interestingly, in preparing this chapter, there was comparably little found to suggest the cognitive theorists who formulated the clinical interventions that forms the basis of cognitive therapy were influenced by linguistic models of language and thought. The closest found was in Ellis (2001), who advocated a specific mode of speaking, called E-Prime (or E′). E′ emphasizes that, by eliminating the verb *to be* and all its conjugations, one can think and write with greater clarity. It also, according to Ellis, removes the possessive qualities on an individual's identity, freeing them for a wider range of personal understanding and growth. To illustrate, if one says, "I cannot do that because it is not in my nature," the verb *to be* (the word "is" in this case) is doing the emotional work in the self-statement and serves as a behavioral inhibitor. Editing the self-statement phrase to eliminate *is* would lead to a statement more about preferences rather than a veridical and defining quality. To be clear, the E′ movement aims to minimize the use of the verb "to be" and to narrow the way personal pronouns lead to possessive qualities. This would not include necessarily specific personal pronoun references or physical attributes. It demands of the speaker that language rely on situational grammar rather than possessive qualities. To further illustrate, assume someone feels anxious in a situation. They might be inclined to state "I am an anxious person," which gives them the overriding quality of being anxious. Regardless of the frequency with which one might feel anxious, E′ would recommend the speaker refer to their anxiety state as being a result of a situation, rather than due to an enduring quality.

The E′ approach to addressing emotional distress has been investigated in a small body of research. For example, Oltean and David (2020) found that the more individuals relied on the verb *to be*, the more they endorsed general negative affectivity. In a laboratory investigation of anger reactions, participants who had anger induction with greater frequency of the verb *to be* (i.e., qualities of the perpetrator) showed greater levels of anger responses and more difficulties in recovering from anger than those with an E-Prime-based induction (David, 2013). More work is called for to further determine the emotion eliciting and maintaining features of this highly specific language concept, but it suggests that it is not merely semantics to address how one "speaks to themselves" when it comes to therapy.

Highlighting the dimensions of language itself in shaping thought calls attention to granular elements of how a client might talk to themselves (i.e., think) that therapists could harness in treatment. As cognitive therapy is, in the end, highly oriented toward self-talk, drawing on the science of linguistics appears to be an essential component. Rational Emotive Behavior Therapy (REBT), a form a cognitive therapy, has emphasized that emotional distress emerges from demanding inner language, such as the use of the words "should," "ought," and "must" (Ellis & Harper, 1975). To address this problem, Ellis directly targeted these specific words and urged clients to re-state their inner talk. So, a client might say "Well, drivers really should stick to the speed limit!" to which a REBT therapist might recommend the client reword to "It would be preferable that drivers stick to the speed limit." This highly structured targeting of inner language forms the basis of cognitive disputation in the REBT model. In a more general way, Beck's approach to cognitive therapy emphasized identifying the specific beliefs that would correspond to emotional distress and challenge the central premises of that thought. Sticking with the speed limit example from above, in cognitive therapy derived from Beck's model, the therapist might urge the client to ask themselves whether it is absolutely required to adhere to the speed limit, or could there be a band of acceptable violations to this rule (such as emergency personnel, or maintaining the flow of traffic even if it is slightly above the limit). These general approaches to disputation have been the basis for cognitive therapy. However, these also assume that specific words, and their use in some sentences, evoke emotional reactivity.

The aforementioned analysis of cognitive therapy assumes a primarily language-based emotional experience, and implies deliberate thought. However, even linguists note that some thoughts are so immediate that there is limited language-based mediation (Pederson, 2010). If cognitive therapy is to continue to advance, it appears that a necessary direction will be to address the fact it has always been a targeted inner-language-based intervention, one whose primary aim is to help clients "edit" their spontaneous and more carefully reasoned thoughts to alleviate emotional distress. Ellis was the most explicit in the extent that treatment was aimed at targeting inner language, including through exercises that directed the client from external statements to inner language with the "rational barb." This exercise involves instructing collaboration between therapist and client in determining a rational alternative to the inner dysfunctional belief. Following this, the therapist states the original belief out loud, and the client counters that belief out loud. After several trials, the therapist continues to state the belief out loud while the client merely whispers the rational counter. Finally, the exercise ends with the therapist stating the belief and the client reciting their rational alternative silently.

There are some mini-movements in mental health care broadly that have attempted to harness linguistic science by shaping emotional experiences through metaphors and metonymy (Eynon, 2002). These movements have not yet caught on, however, possibly given the high degree of conceptual complexity. The delivery of cognitive therapy employing a method reliant on linguistic science would necessarily demand clinicians be capable to monitor the self-directed statements of their clients far more closely than they may already and guide them through a painstaking process of self-editing, both within and between sessions. However, as it appears the basic emotional demands resulting from the everyday use of the verb *to be* appear to have, heading in this direction would be in keeping with the broad philosophical underpinnings of cognitive therapy and would represent an important refinement in the practice. This would tie cognitive therapy directly to recent movements in psychotherapy research and also potentially serve as a unifying framework with other approaches in psychotherapy where language has been examined based on content and emotional processes (i.e., Russell & Stiles, 1979) rather than solely on assumed generalized words and phrases.

Psychotherapy research has emphasized language processes between therapist and client, and that language can be predictive of effective therapeutic processes (discussed in Wiltshire et al., 2020). It would also directly highlight cross-cultural dimensions of how cognitive therapy might be practiced. By expressly and consistently acknowledging the direct interaction between language and thought, clinicians would be sensitized to the unique characteristics of their clients' inner language and associated emotional responses. At the present time, the application of cognitive therapy is often far more general and assumes that clients are likely to experience emotional unrest through a specific set of common words, or the insertion of those words into phrases, such as the aforementioned "should," "ought," and "must" in REBT. However, a more nuanced application of cognitive therapy would assess for putative idiographic words and phrases that might be part of a client's inner language that is in turn the target of disputation.

Recent research would suggest that this linguistic analysis in cognitive therapy has unique predictive value for symptom change. Hernandez-Ramos et al. (2022), using text message content analyses, showed that depression-oriented language diminished as symptoms remitted among Latino participants. Further, the specificity of text content associated with depressed language was associated with level of participant fluency in an English-language society. Research of this sort could be relied upon to expand the ways to guide therapists in how to help clients edit their inner language in order to better address their emotional experiences.

Language and Thought in Cognitive Therapy—Clinician Targets

As noted here, one aspect of the future of cognitive therapy involves focusing on the interplay between language and thought through what we have termed "self-editing." How the client gets to the point of self-editing to a degree that alleviates emotional distress and leads to behavior change is at the mercy of how the clinician conceptualizes and draws out the self-talk. It has long been recognized that the questions asked by clinicians can lead to conclusions that were presupposed by the therapist rather than represent the presenting clinical problem. This was most evident during the early 2000s when false memory syndrome (FMS) was recognized as a problem spurred by the lines of questions from therapists who assumed their client's psychopathology was due to repressed memory of trauma (discussed in McNally, 2003). The presence of FMS, and how it comes about, suggests that clinicians may fall prey to a range of logical fallacies that interfere with clinical judgment. Confirmation bias is probably the most salient logical fallacy to apply in understanding FMS. Below, confirmation bias, as well as several others, is highlighted in how cognitive therapy may be best advanced.

Scott Lilienfeld recognized the hazards of logical fallacies in everyday practice, as many pseudoscientific practices emerged from problematic assumptions of clinicians. Understanding how our own logical fallacies interfere in treatment decisions was deemed essential and considered an important component of training therapists (Bowes et al., 2020) and for students of psychology generally (Lilienfeld et al., 2009).

There is a plethora of logical fallacies, some which are formally identified and others which represent patterns of thinking that fall into categories (discussed in Risen & Gilovich, 2007). There are several candidate fallacies that would appear ideal for therapists to have top of mind when engaged in treatment.

Confirmation Bias In the course of initial assessment, therapists identify symptoms to be targeted in treatment. In order to craft interventions, this demands identification of putative mechanisms that would inform the treatment conceptualization. In the case of cognitive therapy, this means that therapists must elicit, and possibly infer, beliefs that may result in emotional distress and problematic behavior. In doing so, clinicians are in a position to guide the client to some beliefs that might be viewed as problematic, thus confirming the a priori *beliefs of the clinician* about the underlying cognitive dimensions that might contribute to the presenting problem. This would be an illustration of how confirmation bias might lead clinicians to pursue treatment plans that center of specific beliefs in the client. Training clinicians to be aware of the risks of forming beliefs regarding the client's inner language without adequate support would be useful in guarding against this.

False Dilemma/False Dichotomy In the course of treatment, clients are guided to evidence for or against their primary underlying cognitions that are associated with distressing emotions and behaviors. In this guidance, it would be easy for a clinician to present two opposing situations or concepts, with seemingly few alternatives. For some pliable clients, this could leave out other plausible scenarios that could also be fruitfully employed in alleviating distress. In training cognitive therapists, it would be necessary to demonstrate cognitive flexibility in conceptualizing the presenting client problem and present scenarios in ways that are not rigidly constructed (such as "this, or that" format).

Straw Man Argument This fallacy occurs when someone distorts the position of another person, and then attacks that position as though it were the same as the one stated by the other person. For example, a common clinical situation for individuals with generalized anxiety is that they do not tolerate uncertainty well (Shihata et al., 2016). If a client identifies an area where they may find uncertainty hard to tolerate, a clinician might employ the straw man argument to suggest that additional situations are hard to tolerate and begin to guide the client to challenge those, on an assumption these are applicable. This point might easily fail later when applied by the client, but successive sessions could then be devoted to how the client needs to apply the concepts more rigorously/thoroughly/frequently in the service of alleviating distress. The straw man argument might be employed when clients present problems that clinicians struggle to understand, or how to develop disputation strategies. In order to alleviate the cognitive demand on the clinician, the straw man is a handy method for constructing an argument the therapy can actually dispute. It fails the client, but provides the clinician a way to feel that an intervention was administered. In training clinicians in cognitive therapy, avoiding the straw man argument would involve practice in maintaining focus on the ways problem situations emerge for the clients while avoiding the temptation to stray from the data into areas that would support pre-conceived hypotheses entertained by the clinician.

Confusing Correlations with Causation This occurs when a clinician assumes a causal relation between two events when they merely covary with one another. For instance, it is possible that contamination fear associated with obsessive-compulsive disorder is based on the belief that contaminants are all around, and thus washing must be vigorous to remove the contaminants. That is, the washing is caused by the perception of contaminants. On the other hand, it is also possible the individual was taught that washing vigorously was necessary, without explanation, and later on the justification for the extreme washing was constructed. Thus, the washing and the belief are merely correlated, and the thought is not directly related to the action.

The entire cognitive therapy enterprise is based on training clients to serve as their own scientists to appraise situations for their evidence. It assumes that cognitions have a causal impact on mood and emotion. Therefore, in the cognitive therapy model, the aforementioned washing behavior due to contamination fear would be defined as emerging from a belief regarding the means to remove perceived contaminants. However, this relation is not always present, regardless of how strongly the cognitive therapist adheres to the theory. Thus, understanding the causal fallacy in addressing client needs is essential for sound and comprehensive care. Training and supervision of therapists to address this fallacy would thus involve strengthening their understanding of correlative relationships, and how to assess for these in lieu of assuming causal relations.

These are some leading logical fallacies for clinicians to guard against, although hardly an exhaustive consideration of the topic. In training future cognitive therapists, it would be instructive to include detailed knowledge and understanding of how an introspective cognitive therapist might watch for these fallacies and consider alternative approaches.

It appears, however, that attention is being paid to the importance of logical fallacies in cognitive therapy, just not by clinicians. Instead, philosophers have turned their attention to errors in thinking and judgment by clinicians (i.e., Irwin & Bassham, 2003; Murguia & Diaz, 2015). It is probably fitting that philosophy has begun to critically examine the central tenets of cognitive therapy from the therapist's side of the room. After all, Ellis drew heavily on the philosophy of Epictetus in shaping his rational-emotive therapy methods, specifically through the statement, "Nothing is good or bad. Only saying so makes it so."

Conclusions

In this chapter honoring the memory of Scott Lilienfeld, we focused on two important directions that might represent the future of cognitive therapy—formal attention to nuances of language in shaping thought and logical fallacies committed by clinicians. Scott's scholarship demanded rigorous thinking and was carefully considered in its development. Thus, these two areas would also truly honor his memory by demanding greater rigor in thought and treatment implementation. Indeed, Scott so carefully considered the innumerable ways clinicians might commit errors in execution and conclusions about treatment benefits that he and his colleagues developed a taxonomy of explanations for describing ineffective therapies and their seeming benefits (Lilienfeld et al., 2014). We hope this chapter impels further work that is inspired by the legacy Scott left behind.

References

Abramowitz, J., Taylor, S., & McKay, D. (2005). Potentials and limitations of cognitive treatments for obsessive-compulsive disorder. *Cognitive Behaviour Therapy, 34*, 140–147.

Alloy, L. B., Peterson, C., Abramson, L. Y., & Seligman, M. E. (1984). Attribution style and the generality of learned helplessness. *Journal of Personality and Social Psychology, 46*, 681–687.

Beck, A. T., Rush, A. J., Shaw, B. F., & Emery, G. (1979). *Cognitive therapy of depression*. Guilford.

Bennett-Levy, J., Butler, G., Fennell, M., Hackman, A., Mueller, M., & Westbrook, D. (2004). *Oxford guide to behavioral experiments in cognitive therapy*. Oxford Press.

Bowes, S. M., Ammirati, R. J., Costello, T. H., Basterfield, C., & Lilienfeld, S. O. (2020). Cognitive biases, heuristics, and logical fallacies in clinical practice: A brief field guide for practicing clinicians and supervisors. *Professional Psychology: Research and Practice, 51*, 435–445.

Brown, H. (2013, March 25). Looking for evidence that therapy works. *New York Times*. https://well.blogs.nytimes.com/2013/03/25/looking-for-evidence-that-therapy-works/

Cisler, J. M., & Koster, E. H. W. (2010). Mechanisms of attentional biases toward threat in anxiety disorders: An integrative review. *Clinical Psychology Review, 30*, 203–216.

David, D. (2013). E-prime/R-prime and emotion regulation in the context of the binary model of distress: An experimental investigation based on the general semantics framework. *Journal of Cognitive and Behavioral Psychotherapies, 13*, 1–11.

Ellis, A. (1962). *Reason and emotion in psychotherapy*. Penguin.

Ellis, A. (2001). *Feeling better, getting better, staying better: Profound self-help therapy*. Impact Publishers.

Ellis, A., & Harper, R. A. (1975). *A guide to rational living*. Wilshire Publishing.

Eynon, T. (2002). Cognitive linguistics. *Advances in Psychiatric Treatment, 8*, 399–407.

Farrell, N. R., Kemp, J. J., Blakey, S. M., Meyer, J. M., & Deacon, B. J. (2016). Targeting clinician concerns about exposure therapy: A pilot study comparing standard vs. enhanced training. *Behaviour Research and Therapy, 85*, 53–59.

Furukawa, T. A., Suganuma, A., Ostinelli, E. G., Andersson, G., Beevers, C. G., Shumake, J., Berger, T., et al. (2021). Dismantling, optimizing, and personalizing internet cognitive behavioural therapy for depression: A systematic review and component network meta-analysis using individual participant data. *Lancet Psychiatry, 8*, 500–511.

Greenwood, J. D. (1999). Understanding the 'cognitive revolution' in psychology. *Journal of the History of the Behavioral Sciences, 35*, 1–22.

Hallion, L. S., & Ruscio, A. M. (2011). A meta-analysis of the effect of cognitive bias modification on anxiety and depression. *Psychological Bulletin, 137*, 940–958.

Hernandez-Ramos, R., Altszyler, E., Figeroa, C., Avila-Garcia, P., & Aguilera, A. (2022). Linguistic analysis of Latinx patients' responses to a text messaging adjunct during cognitive behavioral therapy for depression. *Behaviour Research and Therapy, 150*, 104027.

Hollon, S. D., & Beck, A. T. (2013). Cognitive and cognitive-behavioral therapies. In M. J. Lambert (Ed.), *Bergin and Garfield's handbook of psychotherapy and behavior change* (pp. 393–441). Wiley.

Irwin, W., & Bassham, G. (2003). Depression, informal fallacies, and cognitive therapy: The critical thinking cure? *Inquiry: Critical Thinking Across the Disciplines, 21*, 15–21.

Joseph, J. E. (1996). The immediate sources of the 'Sapir-Whorf Hypothesis'. *Historiographia Linguistica, 23*, 365–404.

Kim, E. H., Hollon, S. D., & Olatunji, B. O. (2016). Clinical errors in cognitive-behavior therapy. *Psychotherapy, 53*, 325–330.

Knowles, M. M., Foden, P., El-Deredy, W., & Wells, A. (2016). A systematic review of efficacy of the attention training technique in clinical and nonclinical samples. *Journal of Clinical Psychology, 72*, 999–1025.

Lilienfeld, S. O. (2007). Psychological treatments that cause harm. *Perspectives on Psychological Science, 2*, 53–70.

Lilienfeld, S. O., Lohr, J. M., & Morier, D. (2009). The teaching of courses in the science and pseudoscience of psychology: Useful resources. *Teaching of Psychology, 28*, 182–191.

Lilienfeld, S. O., Ritschel, L. A., Lynn, S. J., Cautin, R. L., & Latzman, R. D. (2014). Why ineffective psychotherapies appear to work: A taxonomy of causes of spurious therapeutic effectiveness. *Perspectives on Psychological Science, 9*, 355–387.

Lilienfeld, S. O., Lynn, S. J., & Lohr, J. M. (2015). *Science and pseudoscience in clinical psychology* (2nd ed.). Guilford.
MacLeod, C. M., Watts, F., Mathews, A., & Williams, J. M. G. (1999). *Cognitive psychology and emotional disorders* (2nd ed.). Wiley.
Marino, L., & Lilienfeld, S. O. (1998). Dolphin-assisted therapy: Flawed data, flawed conclusions. *Anthrozoös, 11*, 194–200.
McKay, D. (2014). Awareness and dissemination. *The Behavior Therapist, 37*, 77–79.
McNally, R. J. (2003). *Remembering trauma*. Harvard University Press.
McQuaid, J. R., Lin, E. N., Barber, J. P., Breland-Noble, A. M., Cuijpers, P., Greenberg, L. S., Jones, V. Y., et al. (2019). *APA clinical practice guidelines for the treatment of depression across three age cohorts*. American Psychological Association.
Meichenbaum, D. (1977). *Cognitive-behavior modification*. Springer.
Murguia, E., & Diaz, K. (2015). The philosophical foundations of cognitive behavioral therapy: Stoicism, Buddhism, Taoism, and Existentialism. *Journal of Evidence-based Psychotherapies, 15*, 37–50.
Newman, M. G., Agras, W. S., Haaga, D. A. F., & Jarrett, R. B. (2021). Cognitive, behavioral, and cognitive behavioral therapy. In M. Barkham, W. Lutz, & L. Castonguay (Eds.), *Bergin and Garfield's handbook of psychotherapy and behavior change* (pp. 469–506). Wiley.
Oltean, H. R., & David, D. O. (2020). Affective and cognitive correlates of the frequency of the verb "to be": An empirical test of E-prime theory. *Journal of Rational-Emotive and Cognitive-Behavior Therapy, 38*, 143–154.
Pederson, E. (2010). Cognitive linguistics and linguistic relativity. In D. Geeraerts & H. Cuyckens (Eds.), *The Oxford handbook of cognitive linguistics*. Oxford Press. https://doi.org/10.1093/oxfordhb/9780199738632.013.0038
Price, R. B., Wallace, M., Kuckertz, J. M., Amir, N., Graur, S., Cummings, L., Popa, P., Carlbring, P., & Bar-Haim, Y. (2016). Pooled patient-level meta-analysis of children and adults completing a computer-based anxiety intervention targeting attentional bias. *Clinical Psychology Review, 50*, 37–49.
Richard, D. C. S., & Lauterbach, D. (2006). *Handbook of exposure therapies*. Academic Press.
Risen, J., & Gilovich, T. (2007). Informal logical fallacies. In R. J. Sternberg & H. L. Roediger (Eds.), *Critical thinking in psychology* (pp. 110–130). Cambridge Press.
Russell, R. L., & Stiles, W. B. (1979). Categories for classifying language in psychotherapy. *Psychological Bulletin, 86*, 404–419.
Shihata, S., McEvoy, P. M., Mullan, B. A., & Carleton, R. N. (2016). Intolerance of uncertainty in emotional disorders: What uncertainties remain? *Journal of Anxiety Disorders, 41*, 115–124.
Wiltshire, T. J., Philipsen, J. S., Trasmundi, S. B., Jensen, T. W., & Steffensen, S. V. (2020). Interpersonal coordination dynamics in psychotherapy: A systematic review. *Cognitive Therapy and Research, 44*, 752–773.

When Psychotherapy Fails

Brechje Dandachi-FitzGerald, Henry Otgaar, and Harald Merckelbach

In a landmark paper about harmful treatments, Scott Lilienfeld (2007) argued that the field of psychology should prioritize its efforts to identify adverse therapy effects. He summarized research showing that a sizeable minority of individuals deteriorate during the course of certain psychological interventions. However, as Lilienfeld eloquently pointed out, symptom escalation during psychological treatment is not the same as symptom escalation *due* to psychological treatment.

To determine whether a psychological intervention is beneficial, clinical researchers generally use the methodology of the Randomized Control Trial (RCT), meaning that patients are randomly assigned to either treatment or control groups. When multiple independent studies conclude that treated patients exhibit considerably more symptom decline than control patients, it is safe to assume that the improvement is due to the psychological intervention. This way, empirically supported treatments have been established for specific psychological conditions (Kendall, 1998), which formed a major impetus for, for example, the Improving Access to Psychological Therapies movement in the United Kingdom (e.g., Wakefield et al., 2021).

Understandably, the empirical literature on psychological treatment effects focuses on what works and why. However, Lilienfeld (2007) rightly pointed out that by using the RCT approach, not only successes and victories, but also potentially harmful treatments (PHTs) can be identified. Based on the scarce literature that was available at the time he was writing his paper, Lilienfeld compiled a provisional list of PHTs (see also Teachman et al., 2021). More generally, he argued that in

B. Dandachi-FitzGerald · H. Merckelbach (✉)
Faculty of Psychology and Neuroscience, Maastricht University, Maastricht, The Netherlands
e-mail: h.merckelbach@maastrichtuniversity.nl

H. Otgaar
Faculty of Psychology and Neuroscience, Maastricht University, Maastricht, The Netherlands

Faculty of Law and Criminology, KU Leuven, Leuven, Belgium

C. L. Cobb et al. (eds.), *Toward a Science of Clinical Psychology*,
https://doi.org/10.1007/978-3-031-14332-8_16

treatment outcome research, safety assessments should take precedence over benefits assessments, as clinicians have the primary responsibility to do no harm.

Lilienfeld's message had a tremendous impact in the field of psychology and promoted research on psychotherapeutic expertise and how it may help clinicians to recognize adverse side effects and reduce the risk of therapy failure. In this chapter, we discuss therapeutic failures, adverse events, and therapy side effects (see Table 1 for operational definitions of the main concepts in this chapter). We first address the issue of expertise in psychotherapy. Then we take a historical perspective and briefly

Table 1 Operational definition of main concepts in this chapter

Concept	Definition	Source
Treatment Failure	Treatment non-response, premature treatment termination out of dissatisfaction, or deterioration over the course of psychotherapy	Lilienfeld (2007)
Adverse Event (AE)/Unwanted Event (UE)	Any negative change in physical or mental health, in the social or professional environment as relevantly experienced by the patient or a significant other/close family member or as observed by the treating therapist (since last treatment session/previously asked).	Klatte et al. (2022)
	All negative events that occur in parallel with or after psychological treatment	Linden (2013)
Serious Adverse Event (SAE)	(a) a non–life-threatening event, such as (re-) hospitalization or prolongation of existing hospitalization, (significant) enduring severe impairment and dysfunction, permanent damage, severe or medically significant but not immediately life-threatening events, any medical event that might jeopardize the patient or require intervention to prevent it, or deterioration of symptoms for two weeks or longer or	Klatte et al. (2022)
	(b) a life-threatening event, including suicidality or	
	(c) (sudden) death.	
Adverse Side Effects/Adverse Treatment Reactions	(serious) adverse events caused by correctly applied treatment; i.e., treatment adhering to standard of care.	Linden (2013)
Negative Effects/Negative Experiences	Adverse/unwanted events attributed by the patient to their treatment, for example, in self-report questionnaires such as the Negative Effects Questionnaire (Rozental et al., 2016). For survey studies we prefer the term "experience" because the term "effects" suggests a causal relationship that cannot be established in these study designs.	Dandachi-FitzGerald et al. (2022)
Potentially Harmful Treatments	treatments that have:	Lilienfeld (2007)
	(a) demonstrated harmful psychological or physical effects in clients or others (e.g., relatives)	
	(b) the harmful effects are enduring and do not merely reflect a short-term exacerbation of symptoms during treatment	
	(c) the harmful effects have been replicated by independent investigative teams	

discuss how the two oldest psychotherapeutic orientations—psychoanalysis and behavioral therapy—have dealt with therapeutic failures and harm. Subsequently, we will focus on patient deterioration in clinical practice and discuss how to recognize patients who deteriorate during the course of treatment, how to conceptualize factors that contribute to such worsening, and how to minimize the risk of therapeutic failure or harm. This chapter ends with a list of six recommendations to improve the safety and effectiveness of psychological care.

Expertise in Psychotherapy

What is an expert? What makes a person a good physician, engineer, judge, or—what matters here—a good psychotherapist? Scientists who are interested in these questions often take the following stance: One can recognize experts not so much by their successes, but rather by the degree to which they follow their profession's rules and insights (e.g., professional practice guidelines) (Lerner & Tetlock, 1999). This emphasis on professional rules and insights allows for defining and detecting failures. For example, there are protocols in place for surgical amputations (e.g., "sign your site") and not following them is considered to raise the risk of preventable wrong-site surgery (e.g., Canale, 2005). On the other hand, a physician may treat their patient according to the standard of care, and the patient may nevertheless die due to an unpreventable complication (e.g., pulmonary thromboembolism; Mobilia et al., 2014). Such a negative outcome reflects the profession's limits rather than the physician's lack of expertise.

Feedback on adherence to evidence-based protocols and guidelines is considered essential for acquiring expertise (Ericsson, 2009). However, for feedback to be useful, it must be correct. Biased feedback may increase confidence in the absence of genuine expertise. Circumstances that encourage biased feedback constitute, what is called, *wicked learning environments*, because they promote pseudo-expertise. Consider, as an example, the nineteenth century New York physician, who had the reputation of being an expert on typhoid fever (Hogarth, 2001). His diagnoses were said to be error-free, and in a way they were. With his contaminated fingers, he used to palpate the tongues of his patients, so that they contracted the dreaded disease, which the physician and his circle, in turn, took as a sign of eminent expertise.

The conditions under which psychological treatments are given may easily amount to a wicked learning environment. In general, clinicians do not receive objective, consistent, and immediate feedback on their interventions (Lilienfeld et al., 2014; Tracey et al., 2014). As Lilienfeld (2007) noted, awareness that critical feedback on failures is essential for growth in expertise was for a long time largely absent in the domain of psychotherapy. Indeed, looking at the period from 1964 to 2011, Linden (2013) identified only a handful of scientific papers on adverse side effects (see Table 1) in this domain.

Freud and His Successes

The lack of interest in therapeutic failure has its historical precursors. Sigmund Freud and Joseph Breuer (1885; 1970) claimed in *StudienÜberHysterie* (Studies on Hysteria) that the treatment of patient Anna O. with hypnosis had been a tremendous success. However, Freud knew very well that Anno O. had not become better after the treatment had ended. On the contrary, she had been admitted to a psychiatric institution repeatedly. Freud ignored this information. This insensitivity to treatment fiasco is intertwined with the Freudian notion that a struggling patient is someone who resists because the psychoanalyst exposes them (or more technically their consciousness) to a painful, but previously hidden, truth (Ellenberger, 1972). Protest, contradiction, and symptomatic escalation are seen by Freud and his intellectual heirs as signs of treatment response. The more miserable the patient feels, the more the psychoanalyst's interpretations are apparently uncovering a deeply hidden conflict. In a way, the psychoanalyst can never be wrong in their interpretation, hindering critical reflection on the role of therapists and their interventions as possible contributing factors to adverse events and treatment failure (but see Peebles, 2018).

Behavioral Therapy and Its Failures

Unlike Freud and his intellectual descendants, the pioneers of behavioral therapy were determined to study therapy failures and ways to reduce them (Barlow, 1980). For example, Foa and Emmelkamp edited an influential book on the topic, *Failures in Behavior Therapy* (1983). It is no coincidence that behavioral therapists wrote—and write (e.g., Janse et al., 2017)—about what can be learned from failures. After all, the Freudians had proclaimed that behavioral therapy is only symptom treatment (e.g., Bookbinder, 1962). By their view, patients who are treated with behavioral therapy will sooner or later develop new complaints, because their inner conflicts remain dormant for a while, but then will resurface, a phenomenon called "symptom substitution," which would be a form of treatment fiasco. But does the phenomenon exist at all? Behavioral therapists searched diligently, but found no evidence for it. Tryon (2008, p. 967) listed 35 years of empirical research on symptom substitution and concluded that "no clear evidence of symptom substitution could be found." Lilienfeld et al. (2011) listed symptom substitution as one of the myths in psychology. Admittedly, some patients appear to suffer from new symptoms during behavioral therapy, but in those cases, other explanations (e.g., symptom over-reporting for financial reasons) than symptom substitution seem more likely (Blanchard & Hersen, 1976; but see also Schermuly-Haupt et al., 2018).

It was not only Freudian notions about symptom substitution, but also critical points raised in their own ranks that fostered the interest of some behavioral therapists in therapy failure. For example, Pavlovians had argued that a sudden confrontation with a phobic object—so-called flooding—will fuel the phobic fear because of sensitization (Barlow, 2010). That idea did not stand up to empirical testing either (Barlow, 2010; but see Moritz et al., 2015).

Worse During Psychotherapy

Bystedt et al. (2014) conducted a survey among 1,400 therapists about their experiences with patients getting worse as a result of psychotherapy. Only 74 respondents (<6%) completed the survey. Of this select group, 95% said that therapeutic failures do occur, while 75% reported having observed it themselves as a therapist.

Hardy et al. (2019) interviewed both patients and therapists about adverse events during psychotherapy. Strikingly, patients rated their negative therapy experience as much more harmful than therapists. Other authors have also noted that psychotherapists often underestimate the negative experiences of their patients during treatment (Kächele & Schachter, 2014), a point to which we return below.

Another indication for the low priority given to the topic of therapeutic failures can be found in research on psychotherapeutic outcome (so-called "trials"; Berk & Parker, 2009; Nutt & Sharpe, 2008). Often, trials in the domain of psychotherapy do not monitor adverse events (Holmes et al., 2018; Parry et al., 2016). It is an omission that *The Lancet Psychiatry Commission on Psychological Treatment Research in Tomorrow's Science* also observes: "Historically, psychological therapy trials have been poor at both monitoring hypothesized side effects and deterioration, and reporting serious adverse effects" (Holmes et al., 2018, p. 257).

Negative experiences related to psychotherapy are far from rare. For example, as part of an ongoing research project (Dandachi-FitzGerald et al., 2022), we asked 200 former patients whether they had experienced negative effects (see Table 1) related to psychological treatment. In total, 90% indicated that they had experienced at least one adverse treatment effect, with a median of six reported negative treatment experiences for the total sample. The five most frequently reported negative treatment experiences were: an increase in negative thoughts and memories (55%), feeling overwhelmed by emotions (50%), an upsurge in stress (47%), feeling vulnerable and unprotected (38%), and escalation of symptoms for which help was sought (33%). A sizeable proportion (14%) reported the emergence of suicidal thoughts. Seven participants (4%) reported boundary violations (see Fig. 1) such as verbal abuse, mockery, coercion, or sexual harassment. The self-reported intensity of negative experiences varied. To illustrate, of the participants who said that they had noticed an increase in negative thoughts and memories, 25% evaluated this as *somewhat negative*, 46% as *quite negative*, and 30% as *very negative*. The self-reported duration also varied: 13% of the respondents indicated that they had suffered from this for *a short time*; 28% for *several days to weeks*; 45% for *months*; and 15% suffered from this *permanently* (until the end of the therapy).

Crawford et al. (2016) queried nearly 15,000 patients who had received treatment for an anxiety disorder or depression. The treatments varied from psychodynamically oriented interventions to cognitive behavioral therapy. Patients were asked whether they had "lasting bad effects from the treatment." Five percent answered affirmatively. Interestingly, patients who said they had received sufficient information about the therapy prior to the beginning of therapy reported fewer adverse events than those who said that they had not been well informed during the

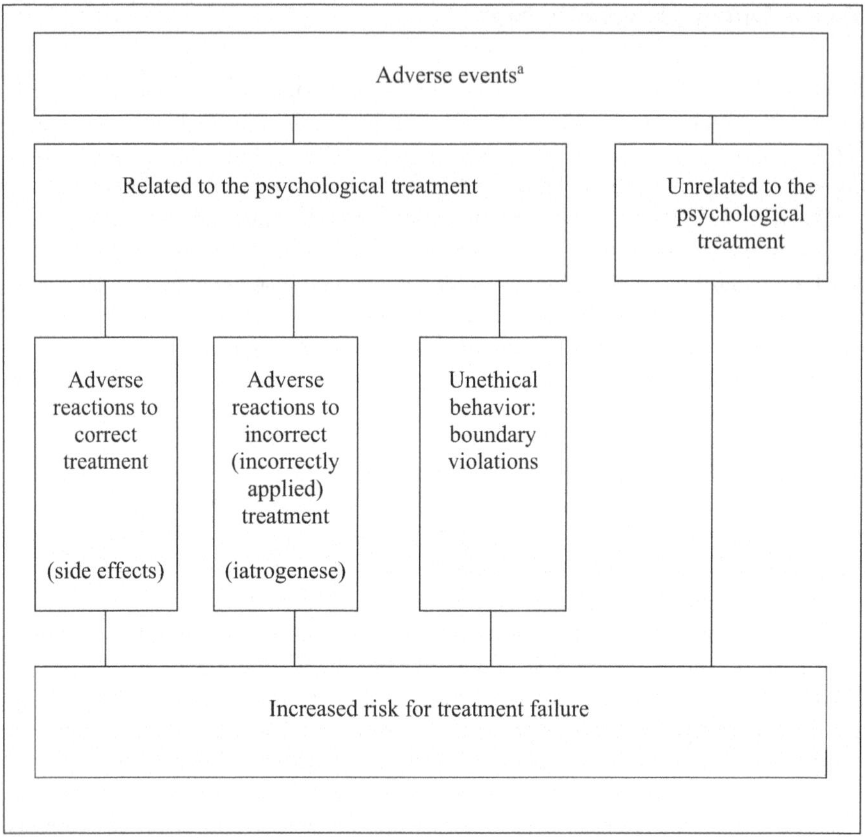

Fig. 1 Linden's taxonomy of adverse events (2013)
[a]Adverse events are defined by Linden as all negative events that occur in parallel with or after psychological treatment. Some examples are: increase in severity of symptoms, new symptoms, tensions within the partner relationship, stigmatization, loss experiences, sick leave from work.

informed consent procedures. Informed consent procedures are an important avenue for future research, because we know little about how information leaflets and informed consents shape expectancies and potential negative effects of people undergoing psychotherapy (see also Blease et al., 2016).

Predicting Failures

Psychotherapists are not accurate in predicting treatment failures (Tracey et al., 2014). For example, Hannan et al. (2005) asked 48 therapists to provide a prognosis for 550 patients. Therapists were provided with the base rate of client deterioration (i.e., 8%) and informed about the independent criterion for measuring treatment outcome: the Outcome Questionnaire-45 (OQ-45, Lambert et al., 2004). The weekly outcome scores on the OQ-45 were not shared with the therapist during the study. Only 3 (0.01%) of 550 patients were predicted to deteriorate, but only 1 of those predicted to deteriorate had, in actuality, deteriorated at the end of therapy. Actual outcome data indicated that 40 patients (7.3%) deteriorated by the end of therapy. Hannan et al. (2005, p. 161) interpreted these findings "as indicating that therapists tend to overpredict improvement and fail to recognize patients who worsen during therapy" (Hannan et al., 2005, p. 161).

To predict treatment response is notoriously difficult. One key question is whether therapists notice when their patients are getting worse over the course of psychotherapy so that they can intervene to reduce the risk of therapy failure. Hatfield et al. (2010) examined notes that psychotherapists compiled concerning their patients. The researchers found that based on the OQ-45 treatment progress scores, 380 (9%) patients deteriorated during treatment. However, this deterioration was often overlooked in therapists' notes. The authors concluded that: "therapists did not indicate client worsening in their notes close to 70% of the time. It appears that often, therapists simply have difficulty noticing client deterioration" (Hatfield et al., 2010, p. 30).

Some authors have speculated that therapists are hindered by a self-serving bias, which would make it difficult for them to predict treatment failure and premature treatment termination. Although the notion of self-serving bias possesses much prima facie validity, the empirical evidence that it plays a critical role in therapists' underestimation of treatment failure is weak at best (see Dandachi-FitzGerald et al., 2021).

Potentially Harmful Treatments

Researchers have estimated that deterioration occurs in about 5–20% of psychotherapy patients (Linden & Schermuly-Haupt, 2014). However, not all negative experiences are causally related to therapy. Feeling worse *during* or *after* psychotherapy is not the same as feeling worse *because* of psychotherapy. There are, however, interventions that are demonstrably iatrogenic (Barlow, 2010; Lilienfeld, 2007; Williams et al., 2021; see Table 1 for a definition of potentially harmful treatments). Examples are *Critical Incident Stress Debriefing* interventions (Mitchell, 1983) in which people are confronted with their traumatic experience, *Scared Straight* interventions (Shapiro, 1978) for conduct-disordered adolescents, or suggestive interventions in which repressed memories of abuse are uncovered (Otgaar et al., 2019).

Interventions to recover memories are particularly problematic because such memories may be inaccurate and are often experienced as highly disturbing. For example, Rozental et al. (2016) noted that 38% of the patients they surveyed (N = 653) mentioned "unpleasant memories [that] surfaced" during treatment explicitly as a negative experience. Fetkewicz et al. (2000) examined 20 patients seeking help for depressive symptoms. These patients were eventually diagnosed with multiple personality disorder (currently dissociative identity disorder). During treatment, uncovering traumatic childhood memories became a prominent goal, whereas less attention was paid to patients' depressive symptoms. Depressive symptoms often became worse, possibly because of the distress caused by the recovered trauma memories. Tragically enough, 60% ($n = 12$) of patients attempted suicide.

In a recent Italian legal case, a therapist was sentenced to four years in prison because of implanting false memories of abuse in a young girl. Studying therapeutic excerpts, Otgaar et al. (2022) found evidence that the therapist had used highly suggestive questions and relied on improper therapeutic techniques making the young girl falsely remember to have been abused by her father. This case illustrates that harmful treatments are not only perilous for the patient, but can be for the therapist as well.

A Taxonomy

Arguably, the scarcity of systematic research on therapeutic failures is linked to the absence of a classification scheme for adverse events during treatment. The lack of such a classification scheme obfuscates talking about potential adverse events and discussing whether they can plausibly be linked to therapy, natural course, or external factors. With this consideration in mind, Linden (2013) developed a first draft of a taxonomy that might help therapists to reflect on (1) adverse events, (2) the extent to which they are caused by treatment, and (3) whether they can best be conceptualized as adverse reactions to correct treatment or as the result of incorrect treatment. Linden's taxonomy ranges from factors external to therapy that cause setbacks (e.g., being fired because of a reorganization) through inevitable side effects due to correctly applied therapeutic interventions (e.g., increase of anxiety during exposure) to iatrogenic effects of ill-applied treatments (e.g., false memories after hypnosis). Figure 1 shows a simplified version of Linden's taxonomy. We think that taxonomies such as this one may help therapists to provide and receive critical feedback during, for example, supervision sessions.

Whereas Linden's taxonomy is a tool for therapists and focuses on events, Rozental et al. (2016) developed the Negative Effects Questionnaire (NEQ) that patients can complete to indicate negative experiences during psychotherapy. The NEQ contains 32 items (e.g., "unpleasant memories resurfaced") that are scored on a 5-point Likert scale (anchors: not all; extremely). Furthermore, patients indicate whether they believe that the negative experiences are related to their treatment. Over the past years, several researchers have employed the NEQ or similar instruments to study negative experiences systematically and whether they are—according to patients—related to therapy. Table 2 summarizes these studies. As can be seen, between 22% and 93% of patients across the studies reported at least one negative treatment experience. This wide range is likely the result of heterogeneity in patient samples and differences in assessment methods (e.g., questionnaires used,

Table 2 Frequency of negative treatment experiences reported by patients

Study	Sample	*N*	Questionnaire	Pertaining to	≥1 negative treatment experience (% sample)	Most frequently endorsed items
Moritz et al. (2015)	Patients with OCD	85	SEPS (97 items)	Previous individual treatment for OCD, preferably last treatment	93	Disappointment about not feeling better at the end of therapy
						Most of the therapeutic content was already familiar
						Therapy was too much talking, and too few exercises
Holsting et al. (2017)	Patients with functional somatic syndromes	80	INEP (21 items)	Current treatment upon completion	31	Feeling addicted to the therapist
						Difficulties in finding health insurance, or feeling anxious to apply for insurance
						Feeling down after therapy
Rheker et al. (2017)	*Sample 1*: Mixed sample psychiatric hospital patients	93	INEP (21 items)	Current treatment upon completion	59	Experiencing more downs during or just before the end of therapy
	Sample 2: Mixed sample psychosomatic rehabilitation hospital patients	63			54	Difficulty making important decisions without the therapist
						Concerns that others might find out about the therapy

(continued)

Table 2 (continued)

Study	Sample	*N*	Questionnaire	Pertaining to	≥1 negative treatment experience (% sample)	Most frequently endorsed items
Moritz et al. (2019)	Patients with depressive disorder	135	PANEPS[a] (43 items)	Last treatment on average 3 years after therapy ended	53	Feeling exhausted after the therapy session
						Feeling worse after therapy ended, because missing conversations with the therapist
						Being fearful that others find out about the therapy
Rozental et al. (2019)	Patients in five clinical CBT trials for specific disorders (e.g., spider phobia, social anxiety disorders)	564	NEQ short form (20 items)	Current treatment upon completion	51	Experiencing more stress
						Resurfacing of unpleasant memories
						Experiencing more anxiety

(continued)

Table 2 (continued)

Study	Sample	*N*	Questionnaire	Pertaining to	≥1 negative treatment experience (% sample)	Most frequently endorsed items
Reins et al. (2019)	Patients following Internet CBT intervention for depression	47	INEP, adapted version (15 items)	Current treatment	26	During the training or since completing the training there were phases I was feeling mentally unwell.
						Since completing the training I have suffered more from past events than I did before.
						During the training or since completing the training I got in trouble regarding my insurances or I fear that problems may appear in the future.
						Since completing the training I experience more conflicts with my partner than before.

(continued)

Table 2 (continued)

Study	Sample	*N*	Questionnaire	Pertaining to	≥1 negative treatment experience (% sample)	Most frequently endorsed items
Gerke et al. (2020)[b]	*Sample 1*: Mixed sample outpatient treatment	197	INEP (21 items)	Last treatment	22	Feeling hurt by the therapist's remarks (e.g., feeling misunderstood).
				Sample 1: on average 4 years after therapy ended		Insurance problems/worries
	Sample 2: Mixed sample inpatient treatment	118		*Sample 2*: on average 9 months after therapy ended	66	Experiencing more downs since the end of therapy
						Experiencing force by therapist to do things (e.g., confrontations, role-plays)
Oehler et al. (2021)	Patients with mild to moderate depression	260	INEP, adapted version (18 items)	RCT	30	Dependent on content of program
				Treatment condition ($n = 130$): Internet intervention Fight Depression		Long periods of feeling bad
				Active control condition ($n = 130$): progressive muscle relaxation	31	Felt not taken seriously

Note. *INEP* Inventory for the assessment of negative effects of psychotherapy, *NEQ* negative effects questionnaire, *OCD* obsessive-compulsive disorder, *PANEPS* positive and negative effects of psychotherapy, *SEPS* side-effects of psychotherapy scale, *SE* side effects

[a]PANEPS is a short version of the SEPS; [b]This study reported the frequency for ≥1 negative treatment experiences for the two subscales, Side Effects and Malpractice-Unethical Behavior, separately. Here we added the two subscale percentages as an indication of the overall frequency

completed for current treatment versus prior treatment, anonymous or not). Nonetheless, even the lower bound percentage is non-trivial and underlines the need for psychotherapy trials to monitor negative experiences to determine the safety and tolerability of interventions.

Monitoring and Feedback of Symptomatology

Instruments such as the NEQ can provide therapists with feedback about a looming therapy failure and in this way promote clinical expertise (Goldberg et al., 2016). There is much to recommend a therapeutic approach that monitors patients' symptom levels during treatment so that therapists can use feedback information about these levels to terminate, amend, or intensify treatment. Lambert et al. (2005), for example, examined the effects of feedback on therapists' ability to prevent or minimize deterioration during therapy. In a large-scale research project, these researchers demonstrated that feedback benefits the quality of psychotherapeutic treatment. When no feedback system was provided, 21% of the patients ($n = 61$) had deteriorated at the end of treatment. However, the percentage of deteriorating patients was 13% ($n = 40$) when therapists were provided with feedback about the risk of treatment failure of their patients, and it was 9% ($n = 5$) when this feedback was expanded with advice to the therapist on how to act.

As another example, Janse et al. (2017) examined whether monitoring and feedback would increase the therapeutic potential of cognitive behavioral therapy. They included 1006 patients and 84 therapists in their study. The researchers monitored treatment with the *Outcome Rating Scale* at the start of each session and the *Session Rating Scale* at the end of each session (Miller & Duncan, 2000). Overall, therapists who received feedback about patients' symptom levels were as effective as those not provided with feedback. However, within the subgroup of depressive patients, therapists provided with feedback were more successful in terms of symptom reduction than those not provided with feedback. Also, those who received feedback needed fewer sessions to obtain a similar treatment outcome as therapists not provided with feedback. In their multi-level meta-analysis including 58 studies and 21.699 patients, de Jong et al. (2021) found a small, but significant effect of progress feedback on reducing symptoms and dropout rates, supporting the general idea that providing therapists with feedback increases the positive impact of their interventions.

Monitoring symptom levels of patients over the course of therapy and feeding this information back to therapists might help these professionals to understand which elements in their treatment are productive and which are not. Without such monitoring and feedback, therapists are vulnerable to the hello-goodbye bias (Tracey et al., 2014). That is, at the start of the treatment, patients may over-report symptoms hoping to be eligible for treatment, whereas at the end of the treatment, they might under-report symptoms to make a good impression on the therapist. Without a detailed monitoring of how symptomatology evolves over the course of therapy, therapists might erroneously conclude that their intervention was more successful than warranted by objective indicators. Lilienfeld et al. (2014) discussed the hello-goodbye bias as one of the many sources of spurious therapy gains that lead clinicians to "perceive improvements in patients in their absence and fail to perceive deterioration in their presence" (p. 360).

Final Thoughts

In general, people are poor at determining causal dynamics, which also holds for therapists understanding the causal agents of symptom escalation or reduction in patients undergoing therapy. The evidence summarized by Lilienfeld et al. (2014) suggests that therapist often overestimate their ability to influence events. Specifically, people who take on the role of therapist tend to associate their interventions with positive outcomes in a biased way such that they exhibit an "illusion of control." For example, Matute et al. (2015) had participants read case vignettes of patients. Several conditions were manipulated and presented in conjunction arbitrarily: fictitious patients could get better or not; they could receive medication or not; and participants in their role of clinician could indicate that they would administer medication or not. Whenever medication was paired with symptomatic relief, participants tended to attribute this to a meaningful connection rather than chance. Perceiving such an illusory correlation (i.e., perceiving a connection between two events—here: medication and symptom reduction—that are actually unrelated) was particularly strong when participants played the role of clinician. Apparently, initiating interventions promotes a bias to perceive therapy-related improvements that are not necessarily present.

The illusion of control conspires against therapists' awareness of harmful therapy interventions. Precisely because the topic can be easily overlooked, adverse therapy effects deserve to be prioritized on the research agenda. This is all the more important given the following two considerations. First, ideally, psychotherapeutic interventions are evaluated in randomized controlled trials (RCTs). RCTs generate solid evidence-based knowledge about optimal patient-treatment combinations. However, there are important differences between RCTs in the psychotherapeutic and pharmacological domain. For pharmacological RCTs, it is standing policy to preregister in advance a host of details (e.g., number of patients included, types of outcome measurements, monitoring of adverse events). Prospective registration is often a prerequisite for publication of the RCT results in a high-impact journal. In contrast, only about 15% of psychotherapeutic RCTs are based on prospective registration (Cybulski et al., 2016; see also Sakaluk et al., 2019), which in part explains the lack of interest in adverse side effects of psychotherapy: Researchers in this field often do not anticipate such effects and have no system in place to systematically monitor these effects when they do occur. To illustrate, in 2010, only 21% of the published trials (N = 132) included any monitoring of adverse effects reported by patients (Cuijpers, 2021; Jonsson et al., 2014; but see Klatte et al., 2022). This neglect fits well with the general impression that many psychotherapy researchers are motivated by the intention to document the beneficial effects of therapy without regard for potential adverse effects of therapy (Cuijpers et al., 2010; Dragioti et al., 2017). Financial incentives may contribute to this tendency, as Cuijpers et al. (2010, p. 177) explained: "Researchers of psychological treatments do have personal interest in publication of (larger) effects, as these are more likely to lead to tenure and lucrative workshop fees."

A second consideration is the imperative to systematically study the adverse side effects of psychotherapy in order to clarify whether specific groups of patients are particularly vulnerable to such effects. Psychotherapy will benefit many patients, but will harm some of them (Barlow, 2010). Collapsing the outcome data of both groups of patients will preclude a clear interpretation of the effectiveness of psychotherapy. It is more informative to identify which patients deteriorate in response to a particular intervention and whether they would profit from another type of treatment, a question that can better be addressed by single case experimental designs than by RCTs.

These considerations are certainly not new; they are, in fact, strongly present in the work of Lilienfeld (2007; Blease et al., 2016; Lilienfeld et al., 2014). With his intellectual heritage in mind, we provide the following recommendations for policymakers, clinicians, and researchers in the domain of psychotherapy:

1. Invest in research that focuses on psychotherapeutic failures and adverse side effects.
2. Monitor and report adverse events in RCTs (e.g., Ellet & Chadwick, 2021). Monitoring of adverse events should also be done in the context of single-case experimental designs (Vlaeyen et al., 2022), which may shed light on causality issues (e.g., Are certain interventions causing harm in certain individuals?).
3. In designing intervention protocols and training psychotherapists, include a taxonomy of adverse events (e.g., Linden, 2013).
4. Optimize information pamphlets and websites for patients, and do mention explicitly potential adverse effects (Blease et al., 2016);
5. Monitor and provide feedback to therapists and patients regarding therapy processes and outcomes over the course of treatment (de Jong et al. 2021).
6. Give the topic of therapeutic failure a prominent place in the curriculum of psychology graduate schools and psychotherapy courses (see, for example, in the medical curriculum; Mohsin et al., 2019).

To be sure, psychotherapy is human work and can never be free of failures. Still, the therapist plays the role of a catalyst that will become more powerful to the extent that errors, failures, mismatches, complications, drawbacks, and disappointments are explicitly recognized and are followed up with constructive and ameliorative actions.

References

Barlow, D. H. (1980). Behavior therapy: The next decade. *Behavior Therapy, 11*, 315–328.

Barlow, D. H. (2010). Negative effects from psychological treatments. *American Psychologist, 65*, 13–20.

Berk, M., & Parker, G. (2009). The elephant on the couch: Side effects of psychotherapy. *The Australian and New Zealand Journal of Psychiatry, 43*, 787–794.

Blanchard, E. B., & Hersen, M. (1976). Behavioural treatment of hysterical neurosis: Symptom substitution and symptom return reconsidered. *Psychiatry: Interpersonal and Biological Processes, 39*, 118–129.

Blease, C. R., Lilienfeld, S. O., & Kelley, J. M. (2016). Evidence-based practice and psychological treatments: The imperatives of informed consent. *Frontiers in Psychology, 7*, 1170.

Bookbinder, L. J. (1962). Simple conditioning versus the dynamic approach to symptoms and symptom substitution: A reply to Yates. *Psychological Reports, 10*, 71–77.

Bystedt, S., Rozental, A., Andersson, G., Boettcher, J., & Carlbring, P. (2014). Clinicians' perspectives on negative effects of psychological treatments. *Cognitive Behaviour Therapy, 43*, 319–331.

Canale, S. T. (2005). Wrong-site surgery: A preventable complication. *Clinical Orthopaedics and Related Research, 433*, 26–29.

Crawford, M. J., Thana, L., Farquharson, L., Palmer, L., Hancock, E., Bassett, P., Clarke, J., & Parry, G. D. (2016). Patient experience of negative effects of psychological treatment: Results of a national survey. *The British Journal of Psychiatry, 208*, 260–265.

Cuijpers, P. (2021). Research on negative effects of psychotherapies: The next steps. *Clinical Psychology: Science and Practice, 28*, 142–144.

Cuijpers, P., Smit, F., Bohlmeijer, E., Hollon, S. D., & Andersson, G. (2010). Efficacy of cognitive–behavioural therapy and other psychological treatments for adult depression: Meta-analytic study of publication bias. *British Journal of Psychiatry, 196*, 173–178.

Cybulski, L., Mayo-Wilson, E., & Grant, S. (2016). Improving transparency and reproducibility through registration: The status of intervention trial published in clinical psychology journals. *Journal of Consulting and Clinical Psychology, 84*, 753–767.

Dandachi-FitzGerald, B., Meijs, L., Moonen, I. M., & Merckelbach, H. (2021). No self-serving bias in therapists' evaluations of clients' premature treatment termination: An approximate replication of Murdock et al. (2010). *Clinical Psychology & Psychotherapy.* Advance Online Publication.

Dandachi-FitzGerald, B., Houben, S., Otgaar, H., van den Hout, M., & Merckelbach, H. (2022). De schaduwkant van psychotherapie: Hoe vaak rapporteren patiënten negatieve ervaringen? [The shadow side of therapy: How often do patients report negative experiences?]. *Tijdschrift voor Psychotherapie, 48*, 12–23.

de Jong, K., Conijn, J. M., Gallagher, R. A., Reshetnikova, A. S., Heij, M., & Lutz, M. C. (2021). Using progress feedback to improve outcomes and reduce drop-out, treatment duration, and deterioration: A multilevel meta-analysis. *Clinical Psychology Review, 85*, 102002.

Dragioti, E., Karathanos, V., Gerdle, B., & Evangelou, E. (2017). Does psychotherapy work? An umbrella review of meta-analyses of randomized controlled trials. *Acta Psychiatrica Scandinavica, 136*, 236–246.

Ellenberger, H. F. (1972). The story of "Anna O": A critical review with new data. *Journal of the History of the Behavioral Sciences, 8*, 267–279.

Ellet, L., & Chadwick, P. (2021). Recommendations for monitoring and reporting harm in mindfulness for psychosis reseach. *The British Journal of Psychiatry, 219*, 629–631.

Ericsson, K. A. (2009). *Development of professional expertise*. Cambridge University Press.

Fetkewicz, J., Sharma, V., & Merskey, H. (2000). A note on suicidal deterioration with recovered memory treatment. *Journal of Affective Disorders, 58*, 155–159.

Foa, E. B., & Emmelkamp, P. M. (1983). *Failures in behavior therapy*. Wiley.

Freud, S., & Breuer, J. (1885; 1970). *StudienÜberHysterie* [Studies on hysteria]. Fischer.

Gerke, L., Meyrose, A.-K., Ladwig, I., Rief, W., & Nestoriuc, Y. (2020). Frequencies and predictors of negative effects in routine inpatient and outpatient psychotherapy: Two observational studies. *Frontiers in Psychology, 11*, 2144.

Goldberg, S. B., Rousmaniere, T., Miller, S. D., Whipple, J., Nielsen, S. L., Hoyt, W. T., & Wampold, B. E. (2016). Do psychotherapists improve with time and experience? A longitudinal analysis of outcomes in a clinical setting. *Journal of Counseling Psychology, 63*, 1–11.

Hannan, C., Lambert, M. J., Harmon, C., Nielsen, S. L., Smart, D. W., Shimokawa, K., & Sutton, S. W. (2005). A lab test and algorithms for identifying clients at risk for treatment failure. *Journal of Clinical Psychology, 61*, 155–163.

Hardy, G. E., Bishop-Edwards, L., Chambers, E., Connell, J., Dent-Brown, K., Kothari, G., et al. (2019). Risk factors for negative experiences during psychotherapy. *Psychotherapy Research, 29*, 403–414.

Hatfield, D., McCullough, L., Frantz, S. H., & Krieger, K. (2010). Do we know when our clients get worse? An investigation of therapists' ability to detect negative client change. *Clinical Psychology & Psychotherapy, 17*, 25–32.

Hogarth, R. M. (2001). *Educating intuition*. The University of Chicago Press.

Holmes, E. A., Ghaderi, A., Harmer, C. J., Ramchandani, P. G., Cuijpers, P., Morrison, A. P., et al. (2018). The Lancet Psychiatry commission on psychological treatments research in tomorrow's science. *The Lancet Psychiatry, 5*, 237–286.

Holsting, A. F., Pedersen, H. F., Rask, M. T., Frostholm, L., & Schröder, A. (2017). Is psychotherapy for functional somatic syndromes harmful? A mixed methods study on negative effects. *Journal of Psychosomatic Research, 98*, 113–121.

Janse, P. D., De Jong, K., Van Dijk, M. K., Hutschemaekers, G. J., & Verbraak, M. J. (2017). Improving the efficiency of cognitive-behavioural therapy by using formal client feedback. *Psychotherapy Research, 27*, 525–538.

Jonsson, U., Alaie, I., Parlin, T., & Arnberg, F. K. (2014). Reporting of harms in randomized controlled trials of psychological interventions for mental and behavioral disorders: A review of current practice. *Contemporary Clinical Trials, 38*, 1–8.

Kächele, H., & Schachter, J. (2014). On side effects, destructive processes, and negative outcomes in psychoanalytic therapies: Why is it difficult for psychoanalysts to acknowledge and address treatment failures? *Contemporary Psychoanalysis, 50*, 233–258.

Kendall, P. C. (1998). Empirically supported psychological therapies. *Journal of Consulting and Clinical Psychology, 66*, 3–6.

Klatte, R., Strauss, B., Flückiger, C., Färber, F., & Rosendahl, J. (2022). *Defining and assessing adverse events and harmful effects in psychotherapy study protocols: A systematic review. Psychotherapy*. Advance Online Publication.

Lambert, M. J., Morton, J. J., Hatfield, D. R., Harmon, C., Hamilton, S., Reid, R. C., & Burlingame, G. M. (2004). *Administration and scoring manual for the OQ-45.2 (Outcome Questionnaire)*. American Professional Credentialing Services.

Lambert, M. J., Harmon, C., Slade, K., Whipple, J. L., & Hawkins, E. J. (2005). Providing feedback to psychotherapists on their patients' progress: Clinical results and practice suggestions. *Journal of Clinical Psychology, 61*, 165–174.

Lerner, J. S., & Tetlock, P. E. (1999). Accounting for the effects of accountability. *Psychological Bulletin, 125*, 255–275.

Lilienfeld, S. (2007). Psychological treatments that cause harm. *Perspectives on Psychological Science, 2*, 53–70.

Lilienfeld, S. O., Lynn, S. J., Ruscio, J., & Beyerstein, B. L. (2011). *50 great myths of popular psychology: Shattering widespread misconceptions about human behavior*. Wiley.

Lilienfeld, S. O., Ritschel, L. A., Lynn, S. J., Cautin, R. L., & Latzman, R. D. (2014). Why ineffective psychotherapies appear to work: A taxonomy of causes of spurious therapeutic effectiveness. *Perspectives on Psychological Science, 9*, 355–387.

Linden, M. (2013). How to define, find and classify side effects in psychotherapy: From unwanted events to adverse treatment reactions. *Clinical Psychology and Psychotherapy, 20*, 286–296.

Linden, M., & Schermuly-Haupt, M. L. (2014). Definition, assessment and rate of psychotherapy side effects. *World Psychiatry, 13*, 306–309.

Matute, H., Blanco, F., Yarritu, I., Díaz-Lago, M., Vadillo, M. A., & Barberia, I. (2015). Illusions of causality: How they bias our everyday thinking and how they could be reduced. *Frontiers in Psychology, 6*, 888.

Miller, S. D., & Duncan, B. L. (2000). *The outcome and session rating scales: Administration and scoring manuals*. Retrieved 21 January 2021, from: https://scott-d-miller-ph-d.myshopify.com/collections/performance-metrics/products/performance-metrics-licenses-for-the-ors-and-srs

Mitchell, J. T. (1983). When disaster strikes: The critical incident stress debriefing process. *Journal of Emergency Medical Services, 13*, 49–52.

Mobilia, F., Casali, M. B., Gallieni, M., & Genovese, U. R. (2014). Lethal pulmonary thromboembolism: An autopsy-based study on a rare but legally relevant event. *Medicine, Science and the Law, 54*, 78–83.

Mohsin, S. U., Ibrahim, Y., & Levine, D. (2019). Teaching medical students to recognise and report errors. *BMJ Open Quality, 8*, e000558.

Moritz, S., Fieker, M., Hottenrott, B., Seeralan, T., Cludius, B., Kolbeck, K., et al. (2015). No pain, no gain? Adverse effects of psychotherapy in obsessive–compulsive disorder and its relationship to treatment gains. *Journal of Obsessive-Compulsive and Related Disorders, 5*, 61–66.

Moritz, S., Nestoriuc, Y., Rief, W., Klein, J. P., Jelinek, L., & Peth, J. (2019). It can't hurt, right? Adverse effects of psychotherapy in patients with depression. *European Archives of Psychiatry and Clinical Neuroscience, 269*, 577–586.

Nutt, D. J., & Sharpe, M. (2008). Uncritical positive regard? Issues in the efficacy and safety of psychotherapy. *Journal of Psychopharmacology, 22*, 3–6.

Oehler, C., Görges, F., Hegerl, U., & Rummel-Kluge, C. (2021). A closer look at negative effects in a guided web-based intervention for mild to moderate depression. *Clinical Psychology: Science and Practice, 28*, 131.

Otgaar, H., Howe, M. L., Patihis, L., Merckelbach, H., Lynn, S. J., Lilienfeld, S. O., & Loftus, E. F. (2019). The return of the repressed: The persistent and problematic claims of long-forgotten trauma. *Perspectives on Psychological Science, 14*, 1072–1095.

Otgaar, H., Curci, A., Mangiulli, I., Battista, F., Rizzotti, E., & Sartori, G. (2022). A court ruled case on therapy-induced false memories. *Journal of Forensic Sciences*. Advance Online Publication.

Parry, G. D., Crawford, M. J., & Duggan, C. (2016). Iatrogenic harm from psychological therapies – Time to move on. *The British Journal of Psychiatry, 208*, 210–212.

Peebles, M. J. (2018). Harm in hypnosis: Three understandings from psychoanalysis that can help. *American Journal of Clinical Hypnosis, 60*, 239–261.

Reins, J. A., Boß, L., Lehr, D., Berking, M., & Ebert, D. D. (2019). The more I got, the less I need? Efficacy of Internet-based guided self-help compared to online psychoeducation for major depressive disorder. *Journal of Affective Disorders, 246*, 695–705.

Rheker, J., Beisel, S., Kräling, S., & Rief, W. (2017). Rate and predictors of negative effects of psychotherapy in psychiatric and psychosomatic inpatients. *Psychiatry Research, 254*, 143–150.

Rozental, A., Kottorp, A., Boettcher, J., Andersson, G., & Carlbring, P. (2016). Negative effects of psychological treatments: An exploratory factor analysis of the negative effects questionnaire for monitoring and reporting adverse and unwanted events. *PLoS One, 11*, e0157503.

Rozental, A., Kottorp, A., Forsström, D., Månsson, K., Boettcher, J., Andersson, G., et al. (2019). The Negative Effects Questionnaire: Psychometric properties of an instrument for assessing negative effects in psychological treatments. *Behavioural and Cognitive Psychotherapy, 47*, 559–572.

Sakaluk, J. K., Williams, A. J., Kilshaw, R. E., & Rhyner, K. T. (2019). Evaluating the evidential value of empirically supported psychological treatments (ESTs): A meta-scientific review. *Journal of Abnormal Psychology, 128*, 500.

Schermuly-Haupt, M. L., Linden, M., & Rush, A. J. (2018). Unwanted events and side effects in cognitive behavior therapy. *Cognitive Therapy and Research*. in druk.

Shapiro, A. (Director). (1978). *Scared Straight!* [Motion Picture]. Golden West Television.

Teachman, B. A., White, B. A., & Lilienfeld, S. O. (2021). Identifying harmful therapies: Setting the research agenda. *Clinical Psychology: Science and Practice, 28*, 101–106.

Tracey, T. J. G., Wampold, B. E., Lichtenberg, J. W., & Goodyear, R. K. (2014). Expertise in psychotherapy: An elusive goal? *American Psychologist, 69*, 218–229.

Tryon, W. W. (2008). Whatever happened to symptom substitution? *Clinical Psychological Review, 28*, 963–968.

Vlaeyen, J. W. S., Onghena, P., Vannest, K. J., & Kratochwill, T. R. (2022). Single-case experimental designs: Clinical research and practice. In G. J. G. Asmundson (Ed.), *Comprehensive clinical psychology* (Vol. 3, 2nd ed., pp. 1–28). Elsevier.

Wakefield, S., Kellett, S., Simmonds-Buckley, M., Stockton, D., Bradbury, A., & Delgadillo, J. (2021). Improving Access to Psychological Therapies (IAPT) in the United Kingdom: A systematic review and meta-analysis of 10-years of practice-based evidence. *British Journal of Clinical Psychology, 60*, 1–37.

Williams, A. J., Botanov, Y., Kilshaw, R. E., Wong, R. E., & Sakaluk, J. K. (2021). Potentially harmful therapies: A meta-scientific review of evidential value. *Clinical Psychology: Science and Practice, 28*, 5.

Part V
Controversies, Issues, and Future Directions

Multiculturalism and Applied Psychological Science: Critical Considerations and Future Directions

Cory L. Cobb, Seth J. Schwartz, and Sagrario Uriostegui Jaramillo

Beginning in the early 1970s after the advent of the civil rights movement, along with the shifting demographics of the US population, multiculturalism emerged as a powerful sociopolitical movement that has influenced nearly every facet of American psychology, including the disciplines of applied psychology. Such influence is illustrated by the American Psychological Association's (APA) formal endorsement of multiculturalism: "Psychologists are in a position to provide leadership as agents of prosocial change, advocacy, and social justice, thereby promoting societal understanding, affirmation, and appreciation of multiculturalism". The more recent document *Multicultural Guidelines: An Ecological Approach to Context, Identity, and Intersectionality* (APA, 2017) further states:

> These guidelines … speak to the profession's recognition of the important role that diversity and multiculturalism play, both in terms of how individuals and groups define themselves, and how they approach others within the United States … and globally. (p. 6)

The influence of multiculturalism is further evidenced by advocacy efforts to institutionalize the movement in several dimensions in the field. Such efforts include the establishment of APA's Minority Fellowship Program in 1973 designed to increase the number of ethnic and racial minority psychologists (Jones & Austin-Dailey, 2009); the formation of the Office of Ethnic Minority Affairs to address issues faced by ethnic minorities (APA, 1993); the provision of multicultural competence

C. L. Cobb (✉)
College of Human Sciences, Department of Human Development and Family Science, Auburn University, Auburn, AL, USA
e-mail: clc0178@auburn.edu

S. J. Schwartz
College of Education, Department of Kinesiology and Health Education, University of Texas at Austin, Auztin, TX, USA

S. U. Jaramillo
Austin Community College, Austin, TX, USA

C. L. Cobb et al. (eds.), *Toward a Science of Clinical Psychology*,
https://doi.org/10.1007/978-3-031-14332-8_17

guidelines for counseling culturally diverse clients (APA, 2003, 2017); the requirement that training programs give ample attention to issues of cultural diversity as a condition for accreditation (APA, 2015); and the recent adoption of the *APA guidelines on Race and Ethnicity in Psychology: Promoting Responsiveness and Equity* (APA, 2019). Multiculturalism is clearly a powerful movement that has penetrated nearly every domain of psychology.

Given the profound influence of multiculturalism on shaping psychology as a field, some scholars have labeled it as the defining issue of contemporary psychology. For example, Pedersen (1991, 2013) advanced the perspective held by many scholars that multiculturalism represents the "fourth force" of psychology. From this label, multiculturalism is implicitly contrasted against three prior movements that were considered to be the dominant paradigms of their respective areas: psychoanalysis (first force), behaviorism (second force), and humanistic psychology (third force; Bugental, 1964). In this sense, multiculturalism represents a key shift in emphasis within contemporary applied psychology, but one that is distinct from its predecessors. Specifically, whereas both behaviorism and humanistic psychology arose as a fundamental challenge to psychoanalysis, the aim of multiculturalism is not to discredit or replace any of the first three forces. Rather, multiculturalism is a philosophical approach to psychology that presumably improves existing models by promoting awareness of and sensitivity to how such models can be applied to individuals from diverse cultural backgrounds (Mio et al., 2012).

For instance, since the emergence of the multiculturalism movement, clinical psychology has experienced a push to move beyond general classifications and treatment of psychopathology to consider how clinical diagnostic and treatment systems are themselves products of culture (Gone & Kirmayer, 2010; Lewis-Fernandez & Kleinman, 1994; Lopez & Guarnaccia, 2000; Tseng, 2006). From this perspective, all humans exist within a cultural context, as do the systems they create to classify and treat psychological phenomena. Similarly, there has been an increasing emphasis by some scholars on the need to adapt existing preventive interventions to be more culturally sensitive (Bernal, 2006; Hall et al., 2016). The assumption underlying these efforts is that current interventions may be ineffective for culturally diverse individuals because they were designed by and for individuals from the majority culture (e.g., Whites). Although these are but a few examples, multiculturalism represents a highly debated and increasingly pervasive force impacting the research and practice of clinical psychologists.

Our position in the present chapter is that multiculturalism has both made progress *and* resulted in several unappreciated issues that continue to impact research and practice within the field of applied psychology. From this perspective, not all aspects of multiculturalism are beneficial, and not all are problematic. Indeed, one major advancement inherent within multiculturalism is that it has directed much-needed attention to marginalized minority populations that have historically been neglected within American psychology. Another contribution of multiculturalism is that it has encouraged psychologists to move away from one-size-fits-all approaches to consider how psychological phenomena might operate differently across various cultural groups and contexts.

However, despite its prominence, multiculturalism is not without its critics and has been critiqued on several grounds. Many scholars argue that multiculturalism is a pseudoscientific paradigm rooted in identity politics and that it does the field more harm than good. These scholars (e.g., Barry, 2001; Brewer, 1997; Frisby, 2013; Reich, 2002; Wilton et al., 2019) contend that multiculturalism represents a divisive sociopolitical ideology that fosters essentialist group attitudes, reifies group differences, contributes to adverse group stereotypes and divisions, results in negative intergroup feelings, and increases psychological distance between groups. Multiculturalism has been further criticized on several other grounds ranging from its propensity to undermine reason, freedom, and individuality (Adamson, 2017); characterizations as an unworkable and divisive governing principle in societies (Garcea, 2008; Malik, 2015; Townsend, 2018); undermining cohesive communities (Putnam, 2007); its influence in undermining critical thinking (Webster, 1997); characterization as political indoctrination in higher education (Ashenfelter, 2010); allegations that it does not contribute much to effective interventions for minority students in schools (Frisby, 2013); lack of consistently improved outcomes in culturally tailored psychotherapies versus generic therapy models (Benuto & O'Donohue, 2015; Huey & Polo, 2008; Huey et al., 2014), and its strong devotion to contemporary notions of political correctness (Wright & Cummings, 2005).

Given the large range of criticisms, it would be impossible in any single chapter to provide a detailed discussion of every issue prevalent within multiculturalism. Therefore, in the present chapter, we selectively focus on three aspects of multiculturalism that we believe to be most relevant to applied psychologists and that tend to receive considerably less attention in academic circles relative to its proposed benefits. These reasons include: (1) definitional and conceptual issues that lead to considerable confusion in discussions and debates surrounding multiculturalism; (2) an overriding and nearly exclusive emphasis on intergroup differences at the expense of intergroup commonalities; and (3) perceptions of multiculturalism as an exclusive rather than inclusive ideology. Our hope in outlining these issues is to raise awareness among psychologists to the potential harm that could result if some of the pitfalls and boundary conditions of multicultural education, research, and interventions in contemporary psychology are not acknowledged and considered (Cobb et al., 2020; Lilienfeld, 2007).

The perspective advanced in this chapter is based on the understanding that most, if not all, psychological phenomena involve a complex set of tradeoffs—few are 100% beneficial with no negative costs, and few are 100% detrimental with no benefits. Evaluating and weighing costs and benefits is largely a values question that goes beyond science. However, well-corroborated theory and empirical evidence have the potential to inform psychologists regarding the nature of such costs and benefits.

Definitional Issues Within Multiculturalism

When engaging in analysis of any construct, it is critical to define explicitly the construct under investigation. Broadly, multiculturalism is a general label referring to a sociopolitical ideology frequently found in social discourse and scholarship related to civic/governmental affairs, the social sciences, and specific areas of research and teaching within applied psychology (Frisby, 2013). In this sense, and arguably like all constructs in psychology, multiculturalism is an open concept (Pap, 1953) that lacks an explicit or strict definition (Schalk-Soekar & van de Vijver, 2008). Indeed, multiculturalism is a decades-old term that gained considerable popularity in the 1980s but that has been particularly difficult to define. As such, a central challenge to scientifically evaluating assertions and practices within multiculturalism is that many well-known scholars have defined it in considerably different ways (e.g., Hollinger, 2000; Sarmento, 2014; Turner, 1993).

For example, scholars have variously characterized multiculturalism as a political ideology (Kymlicka, 2018), a moral philosophy (Fowers & Davidov, 2006), a social justice ideology that entails acceptance of cultural diversity (Vera & Speight, 2003), and an approach to managing immigration-related diversity (Berry & Kalin, 2002). Such definitional variation creates difficulties in assessing critically assertions made within multiculturalism and generates considerable confusion when engaging in discussions about multiculturalism because individuals tend to employ the same term but use a "different dictionary" when defining it. When researchers fail to clearly define and operationalize multiculturalism, they contribute to this confusion because clear definitions and operationalizations enable researchers to improve communication such that people accurately and consistently use the same terms to refer to the same constructs (Ginsberg, 1955; Sell, 2018). Clear definitions and operationalizations also allow us to specify the criteria needed to determine whether a hypothesis about multiculturalism is supported (Popper, 1957). When such criteria are not provided, researchers do not subject their hypotheses to the risk of falsification and thus run the risk of confirmation bias.

General Challenges to Defining Multiculturalism Words have both denotative and connotative elements. The *denotation* of a word refers to its precise, literal definition, such as what may be found in a dictionary. In contrast, the *connotation* of a word refers to positive or negative emotional and/or attitudinal valences that are attached to words. Thus, one way to understand word meanings is to break down a multisyllabic word into its constituent elements, define each element, and then use this as a basis for reconstructing the word's meaning.

An analysis of the term "multiculturalism" can begin with the prefix "*multi*"—which simply means "more than one," or "many." "*Cultural*" is an adjective that denotes a relationship to the way of life of a particular group of people (e.g., their behavior, habits, attitudes, and/or moral/religious beliefs), or refers to the literature, art, music, or intellectual achievements that represent the traditions or way of life among a particular group of people (Cambridge Dictionary, 2018). The root word of cultural is "*culture,*" which can be succinctly defined in dictionaries but that has accrued multiple definitions throughout the history of various branches of the anthropological sciences—which arguably devote the most serious study to the concept of culture. Among anthropologists, working definitions for "culture" have grown from 150 separate definitions (Kroeber & Kluckhohn, 1952) to 200 separate definitions (Baldwin & Lindsley, 1994), to more than 300 separate definitions (Baldwin et al., 2006).

Most knowledgeable observers note that "culture" is an extremely difficult concept on which to forge a professional consensus, as "culture is viewed as a constantly evolving and fluid entity which requires definitions to adaptively shift over time in concert with emerging developments in particular disciplines" (Frisby, 2018, p. 58). As such, efforts to define culture become increasingly more abstract. As examples:

> Cultures … are not material phenomena; they are cognitive organizations of material phenomena (Tyler, 1976, p. 177).

> One useful way to think about culture is to think of unstated assumptions, standard operating procedures, ways of doing things that have been internalized to such an extent that people do not argue about them (Triandis, 1994, p. 16).

> By approaching culture through the use of the idea of hegemony, culture can be conceptualized as a space within which struggles between social forces are conducted (Smith, 2000, p. 81).

Finally, the suffix "*ism*" modifies root words to denote an ideology that is seeded in social, economic, political, or religious doctrines, or in theories, systems, practices, or sets of principles. Common examples of root words modified by the "ism" suffix are Buddhism, capitalism, communism, Eurocentrism, fascism, feminism, Marxism, progressivism, sexism, and racism—to name a few. From the aforementioned semantic analysis, we can extrapolate a general definition of multiculturalism: It is some sort of abstract ideology with an assumed set of underlying doctrines that entail a focus on many cultures which are never clearly defined. This exercise suggests that multiculturalism is a loosely defined term where there is no real consensus regarding its actual meaning, much less its validity as an established scientific construct.

Defining Multiculturalism in Psychology In contrast to the anthropological tradition, applied psychology drastically oversimplifies and concretizes the concept of culture to denote racial, gender, religious, sexual orientation, or ethnic group membership (e.g., see Lott, 2010). Thus, a collection of persons who can be easily identified as belonging to different subcategories within these broad groupings are commonly described as "multicultural." Although such oversimplified definitions may improve communication within applied psychology, scholars have noted that they do not accurately depict the complexities of human life and experience (e.g., Frisby, 2013; Naylor, 1998; Wood, 2003). As noted by Triandis (2007):

> Attributes such as nationality, religion, race, or occupation are not appropriate criteria for defining cultures. The use of a single criterion is likely to lead to confusion, as would happen if all people who eat pizza were placed in one category. Culture is a complex whole, and it is best to use many criteria to discriminate between one culture and another (p. 65).

Writing from a developmental perspective, Stuart (2004) further argues this point using parents and their children as examples:

> Parenting is the ultimate form of socialization, through which children learn how to function in society. But parents vary in their ability and desire to transmit cultural beliefs to their children, and children are not passive recipients of their parents' values and practices. This explains the fact that the culture with which young adults leave their families of origin is rarely a carbon copy of parental beliefs, making for a diversity of characters at every family reunion. (p. 4)

In a similar fashion, the APA Task Force on Evidence-Based Practice (2006) noted the complex nature of and difficulty in defining culture:

> Culture, in this context, is understood to encompass a broad array of phenomena (e.g., shared values, history, knowledge, rituals, customs) that often result in a shared sense of identity. Racial and ethnic groups may have a shared culture, but those personal characteristics are not the only characteristics that define cultural groups (e.g., deaf culture, inner-city culture). Culture is a multifaceted construct, and cultural factors cannot be understood in isolation from social, class, and personal characteristics that make each patient unique. (p. 278)

Although there are several more examples that illustrate the complexity of defining culture, the point here is that "culture" and "cultural differences" are multidimensional and cannot be adequately characterized by a selective subset of one or two cultural dimensions. In this sense, individuals can be culturally similar on one dimension but quite different on other dimensions. For example, two Black and White friends who grow up in the same neighborhood can be culturally different according to their ethnic/racial group membership but culturally similar in terms of their formative neighborhood and educational socialization. Thus, by assuming that two individuals are different in most or all areas because they differ in their ethnic group membership is an oversimplification of complex realities. As noted by Stuart (2004):

> … [E]very individual is a unique blend of many influences. Whereas culture helps to regulate social life, specific beliefs are products of individuals' minds. Because of this complexity, it is never safe to infer a person's cultural orientation from knowledge of any group to which he or she is believed to belong (p. 5)

Given the complexity of defining culture, the discussion as to what aspects of culture should receive attention within psychology remains a topic of vigorous debate. The discussion typically centers on whether culture should be limited to the study of race and ethnicity (the exclusive position) or whether it should encompass the vast myriad of dimensions that constitute the human experience (the inclusive position; Sue & Sue, 2003). According to the exclusive position, there is general concern that expanding the definition of culture will result in dilution of the term. As Sue and Sue (2003) argue, broad definitions of culture permit individuals who experience discomfort about issues related to race and racism to discount the importance of these issues within multicultural theory and practice. On the other hand, some scholars (Frisby, 2013; Stuart, 2004; Triandis, 2007) contend that exclusive approaches to the study of culture ignore important life domains that are critical to an adequate understanding of human experience. As noted earlier in this chapter, to date, there is no consensus about how culture should be defined or studied.

The debate between the need to provide a specific operationalization of culture (exclusive)—weighed against the need to incorporate all its complexity (inclusive)—creates a definitional quagmire. When researchers define culture so specifically as to focus only on race and ethnicity, they drastically oversimply the complex nature of human reality. However, if they define culture so broadly as to encompass everything, then the concept becomes essentially meaningless.

Despite a lack of scientific consensus on what constitutes culture, and even less a clear understanding as to what constitutes multiculturalism, governing bodies within the field of psychology (APA, 2003, 2015, 2017, 2019) nevertheless emphasize imperatively the importance of incorporating multiculturalism into every aspect of research, advocacy, teaching, practice, and activism. That is, psychologists are strongly encouraged to adopt and promote multiculturalism, despite a lack of clarity vis-à-vis what multiculturalism entails.

Consider APA's *Report of the Task Force on the Implementation of the Multicultural Guidelines* (American Psychological Association, 2008). The term "multiculturalism" is mentioned 15 times but is never defined. As inferred from the context in which this word is used, multiculturalism is referred to as a four-decades old movement in psychology (p. 1) that is an "integral and driving force in the field" (p. 18); a concept that includes core assumptions (though never explicitly stated, p. 2) about which psychologists have expertise (p. 15); a concept that psychological trainers are encouraged to employ in the education of psychologists (pp. 3, 10), which includes activities and programs (p. 8) that should be infused into training curriculum across multiple courses and accreditation standards (p. 11). Multiculturalism is also portrayed as an organizational initiative for which internal APA directorates and outside organizations should be rewarded with incentives for its significant infusion into theory and practice (p. 17). Such actions are depicted as addressing a need related to training, research, and organizational change (p. 3), for which APA is encouraged to provide national leadership (p. 4) and continuing education (p. 7). Thus, multiculturalism in professional psychology is consistently portrayed as possessing the inherent power to improve psychology research and practice. Such a portrayal persists despite the field's inability to provide an agreed-upon definition of multiculturalism, operationalization of the construct, or consistent empirical evidence that it improves psychological science.

So, what is multiculturalism? Unfortunately, there is no clear answer, and the answer one receives depends largely on who is asked. All one can really conclude is that multiculturalism remains an umbrella term that represents a heterogeneous mixture of practices and approaches related to "culture," however defined, that differ significantly in both quality and content. This lack of definitional clarity naturally extends to other concepts related to multiculturalism such as social justice, multicultural competence, and cultural sensitivity.

For example, there has been nearly two decades worth of research and policy regarding the need for psychologists to become culturally sensitive; yet, we still know very little regarding what cultural sensitivity (or competence) actually entails, and even less regarding how to achieve it. Critical questions remain unanswered such as: Who is culturally sensitive? What criteria exist to determine whether one has become culturally sensitive and for whom? What information about which groups should psychologists know to become culturally sensitive? Can one ever fully achieve cultural sensitivity? If so, at what point would one be considered competent to work with a certain cultural group? Although these questions are but a few among many, the fact that they remain unanswered after nearly 20 years demonstrates that key definitional issues regarding multiculturalism are far from settled (see Frisby et al., 2018; O'Donohue & Benuto, 2010, for more detailed discussions).

Thus, when considered together, the large body of research and practices associated with multiculturalism likely include a conglomeration of rigorous, high-quality research; mediocre research; evidence-based practices; sociopolitical advocacy; and ideological pseudoscience masquerading as science (Frisby, 2013). The ambiguity in what constitutes multiculturalism and related practices is captured by Lynch (1997), who stated that "the diversity machine indiscriminately blends social science and ideology, serious substance with silly platitudes. Often it is easy to tell the difference; sometimes it is not. Therein lies one of many dangers" (pp. 17–18).

Such an insight raises an important question: If applied psychology as a discipline is to be considered a legitimate science (Lilienfeld 2010, 2012), why do its governing bodies continue to advance the concept of multiculturalism without a clear delineation of what it is, and before there is well-corroborated evidence that it works? Indeed, in the earliest stages of the movement, before virtually any evidence had accumulated, multiculturalism was already being widely adopted and implemented within the field (e.g., Fowers & Richardson, 1996; Pederson, 1991; Stone, 1997; Sue et al., 1992). This tendency to adopt prematurely certain constructs in the field of psychology also applies to prominent concepts in applied psychology that flow from multiculturalism, such as multicultural sensitivity and microaggressions, both of which were quickly accepted within applied psychology before adequate evidence existed to support their validity (Lilienfeld, 2017a, b, 2020; O'Donohue & Benuto, 2010). By prematurely advancing multiculturalism as a guiding philosophy for applied psychologists, it appears that the field put the proverbial "cart before the horse." Such a leap within psychology to advance prematurely the tenets and practices of multiculturalism before adequate evidence had accumulated should be regarded as a cautionary note for the field (Lilienfeld, 2010, 2012).

Dogmatic Emphasis on Group Differences Within Multiculturalism

Although there is no consensus as to what constitutes multiculturalism, virtually all definitions, regardless of their variations, share a common theme: *a strong philosophical emphasis on group differences and diversity* (Deaux & Verkuyten, 2014; Fowers & Richardson, 1996; Frisby, 2013; Verkuyten, 2007). To understand why a strong, and in many cases, dominant emphasis on group differences can result in negative intergroup outcomes, one must consider the scientific literature regarding some of the most prominent cognitive processes at work in group interactions.

Well-established social psychological literatures have consistently documented that human beings organize their perceptions of the social world according to discrete categories (e.g., groups) that minimize within-group (ingroup) differences and accentuate between-group (outgroup) differences (e.g., Macrae & Bodenhausen, 2000; Tajfel & Turner, 1986; Turner et al., 1987). When between-group differences are emphasized, intergroup commonalities tend to be neglected, resulting in strong ingroup–outgroup (us–them) distinctions. Such us–them categorizations form a central basis for intergroup conflicts (Brewer, 1997; Deaux & Verkuyten, 2014). Accordingly, the overriding emphasis on group differences inherent in multiculturalism risks reifying already naturally occurring, contentious group differences (Moshman, 2011).

More precisely, as group differences are emphasized and become increasingly salient, an intergroup schema emerges among group members with the following characteristics: (a) ingroup favoritism (trust, compassion, etc.) develops where positive attributes are extended to ingroup members but not to outgroup members; (2) divisive intergroup social comparisons emerge as groups compete for social resources; and (3) ingroup members perceive one another to be similar whereas outgroup members are perceived to be different (Abrams et al., 2005; Tajfel & Turner, 1986; Turner et al., 1987). This intergroup schema often carries several negative consequences, such as the perception that ingroups and outgroups constitute homogenous entities; mutual distrust between groups; intergroup competition; and increased preferential treatment of ingroup members (Brewer, 1997; Hogg et al., 2017). Research shows that such ingroup favoritism, often coupled with outgroup hostility, is strongly associated with discrimination toward outgroup members and with viewing one's ingroup as superior to a relevant outgroup (Greenwald & Pettigrew, 2014).

Of course, the extent to which this intergroup schema results in adverse consequences is likely contingent on myriad personality (e.g., negative emotionality) and contextual (e.g., power differences) factors. Nevertheless, there is good reason to believe that human beings have been shaped by evolutionary pressures to be tribal in nature, and so ingroup favoritism, outgroup hostility, and similar cognitive biases are likely characteristics of all groups (Caporael, 1997; Clark et al., 2019; Liberman et al., 2017; Wilson, 2014).

A strong emphasis on group differences may also lead to race essentialism, the notion that racial differences are rooted in biology and thus immutable (Haslam & Whelan, 2008). In two experiments, Wilton et al. (2019) found that, compared to colorblind conditions, individuals who were exposed to the multiculturalism condition—operationalized by an emphasis on intergroup differences—reported stronger race essentialists beliefs on items such as: "*The physical features of different racial groups haven't really changed much over the centuries*" and "*Siblings born to the same parents will always be of the same race as each other*" (Study 1). These authors also reported reduced endorsement of belief in racial inequality as an important issue (Study 2). These findings suggest that an emphasis on group differences is directly associated with race-essentialist beliefs and may be explained by the fact that multiculturalism and race essentialism are rooted in similar social categorization processes.

For example, for individuals to appreciate intergroup differences, they must first identify and categorize individuals as belonging to different groups. Accordingly, a strong emphasis on group differences within multiculturalism, in part, provides the platform for race essentialism because it begins with recognizing racial differences as a legitimate basis for identifying and classifying people. In addition to promoting race essentialism, this tendency within multiculturalism to classify people into homogenous racial groups has been directly linked with group stereotyping (e.g., Gutiérrez & Unzueta, 2010; No et al., 2008; Wolsko et al., 2000).

Overemphasizing group differences can also lead to collective identities that are associated with ethnocentrism. According to the theory of optimal distinctiveness (Leonardelli et al., 2010), human beings possess two competing needs for: (a) group inclusion and (b) group differentiation. Identification with a relevant social group provides both needs simultaneously, such that inclusion is satisfied through belonging to an ingroup, and differentiation is satisfied through drawing distinctions between the ingroup and outgroups (Vignoles, 2011). In this sense, groups provide explicit rules regarding who is included and who is excluded. Because of these rules for inclusion and exclusion, group processes that promote allegiance and social cooperation do not necessarily generalize to outgroups, resulting in a type of "*clique selfishness*" that often results in hostility toward outgroups when interests of one's ingroup are pitted against those of an outgroup (Brewer, 1997; Campbell, 1982). Other scholars have echoed concerns about segregating individuals into noninteracting and distrusting groups, particularly because such segregation can lead to reduced social cohesion, can diminish a community's social capital, and can undermine the trust and common goals that are necessary to maintain stable, cohesive, and unified communities (Coleman, 1988; Lancee & Dronkers, 2010; Putnam, 2007).

There is also a tendency within multiculturalism to focus selectively on a small subset of "cultural" groups and their differences. Such a narrow focus is disconcerting because multiculturalism is argued to be an ideology that values and respects all groups. For example, groups that tend to receive the most attention within multiculturalism include certain ethnic minority groups including African Americans, Native Americans, and Latinos; various sexual and gender minority groups such as those identifying as lesbian, gay, bisexual, transgender, and queer (LGBTQ+); and certain religious groups such as Muslims. The purported rationale for this selective focus is generally that these groups represent those that were both historically and currently marginalized or oppressed (Sue, 2004; Sue et al., 1999). Although such a rationale is well founded, it is unclear why scholars of multiculturalism largely ignore other historically stigmatized minority groups such as Jews—who have a long history of oppression in the United States and abroad—or certain Asian groups such as the Japanese who also share an oppressed history in the United States, to name a few. In contrast, there is a strong tendency among multiculturalism scholars to avoid criticism of their preferred cultural groups on virtually any dimension while selectively critiquing other groups such as heterosexuals, males, Whites, Christians, and conservatives, usually with little to no consideration for the diversity that comprises these groups (O'Donohue, 2018).

Because an overriding emphasis on group differences often results in adverse outcomes, intergroup relation scholars have developed several prominent models to reduce the negative processes that stem from the aforementioned intergroup schema. Although these models propose different paths toward improving intergroup relations, they share a common element: to change how ingroups and outgroups perceive one another by minimizing negative intergroup schemata. Inherent in each of these models is an attempt to minimize the reification of an overriding and almost exclusive emphasis on group differences through cognitively restructuring how groups view one another.

Four prominent models currently dominate the literature, each of which is grounded in intergroup contact theory (Allport, 1954; Pettigrew & Tropp, 2006). The *decategorization model* suggests that contact between groups should be organized in a way such that opportunities are provided for ingroup and outgroup members to become acquainted at the individual level, thus reducing the salience of strict categorizations while breaking down ingroups' and outgroups' perceptions of one another as homogenous entities (Brewer & Miller, 1984). The *recategorization model* suggests arranging intergroup contact to center on a superordinate social identity, in which both ingroup and outgroup members perceive themselves as belonging to a common social group (Gaertner et al., 1993). This model is based on the notion that increasing perceptions of a shared, common social identity will minimize intergroup prejudice because ingroup and outgroup members no longer view themselves as competing against one another and representing two separate entities.

Moreover, the *dual identity model* suggests that it is important for group members both to retain their unique ingroup identity *and* to recognize their membership in shared, superordinate social identities. This model is based on research showing that an overriding emphasis on intergroup similarities at the expense of one's ingroup identity can carry the unintentional consequence of reducing ingroup group members' motivation for social change (Saguy et al., 2009). Finally, the *ingroup projection model* suggests that intergroup prejudice is lessened when a shared, superordinate category is defined by the diversity of individuals who inhabit that category (Mummendey & Wenzel, 1999). For example, if Canadians are defined as valuing Canada for being multicultural, White Canadians may be less likely to judge non-White Canadians negatively for behaving differently because they view such behavior as a manifestation of Canadian diversity.

Considered together, these four social-cognitive models designed to improve intergroup relations, although taking different approaches, tend to *deemphasize rather than emphasize intergroup differences* that are at the heart of divisive "us–them" social categorizations. The more recent of the four models, particularly the dual identity and ingroup projection models, underscore the importance of ingroup members retaining their unique social identities. This is an important point, because a critical boundary condition of these models holds that, if ingroup members feel pressured to assimilate into a larger superordinate group at the expense of their ingroup identity, they may rebel against rather than support such initiatives. This is because identification with a social group confers several psychological benefits to group members, including social support, feelings of inclusion, pride, shared social realities, and protection from outgroup discrimination (Branscombe et al., 1999; Greenaway et al., 2015; Jetten et al., 2015).

In sum, multiculturalism in its various forms entails an emphasis on group differences, despite the large body of evidence cautioning against such a heavy emphasis (Cobb et al., 2020). This is not to say that group differences should not be highlighted. Rather, it suggests that it may be harmful for intergroup relations to focus constantly and exclusively on how groups differ from one another. Although multiculturalism is characterized largely by its celebration of group differences, this legitimate focus need not exclude a similar focus on intergroup commonalties. To assume that these positions are mutually exclusive would be to commit what logicians call the "either-or fallacy," that is, to assume that the best solution to a problem is to select one perspective over another rather the simultaneous adoption of both perspectives.

Multiculturalism as a Perceived Exclusive Ideology

Another issue with multiculturalism is that it is often perceived to be an ideology that includes members from minority groups while excluding members of majority groups. Whereas members of minority groups tend to view multiculturalism as identity-supporting, many members of majority groups tend to view it as identity-threatening (Deaux et al., 2006). Such divergence in perceptions regarding the inclusiveness versus exclusiveness of multiculturalism is greatest among minority and majority group members who more strongly identify with their ingroups (Verkuyten & Brug, 2004; Verkuyten & Martinovic, 2006). These discrepancies in attitudes toward issues of diversity, particularly as presented in multiculturalism, may arguably lead to a less cohesive society and to greater intergroup conflict.

To account for such divergence in attitudes, several scholars have legitimately argued that many majority group members (e.g., Whites) may reject multiculturalism due to ingroup bias, identity threat, and racism (e.g., Sanchez-Burks et al., 2000; Sidanius, 1993; Stephan & Stephan, 2013; Verkuyten & Martinovic, 2006). In addition, there is a large body of evidence suggesting that majority group members often perceive efforts geared toward addressing racial inequality as leading to a potential loss of group status, dominance, and power (Eibach & Keegan, 2006; Jardina, 2019; Knowles et al., 2009). These points are important to consider as majority group members have held the most power in Western countries for several centuries, and many majority group members have oppressed, and continue to oppress, minority group members. In addition, there is evidence that pockets of overt racism still exist in some US communities (Gallup, 2020).

These legitimate explanations notwithstanding, one issue that has received considerably less attention in discussions surrounding multiculturalism is that many majority group members perceive multiculturalism as a sociopolitical ideology that excludes their group. Even some scholars who are more sympathetic to multiculturalism echo this concern: "Multiculturalism can also be considered as being asymmetrical because it focuses on ethnic minority groups and neglects the majority, which encourages resentment and fragmentation" (Verkuyten & Yogeeswaran, 2020, p. 2). As noted by most social-psychological perspectives (see Baumeister & Leary, 1995, for a review), humans possess an innate need for belonging, and feeling excluded may represent an attack on one's central need to belong. If majority group members feel that multiculturalism is primarily directed toward minority groups, it is less likely that they will be supportive of multiculturalism as an ideology worth adopting.

Experimental evidence supports the notion that some Whites' perceptions of social exclusion may explain, in part, why some of them reject multiculturalism. In a series of controlled studies, Plaut et al. (2011) found that (a) Whites implicitly associate multiculturalism with exclusion (Study 1); Whites do not associate multiculturalism with exclusion when they are included in conceptualizations of multiculturalism (Study 2); multiculturalism is less central to Whites' self-concept than to minority group members' self-concepts (Study 3); feelings of being included mediate the relationship between group status (Whites vs. racial/ethnic minorities) and endorsement of diversity (Study 4); and Whites with greater need for belonging report being less interested in working for organizations that endorse a multiculturalism-based approach (Study 5). These findings suggest that, across samples, methodologies, and conceptualizations of multiculturalism, many Whites consistently consider multiculturalism to be an exclusive ideology that does not include them.

Other studies have also found that many majority group members consider multiculturalism to be targeted toward non-White minority groups (Unzueta & Binning, 2010). In a content analysis of multicultural syllabi in counseling psychology, Pieterse et al. (2009) found that, although 87% of courses focused on racial identity, only 11% considered Whites as a racial group. Samson (2018) found that both Whites and Hispanics reported increased psychological distress (hopelessness, depression, and worthlessness) when they more strongly disagreed with multiculturalism. Thus, despite well-intentioned efforts to be inclusive, the emphatic and exclusive theme of group differences within multiculturalism ironically elicits feelings of distress and exclusion for many majority (and some minority) group members.

There is also cross-disciplinary evidence, including among minority group members, that multiculturalism represents an exclusive ideology. Academics, bloggers, historians, and other writers have expressed concern that multiculturalism subjugates majority groups in exchange for inclusion and acceptance of minority groups (e.g., Auster, 2004; Fowers & Richardson, 1996; Michaels, 2006; Schlesinger, 1998; Shepherd, 2019). For example, Bhikhu Parekh (2000), a well-known political theorist, stated that "in no theory of multiculturalism is the explicit act of 'recognition' reciprocal, denoting instead an act that goes from the majority to the minority" (p. 272). Sociologist Christian Joppke (2004) echoed similar sentiments: "it evokes and mobilizes around involuntary and mutually exclusive statuses and tends to render 'recognition' a one-sided act by the majority society only" (p. 238). The Indian-born writer Kenan Malik (2015) opined,

> Multiculturalism as a political tool has functioned as not merely a response to diversity but also a means of constraining it. And that insight reveals a paradox. Multicultural policies accept as a given that societies are diverse, yet they implicitly assume that such diversity ends at the edge of minority communities. (p. 21)

Although these excerpts are but a few of many examples, they represent a perspective held by many scholars that multiculturalism exists primarily for inclusion of minority groups at the expense of excluding majority groups.

Finally, another reason many majority group members may perceive multiculturalism to be exclusive is that majority group members are often one-sidedly portrayed in a pejorative way by several multicultural advocates. For instance, in one of the most widely used texts in applied psychology programs, Sue and Sue (1990) advanced a negative view toward majority group members that is indicative of perspectives held by many multicultural advocates: "Racism is a basic and integral part of U.S. life and … all Whites are racist whether knowingly or unknowingly" (p. 113). In their 2017 revision of *Counseling the Culturally Diverse*—perhaps the standard textbook used in multicultural courses and programs—Sue and Sue suggested that:

> as members of a White Euro-American group, what responsibility do you hold for the racist, oppressive, and discriminating manner by which you personally and professionally deal with people of color? This is a threatening question for White people. However, to be effective in MCT (multicultural counseling/therapy) means that one has adequately dealt with this question and worked through the biases, feelings, fears, and guilt associated with it. (pp. 56–57)

In recent calls for Whites to become allies with minorities in the struggle for equality, the predominant focus of much literature in applied psychology has been almost exclusively what Whites must do to addresses their biases minority groups, with little to no attention to what minority groups must also do to overcome their biases against Whites (e.g., Atkins et al., 2017; Smith et al., 2017; Spanierman & Smith, 2017; Sue, 2017). As a final example, in their description of a White ally, Spanierman and Smith (2017b) opined: "We acknowledge … that, regardless of their commitment and dedication to racial justice, White individuals likely cannot completely purge the impact of racist socialization from the deepest levels of their consciousness" (p. 609). These excerpts illustrate a widely held and prevailing multicultural perspective held in most circles of applied psychology: Whites are inevitably racist individuals who can never fully rid themselves of their prejudice, and they can never become effective counselors until they have addressed their biases, fears, guilt, and complicity in racism.

It is not difficult to appreciate the many issues inherent in these perspectives that are so prevalent in applied psychology. First, such statements are unfalsifiable and thus have no place in a scientific discipline, and it is questionable (at best) whether these statements should be included in prominent journals and in textbooks used to educate the next generation of practitioners (Popper, 1957). Second, they ignore evidence that humans have evolved to be tribal in nature, and that racism and prejudice are characteristic of all groups—not just majority groups. As noted by Fowers and Richardson (1996), within multiculturalism, ethnocentricity, and racism are nearly always regarded as characteristics of Whites. Third, the claim that White psychologists cannot be effective when working with ethnically and racially diverse individuals until they have addressed their racism is based on a selective review of the evidence. In reality, therapy outcome research associated with counselors' multicultural competence has been mixed, with some research (143 clients and 31 therapists) indicating that clients' ratings of their counselors' multicultural competence are not significantly associated with more favorable therapeutic outcomes (Owen et al., 2011). Fourth, if majority group members continue to be characterized as the helplessly racist group in society, it is unlikely that multiculturalism will ever become the uniting force that it could be if all groups were portrayed with the same degree of moral legitimacy.

The Future of Multiculturalism in Psychology: Some Concluding Thoughts

What is the future of multiculturalism in applied psychology? Given the longstanding and contentious debate surrounding multiculturalism, it is difficult to say with any degree of certainty. Whereas some scholars believe that multiculturalism is a morally good ideology that is effective at managing the increasing diversity within US society, other scholars contend that it represents an unworkable sociopolitical doctrine that results in more harm than good.

Our position, however, falls somewhere in the middle. On the one hand, we recognize the myriad issues with contemporary presentations of multiculturalism, as well as the potential harm it can produce if not implemented in a theoretically informed and empirically based manner. On the other hand, the emergence of multiculturalism within psychology has sparked a large body of much-needed research on historically neglected minority groups in the United States. It has also informed some areas of psychological science with respect to how certain psychological phenomena may operate differently for minority groups whose sociocultural experiences differ drastically from those of majority groups.

Thus, we do not believe that the field should throw out the proverbial "baby with the bath water" when it comes to multiculturalism. Most research, with some exceptions, indicates that approaches rooted in multiculturalism tend to outperform colorblind approaches with respect to managing diversity (see Plaut et al., 2018; Verkuyten & Yogeeswaran, 2020, for reviews). Rather, we suggest that, if the field of applied psychology wishes to establish itself as a credible scientific discipline, then it must begin to grapple seriously with the many concerns raised by critics of multiculturalism and not reflexively dismiss them as illegitimate or racist.

The field would increase its credibility as a scientific discipline if its governing bodies (e.g., APA) would refrain from institutionalizing questionable sociopolitical frameworks and policies before adequate evidence has accumulated that they are scientifically supported. As noted earlier, the APA prematurely adopted multiculturalism as a governing philosophy, including its corresponding ethical codes and clinical multicultural competencies, despite a lack of extant initial evidence to support their validity. Twenty years later, there remains no consensus regarding what multiculturalism is, what it entails, or whether it works. Such premature leaps with the field undermine its credibility as a serious science (Lilienfeld, 2010).

In addition, applied psychology researchers should investigate how to address the plethora of negative intergroup outcomes associated with a strong, albeit well-intentioned, emphasis on intergroup differences. There have been recent calls (Cobb et al., 2020) to balance the current emphasis on group differences with a simultaneous emphasis on intergroup similarities. However, to our knowledge, approaches that balance group differences with commonalities have yet to be developed and tested against alternative approaches, such as downplaying (colorblind) or emphasizing (multiculturalism) group differences. Further, most research on multiculturalism has been limited to laboratory experiments, and research is needed that tests various approaches in more naturalistic settings across diverse populations.

Moreover, contrary to popular opinion, the scientific literature on multiculturalism has yielded largely mixed results. Thus, it remains unknown which intergroup differences, when emphasized, result in more positive versus negative outcomes. As noted by most social identity perspectives (e.g., Deaux et al., 2006; Tajfel et al., 1986), social identities generally become more salient in some contexts than others. In this sense, emphasizing certain group differences may in some cases contribute to positive outcomes, such as heightened awareness of and empathy for minority group members' struggle for equal rights. However, there is little to no theoretical or empirical guidance regarding whether positive or negative outcomes will emerge when certain differences are emphasized, or which specific multiculturalism-based interventions will elicit them. Pursuing these directions would represent a much-needed area of research that is ripe for the picking.

Finally, as discussed earlier, evidence across disciplines suggests that multiculturalism is often perceived by many majority group members as an ideology that excludes their group. When majority group members were explicitly included in multicultural discussions, they no longer associated multiculturalism with exclusion. Accordingly, it is important to value and include both majority and minority group members in discussions of initiatives and policies grounded in multiculturalism. Unfortunately, there is little to no research regarding how to effectively structure conversations and interventions to be perceived by both majority and minority groups as inclusive and accommodating. Thus, a helpful future line of research would involve designing and testing inclusive and efficacious multicultural initiatives that could be implemented in multicultural coursework, practice, diversity training, and multicultural workshops.

In sum, science thrives on criticism, both conceptual and empirical (Lilienfeld; 2010, 2012; Popper, 1963). In the present chapter, we have outlined several prominent issues within multiculturalism that receive little attention in most academic circles. Our goal in highlighting these issues is to increase awareness among students, educators, and researchers within applied psychology of many of the pitfalls in multiculturalism that could result in more harm than good if unaddressed. It is our belief that psychological science advances most effectively when authors from differing perspectives engage in critical research and respectful conversations regarding salient issues in the field—including contentious issues such as the legitimacy of widely held, and often-cherished, sociopolitical perspectives such as multiculturalism. We hope that this chapter serves as a step toward advancing such work.

References

Abrams, D., Hogg, M. A., & Marques, J. M. (2005). *The social psychology of inclusion and exclusion*. Psychology Press.

Adamson, G. (2017). *The Trojan horse: A leftist critique of multiculturalism in the West.* PostDiversity Press.

Allport, G. W. (1954). *The nature of prejudice*. Addison Wesley.

American Psychological Association. (2003). Guidelines on multicultural education, training, research, practice, and organizational change for psychologists. *American Psychologist, 58*, 377–402.

American Psychological Association. (2017). *Multicultural guidelines: An ecological approach to context, identity, and intersectionality*. Retrieved from https://www.apa.org/about/policy/multicultural-guidelines.

American Psychological Association. (2008). *Report of the Task Force on the Implementation of the Multicultural Guidelines*. Author. Accessed November 2020 from https://www.apa.org/about/policy/multicultural-report.pdf

American Psychological Association, Commission on Accreditation. (2015). *Standards of accreditation for health service psychology*. Retrieved from http://www.apa.org/ed/accreditation/about/policies/standards-of-accreditation.pdf

American Psychological Association, Office of Ethnic Minority Affairs. (1993). Guidelines for providers of psychological services to ethnic, linguistic, and culturally diverse populations. *American Psychologist, 48*, 45–48.

American Psychological Association. (2019). *APA guidelines on race and ethnicity in psychology*. Retrieved on November 17th, 2020 from https://www.apa.org/about/policy/guidelines-race-ethnicity.pdf

Ashenfelter, M. (2010). Multicultural classes criticized as indoctrination. *The Nation*. Accessed October 2018 from https://www.thenation.com/article/multicultural-classes-criticizedindoctrination/
Atkins, S. L., Fitzpatrick, M. R., Poolokasingham, G., Lebeau, M., & Spanierman, L. B. (2017). Make it personal: A qualitative investigation of White counselors' multicultural awareness development. *The Counseling Psychologist, 45*, 669–696.
Auster, L. (2004). How the multicultural ideology captured America. *Social Contract, 14*, 197–208.
Baldwin, J. R., Faulkner, S. L., Hecht, M. L., & Lindsley, S. L. (2006). A moving target: The illusive definition of culture. In J. R. Baldwin, S. L. Faulkner, M. L. Hecht, & S. L. Lindsley (Eds.), *Redefining culture: Perspectives across the disciplines* (pp. 3–26). Routledge.
Baldwin, J. R., & Lindsey, S. L. (1994). *Conceptualization of culture*. Urban Studies Center.
Barry, B. (2001). *Culture and Equality*. Polity Press.
Berry, J. W., & Kalin, R. (2002). Multicultural policy and social psychology: The Canadian experience. In S. Rehnson & J. Duckitt (Eds.), *Political psychology: Cultural and cross-cultural foundations* (pp. 263–284). Macmillan.
Baumeister, R. F., & Leary, M. R. (1995). The need to belong: Desire for interpersonal attachments as a fundamental human motivation. *Psychological Bulletin, 117*, 497–529.
Benuto, L. T., & O'Donohue, W. (2015). Is culturally sensitive cognitive behavioral therapy an empirically supported treatment?: The case for Hispanics. *International Journal of Psychology and Psychological Therapy, 15*, 405–421.
Bernal, G. (2006). Intervention development and cultural adaptation research with diverse families. *Family Process, 45*, 143–151.
Branscombe, N. R., Schmitt, M. T., & Harvey, R. D. (1999). Perceiving pervasive discrimination among African Americans: Implications for group identification and well-being. *Journal of Personality and Social Psychology, 77*, 135–149.
Brewer, M. B. (1997). The social psychology of intergroup relations: Can research inform practice? *Journal of Social Issues, 53*, 197–211.
Brewer, M. B., & Miller, N. (1984). Beyond the contact hypothesis: Theoretical perspectives on desegregation. In N. Miller & M. Brewer (Eds.), *Groups in contact: The psychology of desegregation* (pp. 281–302). Academic Press.
Cambridge Dictionary. (2018). *Definition of "cultural"*. Accessed October 2018 from https://dictionary.cambridge.org/us/dictionary/english/cultural
Caporael, L. R. (1997). The evolution of truly social cognition: The core configurations model. *Personality and Social Psychology Review, 1*(4), 276–298.
Clark, C. J., Liu, B. S., Winegard, B. M., & Ditto, P. H. (2019). Tribalism is human nature. *Current Directions in Psychological Science, 28*, 587–592.
Cobb, C. L., Lilienfeld, S. O., Schwartz, S. J., Frisby, C., & Sanders, G. L. (2020). Rethinking Multiculturalism: Toward a Balanced Approach. *The American Journal of Psychology, 133*, 275–293.
Coleman, J. S. (1988). Social capital in the creation of human capital. *American Journal of Sociology, 94*, 95–120.
Deaux, K., Reid, A., Martin, D., & Bikmen, N. (2006). Ideologies of diversity and inequality: Predicting collective action in groups varying in ethnicity and immigrant status. *Political Psychology, 27*, 123–146.
Deaux, K., & Verkuyten, M. (2014). The social psychology of multiculturalism: Identity and intergroup relations. In V. Benet-Martínez & Y.-Y. Hong (Eds.), *Oxford library of psychology: The Oxford handbook of multicultural identity* (pp. 118–138). Oxford University Press.
Eibach, R. P., & Keegan, T. (2006). Free at last? Social dominance, loss aversion, and white and black Americans' differing assessments of racial progress. *Journal of Personality and Social Psychology, 90*, 453–467.
Fowers, B. J., & Davidov, B. J. (2006). The virtue of multiculturalism: Personal transformation, character, and openness to the other. *American Psychologist, 61*, 581–594.
Fowers, B. J., & Richardson, F. C. (1996). Why is multiculturalism good? *American Psychologist, 51*, 609–621.

Frisby, C. L. (2013). Chapter 2: The Problem of Quack Multiculturalism. In C. L. Frisby (Ed.), *Meeting the psychoeducational needs of minority students: Evidence-based guidelines for school psychologists and other school personnel* (pp. 9–72). Wiley.

Frisby, C. L. (2018). History and development of cultural competence evaluation in applied psychology. In C. L. Frisby & W. T. O'Donohue (Eds.), *Cultural Competence in Applied Psychology: An Evaluation of Current Status and Future Directions* (pp. 57–94). Springer.

Frisby, C. L., O'Donohue, W., Benuto, L. T., & Casas, J. B. (2018). Conceptual and empirical issues in training culturally competent psychologists. In *Cultural competence in applied psychology* (pp. 95–102). Springer.

Gaertner, S. L., Dovidio, J. F., Anastasio, P. A., Bachman, B. A., & Rust, M. C. (1993). The common ingroup identity model: Recategorization and the reduction of intergroup bias. *European Review of Social Psychology, 4*, 1–26.

Gallup. (2020). *Race relations*. Retrieved from https://news.gallup.com/poll/1687/Race-Relations.aspx

Garcea, J. (2008). Postulations on the fragmentary effects of multiculturalism in Canada. *Canadian Ethnic Studies, 40*(1), 141–160.

Ginsberg, A. (1955). Operational definitions and theories. *The Journal of General Psychology, 52*, 223–245.

Gone, J. P., & Kirmayer, L. J. (2010). On the wisdom of considering culture and context in psychopathology. In T. Millon, R. F. Krueger, & E. Simonsen (Eds.), *Contemporary Directions in Psychopathology: Scientific Foundations of the DSM-V and ICD-11* (pp. 72–96). Guilford.

Greenwald, A. G., & Pettigrew, T. F. (2014). With malice toward none and charity for some: Ingroup favoritism enables discrimination. *American Psychologist, 69*, 669–684.

Greenaway, K. H., Haslam, S. A., Cruwys, T., Branscombe, N. R., Ysseldyk, R., & Heldreth, C. (2015). From "we" to "me": Group identification enhances perceived personal control with consequences for health and well-being. *Journal of Personality and Social Psychology, 109*, 53–74.

Gutiérrez, A. S., & Unzueta, M. M. (2010). The effect of interethnic ideologies on the likability of stereotypic vs. counterstereotypic minority targets. *Journal of Experimental Social Psychology, 46*, 775–784.

Jones, J. M., & Austin-Dailey, A. T. (2009). The Minority Fellowship Program: A 30-year legacy of training psychologists of color. *Cultural Diversity and Ethnic Minority Psychology, 15*, 388–399.

Hall, G. C. N., Ibaraki, A. Y., Huang, E. R., Marti, C. N., & Stice, E. (2016). A meta-analysis of cultural adaptations of psychological interventions. *Behavior Therapy, 47*, 993–1014.

Haslam, N., & Whelan, J. (2008). Human natures: Psychological essentialism in thinking about differences between people. *Social and Personality Psychology Compass, 2*, 1297–1312.

Hogg, M. A., Abrams, D., & Brewer, M. B. (2017). Social identity: The role of self in group processes and intergroup relations. *Group Processes & Intergroup Relations, 20*, 570–581.

Hollinger, D. (2000). *Postethnic America: Beyond multiculturalism*. Harper Collins.

Huey, S. J., Jr., & Polo, A. J. (2008). Evidence-based psychosocial treatments for ethnic minority youth. *Journal of Clinical Child & Adolescent Psychology, 37*(1), 262–301.

Huey, S. J., Jr., Tilley, J. L., Jones, E. O., & Smith, C. A. (2014). The contribution of cultural competence to evidence-based care for ethnically diverse populations. *Annual Review of Clinical Psychology, 10*, 305–338.

Jardina, A. (2019). *White identity politics*. Routledge.

Jetten, J., Branscombe, N. R., Haslam, S. A., Haslam, C., Cruwys, T., Jones, J. M., et al. (2015). Having a lot of a good thing: Multiple important group memberships as a source of self-esteem. *PLoS One, 10*, 1–29.

Joppke, C. (2004). The retreat of multiculturalism in the liberal state: theory and policy 1. *The British Journal of Sociology, 55*, 237–257.

Knowles, E. D., Lowery, B. S., Hogan, C. M., & Chow, R. M. (2009). On the malleability of ideology: Motivated construals of color blindness. *Journal of Personality and Social Psychology, 96*, 857–869.

Kroeber, A. L., & Kluckhohn, C. (1952). Culture: A critical review of concepts and definitions. *Papers. Peabody Museum of Archaeology & Ethnology, Harvard University*.

Kymlicka, W. (2018). Liberal multiculturalism as a political theory of state–minority relations. *Political Theory, 46*(1), 81–91.

Lancee, B., & Dronkers, J. (2010). Ethnic diversity in the neighborhood and social trust of immigrants and natives: A replication of Putnam (2007) in a West-European country. In M. Hooghe (Ed.), *Social cohesion: Contemporary theoretical perspectives on the study of social cohesion and social capital* (pp. 77–103). Royal Academy of Belgium.

Leonardelli, G. J., Pickett, C. L., & Brewer, M. B. (2010). Optimal distinctiveness theory: A framework for social identity, social cognition, and intergroup relations. *Advances in Experimental Social Psychology, 43*, 63–113.

Lewis-Fernandez, R., & Kleinman, A. (1994). Culture, personality, and psychopathology. *Journal of Abnormal Psychology, 103*, 67–71.

Liberman, Z., Woodward, A. L., & Kinzler, K. D. (2017). The origins of social categorization. *Trends in Cognitive Sciences, 21*, 556–568.

Lilienfeld, S. O. (2007). Psychological treatments that cause harm. *Perspectives on Psychological Science, 2*(1), 53–70.

Lilienfeld, S. O. (2010). Can psychology become a science? *Personality and Individual Differences, 49*(4), 281–288.

Lilienfeld, S. O. (2012). Public skepticism of psychology: why many people perceive the study of human behavior as unscientific. *American Psychologist, 67*, 111–129.

Lilienfeld, S. O. (2017a). Microaggressions: Strong claims, inadequate evidence. *Perspectives on Psychological Science, 12*(1), 138–169.

Lilienfeld, S. O. (2017b). Through a glass, darkly: Microaggressions and psychological science. *Perspectives on Psychological Science, 12*(1), 178–180.

Lilienfeld, S. O. (2020). Microaggression research and application: Clarifications, corrections, and common ground. *Perspectives on Psychological Science, 15*(1), 27–37.

Lopez, S. R., & Guarnaccia, P. J. (2000). Cultural psychopathology: Uncovering the social world of mental illness. *Annual Review of Psychology, 51*(1), 571–598.

Lott, B. (2010). *Multiculturalism and diversity: A social psychological perspective*. Blackwell.

Lynch, F. R. (1997). The diversity machine. *Society, 34*, 32–44.

Macrae, C. N., & Bodenhausen, G. V. (2000). Social cognition: Thinking categorically about others. *Annual Review of Psychology, 51*, 93–120.

Malik, K. (2015). The failure of multiculturalism: Community versus society in Europe. *Foreign Affairs, 94*, 21–32.

Michaels, W. B. (2006). *The trouble with diversity: How we learned to love identity and ignore inequality*. Metropolitan Books.

Mio, J. S., Barker, L. A., & Tumambing, J. S. (2012). *Multicultural psychology: Understanding our diverse communities*. Oxford University Press.

Moshman, D. (2011). Identity, genocide, and group violence. In S. J. Schwartz, K. Luyckx, & V. L. Vignoles (Eds.), *Handbook of identity theory and research* (pp. 917–932). Springer.

Mummendey, A., & Wenzel, M. (1999). Social discrimination and tolerance in intergroup relations: Reactions to intergroup difference. *Personality and Social Psychology Review, 3*, 158–174.

Naylor, L. L. (1998). *American culture: Myth and reality of a culture of diversity*. Greenwood Publishing Group.

No, S., Hong, Y. Y., Liao, H. Y., Lee, K., Wood, D., & Chao, M. M. (2008). Lay theory of race affects and moderates Asian Americans' responses toward American culture. *Journal of Personality and Social Psychology, 95*, 991–1004.

O'Donohue, W. (2018). Cultural competence and sensitivity in applied psychology: Ethical and scientific problems. In *Cultural competence in applied psychology* (pp. 103–122). Springer.

O'Donohue, W., & Benuto, L. (2010). The many problems of cultural sensitivity. *Scientific Review of Mental Health Practice, 7*, 34–37.

Owen, J., Leach, M. M., Wampold, B., & Rodolfa, E. (2011). Client and therapist variability in clients' perceptions of their therapists' multicultural competencies. *Journal of Counseling Psychology, 58*(1), 1–9.

Pap, A. (1953). Reduction-sentences and open concepts. *Methodos, 5*, 3–30.

Parekh, B. (2000). *Rethinking multiculturalism*. Palgrave Macmillan.

Pedersen, P. B. (1991). Introduction to the special issue on multiculturalism as a fourth force in counseling. *Journal of Counseling & Development, 70*(1), 4–4.

Pedersen, P. (Ed.). (2013). *Multiculturalism as a fourth force*. Brunner/Mazel.

Pettigrew, T. F., & Tropp, L. R. (2006). A meta-analytic test of intergroup contact theory. *Journal of Personality and Social Psychology, 90*, 751–783.

Pieterse, A. L., Evans, S. A., Risner-Butner, A., Collins, N. M., & Mason, L. B. (2009). Multicultural competence and social justice training in counseling psychology and counselor education: A review and analysis of a sample of multicultural course syllabi. *The Counseling Psychologist, 37*(1), 93–115.

Plaut, V. C., Garnett, F. G., Buffardi, L. E., & Sanchez-Burks, J. (2011). "What about me?" Perceptions of exclusion and Whites' reactions to multiculturalism. *Journal of Personality and Social Psychology, 101*, 337–353.

Plaut, V. C., Thomas, K. M., Hurd, K., & Romano, C. A. (2018). Do colorblindness and multiculturalism remedy or foster discrimination and racism? *Current Directions in Psychological Science, 27*, 200–206.

Popper, K. R. (1957). The aim of science. *Ratio, 1*(1), 24–35.

Reich, R. (2002). *Bridging liberalism and multiculturalism in American education*. University of Chicago Press.

Popper, K. R. (1963). *Conjectures and refutations: The growth of scientific knowledge*. Routledge.

Putnam, R. D. (2007). E Pluribus Unum: Diversity and community in the twenty-first century. The 2006 Johan Skytte prize lecture. *Scandinavian Political Studies, 30*, 137–174.

Saguy, T., Tausch, N., Dovidio, J. F., & Pratto, F. (2009). The irony of harmony: Intergroup contact can produce false expectations for equality. *Psychological Science, 20*, 114–121.

Samson, F. L. (2018). An association between multiculturalism and psychological distress. *PLoS One, 13*(12), e0208490.

Sanchez-Burks, J., Nisbett, R. E., & Ybarra, O. (2000). Cultural styles, relationship schemas, and prejudice against out-groups. *Journal of Personality and Social Psychology, 79*, 174–189.

Sarmento, C. (2014). Interculturalism, multiculturalism, and intercultural studies: Questioning definitions and repositioning strategies. *Intercultural Pragmatics, 11*, 603–618.

Schalk-Soekar, S., & van de Vijver, F. J. R. (2008). The concepts of multiculturalism: A study among Dutch majority members. *Journal of Applied Social Psychology, 38*, 2152–2178.

Schlesinger, A. M., Jr. (1998). *The disuniting of America: Reflections on a multicultural society* (2nd ed.). Norton.

Sell, J. (2018). Definitions and the development of theory in social psychology. *Social Psychology Quarterly, 81*(1), 8–22.

Shepherd, S. M. (2019). Cultural awareness workshops: limitations and practical consequences. *BMC Medical Education, 19*(1), 14–24.

Smith, M. J. (2000). *Culture: Reinventing the social sciences*. Open University Press.

Sidanius, J. (1993). The psychology of group conflict and the dynamics of oppression: A social dominance perspective. In S. Iyengar & W. J. McGuire (Eds.), *Explorations in political psychology* (pp. 183–219). Duke University Press.

Smith, L., Kashubeck-West, S., Payton, G., & Adams, E. (2017). White professors teaching about racism: Challenges and rewards. *The Counseling Psychologist, 45*, 651–668.

Spanierman, L. B., & Smith, L. (2017). Confronting White hegemony: A moral imperative for the helping professions. *The Counseling Psychologist, 45*, 727–736.

Spanierman, L. B., & Smith, L. (2017b). Roles and responsibilities of White allies: Implications for research, teaching, and practice. *The Counseling Psychologist, 45*, 606–617.
Stephan, W. G., & Stephan, C. W. (2013). Anintegrated theory of prejudice. In S. Oskamp (Ed.), *Reducing prejudice and discrimination: The Claremont Symposium on applied social psychology* (pp. 23–45). Lawrence Erlbaum Associates.
Stone, G. L. (1997). Multiculturalism as a context for supervision: Perspectives, limitations, and implications. In D. B. Pope-Davis & H. L. K. Coleman (Eds.), *Multicultural aspects of counseling series, Vol. 7. Multicultural counseling competencies: Assessment, education and training, and supervision* (pp. 263–289). Sage.
Stuart, R. B. (2004). Twelve practical suggestions for achieving multicultural competence. *Professional Psychology: Research and Practice, 35*(1), 3–9.
Sue, D. W. (2004). Whiteness and Ethnocentric Monoculturalism: Making the" Invisible" Visible. *American Psychologist, 59*, 761–769.
Sue, D. W. (2017). The challenges of becoming a White ally. *The Counseling Psychologist, 45*, 706–716.
Sue, D. W., Arredondo, P., & McDavis, R. J. (1992). Multicultural counseling competencies and standards: A call to the profession. *Journal of Counseling & Development, 70*(4), 477–486.
Sue, D. W., Bingham, R. P., Porché-Burke, L., & Vasquez, M. (1999). The diversification of psychology: A multicultural revolution. *American Psychologist, 54*, 1061–1069.
Sue, D. W., & Sue, S. (1990). *Counseling the culturally different*. Wiley.
Sue, D. W., & Sue, D. S. (2003). *Counseling the culturally diverse: Theory and practice* (4th ed.). Wiley.
Sue, D. W., & Sue, D. (2017). *Counseling the culturally diverse: Theory and practice* (7th ed.). Wiley.
Tajfel, H., & Turner, J. (1986). The social identity theory of intergroup behavior. In S. Worchel & W. Austin (Eds.), *Psychology of intergroup relations* (pp. 7–24). Nelson-Hall.
Townsend, M. (2018, April 14). Multiculturalism has failed, believe substantial minority of Britons. *The Guardian*. Accessed October 2018 from https://www.theguardian.com/world/2018/apr/14/multiculturalism-failed-substantial-minority-britons-integration-rivers-blood-enoch-powell
Triandis, H. C. (1994). *Culture and social behavior*. McGraw-Hill.
Triandis, H. C. (2007). Culture and psychology: A history of the study of their relationship. In S. Kitayama & D. Cohen (Eds.), *Handbook of cultural psychology* (pp. 59–76). Guilford Press.
Tseng, W. S. (2006). From peculiar psychiatric disorders through culture-bound syndromes to culture-related specific syndromes. *Transcultural Psychiatry, 43*, 554–576.
Turner, T. (1993). Anthropology and multiculturalism: What is anthropology that multiculturalists should be mindful of it? *Cultural Anthropology, 8*, 411–429.
Turner, J. C., Hogg, M., Oakes, P., Reicher, S., & Wetherell, M. (1987). *Rediscovering the social group: A self-categorization theory*. Basil Blackwell.
Tyler, S. A. (1976). Introduction to cognitive anthropology. In F. F. C. Gamst & E. Norbeck (Eds.), *Ideas of culture: Sources and uses* (pp. 177–186). Holt, Rinehart & Winston.
Unzueta, M. M., & Binning, K. R. (2010). Which racial groups are associated with diversity? *Cultural Diversity and Ethnic Minority Psychology, 16*, 443–446.
Vera, E. M., & Speight, S. L. (2003). Multicultural competence, social justice, and counseling psychology: Expanding our roles. *The Counseling Psychologist, 31*, 253–272.
Verkuyten, M. (2007). Social psychology and multiculturalism. *Social and Personality Psychology Compass, 1*(1), 280–297.
Verkuyten, M., & Brug, P. (2004). Multiculturalism and group status: The role of ethnic identification, group essentialism and protestant ethic. *European Journal of Social Psychology, 34*, 647–661.
Verkuyten, M., & Martinovic, B. (2006). Understanding multicultural attitudes: The role of group status, identification, friendships, and justifying ideologies. *International Journal of Intercultural Relations, 30*(1), 1–18.

Verkuyten, M., & Yogeeswaran, K. (2020). Cultural diversity and its implications for intergroup relations. *Current Opinion in Psychology*.

Vignoles, V. L. (2011). Identity motives. In S. J. Schwartz, K. Luyckx, & V. L. Vignoles (Eds.), *Handbook of identity theory and research* (pp. 403–432). Springer.

Webster, Y. O. (1997). *Against the multicultural agenda: A critical thinking alternative*. Praeger.

Wilton, L. S., Apfelbaum, E. P., & Good, J. J. (2019). Valuing differences and reinforcing them: Multiculturalism increases race essentialism. *Social Psychological and Personality Science, 10*, 681–689.

Wilson, E. O. (2014). *The meaning of human existence*. WW Norton & Company.

Wolsko, C., Park, B., Judd, C. M., & Wittenbrink, B. (2000). Framing interethnic ideology: Effects of multicultural and color-blind perspectives on judgments of groups and individuals. *Journal of Personality and Social Psychology, 78*, 635–654.

Wood, R. T. (2003). The straightedge youth sub-culture: Observations on the complexity of sub-cultural identity. *Journal of Youth Studies, 6*(1), 33–52.

Wright, R. H., & Cummings, N. A. (Eds.). (2005). *Destructive trends in mental health: The well intentioned path to harm*. Routledge.

Controversies in Posttraumatic Stress Disorder

Richard A. Bryant

One of the fundamental controversies regarding PTSD involves the conceptualization of the syndrome. Specifically, does it reflect a disease state or is it better understood as a construct reflecting one dimension of human stress response? Put another way, is PTSD qualitatively or quantitatively distinct from normal stress reactions? The DSM nosology functions under the assumption that PTSD is a distinct diagnostic entity. However, research has shown that the severity and number of PTSD symptoms both have linear relationships with impairment in both role functioning and psychopathology (Blanchard et al., 1994; Kulka et al., 1990). PTSD symptoms have been shown to emerge in response to minor oral surgery (de Jongh et al., 2008), routine childbirth (Olde et al., 2006), and bad movies (Lees-Haley et al., 2001). These findings make sense if we consider that many of the symptoms of PTSD, such as nightmares and sleep disturbances, represent common non-descript stress symptoms (Bonanno et al., 2006). This may indicate that PTSD symptoms are best represented and studied as a single dimension of severity. Over 50 years ago, Meehl popularized an important line of inquiry that attempted to distinguish between taxometric and dimensional approaches to understanding psychological disorders (Meehl, 1965). Over the years this approach has led to a range of statistical methods to understand if psychological disorders are better understood as categorical entities or dimensions of a phenotype (Haslam, 2011). Although a gross over-simplification, it may be said that those trained in medical sciences tend to adopt a categorical approach and view psychiatric disorders in a dichotomous manner in which it is either present or absent. Those trained in psychology may be more likely to view psychological states in a dimensional framework and conceptualize PTSD on a continuum of stress symptoms.

R. A. Bryant (✉)
School of Psychology, University of New South Wales, Sydney, Australia
e-mail: r.bryant@unsw.edu.au

C. L. Cobb et al. (eds.), *Toward a Science of Clinical Psychology*,
https://doi.org/10.1007/978-3-031-14332-8_18

The underlying challenge for the PTSD diagnosis (as well as other psychiatric disorders) is that it attempts to differentiate those who function well and those who do not. There is abundant evidence that people who experience subsyndromal levels of PTSD experience comparable levels of impairment as those with sufficient symptoms to meet the full criteria for the PTSD diagnosis (Marshall et al., 2001; Stein et al., 1997). The importance of this pattern is indicated by studies showing that subsyndromal PTSD is associated with marked impairment and comorbidity and apparently would benefit from mental health assistance (Mylle & Maes, 2004; Pietrzak et al., 2012). From an epidemiological point of view, this is problematic because reported rates of PTSD do not account for people who do not meet the cut-off for the requisite for the PTSD diagnosis by one or two symptoms. The limitation of categorizing people into either having or not having PTSD assumes that these groups are actually different groups, when in fact this is an artificial distinction imposed by definitions developed by diagnostic committees (MacCallum et al., 2002).

Perusal of studies of large cohorts that utilize taxometric analyses to examine if PTSD represents a distinct clinical syndrome has concluded that PTSD does not form a taxon, and that PTSD symptomatology is difference in degree rather than in kind from lesser stress responses (Broman-Fulks et al., 2006; Ruscio et al., 2002). This finding does not discount the value of diagnostic categorizations because they do provide a range of benefits, and most importantly allowing clinicians and researchers to simply identify people as having PTSD, promoting treatments, and classifying people into groups to facilitate analyses (DeCoster et al., 2009). It is important, however, to keep in mind that this categorization of PTSD is not reflective of an underlying qualitatively distinct disease.

How Common Is PTSD?

The problems of how PTSD is conceptualized diagnostically are reflected in epidemiological studies. There is a wide range in prevalence rates of PTSD in standardized studies of PTSD. For example, the World Mental Health Survey used the Composite International Diagnostic Interview that is based on DSM-IV and ICD-10 (Kessler & Üstün, 2004). This study found that 12-month prevalence rates of PTSD varied from 0.3% in Mexico to 3.8% in Northern Ireland (Karam et al., 2014). Interestingly, there were lower rates of PTSD in low- (0.8%) and middle-income (0.7%) countries relative to high-income (1.5%) countries. This is a somewhat surprising pattern considering that traumatic and adverse events are experienced more frequently in low- and middle-income countries as a result of humanitarian crises, war, and civil conflict (Charlson et al., 2019).

One salient example of how the PTSD diagnosis can lead to problems in estimating prevalence of PTSD can be seen in the prevalence rates of PTSD in Vietnam veterans. In an early estimate of PTSD in this population, the National Vietnam Veteran Readjustment Study (NVRRS) reported that the point prevalence in the late

1980s of PTSD was 15.2% of veterans (Kulka et al., 1990). A subsequent re-analysis of the study that adjusted for several factors, including a more stringent test of satisfaction of the stressor criterion and requiring cases to have more than mild levels of functional impairment, found that the rate of PTSD decreased to 9.1%, which represented a 40% decrease in prevalence relative to the initial estimate (Dohrenwend et al., 2006). When this analysis was adjusted to recognize only those cases with clinically significant functional impairment, the rate of PTSD fell further to 5.4% (McNally, 2007). This re-analysis of the NVVRS led to a major debate among PTSD researchers as they argued over the different ways in which PTSD could be operationalized and the impacts these variants had on the observed prevalence rates of PTSD in Vietnam veterans (McNally, 2007; Schlenger et al., 2007). This example highlights one of the key problems in how we define the diagnosis of PTSD.

In this context the PTSD diagnosis was introduced in DSM-III primarily in reaction to the need to classify the psychological problems experienced by Vietnam veterans (Helzer et al., 1987). In this iteration of DSM the diagnosis required that a person report a minimum number of symptoms from three groupings of symptoms; this approach has been used consistently since then with the diagnosis requiring a minimum number of symptoms from a specified number of symptom types. This approach makes certain assumptions that may not be necessarily justified. For example, by tallying the symptoms to arrive at the necessary number, it assumes that each symptom is of equal weight in contributing to the disorder. This assumption is not necessarily justified. Moreover, the assumption that the contribution of each cluster is equally weighted may also not be justified.

Though clusters and symptoms have always ultimately been decided by committees (Buckley et al., 1998), in an attempt to put this practice on strong empirical footing, numerous factor analytic studies have been conducted to empirically identify the correct dimensions of PTSD. Factor analyses have most commonly revealed two (Buckley et al., 1998; Taylor et al., 1998), three (Larsson, 2005), and four symptom factors (Asmundson et al., 2000; King et al., 1998; Palmieri & Fitzgerald, 2005). The symptoms within a factor often vary across these studies even if the number of factors did not. The DSM-5 task force has come out in favor of four clusters because this converges with findings from most factor analytic studies (American Psychiatric Association, 2011). The reason for the different factor solutions remains unknown. However, recent findings indicate that the factor structure, including the number of factors and symptoms that comprise those factors, is population dependent (Shevlin & Elklit, 2012). This indicates that a true universal factor structure may not exist, although this conclusion requires further replication.

The Diagnostic Definition Conundrum

Another issue in how PTSD is defined is how the core symptoms are identified. One of the major controversies in recent years was expansion of the PTSD definitional criteria in DSM-5 (American Psychiatric Association, 2013). There was a major shift in DSM-5 to increase the number of potential symptoms that one could have as part of the PTSD syndrome from 17 in DSM-IV to 20 in DSM-5. Moreover, DSM-5 introduced a new cluster of symptoms called *Negative Alterations in Mood and Cognition*. New symptoms included risky behavior, distorted negative beliefs about oneself or the trauma, self-blame, and general negative emotional states. These additional symptoms were included because of increasing evidence of the role of cognitive processes in the development and maintenance of PTSD (Ehlers & Clark, 2000). However, another major reason for introducing symptoms, such as risk-taking and negative emotional states, was that it was considered to reflect certain groups of trauma-exposed people, such as the military and victims of crime (Friedman et al., 2011). This approach was strongly criticized by some commentators because it was perceived that the attempt to have a more all-embracing diagnosis that addressed the range of psychological reactions people may experience after trauma undermined much of the evidence pertaining to the fear-based disorder that has traditionally characterized PTSD (Hoge et al., 2016). Potentially supporting this argument is one report that calculated that, considering the 20 PTSD symptoms in PTSD across the four clusters, there were 636,120 different permutations that could make up the PTSD diagnosis (Galatzer-Levy & Bryant, 2013).

Apart from highlighting the manner in which the PTSD diagnosis reflects changing views about the purpose of the diagnosis rather than an underlying disease state, the expansion of symptoms in the DSM-5 raises an old question regarding PTSD: Should it encompass the range of common stress reactions or should it be restricted to those that are most distinctive of disorder? This issue is particularly pertinent to PTSD because stress reactions are common in the population as people are faced with life stressors (Bonanno et al., 2006), and indeed numerous PTSD symptoms can occur in the wake of common stressors such as childbirth (Olde et al., 2006). It has been argued that a purer way to identify true disorder is to focus on people with symptoms that are distinctive of PTSD rather than those that are common to more normative forms of stress reaction (McNally, 2009). It is possible that less common symptoms, such as emotional numbing, may be more distinctive of PTSD (Foa et al., 1995). It is possible that focusing on constellations of symptoms that identify people with key functional impairment and distress may optimally define PTSD. In adopting such a position, however, one could sacrifice the clinical utility of the disorder because many people who would otherwise benefit from evidence-based treatments for PTSD may not be identified with a highly restrictive definition.

The underlying premise of many conceptualizations of PTSD is that the symptoms defined by diagnostic definitions reflect an underlying core pathology. One of the ongoing challenges in the field of PTSD is that because the PTSD diagnosis is used widely by clinicians, researchers, and the public, it is easy to begin to accept that it is a distinct illness. It is always worth remembering that psychiatric diagnoses are determined by committees that interpret the available literature in a way that allows groups of symptoms to be clustered into a discrete syndrome and that purportedly identifies people with and without the illness. Today the two most widely used systems are the American Psychiatric Association's DSM and the World Health Organization's *International Classification of Diseases* (ICD). Rather than being mechanistically based, psychiatric diagnoses in the systems were initially intended to simply provide a method for pragmatic use of counting people in health systems that had a designated disorder (Kraemer, 2007). In the early iterations of these systems, the diagnostic categories were very broad and did not accurately distinguish among patients with different psychological presentations (Wilson, 1993). DSM-III marked a shift in emphasis in which the diagnostic system strove for greater specificity, placed emphasis on observable symptoms to achieve greater reliability in diagnostic decisions, and made an explicit link with biological bases of disorders (Spitzer et al., 1975, 1978). This highlights a long-standing debate in the field of PTSD in which some people have argued that PTSD reflects a biological entity (Yehuda & McFarlane, 1997), whereas others have suggested it is a socially constructed construct that is shaped by cultural factors (Young, 1995). Although it is often stated that PTSD does reflect an extreme form of normal stress (Ruscio et al., 2002), there is a persistent assumption that PTSD is a qualitatively distinct set of symptoms that are a consequence of an underlying biological (typically it is considered a neural dysfunction) disorder. That is, in the same way as a fever may reflect an infection, underpinning the extreme stress symptoms that are defined as PTSD there is a pathological stress disease (Borsboom & Cramer, 2013).

In recent years this issue has led to an explosion of work that has adopted a statistical approach to studying PTSD termed network analyses. This method assumes that symptoms of PTSD, or any disorder, do not covary because they are a consequence of an underlying latent disease; rather, they are linked with each other in potentially causal ways (Cramer et al., 2010; Kendler et al., 2011). Put another way, the network analysis approach regards symptoms as constituting a disorder rather than being reflective of an underlying disease, and in this sense, the symptoms can perpetuate each other (McNally et al., 2015). For example, nightmares in PTSD may contribute to sleep disturbance, which can lead to irritability, which can influence social withdrawal, which can lead to rumination, which can further contribute to sleep disturbance. In this way, these symptoms can potentially feedback on each other and perpetuate the syndrome. From a clinical perspective, this approach presumes that the causal direction embedded in network analyses allows for the possibility of a symptom to be targeted in an intervention with the expectation that there may be benefits in reductions in symptoms that are impacted by the targeted symptom. If intrusive memories were observed to be causally related to sleep disturbance, which was associated with concentration deficits, one could expect an intervention specifically addressing intrusive memories to result in consequent improvements in concentration.

Recent years have seen several network studies conducted with PTSD samples. These have observed a range of patterns across many different samples of trauma-exposed people. These studies have shown strong connections between hypervigilance and startle (Armour et al., 2017; McNally et al., 2015; Birkeland & Heir, 2017), nightmares and intrusions (Birkeland & Heir, 2017; Knefel et al., 2016), flashbacks and intrusive memories (McNally et al., 2017), and intrusive thoughts and irritability (Phillips et al., 2018). Studies have also identified those PTSD symptoms that are highly central, meaning they have strong links to many other PTSD symptoms, including physiological and psychological reactivity (McNally et al., 2017), negative trauma-related emotions, flashbacks, and detachment (Armour et al., 2017), emotional numbing (Birkeland & Heir, 2017), and intrusion, social detachment, nightmares, concentration deficits, and startle response (Fried et al., 2018). This approach has also investigated how symptom networks change over time (Bryant et al., 2017). Interestingly, these studies have also shown how PTSD symptoms are related to other symptoms associated with related disorders, including depression and prolonged grief disorder (Malgaroli et al., 2018). The growing literature using network analyses is strongly indicating that PTSD does reflect several symptoms that are, to varying degrees, reliant on each other. This is a robust indication that the PTSD diagnosis should not be understood as reflecting an underlying disease state.

The Role of Dissociation in PTSD

One of the most persistent controversies in PTSD has been the nature of dissociation and how it fits into our understanding of PTSD. The notion of dissociation is based on the premise that traumatized people can regulate their distress by dissociating awareness of the experience and its associated emotions, and in this way, they can cope more effectively in the short term. From a historical perspective, this perspective can be traced back to the end of the nineteenth century when Jean-Martin Charcot studied the dissociative reactions in traumatized patients he treated at the Salpêtrière Hospital in Paris (Micale, 2001). Charcot documented the disturbances in perception, cognition, or motor ability in patients without commensurate physical injuries. Charcot proposed that these patients experienced a dissociation of the ego, in which one is suggestible to representations of the accident or experience and could result in physical or sensory dysfunctions (Charcot, 1877). One of Charcot's students, Pierre Janet, expanded on this view and proposed that people attempt to cope with aversive experiences by dissociating from awareness, but that this resulted in much psychological energy being expended that led to poor psychological functioning (Janet, 1907). Although the attention given to dissociation was largely overshadowed by behaviorism and biological models in the following years, it had a resurgence in the later part of the twentieth century as psychiatry "re-discovered" the ideas in dissociative models (van der Kolk & van der Hart, 1989).

Consistent with the emerging popularity of dissociative models, models began to emerge of dissociative processes in models of PTSD (Butler et al., 1996). These models reshaped Janet's earlier thinking and suggested that dissociative responses after trauma could take the shape of dissociative amnesia, emotional numbing, derealization, or depersonalization, and that the common factor of these reactions was that they reduced awareness of aversive emotions. Without a great deal of supporting evidence, this influence in North American psychiatry led to the introduction of the new diagnosis of acute stress disorder into DSM-IV, which put much emphasis on dissociative symptoms (American Psychiatric Association, 1994). One goal of this diagnosis was to identify people who would subsequently develop PTSD, and the rationale for the emphasis on dissociative reactions was that they may limit access to trauma memories and associated emotions, which may impede processing of trauma memories and thereby may predict PTSD (Bryant & Harvey, 1997).

There has been indirect evidence of the role of dissociation in trauma response, insofar as there are higher levels of hypnotizability in people with PTSD (Spiegel et al., 1988) and acute stress disorder (Bryant et al., 2001), and people with dissociative disorders have higher rates of traumatic histories (Kluft, 1987). There has been considerable evidence of a relation between dissociative responses during or after a traumatic experience ("peritraumatic dissociation") and subsequent PTSD. Longitudinal studies have consistently demonstrated a statistical association between self-reported dissociative responses and subsequent PTSD (Ehlers et al., 1998; Murray et al., 2002; Shalev et al., 1998).

There is also evidence, however, that questions the predictive role of peritraumatic dissociation. Peritraumatic dissociation has been found in nonsexual assault victims; however, it has been found to be not predictive in rape victims (Dancu et al., 1996). More evidence comes from longitudinal studies of acute stress disorder and subsequent PTSD. One review of longitudinal studies revealed that whereas most studies found that more than half of people with acute stress disorder subsequently developed PTSD, less than half of people who eventually developed PTSD initially met the full criteria for acute stress disorder (Bryant, 2011). A number of these longitudinal studies determined that not requiring the dissociative cluster of symptoms as necessary for a definition of acute stress disorder found more people who developed PTSD were identified by the acute stress disorder diagnosis. This pattern of findings suggests that there are multiple pathways to developing PTSD, and some people may develop the disorder without ever experiencing dissociative reactions. As a result of this accumulating evidence, dissociation was de-emphasized in DSM-5 and was no longer required for one to meet the criteria for a diagnosis of acute stress disorder (Bryant et al., 2011).

It is important to note that despite the fact that the statistical association between peritraumatic dissociation and later PTSD is a robust finding, this relation may occur as a result of dissociation interacting with other factors rather than occurring in a linear manner (Breh & Seidler, 2007; Velden et al., 2006). In other words, dissociation may be an epiphenomenon that is associated with predicting PTSD. It has been suggested that peritraumatic dissociation is a function of hyperarousal in the aftermath of trauma exposure, resulting in dissociation reflecting heightened peritraumatic arousal rather than a distinct cognitive defense mechanism (Friedman, 2000; Gershuny & Thayer, 1999). The notion that dissociation is associated with strong arousal is well documented. Flashbacks, which are dissociative episodes in which a person momentarily loses episodic awareness, can be triggered by administering yohimbine to PTSD individuals (Southwick et al., 1993). People also often dissociate during panic attacks (Krystal et al., 1991). Most importantly, recently trauma-exposed people experience dissociation if asked to hyperventilate (Nixon & Bryant, 2006), which is relevant because panic attacks are very common during trauma, and more than half of trauma-exposed people experience some panic in the period immediately after the event (Nixon & Bryant, 2003). Further, there is evidence that the association between peritraumatic dissociation and acute stress is influenced by levels of peritraumatic panic (Fikretoglu et al., 2006, 2007). Additionally, many people report dissociative experiences during states of high arousal that are not associated with any current or subsequent psychopathology, such as skydiving (Bryant, 2007; Sterlini & Bryant, 2002). The normality of dissociative responses under conditions of high arousal is also reflected in the common reports after trauma of reduced awareness of one's surroundings (Sloan, 1988; Titchener & Kapp, 1976), as well as derealization and depersonalization (Cardeña & Spiegel, 1993; Sloan, 1988).

The notion that dissociative responses are normative in the wake of high arousal would suggest that transient dissociation during a trauma may not be strongly predictive of later PTSD. Consistent with this view, several studies have found that peritraumatic dissociation measured shortly after trauma exposure is not as predictive of ASD (Panasetis & Bryant, 2003) or later PTSD (Briere et al., 2005; Gil et al., 2016) as dissociative responses that are persistent over time. Reinforcing the doubts over the extent that dissociation does predict PTSD, researchers have shown that after controlling for the effects of initial PTSD and depression, peritraumatic dissociation does not predict subsequent PTSD (Zatzick et al., 2006).

It is also possible that peritraumatic dissociation may be associated with subsequent PTSD because dissociation is associated with other known risk factors for PTSD. For example, history of childhood trauma is associated with both subsequent dissociation tendencies (Spiegel & Cardeña, 1991) and adult PTSD (Brewin et al., 2000b). Although not adequately researched, it is possible that psychopathological mechanisms resulting from childhood trauma set in chain a pattern of coping, cognitive styles, and behavioral patterns that are associated with a predisposition to later dissociation and PTSD when confronted by a traumatic experience. This is a different conclusion from the one that emphasizes a causal relation between peritraumatic dissociation and later PTSD.

A key platform of dissociative models is that trauma memories are managed in a way that limits emotional engagement with them. One prevailing perspective on why memories may be formed differently in the context of PTSD is that the high arousal associated with a traumatic experience results in a predominance of sensory information being encoded. Importantly, this perspective does not invoke models of dissociation or defense mechanisms. Ehlers and Clark (2000) postulated a model that emphasizes the "data-driven" nature of encoding of trauma memories, which involves heightened arousal resulting in people encoding sensory impressions of an experience rather than verbal thoughts. In this model, a person may encode images of blood splattered across a windscreen after a car crash but lack the coherent narrative that would normally be encoded into one's autobiographical memory. As a result of this sensory encoding, it is proposed that trauma memories are often consolidated in a fragmented manner and lack a coherent narrative. This model has many similarities with other cognitive models of PTSD, including Brewin's Dual Representation Theory (Brewin et al., 1996, 2010), which holds that flashback memories are encoded via a perceptually processed system that entails fragmented, high detailed sensory information. Extending these models, Holmes has led a series of studies in which completing a visuospatial task interferes with encoding perceptual information and subsequently results in fewer intrusive memories (Davies et al., 2012; Deeprose et al., 2012; Holmes et al., 2004, 2009). Longitudinal studies have also found that self-reported data-driven processing of events during the traumatic event predicts subsequent PTSD (Ehring et al., 2008; Halligan et al., 2002, 2003).

Consistent with models of perceptual processing of traumatic stimuli, some studies indicate that trauma memories tend to be fragmented and lack coherence. These memories tend to be out of sequence or contain gaps in the narrative (Amir et al., 1998; Foa et al., 1995; Foa & Riggs, 1993; van der Kolk & Fisler, 1995). Similar patterns have been observed in the acute phase after trauma; people with acute stress disorder reported more fragmented narratives than those without this presentation (Harvey & Bryant, 1999). It should be noted, however, that other evidence indicates that PTSD is *not* characterized by fragmented memories and should not be considered a robust feature of the disorder (Rubin et al., 2016). Overall, although the evidence regarding trauma memories describes phenomena that are often included as "dissociative," the models that explain this evidence do not presume a defensive mechanism involved in theories of dissociation but rather describe distinctive encoding processes during heightened threat.

Prediction of PTSD

At a clinical level, one of the major goals in the field of traumatic stress for nearly 30 years has been developing accurate means to predict who will develop PTSD in the immediate aftermath of trauma exposure. This effort has sparked much debate among researchers and clinicians, and, as noted above, was a major driver for introducing the acute stress disorder diagnosis (Harvey & Bryant, 2002). Much of the earlier work was conducted on the premise that there was a linear course after trauma, with many people having PTSD symptoms in the immediate aftermath of trauma but for most people these reactions would subside over time. This perspective was supported by evidence that rates of PTSD tended to diminish in the months after trauma with respect to the rates in the acute phase (Riggs et al., 1995; Rothbaum et al., 1992). This pattern was the rationale for PTSD traditionally not being diagnosed in DSM until a month after trauma exposure, as the DSM did not warrant to confuse transient stress reactions as a psychiatric disorder.

The conceptualization of the course of PTSD has changed over the years as researchers have conducted more sophisticated longitudinal studies. In short, studies that have tracked the course of traumatic stress in the same people over time have found that the course of PTSD is very dynamic and fluctuates greatly over time. One longitudinal study that assessed traumatic injury patients in the hospital, and subsequently at periodic times over the course of the following two years, found that the rate of PTSD remained generally consistent; however, the people who displayed no, subsyndromal, or full PTSD shifted by approximately 50% from one assessment to the next (Bryant et al., 2013). This pattern has been noted in other studies with multiple assessments, and it appears that a major influence of worsening PTSD at any point is the extent that current life stressors are affecting a person (Bryant et al., 2021a). The recognition that PTSD fluctuates over time and is moderated by ongoing stressors highlights a major challenge for predicting PTSD from the acute phase because it does not follow a linear course and a major predictor of subsequent PTSD (i.e., subsequent life stressors) is not present in the acute phase.

Arguably, the most interesting shift in how we have changed our understanding of the course of PTSD in more recent times has been the focus on trajectories of severity of PTSD. One of the major limitations of focusing on diagnostic prevalence rates is that it assumes that the diagnostic category properly accounts for the posttraumatic stress associated with impairment and distress. The previously discussed evidence regarding the detrimental impact of subsyndromal PTSD highlights that the PTSD diagnosis fails to adequately capture all those patients who display posttraumatic distress sufficient to contribute to impairment (Stein et al., 1997). To improve on this simplistic and potentially misleading approach, many studies have used a statistical method involving latent growth mixture modeling, which classifies homogeneous groups in a population to identify classes of individual variation over time. Instead of assuming that each person is part of a homogeneous or uniform group, it maps heterogeneous patterns of response that permit distinct trajectories to be mapped over time.

Many studies have now been completed using this technique, and the findings have generally been very consistent, with most studies identifying four major trajectories of posttraumatic stress: (a) a resilient class that consistently shows few PTSD symptoms, (b) a recovery class with initial distress then gradual remission over time, (c) a delayed reaction class with initial low symptom levels but increased symptoms over time, and (d) a chronic distress class with consistently high PTSD levels (Galatzer-Levy et al., 2018a). These patterns have been found in survivors of traumatic injury (Bryant et al., 2015), SARS infection (Bonanno et al., 2008), women diagnosed with breast cancer (Lam et al., 2010), disaster (Pietrzak et al., 2013), and military personnel deployed to the Middle East (Bonanno et al., 2012).

One conclusion from these studies is that in general 75–80% of people are resilient over time and do not require mental health assistance. We have limited knowledge at this time to accurately predict the trajectories that the other 25% of people may follow, which could be chronically stressed, worsening over time, or potentially remitting as time progresses. One approach may be to develop methods to identify those who are likely to follow a resilient trajectory and focus mental health resources on the much smaller proportion of a population who may not be resilient. New approaches are needed to identify probable subsequent psychological outcomes following a traumatic event that allow clinicians to identify a person as being probably resilient or not. The capacity to adequately predict who will develop PTSD requires that we can differentiate in the acute phase between people experiencing a transient stress response and those who display signs of stress that is a precursor of subsequent PTSD. To achieve optimal prediction there is the need for a good balance between sensitivity and specificity, as well as positive and negative predictive power.

In terms of predicting PTSD, sensitivity involves the probability that someone who eventually develops PTSD satisfied the acute predictor, and specificity is the probability that someone who does not develop PTSD did not satisfy the acute predictor. Positive predictive power involves the probability that a person who satisfies the acute predictor subsequently develops PTSD, and negative predictive power is the probability that someone who does not display the acute predictor does not develop PTSD. It would be simple to achieve very strong sensitivity and positive predictive power for predicting PTSD if we used a very low threshold for a predictor in the acute phase, but the trade-off is that this formula would identify too many people who would subsequently not develop PTSD. This would make the utility of such a prediction tool very weak.

Although there have been many attempts to study the capacity to predict PTSD from early stress symptoms, the results have generally been modest in terms of accurate prediction (Bryant, 2003). In more recent years researchers have attempted to use more rigorous approaches to investigating the relation between acute responses and longer-term adaptation. One study used data from a consortium of teams that used comparable methods to predict longer-term PTSD from acute responses and used a pooled sample of 2473 trauma survivors from ten studies using a likelihood estimate approach (Shalev et al., 2019). This study used multiple indicators and found that among people with elevated early symptom severity, being female, having less than secondary-level education, and reporting exposure to prior interpersonal trauma was associated with a 34% greater likelihood of developing PTSD. This approach highlights the utility of looking beyond acute self-reported symptoms and recognizing the predictive role of other risk factors for PTSD. This general approach has also been reported in more recent studies using machine learning with large sets of potential candidate predictors. The advantage of machine learning is that it uses supervised methods to compute many different variables by using mathematical rules to derive best-fitting models (Galatzer-Levy et al., 2018b). One very well-controlled study of patients admitted to an emergency department used both psychological symptoms and biological variables routinely collected in hospital admission (including lymphocytes, blood glucose) (Schultebraucks et al., 2020). This study found that using the algorithm derived by the machine learning model, of the patients that the algorithm predicted would be non-remitting in their stress symptoms, 90% were still non-remitting 12 months after admission; impressively, this finding was replicated in an independent emergency department. We have still not arrived at a point where we can accurately predict who will develop PTSD, but our approaches are becoming more sophisticated. We are now asking more sensible questions rather than who will and will not develop PTSD in a way that assumes people will fall neatly into two distinct categories.

The Definition of a Traumatic Event

One of the factors that have been debated over many years is the specification of the type of stressful event that can precipitate PTSD (Maier, 2007; Weathers & Keane, 2007). People experience many stressors during their lives, and it is normal to have a stress response when these events occur. What exactly are the types of events that can be considered "traumatic" relative to lesser stressors? PTSD is one of the few psychiatric disorders to specify the trigger event, and in this sense the Criterion A cluster in DSM has always served as a "gatekeeper" for considering potential symptoms that a person presents with. The conceptualization of the traumatic event has evolved over time. In DSM-III the trigger stressor was defined as a stressor that would elicit significant symptoms in "almost anyone," and it was presumed that these occurred after events that were "generally outside the range of usual human experiences" (American Psychiatric Association, 1980). As awareness grew that traumatic events actually occur for most people at some time in their lives (Breslau et al., 1991), the criteria were restricted into two subdivisions that described the event itself and the subjective response to it. DSM-IV stipulated that the event was a significant threat to oneself or others (Criterion A1). To limit the definition to more traumatic events, Criterion A2 was included to require the person respond to the event with "fear, helplessness, or horror." These varying definitions highlight some of the vagaries of how we define traumatic events and need to be considered carefully.

The different iterations of DSM have been somewhat loose in the extent to which they consider the traumatic event as being causal in developing PTSD or simply temporally preceding the event (Friedman et al., 2011). As knowledge has accumulated over the years, it has become apparent that the risk of developing PTSD following exposure to a traumatic event is strongly influenced by genetic and characterological factors (Ozer et al., 2003). This pattern reinforces the conclusion that traumatic events are not entirely causative, but they interact with pre-existing factors that lead to the development of PTSD. Much work has been done on the relative influences of these two factors, with delineation between traumatic and non-traumatic stressors (Dohrenwend, 2006). In short, studies have supported the position that PTSD is typically more likely to occur in the aftermath of potentially life-threatening events (e.g., disasters, assaults, war), rather than events such as bullying or sexual harassment (Kilpatrick et al., 2009). Some people will report post-traumatic stress symptoms, including intrusive memories, after non-traumatic stressors such as childbirth and violent movies (Lees-Haley et al., 2001; Olde et al., 2006). However, in these cases, the causal influence tends to involve pre-existing factors more than the triggering event.

Over the years much debate has focused on the so-called bracket-creep that involves the broadening of the definition of eligible traumatic events. In different iterations of DSM, the definition has expanded to include learning about others experiencing threat, and to more recent times, electronic or digital exposure to events (Friedman et al., 2011). This issue was addressed empirically in a study that compared prevalence rates of PTSD when traumatic events were defined variably in a narrow (including combat, rape) versus a more broadly defined (e.g., learning about manner; Breslau & Kessler, 2001). This study found that the prevalence increased by 59.2% when using a broader definition of traumatic event. Some debate has also occurred over the extent to which viewing televised or photographed traumatic material can trigger PTSD. Some studies reported high rates of PTSD on the west coast of the US in people who watched broadcasts of the attacks on the World Trade Towers on 9/11 (Silver et al., 2002); however, other studies found this effect was only evident for those directly affected by the attacks or had been exposed to other disasters (Ahern et al., 2002). Overall, the evidence that this form of indirect exposure is responsible for PTSD is not well supported by evidence (Breslau et al., 2010). One of the major problems is that the causal direction between an observed association of PTSD and amount of viewing of trauma images has yet to be clarified.

The issue of how to define traumatic events continues to be debated, and some commentators have proposed omitting the requirement of exposure to a traumatic event because traumatic events can also trigger other psychiatric disorders, and repeated exposure to less traumatic stressful events can trigger PTSD symptoms (Brewin et al., 2009). This position has never been adopted by DSM because the weight of evidence is on the side of more traumatic events accounting for the vast bulk of PTSD cases. Further, legal experts have often voiced many concerns that excessively broadening or removing the Criterion A would result in excessive litigation arising from minor events that one could not reasonably expect to trigger PTSD (Rosen & Lilienfeld, 2008). Overall, the convergent evidence has resulted in the consensus view that restricting the definition of a traumatic event to those events that are more likely to be experienced as life-threatening or a major threat to a person are those that are more likely to trigger PTSD.

The other contentious feature of the definition of traumatic event has been linking it in DSM-IV to the response of "fear, helplessness, or horror" (Criterion A2). This component of the diagnosis has always been problematic because it confuses the event with the response to it (McNally, 2009). Practical problems with the Criterion A2 include findings that many people can develop PTSD who do not have an immediate emotional response (e.g., first responders who are in "operational mode" during a traumatic event; Creamer et al., 2005; O'Donnell et al., 2010) or may have other emotional responses other than the ones prescribed by DSM (e.g., shame, anger; Brewin et al., 2000a; Rizvi et al., 2008). Interestingly, removing the requirement of the A2 criterion does not markedly affect the prevalence of PTSD: This finding has been observed in community (Breslau & Kessler, 2001), military (Schnurr et al., 2000), and cross-national studies (Karam et al., 2010). It is for these reasons that this feature of the definition of a traumatic event was removed in DSM-5 (Friedman et al., 2011).

Does Delayed-Onset PTSD Exist?

One of the great curiosities in the field of traumatic stress has been delayed-onset PTSD, which has traditionally been defined as PTSD that develops at least six months after exposure to the traumatic event. This subtype of PTSD was introduced into DSM many years ago, initially as a result of historical cases of soldiers who showed no symptoms of PTSD during combat but reported the disorder months or years later (Andreasen, 2004). There are even reported cases of PTSD developing decades after trauma exposure (Ruzich et al., 2005). Many studies have documented the rates of this type of presentation, and systematic reviews suggest that of those people who develop PTSD, approximately 25% may be delayed-onset cases (Andrews et al., 2007; Smid et al., 2009). Despite the pattern of DSM always recognizing this delayed-onset, there has never been clear understanding of the exact definition or mechanisms of this form of PTSD.

The greater knowledge of the course of posttraumatic stress symptoms has produced more insights into delayed-onset PTSD. The available evidence indicates that most cases of delayed-onset experience significant levels of PTSD in the acute phase, but these levels do not meet diagnostic threshold; these stress reactions apparently worsen over time and people subsequently meet the diagnostic criteria (Bryant & Harvey, 2002; Buckley et al., 1996; Carty et al., 2006; Green et al., 1993; O'Donnell et al., 2013). That is, many of the so-called cases of delayed-onset PTSD are more accurately described as worsening of symptoms rather than a sudden onset of PTSD after the absence of symptoms. This pattern accords with latent growth mixture modeling studies of longitudinal data that have reliably identified a worsening class of symptoms in a proportion of trauma survivors (for a review, see Galatzer-Levy et al., 2018a). The conclusion that this form of PTSD may involve worsening mental health is indicated in DSM-5, which unlike previous iterations of DSM states that delayed-onset cases are those in which the person does not fulfill all diagnostic criteria and may experience some level of subsyndromal symptomatology in the acute phase.

It needs to be noted, however, that there is some evidence that true delayed-onset PTSD does occur in some individuals (Smid et al., 2009). This pattern of having minimal apparent symptoms in the acute phase but meeting diagnostic criteria after six months is particularly evident in military cohorts (Andrews et al., 2007). Although we do not have strong evidence for the reasons for how delayed-onset cases develop, there are several mechanisms proposed. Emotion researchers have focused on the central role of denial and numbing in the acute phase, and how this can inhibit PTSD responses for a period of time. This perspective holds that as numbing abates over time, people experience worsening of PTSD symptoms (Horowitz & Solomon, 1975). It should be emphasized that this proposal lacks evidence. Another perspective proposes that people are excessively distracted by competing events that divert attention from stress symptoms to other immediate events, such as relocation, surgery, end of deployments, or legal proceedings (Andreasen, 2004). Indirect evidence comes from many studies that show that worsening PTSD is associated with more posttraumatic stressors (Bryant & Harvey, 2002; Bryant et al., 2013; Horesh et al., 2011; Smid et al., 2012). Finally, cognitive models of PTSD speculate that delayed-onset of PTSD can occur when a person develops interpretations of the experience that lead to more traumatic emotional reactions (Ehlers & Clark, 2000). While logical and plausible, there is a lack of clear evidence to support this potential mechanism.

The Optimal Treatment for PTSD

One of the perennial debates in the field of PTSD surrounds the optimal treatment for the condition. Treatment guidelines around the world converge on recommending a category of treatments, commonly termed "trauma-focused cognitive behavior therapy" (TF-CBT), for treating PTSD. This conclusion is noted in guidelines of the UK National Institute for Clinical Excellence (2005), the USA Institute of Medicine (2008), and the International Society of Traumatic Stress Studies (Foa et al., 2010). This approach has been shown to be effective across many different populations, including survivors of traumatic injury and assault, sexual assault, combat, terrorist attacks, refugees, and child sexual abuse (Foa et al., 1991; McDonagh et al., 2005; Schnurr et al., 2007; Schnurr et al., 2003). We should note that despite this group of therapies being recommended as frontline treatment of PTSD, between 50% and 60% of people with PTSD do not respond adequately to this treatment (Bradley, 2005; Loerinc et al., 2015).

While there is little debate surrounding the superior capacity for TF-CBT to improve PTSD symptoms relative to other treatments, there is more argument about the advantages of the specific treatment packages that are encompassed in this category. The earliest popular variant of TF-CBT was Prolonged Exposure, which has been proven across many controlled trials since the 1990s (McLean et al., 2015). This therapy is heavily based on emotional processing of the trauma memory and typically comprises prolonged focus on reliving of the trauma (often 40 min), followed by a discussion of issues that arose during the exposure session. Over the years other forms of therapies have amended this approach. Since the emergence of Prolonged Exposure, numerous variants have been developed. Cognitive Processing Therapy (CPT) was developed as a variant of Prolonged Exposure and focused specifically on the cognitive reactions of survivors of sexual assault (Resick & Schnicke, 1993). Whereas in the original version of this therapy emotional processing of the trauma memories was done by writing detailed accounts of the trauma, it has evolved over time to remove the writing component, and it focuses much more on altering maladaptive appraisals (Resick et al., 2008). Another variant of TF-CBT is Eye Movement Desensitization and Reprocessing (EMDR), which has been somewhat controversial since its inception. EMDR is distinctive insofar as it requires a person to focus their attention on a traumatic memory while simultaneously visually tracking the therapist's finger as it is moved across their visual field, and then to engage in restructuring of the memory (Shapiro, 1995). The person subsequently identifies more adaptive thoughts about the traumatic memory and again tracks the therapist's fingers while reliving the memory. Although it is alleged that the saccadic eye movements facilitate neural processing of new information that is integrated into trauma memory (Shapiro, 1995), this idea has never been validated with evidence (Davidson & Parker, 2001).

Building on cognitive models of PTSD, Cognitive Therapy emphasizes (a) promoting a coherent narrative of the trauma memory, so it is embedded more in one's normal autobiographical memory and (b) correcting key maladaptive appraisals about the traumatic experience (e.g., "I can never forgive myself because that woman died in the accident") (Ehlers & Clark, 2000). This approach entails addressing the sequence of events in a trauma memory, and integrating corrective information to alter the key mechanisms that this model posits maintains PTSD. The emphasis of this treatment is strongly on altering appraisals and integrating these into the trauma memory (Ehlers et al., 2003, 2014).

Yet another form of TF-CBT, which was developed specifically for refugees, is Narrative Exposure Therapy. In the context of refugees who often experience many traumatic events, this treatment directs the person to narrate an accurate life narrative with the counselor that maps both positive and negative experiences in their lives and elicits exposure to trauma memories during this life story. Numerous trials attest to the efficacy of this treatment for refugees (Ertl et al., 2011; Neuner et al., 2004). In more recent times phase-based treatments have been developed that attempt to prepare people for emotional processing by training emotion regulation and self-organization skills. One such program that has focused on people with more complex reactions is termed Complex PTSD is STAIR (Skills Training in Affect and Interpersonal Regulation), which has support from a controlled trial (Cloitre et al., 2010).

It is interesting to study these variants of TF-CBT because proponents of each treatment tend to emphasize certain components and highlight the advantages of their respective strategies (Schnyder et al., 2015). In reality, however, each of these treatments has two components in common. First, all the treatments contain an element of emotional processing of the trauma memory. Although the treatments elicit emotional processing in marginally different ways, and to varying intensities, they each require the person to activate the trauma memory directly and indirectly with the goal of promoting a sense of safety and mastery of the memory. It is questionable what the exact change mechanism is that underpins this process, although many commentators converge in the belief that it involves extinction learning in which previous associations of memory content with fear and other threat-related emotions become reduced with repeated processing of the memory (Myers & Davis, 2007). The other strategy common to all the TF-CBT treatments is they include strategies that alter maladaptive or catastrophic appraisals about the traumatic experience, oneself, or about how future events may unfold. Again, the different treatments do this to differing extents, but all treatments directly or indirectly modify how people are thinking about their trauma or themselves. When discussing the distinctive role of eye movements in EMDR, McNally summed it up nicely when he said, "what is effective in EMDR is not new, and what is new is not effective" (McNally, 1999). This quote could be applied to most TF-CBT treatments because their distinctive elements do not appear to be the key strategies driving therapy gains but instead the commonalities among them seem to be most pivotal.

The Search for Biomarkers in PTSD

One of the great ambitions over the past decade or two has been to identify biomarkers of PTSD. The assessment of PTSD has often been criticized because clinicians rely primarily on a person's self-reported descriptions of their psychological state and behaviors. Apart from accounts being potentially inaccurate, this situation creates problems in forensic settings where it is important to clarify definitively whether someone has a psychological disorder. Perhaps most importantly, many argue that identifying biomarkers of PTSD will facilitate the underpinning pathology that drives the disorder, facilitate early detection of PTSD, and lead to novel treatments (Harnett et al., 2021). This initiative has led to many studies being undertaken to identify genetic, neural, inflammatory, hormonal, psychophysiological, and other candidate markers that can distinguish people with PTSD from those without PTSD (Michopoulos et al., 2015; Passos et al., 2015).

Despite many attempts to identify these biomarkers, they have yielded no specific reliable markers of PTSD. Perhaps this pattern has been demonstrated most clearly in the case of the search for genetic markers. In the wake of many failed attempts to identify a PTSD gene in smaller samples, an international consortium pooled many people from multiple genomic studies to determine the genetic marker of PTSD. In the initial analysis of this combined data, which comprised 20,000 people, no genetic markers were identified in a genome-wide analysis (Duncan et al., 2018). When subsequent data were collected that included more than 30,000 people with PTSD and more than 170,000 controls, some genetic loci were identified in different ethnicities, as well as some associated with sex; notably, even with this number of people it was acknowledged that this number was insufficient to detect potential specific loci associated with PTSD relative to other disorders (Nievergelt et al., 2019).

More recently, there have been potentially more promising approaches to finding a marker of PTSD. Genetic studies have moved toward polygenetic scores to identify markers of PTSD, which appears to yield greater success (Swart et al., 2021). As discussed earlier in this chapter, some of these studies have focused on early detection of PTSD using machine learning methods that have incorporated multiple candidate factors encompassing biological and non-biological markers (Schultebraucks & Chang, 2021). For example, one study that recruited patients in an emergency department used psychophysiological, endocrine, prescribed pharmacotherapy from the hospital, and psychological measures used machine learning to predict subsequent severe PTSD levels. This study impressively found strong accuracy in predicting severe stress at 12 months (area under the curve, 0.89; Schultebraucks et al., 2021b). An increasing number of studies are not simply focusing on PTSD cases, at some arbitrary timepoint after trauma, but have linked acute predictors with trajectories of posttraumatic stress (derived by growth mixture modeling) and demonstrated solid predictive ability (Lori et al., 2021; Schultebraucks et al., 2021a, b). In an important step forward, some studies are also reporting replication of observed markers of PTSD across independent samples (Lori et al.,

2021; Schultebraucks et al., 2020; Ziobrowski et al., 2021). These efforts represent a critical advance in how prediction is investigated, because non-replication across studies has been the norm rather than the exception, and the ability to validate candidate predictors identified in machine learning studies is essential.

Despite the gains made in the rigor of studies of biomarkers of PTSD, these attempts to identify a biological marker have been problematic for several reasons. Many of the studies have found that biomarkers tend to be associated more with general psychopathology than with PTSD specifically (Harnett et al., 2021). In fact, some studies have reported optimal markers of PTSD *or* depression in their predictive models (Ziobrowski et al., 2021). These data parallel findings of candidate gene studies have reported shared variance of particular genetic markers for PTSD and depression (Garrett et al., 2021). However, most studies have compared samples of people with PTSD with people without the diagnosis. This approach fails to address the diagnostic specificity needed to distinguish between PTSD and other disorders (Bandelow et al., 2016, 2017).

As noted earlier in this chapter, one of the problems in identifying a biomarker of PTSD is the presumption that an underlying disease causes the symptoms, but this notion is not empirically supported (McNally et al., 2015). For a biological marker to succeed, it needs to provide sufficient specificity and sensitivity in distinguishing PTSD from people without the disorder, as well as those without PTSD but with other psychiatric disorders. This is problematic for PTSD because of the very high rates of comorbidity of PTSD and other disorders. To some extent, the problem of categorizing people as having PTSD or not is addressed in biomarker research that focuses on trajectories of stress response, but this research does not resolve the issue of identifying markers of posttraumatic stress as distinct from other mental health outcomes. This issue has been highlighted recently by studies that have used machine learning to identify markers of depression after major stressful life events, which have identified trajectories of depressed individuals but not distinguished these from other psychiatric disorders that commonly co-exist with depression (Schultebraucks et al., 2021).

Another challenge in identifying PTSD biomarkers is the variability in how PTSD is defined. As highlighted in DSM-5, there are 636,120 different permutations for how PTSD can present, which constitutes a major challenge for expecting a neural, genetic, or hormonal candidate to encompass this heterogeneity (Galatzer-Levy & Bryant, 2013). The current definition is based on the need to capture the range of PTSD reactions rather than identify a mechanism underpinning the disorder, which invariably leads to a problem in biomarker specification. Some recent research has indicated the relevance of paying attention to this issue in that there is evidence of biomarkers of subtypes of PTSD (Bryant et al., 2021b; Esterman et al., 2020; Nicholson et al., 2019). This emerging evidence reflects the need to understand markers of symptom profiles that may map onto underlying mechanisms. No doubt biological researchers will continue to seek the "holy grail" of the biomarker of PTSD, but it is imperative that a more sophisticated and mechanism-driven approach is needed if advances are to be achieved.

Summary

PTSD has attracted its share of controversy over the years, and it is fair to conclude that the debates about the condition have been more frequent than exist in relation to most other psychological disorders. This review has highlighted that study of PTSD has advanced in recent times, and the early acceptance of assumptions about traumatic stress response has been rightly challenged. Today there is a shift toward striving to replicate findings, transparency about the limitations of diagnostic systems, attempts to identify phenotypes of psychological response to trauma rather than dichotomous categorizations, and the realization that we need to understand mechanisms of change in treatment rather than simply comparing packages of TF-CBT, for example. The more the study of PTSD can embrace these principles, the further the field of traumatic stress will advance as a rigorous science.

References

Ahern, J., Galea, S., Resnick, H., Kilpatrick, D., Bucuvalas, M., Gold, J., & Vlahov, D. (2002). Television images and psychological symptoms after the September 11 terrorist attacks. *Psychiatry, 65*(4), 289–300.

American Psychiatric Association. (1980). *Diagnostic and statistical manual of mental disorders* (3rd ed.). American Psychiatric Association.

American Psychiatric Association. (1994). *Diagnostic and statistical manual of mental disorders* (4th ed.). American Psychiatric Association.

American Psychiatric Association. (2011). *DSM-5 development*. Retrieved from www.dsm-5.org

American Psychiatric Association. (2013). *Diagnostic and statistical manual for mental disorders* (5th ed.). American Psychiatric Association.

Amir, N., Stafford, J., Freshman, M. S., & Foa, E. B. (1998). Relationship between trauma narratives and trauma pathology. *Journal of Traumatic Stress, 11*(2), 385–392.

Andreasen, N. C. (2004). Acute and delayed posttraumatic stress disorders: A history and some issues. *American Journal of Psychiatry, 161*(8), 1321–1323.

Andrews, B., Brewin, C. R., Philpott, R., & Stewart, L. (2007). Delayed-onset posttraumatic stress disorder: A systematic review of the evidence. *American Journal of Psychiatry, 164*(9), 1319–1326.

Armour, C., Fried, E. I., Deserno, M. K., Tsai, J., & Pietrzak, R. H. (2017). A network analysis of DSM-5 posttraumatic stress disorder symptoms and correlates in U.S. military veterans. *Journal of Anxiety Disorders, 45*, 49–59.

Asmundson, G. J., Frombach, I., McQuaid, J., Pedrelli, P., Lenox, R., & Stein, M. B. (2000). Dimensionality of posttraumatic stress symptoms: A confirmatory factor analysis of DSM-IV symptom clusters and other symptom models. *Behaviour Research and Therapy, 38*(2), 203–214.

Bandelow, B., Baldwin, D., Abelli, M., Altamura, C., Dell'Osso, B., Domschke, K., et al. (2016). Biological markers for anxiety disorders, OCD and PTSD – A consensus statement. Part I: Neuroimaging and genetics. *World Journal of Biological Psychiatry, 17*(5), 321–365.

Bandelow, B., Baldwin, D., Abelli, M., Bolea-Alamanac, B., Bourin, M., Chamberlain, S. R., et al. (2017). Biological markers for anxiety disorders, OCD and PTSD: A consensus statement. Part II: Neurochemistry, neurophysiology and neurocognition. *World Journal of Biological Psychiatry, 18*(3), 162–214.

Blanchard, E. B., Hickling, E. J., Taylor, A. E., Loos, W. R., & Gerardi, R. J. (1994). Psychological morbidity associated with motor vehicle accidents. *Behaviour Research and Therapy, 32*(3), 283–290.

Bonanno, G. A., Galea, S., Bucciarelli, A., & Vlahov, D. (2006). Psychological resilience after disaster – New York City in the aftermath of the September 11th terrorist attack. *Psychological Science, 17*(3), 181–186.

Bonanno, G. A., Ho, S. M., Chan, J. C., Kwong, R. S., Cheung, C. K., Wong, C. P., & Wong, V. C. (2008). Psychological resilience and dysfunction among hospitalized survivors of the SARS epidemic in Hong Kong: a latent class approach. *Health Psychology, 27*(5), 659–667.

Bonanno, G. A., Mancini, A. D., Horton, J. L., Powell, T. M., Leardmann, C. A., Boyko, E. J., et al. (2012). Trajectories of trauma symptoms and resilience in deployed U.S. military service members: prospective cohort study. *British Journal of Psychiatry, 200*(4), 317–323.

Borsboom, D., & Cramer, A. O. (2013). Network analysis: An integrative approach to the structure of psychopathology. *Annual Review of Clinical Psychology, 9*, 91–121.

Bradley, R. (2005). A multidimensional meta-analysis of psychotherapy for PTSD. *American Journal of Psychiatry, 162*(4), 832–832.

Breh, D. C., & Seidler, G. H. (2007). Is peritraumatic dissociation a risk factor for PTSD? *Journal of Trauma and Dissociation, 8*(1), 53–69.

Breslau, N., & Kessler, R. C. (2001). The stressor criterion in DSM-IV posttraumatic stress disorder: An empirical investigation. *Biological Psychiatry, 50*(9), 699–704.

Breslau, N., Davis, G., Andreski, P., & Peterson, E. (1991). Traumatic events and posttraumatic stress disorder in an urban population of young adults. *Archives of General Psychiatry, 48*, 216–222.

Breslau, N., Bohnert, K. M., & Koenen, K. C. (2010). The 9/11 terrorist attack and posttraumatic stress disorder revisited. *Journal of Nervous and Mental Disease, 198*(8), 539–543.

Brewin, C. R., Dalgleish, T., & Joseph, S. (1996). A dual representation theory of posttraumatic stress disorder. *Psychological Review, 103*(4), 670–686.

Brewin, C. R., Andrews, B., & Rose, S. (2000a). Fear, helplessness, and horror in posttraumatic stress disorder: Investigating DSM-IV criterion A2 in victims of violent crime. *Journal of Traumatic Stress, 13*(3), 499–509.

Brewin, C. R., Andrews, B., & Valentine, J. D. (2000b). Meta-analysis of risk factors for posttraumatic stress disorder in trauma-exposed adults. *Journal of Consulting and Clinical Psychology, 68*(5), 748–766.

Brewin, C. R., Lanius, R. A., Novac, A., Schnyder, U., & Galea, S. (2009). Reformulating PTSD for DSM-V: Life after Criterion A. *Journal of Traumatic Stress, 22*(5), 366–373.

Brewin, C. R., Gregory, J. D., Lipton, M., & Burgess, N. (2010). Intrusive images in psychological disorders: Characteristics, neural mechanisms, and treatment implications. *Psychological Review, 117*(1), 210–232.

Briere, J., Scott, C., & Weathers, F. (2005). Peritraumatic and persistent dissociation in the presumed etiology of PTSD. *American Journal of Psychiatry, 162*(12), 2295–2301.

Broman-Fulks, J. J., Ruggiero, K. J., Green, B. A., Kilpatrick, D. G., Danielson, C. K., Resnick, H. S., & Saunders, B. E. (2006). Taxometric investigation of PTSD: Data from two nationally representative samples. *Behavior Therapy, 37*(4), 364–380.

Bryant, R. A. (2003). Early predictors of posttraumatic stress disorder. *Biological Psychiatry, 53*(9), 789–795.

Bryant, R. A. (2007). Does dissociation further our understanding of PTSD? *Journal of Anxiety Disorders, 21*(2), 183–191.

Bryant, R. A. (2011). Acute stress disorder as a predictor of posttraumatic stress disorder: A systematic review. *Journal of Clinical Psychiatry, 72*(2), 233–239.

Bryant, R. A., & Harvey, A. G. (1997). Acute stress disorder: A critical review of diagnostic issues. *Clinical Psychology Review, 17*(7), 757–773.

Bryant, R. A., & Harvey, A. G. (2002). Delayed-onset posttraumatic stress disorder: A prospective evaluation. *Australian and New Zealand Journal of Psychiatry, 36*(2), 205–209.

Bryant, R. A., Guthrie, R. M., & Moulds, M. L. (2001). Hypnotizability in acute stress disorder. *American Journal of Psychiatry, 158*(4), 600–604.

Bryant, R. A., Friedman, M. J., Spiegel, D., Ursano, R., & Strain, J. (2011). A review of acute stress disorder in DSM-5. *Depression and Anxiety, 28*(9), 802–817.

Bryant, R. A., O'Donnell, M., Creamer, M., McFarlane, A. C., & Silove, D. (2013). A multisite analysis of the fluctuating course of posttraumatic stress disorder. *JAMA. Psychiatry, 70*, 839–846.

Bryant, R. A., Nickerson, A., Creamer, M., O'Donnell, M., Forbes, D., Galatzer-Levy, I., et al. (2015). Trajectory of post-traumatic stress following traumatic injury: 6-year follow-up. *British Journal of Psychiatry, 206*(5), 417–423.

Bryant, R. A., Creamer, M., O'Donnell, M., Forbes, D., McFarlane, A. C., Silove, D., & Hadzi-Pavlovic, D. (2017). Acute and chronic posttraumatic stress symptoms in the emergence of posttraumatic stress disorder: a network analysis. JAMA Psychiatry, 74, 135–142.

Bryant, R. A., Gibbs, L., Colin Gallagher, H., Pattison, P., Lusher, D., MacDougall, C., et al. (2021a). The dynamic course of psychological outcomes following the Victorian Black Saturday bushfires. *Australian and New Zealand Journal of Psychiatry, 55*(7), 666–677.

Bryant, R. A., Williamson, T., Erlinger, M., Felmingham, K. L., Malhi, G., Hinton, M., et al. (2021b). Neural activity during response inhibition associated with improvement of dysphoric symptoms of PTSD after trauma-focused psychotherapy-an EEG-fMRI study. *Translational Psychiatry, 11*(1), 218. https://doi.org/10.1038/s41398-021-01340-8

Buckley, T. C., Blanchard, E. B., & Hickling, E. J. (1996). A prospective examination of delayed onset PTSD secondary to motor vehicle accidents. *Journal of Abnormal Psychology, 105*(4), 617–625.

Buckley, T. C., Blanchard, E. B., & Hickling, E. J. (1998). A confirmatory factor analysis of posttraumatic stress symptoms. *Behaviour Research and Therapy, 36*(11), 1091–1099.

Butler, L. D., Duran, R. E. F., Jasiukaitis, P., Koopman, C., et al. (1996). Hypnotizability and traumatic experience: A diathesis-stress model of dissociative symptomatology. *American Journal of Psychiatry, 153*(Suppl), 42–63.

Birkeland, M. S., & Heir, T. (2017). Making connections: exploring the centrality of posttraumatic stress symptoms and covariates after a terrorist attack. European Journal of Psychotraumatology, 8, 1333387.

Cardeña, E., & Spiegel, D. (1993). Dissociative reactions to the San Francisco Bay Area earthquake of 1989. *American Journal of Psychiatry, 150*(3), 474–478.

Carty, J., O'Donnell, M. L., & Creamer, M. (2006). Delayed-onset PTSD: A prospective study of injury survivors. *Journal of Affective Disorders, 90*(2-3), 257–261.

Charlson, F., van Ommeren, M., Flaxman, A., Cornett, J., Whiteford, H., & Saxena, S. (2019). New WHO prevalence estimates of mental disorders in conflict settings: A systematic review and meta-analysis. *Lancet, 394*(10194), 240–248.

Charcot, J. M. (1877). *Lectures on the diseases of the nervous system, delivered at La Salpêtrière*. Translated by George Sigerson, G. London: Sydenham Society.

Cloitre, M., Stovall-McClough, K. C., Nooner, K., Zorbas, P., Cherry, S., Jackson, C. L., et al. (2010). Treatment for PTSD related to childhood abuse: A randomized controlled trial. *American Journal of Psychiatry, 167*(8), 915–924.

Cramer, A. O., Waldorp, L. J., van der Maas, H. L., & Borsboom, D. (2010). Comorbidity: A network perspective. *Behavioural Brain Sciences, 33*(2-3), 137–150.

Creamer, M., McFarlane, A. C., & Burgess, P. (2005). Psychopathology following trauma: The role of subjective experience. *Journal of Affective Disorders, 86*(2-3), 175–182.

Dancu, C. V., Riggs, D. S., Hearst-Ikeda, D., Shoyer, B. G., & Foa, E. B. (1996). Dissociative experiences and posttraumatic stress disorder among female victims of criminal assault and rape. *Journal of Traumatic Stress, 9*(2), 253–267.

Davidson, P. R., & Parker, K. C. (2001). Eye movement desensitization and reprocessing (EMDR): A meta-analysis. *Journal of Consulting & Clinical Psychology, 69*(2), 305–316.

Davies, C., Malik, A., Pictet, A., Blackwell, S. E., & Holmes, E. A. (2012). Involuntary memories after a positive film are dampened by a visuospatial task: Unhelpful in depression but helpful in mania? *Clinical Psychology & Psychotherapy, 19*(4), 341–351.

de Jongh, A., Olff, M., van Hoolwerff, H., Aartman, I. H. A., Broekman, B., Lindauer, R., & Boer, F. (2008). Anxiety and post-traumatic stress symptoms following wisdom tooth removal. *Behaviour Research and Therapy, 46*(12), 1305–1310.

DeCoster, J., Iselin, A. M., & Gallucci, M. (2009). A conceptual and empirical examination of justifications for dichotomization. *Psychological Methods, 14*(4), 349–366.

Deeprose, C., Zhang, S., Dejong, H., Dalgleish, T., & Holmes, E. A. (2012). Imagery in the aftermath of viewing a traumatic film: Using cognitive tasks to modulate the development of involuntary memory. *Journal of Behaviour Therapy and Experimental Psychiatry, 43*(2), 758–764.

Dohrenwend, B. P. (2006). Inventorying stressful life events as risk factors for psychopathology: Toward resolution of the problem of intracategory variability. *Psychological Bulletin, 132*(3), 477–495.

Dohrenwend, B. P., Turner, J. B., Turse, N. A., Adams, B. G., Koenen, K. C., & Marshall, R. (2006). The psychological risks of Vietnam for US veterans: A revisit with new data and methods. *Science, 313*(5789), 979–982.

Duncan, L. E., Ratanatharathorn, A., Aiello, A. E., Almli, L. M., Amstadter, A. B., Ashley-Koch, A. E., et al. (2018). Largest GWAS of PTSD (N=20 070) yields genetic overlap with schizophrenia and sex differences in heritability. *Molecular Psychiatry, 23*(3), 666–673.

Ehlers, A., & Clark, D. M. (2000). A cognitive model of posttraumatic stress disorder. *Behaviour Research and Therapy, 38*(4), 319–345.

Ehlers, A., Mayou, R. A., & Bryant, B. (1998). Psychological predictors of chronic posttraumatic stress disorder after motor vehicle accidents. *Journal of Abnormal Psychology, 107*(3), 508–519.

Ehlers, A., Clark, D. M., Hackmann, A., McManus, F., Fennell, M., Herbert, C., & Mayou, R. (2003). A randomized controlled trial of cognitive therapy, a self-help booklet, and repeated assessments as early interventions for posttraumatic stress disorder. *Archives of General Psychiatry, 60*(10), 1024–1032.

Ehlers, A., Hackmann, A., Grey, N., Wild, J., Liness, S., Albert, I., et al. (2014). A randomized controlled trial of 7-day intensive and standard weekly cognitive therapy for PTSD and emotion-focused supportive therapy. *American Journal of Psychiatry, 171*(3), 294–304.

Ehring, T., Ehlers, A., & Glucksman, E. (2008). Do cognitive models help in predicting the severity of posttraumatic stress disorder, phobia, and depression after motor vehicle accidents? A prospective longitudinal study. *Journal of Consulting and Clinical Psychology, 76*(2), 219–230.

Ertl, V., Pfeiffer, A., Schauer, E., Elbert, T., & Neuner, F. (2011). Community-implemented trauma therapy for former child soldiers in Northern Uganda: a randomized controlled trial. *JAMA, 306*(5), 503–512.

Esterman, M., Stumps, A., Jagger-Rickels, A., Rothlein, D., DeGutis, J., Fortenbaugh, F., et al. (2020). Evaluating the evidence for a neuroimaging subtype of posttraumatic stress disorder. *Science Translational Medicine, 12*(568).

Fikretoglu, D., Brunet, A., Best, S., Metzler, T., Delucchi, K., Weiss, D. S., et al. (2006). The relationship between peritraumatic distress and peritraumatic dissociation. *Journal of Nervous and Mental Disease, 194*(11), 853–858.

Fikretoglu, D., Brunet, A., Best, S. R., Metzler, T. J., Delucchi, K., Weiss, D. S., et al. (2007). Peritraumatic fear, helplessness and horror and peritraumatic dissociation: Do physical and cognitive symptoms of panic mediate the relationship between the two? *Behaviour Research and Therapy, 45*(1), 39–47.

Foa, E. B., & Riggs, D. S. (1993). Post-traumatic stress disorder in rape victims. In J. Oldham, M. B. Riba, & A. Tasman (Eds.), *American Psychiatric Press Review of Psychiatry* (Vol. 12, pp. 273–303). American Psychiatric Press.

Foa, E. B., Rothbaum, B. O., Riggs, D. S., & Murdock, T. B. (1991). Treatment of posttraumatic stress disorder in rape victims: A comparison between cognitive-behavioral procedures and counseling. *Journal of Consulting and Clinical Psychology, 59*(5), 715–723.

Foa, E. B., Riggs, D. S., & Gershuny, B. S. (1995). Arousal, numbing, and intrusion: Symptom structure of PTSD following assault. *American Journal of Psychiatry, 152*(1), 116–120.

Foa, E. B., Keane, T. M., Friedman, M. J., & Cohen, J. A. (Eds.). (2010). *Effective treatments for PTSD: Practice guidelines from the International Society of Traumatic Stress Studies* (2nd ed.). Guilford.

Friedman, M. J. (2000). What might the psychobiology of posttraumatic stress disorder teach us about future approaches to pharmacotherapy? *Journal of Clinical Psychiatry, 61*(Suppl 7), 44–51.

Friedman, M. J., Resick, P. A., Bryant, R. A., & Brewin, C. R. (2011). Considering PTSD for DSM-5. *Depression and Anxiety, 28*(9), 750–769.

Fried, E. I., Eidhof, M. B., Palic, S., Costantini, G., Huisman-van Dijk, H. M., Bockting, C. L. H., et al. (2018). Replicability and generalizability of posttraumatic stress disorder (PTSD) networks: a cross-cultural multisite study of PTSD symptoms in four trauma patient samples. Clinical Psychological Science, 6, 335–351.

Galatzer-Levy, I., & Bryant, R. A. (2013). 636,120 ways to have posttraumatic stress disorder: The relative merits of categorical and dimensional approaches to posttraumatic stress. *Perspectives in Psychological Science, 8*, 651–662.

Galatzer-Levy, I. R., Huang, S. H., & Bonanno, G. A. (2018a). Trajectories of resilience and dysfunction following potential trauma: A review and statistical evaluation. *Clinical Psychology Review, 63*, 41–55.

Galatzer-Levy, I. R., Ruggles, K., & Chen, Z. (2018b). Data science in the research domain criteria era: Relevance of machine learning to the study of stress pathology, recovery, and resilience. *Chronic Stress, 2*. https://doi.org/10.1177/2470547017747553

Garrett, M. E., Qin, X. J., Mehta, D., Dennis, M. F., Marx, C. E., Grant, G. A., et al. (2021). Gene expression analysis in three posttraumatic stress disorder cohorts implicates inflammation and innate immunity pathways and uncovers shared genetic risk with major depressive disorder. *Frontiers in Neuroscience, 15*, 678548.

Gershuny, B. S., & Thayer, J. F. (1999). Relations among psychological trauma, dissociative phenomena, and trauma-related distress: A review and integration. *Clinical Psychology Review, 19*(5), 631–657.

Gil, S., Weinberg, M., Shamai, M., Ron, P., Harel, H., & Or-Chen, K. (2016). Risk factors for DSM-5 posttraumatic stress symptoms (PTSS) among Israeli civilians during the 2014 Israel-Hamas war. *Psychological Trauma, 8*(1), 49–54.

Green, M. M., McFarlane, A. C., Hunter, C. E., & Griggs, W. M. (1993). Undiagnosed posttraumatic stress disorder following motor vehicle accidents. *Medical Journal of Australia, 159*(8), 529–534.

Halligan, S. L., Clark, D. M., & Ehlers, A. (2002). Cognitive processing, memory, and the development of PTSD symptoms: Two experimental analogue studies. *Journal of Behavior Therapy & Experimental Psychiatry, 33*(2), 73–89.

Halligan, S. L., Michael, T., Clark, D. M., & Ehlers, A. (2003). Posttraumatic stress disorder following assault: The role of cognitive processing, trauma memory, and appraisals. *Journal of Consulting and Clinical Psychology, 71*(3), 419–431.

Harnett, N. G., van Rooij, S. J. H., Ely, T. D., Lebois, L. A. M., Murty, V. P., Jovanovic, T., et al. (2021). Prognostic neuroimaging biomarkers of trauma-related psychopathology: Resting-state fMRI shortly after trauma predicts future PTSD and depression symptoms in the AURORA study. *Neuropsychopharmacology, 46*(7), 1263–1271.

Harvey, A. G., & Bryant, R. A. (1999). A qualitative investigation of the organization of traumatic memories. *British Journal of Clinical Psychology, 38(4)*, 401–405.

Harvey, A. G., & Bryant, R. A. (2002). Acute stress disorder: A synthesis and critique. *Psychological Bulletin, 128*(6), 886–902.
Haslam, N. (2011). The latent structure of personality and psychopathology: A review of trends in taxometric research. *Scientific Review of Mental Health Practice, 8*(1), 17–29.
Helzer, J. E., Robins, L. N., & McEvoy, L. (1987). Post-traumatic stress disorder in the general population: Findings of the Epidemiologic Catchment Area survey. *New England Journal of Medicine, 317*, 1630–1634.
Hoge, C. W., Yehuda, R., Castro, C. A., McFarlane, A. C., Vermetten, E., Jetly, R., et al. (2016). Unintended consequences of changing the definition of posttraumatic stress disorder in DSM-5: Critique and call for action. *JAMA Psychiatry, 73*(7), 750–752.
Holmes, E. A., Brewin, C. R., & Hennessy, R. G. (2004). Trauma films, information processing, and intrusive memory development. *Journal of Experimental Psychology-General, 133*(1), 3–22.
Holmes, E. A., James, E. L., Coode-Bate, T., & Deeprose, C. (2009). Can playing the computer game "Tetris" reduce the build-up of flashbacks for trauma? A proposal from cognitive science. *PLoS One, 4*(1), e4153.
Horesh, D., Solomon, Z., Zerach, G., & Ein-Dor, T. (2011). Delayed-onset PTSD among war veterans: The role of life events throughout the life cycle. *Social Psychiatry and Psychiatric Epidemiology, 46*(9), 863–870.
Horowitz, M. J., & Solomon, G. F. (1975). A prediction of delayed stress response syndromes in Vietnam veterans. *Journal of Social Issues, 31*, 67–80.
Institute of Medicine. (2008). *Treatment of posttraumatic stress disorder: An assessment of the evidence*. Academic.
Janet, P. (1907). *The major symptoms of hysteria*. Macmillian.
Karam, E. G., Andrews, G., Bromet, E., Petukhova, M., Ruscio, A. M., Salamoun, M., et al. (2010). The role of criterion A2 in the DSM-IV diagnosis of posttraumatic stress disorder. *Biological Psychiatry, 68*(5), 465–473.
Karam, E. G., Friedman, M. J., Hill, E. D., Kessler, R. C., McLaughlin, K. A., Petukhova, M., et al. (2014). Cumulative traumas and risk thresholds: 12-month PTSD in the World Mental Health (WMH) surveys. *Depression and Anxiety, 31*(2), 130–142.
Kendler, K. S., Zachar, P., & Craver, C. (2011). What kinds of things are psychiatric disorders? *Psychological Medicine, 41*(6), 1143–1150.
Kessler, R. C., & Üstün, T. B. (2004). The world mental health (WMH) survey initiative version of the world health organization (WHO) composite international diagnostic interview (CIDI). *International Journal of Methods in Psychiatric Research, 13*(2), 93–121.
Kilpatrick, D. G., Resnick, H. S., & Acierno, R. (2009). Should PTSD criterion a be retained? *Journal of Traumatic Stress, 22*(5), 374–383.
King, D. W., Leskin, G. A., King, L. A., & Weathers, F. W. (1998). Confirmatory factor analysis of the clinician-administered PTSD Scale: Evidence for the dimensionality of posttraumatic stress disorder. *Psychological Assessment, 10*(2), 90–96.
Kluft, R. P. (1987). An update on multiple personality disorder. *Hospital and Community Psychiatry, 38*(4), 363–373.
Kraemer, H. C. (2007). DSM categories and dimensions in clinical and research contexts. *International Journal of Methods in Psychiatric Research, 16*(S1), S8–S15.
Krystal, J. H., Woods, S. W., Hill, C. L., & Charney, D. S. (1991). Characteristics of panic attack subtypes: Assessment of spontaneous panic, situational panic, sleep panic, and limited symptom attacks. *Comprehensive Psychiatry, 32*(6), 474–480.
Kulka, R. A., Schlenger, W. E., Fairbank, J. A., Hough, R. L., Jordan, B. K., Marmar, C. R., & Weiss, D. S. (1990). *The National Vietnam veterans readjustment study: Table of findings and technical appendices*. Brunner/Mazel.
Knefel, M., Tran, U. S., & Lueger-Schuster, B. (2016). The association of posttraumatic stress disorder, complex posttraumatic stress disorder, and borderline personality disorder from a network analytical perspective. Journal of Anxiety Disorders, 43, 70–78.

Lam, W. W., Bonanno, G. A., Mancini, A. D., Ho, S., Chan, M., Hung, W. K., et al. (2010). Trajectories of psychological distress among Chinese women diagnosed with breast cancer. *Psychooncology, 19*(10), 1044–1051.

Larsson, G. (2005). Dimensional analysis of the impact of event scale using structural equation modeling. *Journal of Traumatic Stress, 13*(2), 193–204.

Lees-Haley, P. R., Price, J. R., Williams, C. W., & Betz, B. P. (2001). Use of the impact of events scale in the assessment of emotional distress and PTSD may produce misleading results. *Journal of Forensic Neuropsychology, 2*(2), 45–52.

Loerinc, A. G., Meuret, A. E., Twohig, M. P., Rosenfield, D., Bluett, E. J., & Craske, M. G. (2015). Response rates for CBT for anxiety disorders: Need for standardized criteria. *Clinical Psychology Review, 42*, 72–82.

Lori, A., Schultebraucks, K., Galatzer-Levy, I., Daskalakis, N. P., Katrinli, S., Smith, A. K., et al. (2021). Transcriptome-wide association study of post-trauma symptom trajectories identified GRIN3B as a potential biomarker for PTSD development. *Neuropsychopharmacology, 46*(10), 1811–1820.

MacCallum, R. C., Zhang, S., Preacher, K. J., & Rucker, D. D. (2002). On the practice of dichotomization of quantitative variables. *Psychological Methods, 7*(1), 19–40.

Maier, T. (2007). Weathers' and Keane's, "The criterion a problem revisited: Controversies and challenges in defining and measuring psychological trauma". *Journal of Traumatic Stress, 20*(5), 915–916.

Malgaroli, M., Maccallum, F., & Bonanno, G. A. (2018). Symptoms of persistent complex bereavement disorder, depression, and PTSD in a conjugally bereaved sample: A network analysis. *Psychological Medicine, 48*(14), 2439–2448.

Marshall, R. D., Olfson, M., Hellman, F., Blanco, C., Guardino, M., & Struening, E. L. (2001). Comorbidity, impairment, and suicidality in subthreshold PTSD. *American Journal of Psychiatry, 158*(9), 1467–1473.

McDonagh, A., Friedman, M., McHugo, G., Ford, J., Sengupta, A., Mueser, K., et al. (2005). Randomized trial of cognitive-behavioral therapy for chronic posttraumatic stress disorder in adult female survivors of childhood sexual abuse. *Journal of Consulting and Clinical Psychology, 73*(3), 515–524.

McLean, C. P., Asnaani, A., & Foa, E. B. (2015). Prolonged exposure therapy. In U. Schnyder & M. Cloitre (Eds.), *Evidence based treatments for trauma-related psychological disorders* (pp. 143–159). Springer.

McNally, R. J. (1999). On eye movements and animal magnetism: A reply to Greenwald's defense of EMDR. *Journal of Anxiety Disorders, 13*, 617–620.

McNally, R. J. (2007). Revisiting Dohrenwend et al.'s revisit of the National Vietnam Veterans Readjustment Study. *Journal of Traumatic Stress, 20*(4), 481–486.

McNally, R. J. (2009). Can we fix PTSD in DSM-V? *Depression and Anxiety, 26*(7), 597–600.

McNally, R. J., Robinaugh, D. J., Wu, G. W. Y., Wang, L., Deserno, M. K., & Borsboom, D. (2015). Mental disorders as causal systems: A network approach to posttraumatic stress disorder. *Clinical Psychological Science, 3*, 836–849.

McNally, R. K., Heeren, A., & Robinaugh, D. J. (2017). A Bayesian network analysis of posttraumatic stress disorder symptoms in adults reporting childhood sexual abuse. European Journal of Psychotraumatology, 8, 1341276.

Meehl, P. E. (1965). *Detecting latent clinical taxa by fallible quantitative indicators lacking an accepted criterion*. Retrieved from https://conservancy.umn.edu/bitstream/handle/11299/151479/PR-65-2.pdf?sequence=1.

Micale, M. S. (2001). Jean-Martin Charcot and *les névroses traumatiques*: From medicine to culture in French theory of the late nineteenth century. In *Traumatic pasts: History, psychiatry, and trauma in the modern age, 1870–1930* (pp. 115–139). Cambridge University Press.

Michopoulos, V., Norrholm, S. D., & Jovanovic, T. (2015). Diagnostic biomarkers for posttraumatic stress disorder: Promising horizons from translational neuroscience research. *Biological Psychiatry, 78*(5), 344–353. https://doi.org/10.1016/j.biopsych.2015.01.005

Murray, J., Ehlers, A., & Mayou, R. A. (2002). Dissociation and post-traumatic stress disorder: Two prospective studies of road traffic accident survivors. *British Journal of Psychiatry, 180*, 363–368.

Myers, K. M., & Davis, M. (2007). Mechanisms of fear extinction. *Molecular Psychiatry, 12*(2), 120–150.

Mylle, J., & Maes, M. (2004). Partial posttraumatic stress disorder revisited. *Journal of Affective Disorders, 78*(1), 37–48.

National Institute for Clinical Excellence (2005). *The management of PTSD in adults and children in primary and secondary care*. Retrieved from Wiltshire.

Neuner, F., Schauer, M., Klaschik, C., Karunakara, U., & Elbert, T. (2004). A comparison of narrative exposure therapy, supportive counseling, and psychoeducation for treating posttraumatic stress disorder in an African refugee settlement. *Journal of Consulting and Clinical Psychology, 72*(4), 579–587.

Nicholson, A. A., Densmore, M., McKinnon, M. C., Neufeld, R. W. J., Frewen, P. A., Theberge, J., et al. (2019). Machine learning multivariate pattern analysis predicts classification of posttraumatic stress disorder and its dissociative subtype: A multimodal neuroimaging approach. *Psychological Medicine, 49*(12), 2049–2059.

Nievergelt, C. M., Maihofer, A. X., Klengel, T., Atkinson, E. G., Chen, C. Y., Choi, K. W., et al. (2019). International meta-analysis of PTSD genome-wide association studies identifies sex- and ancestry-specific genetic risk loci. *Nature Communications, 10*(1), 4558.

Nixon, R. D., & Bryant, R. A. (2003). Peritraumatic and persistent panic attacks in acute stress disorder. *Behaviour Research and Therapy, 41*(10), 1237–1242.

Nixon, R. D. V., & Bryant, R. A. (2006). Dissociation in acute stress disorder after a hyperventilation provocation test. *Behavioural and Cognitive Psychotherapy, 34*(3), 343–349.

O'Donnell, M. L., Creamer, M., McFarlane, A., Silove, D., & Bryant, R. A. (2010). Should A2 be a diagnostic requirement for posttraumatic stress disorder in DSM-V? *Psychiatry Research, 176*, 257–260.

O'Donnell, M. L., Varker, T., Creamer, M., Fletcher, S., McFarlane, A. C., Silove, D., et al. (2013). Exploration of delayed-onset posttraumatic stress disorder after severe injury. *Psychosomatic Medicine, 75*(1), 68–75.

Olde, E., van der Hart, O., Kleber, R., & van Son, M. (2006). Posttraumatic stress following childbirth: A review. *Clinical Psychology Review, 26*(1), 1–16.

Ozer, E. J., Best, S. R., Lipsey, T. L., & Weiss, D. S. (2003). Predictors of posttraumatic stress disorder and symptoms in adults: A meta-analysis. *Psychological Bulletin, 129*(1), 52–73.

Palmieri, P. A., & Fitzgerald, L. F. (2005). Confirmatory factor analysis of posttraumatic stress symptoms in sexually harassed women. *Journal of Traumatic Stress, 18*(6), 657–666.

Panasetis, P., & Bryant, R. A. (2003). Peritraumatic versus persistent dissociation in acute stress disorder. *Journal of Traumatic Stress, 16*(6), 563–566.

Passos, I. C., Vasconcelos-Moreno, M. P., Costa, L. G., Kunz, M., Brietzke, E., Quevedo, J., et al. (2015). Inflammatory markers in post-traumatic stress disorder: A systematic review, meta-analysis, and meta-regression. *Lancet Psychiatry, 2*(11), 1002–1012.

Pietrzak, R. H., Schechter, C. B., Bromet, E. J., Katz, C. L., Reissman, D. B., Ozbay, F., et al. (2012). The burden of full and subsyndromal posttraumatic stress disorder among police involved in the World Trade Center rescue and recovery effort. *Journal of Psychiatric Research, 46*(7), 835–842.

Pietrzak, R. H., Van Ness, P. H., Fried, T. R., Galea, S., & Norris, F. H. (2013). Trajectories of posttraumatic stress symptomatology in older persons affected by a large-magnitude disaster. *Journal of Psychiatric Research, 47*(4), 520–526.

Phillips, R. D., Wilson, S. M., Sun, D., Workgroup, V. A., Mid-Atlantic Workgroup, & Morey, R. (2018). Posttraumatic stress disorder symptom network analysis in U.S. military veterans: examining the impact of combat exposue. Frontiers in Psychiatry, 9, 608.

Resick, P. A., & Schnicke, M. K. (1993). *Cognitive processing therapy for sexual assault victims: A treatment manual*. Sage.

Resick, P. A., Galovski, T. E., O'Brien Uhlmansiek, M., Scher, C. D., Clum, G. A., & Young-Xu, Y. (2008). A randomized clinical trial to dismantle components of cognitive processing therapy for posttraumatic stress disorder in female victims of interpersonal violence. *Journal of Consulting and Clinical Psychology, 76*(2), 243–258.

Riggs, D. S., Rothbaum, B. O., & Foa, E. B. (1995). A prospective examination of symptoms of posttraumatic stress disorder in victims of nonsexual assault. *Journal of Interpersonal Violence, 10*(2), 201–214.

Rizvi, S. L., Kaysen, D., Gutner, C. A., Griffin, M. G., & Resick, P. A. (2008). Beyond fear: The role of peritraumatic responses in posttraumatic stress and depressive symptoms among female crime victims. *Journal of Interpersonal Violence, 23*(6), 853–868.

Rosen, G. M., & Lilienfeld, S. O. (2008). Posttraumatic stress disorder: An empirical evaluation of core assumptions. *Clinical Psychology Review, 28*(5), 837–868.

Rothbaum, B. O., Foa, E. B., Riggs, D. S., Murdock, T., & Walsh, W. (1992). A prospective examination of post-traumatic stress disorder in rape victims. *Journal of Traumatic Stress, 5*(3), 455–475.

Rubin, D. C., Deffler, S. A., Ogle, C. M., Dowell, N. M., Graesser, A. C., & Beckham, J. C. (2016). Participant, rater, and computer measures of coherence in posttraumatic stress disorder. *Journal of Abnormal Psychology, 125*(1), 11–25.

Ruscio, A. M., Ruscio, J., & Keane, T. M. (2002). The latent structure of posttraumatic stress disorder: A taxometric investigation of reactions to extreme stress. *Journal of Abnormal Psychology, 111*(2), 290–301.

Ruzich, M. J., Looi, J. C. L., & Robertson, M. D. (2005). Delayed onset of posttraumatic stress disorder among male combat veterans – A case series. *American Journal of Geriatric Psychiatry, 13*(5), 424–427.

Schlenger, W. E., Kulka, R. A., Fairbank, J. A., Hough, R. L., Jordan, B. K., Marmar, C. R., & Weiss, D. S. (2007). The psychological risks of Vietnam: The NVVRS perspective. *Journal of Traumatic Stress, 20*(4), 467–479.

Schnurr, P. P., Ford, J. D., Friedman, M. J., Green, B. L., Dain, B. J., & Sengupta, A. (2000). Predictors and outcomes of posttraumatic stress disorder in World War II veterans exposed to mustard gas. *Journal of Consulting and Clinical Psychology, 68*(2), 258–268.

Schnurr, P. P., Friedman, M. J., Foy, D. W., Shea, M. T., Hsieh, F. Y., Lavori, P. W., et al. (2003). Randomized trial of trauma-focused group therapy for posttraumatic stress disorder: Results from a department of veterans affairs cooperative study. *Archives of General Psychiatry, 60*(5), 481–489.

Schnurr, P. P., Friedman, M. J., Engel, C. C., Foa, E. B., Shea, M. T., Chow, B. K., et al. (2007). Cognitive behavioral therapy for posttraumatic stress disorder in women: A randomized controlled trial. *JAMA, 297*(8), 820–830.

Schnyder, U., Ehlers, A., Elbert, T., Foa, E. B., Gersons, B. P., Resick, P. A., et al. (2015). Psychotherapies for PTSD: What do they have in common? *European Journal of Psychotraumatology, 6*, 28186.

Schultebraucks, K., & Chang, B. P. (2021). The opportunities and challenges of machine learning in the acute care setting for precision prevention of posttraumatic stress sequelae. *Experimental Neurology, 336*, 113526.

Schultebraucks, K., Shalev, A. Y., Michopoulos, V., Grudzen, C. R., Shin, S. M., Stevens, J. S., et al. (2020). A validated predictive algorithm of post-traumatic stress course following emergency department admission after a traumatic stressor. *Nature Medicine, 26*(7), 1084–1088.

Schultebraucks, K., Choi, K. W., Galatzer-Levy, I. R., & Bonanno, G. A. (2021a). Discriminating heterogeneous trajectories of resilience and depression after major life stressors using polygenic scores. *JAMA Psychiatry, 78*(7), 744–752.

Schultebraucks, K., Sijbrandij, M., Galatzer-Levy, I., Mouthaan, J., Olff, M., & van Zuiden, M. (2021b). Forecasting individual risk for long-term posttraumatic stress disorder in emergency medical settings using biomedical data: A machine learning multicenter cohort study. *Neurobiology of Stress, 14*, 100297.

Shalev, A. Y., Freedman, A., Peri, T., Brandes, D., Sahara, T., Orr, S., & Pitman, R. K. (1998). Prospective study of posttraumatic stress disorder and depression following trauma. *American Journal of Psychiatry, 155*(5), 630–637.

Shalev, A. Y., Gevonden, M., Ratanatharathorn, A., Laska, E., van der Mei, W. F., Qi, W., et al. (2019). Estimating the risk of PTSD in recent trauma survivors: Results of the International Consortium to Predict PTSD (ICPP). *World Psychiatry, 18*(1), 77–87.

Shapiro, F. (1995). *Eye movement desensitization and reprocessing: Basic principles, protocols, and procedures*. Guilford.

Shevlin, M., & Elklit, A. (2012). The latent structure of posttraumatic stress disorder: Different models or different populations? *Journal of Abnormal Psychology, 121*(3), 610–615.

Silver, R. C., Holman, E. A., McIntosh, D. N., Poulin, M., & Gil-Rivas, V. (2002). Nationwide longitudinal study of psychological responses to September 11. *JAMA, 288*(10), 1235–1244.

Sloan, P. (1988). Post-traumatic stress in survivors of an airplane crash-landing: A clinical and exploratory research intervention. *Journal of Traumatic Stress, 1*(2), 211–229.

Smid, G. E., Mooren, T. T., van der Mast, R. C., Gersons, B. P., & Kleber, R. J. (2009). Delayed posttraumatic stress disorder: Systematic review, meta-analysis, and meta-regression analysis of prospective studies. *Journal of Clinical Psychiatry, 70*(11), 1572–1582.

Smid, G. E., van der Velden, P. G., Lensvelt-Mulders, G. J., Knipscheer, J. W., Gersons, B. P., & Kleber, R. J. (2012). Stress sensitization following a disaster: A prospective study. *Psychological Medicine, 42*, 1675–1686.

Southwick, S. M., Krystal, J. H., Morgan, C. A., Johnson, D., et al. (1993). Abnormal noradrenergic function in posttraumatic stress disorder. *Archives of General Psychiatry, 50*(4), 266–274.

Spiegel, D., & Cardeña, E. (1991). Disintegrated experience: The dissociative disorders revisited. *Journal of Abnormal Psychology, 100*(3), 366–378.

Spiegel, D., Hunt, T., & Dondershine, H. E. (1988). Dissociation and hypnotizability in posttraumatic stress disorder. *American Journal of Psychiatry, 145*(3), 301–305.

Spitzer, R. L., Endicott, J., & Robins, E. (1975). Clinical criteria for psychiatric diagnosis and DSM-III. *American Journal of Psychiatry, 132*(11), 1187–1192.

Spitzer, R. L., Endicott, J., & Robins, E. (1978). Research diagnostic criteria: Rationale and reliability. *Archives of General Psychiatry, 35*(6), 773–782.

Stein, M. B., Walker, J. R., Hazen, A. L., & Forde, D. R. (1997). Full and partial posttraumatic stress disorder: Findings from a community survey. *American Journal of Psychiatry, 154*, 1114–1119.

Sterlini, G. L., & Bryant, R. A. (2002). Hyperarousal and dissociation: A study of novice skydivers. *Behaviour Research and Therapy, 40*(4), 431–437.

Swart, P. C., van den Heuvel, L. L., Lewis, C. M., Seedat, S., & Hemmings, S. M. J. (2021). A genome-wide association study and polygenic risk score analysis of posttraumatic stress disorder and metabolic syndrome in a South African population. *Frontiers in Neuroscience, 15*, 677800.

Taylor, S., Kuch, K., Koch, W. J., Crockett, D. J., & Passey, G. (1998). The structure of posttraumatic stress symptoms. *Journal of Abnormal Psychology, 107*(1), 154–160.

Titchener, J. L., & Kapp, F. T. (1976). Family and character change at Buffalo Creek. *American Journal of Psychiatry, 133*(3), 295–299.

van der Kolk, B. A., & Fisler, R. (1995). Dissociation and the fragmentary nature of traumatic memories: Overview and exploratory study. *Journal of Traumatic Stress, 8*(4), 505–525.

van der Kolk, B., & van der Hart, O. (1989). Pierre Janet and the breakdown of adaptation in psychological trauma. *American Journal of Psychiatry, 146*(12), 1530–1537.

van der Velden, P. G., Kleber, R. J., Christiaanse, B., Gersons, B. P. R., Marcelissen, F. G. H., Drogendijk, A. N., et al. (2006). The independent predictive value of peritraumatic dissociation for postdisaster intrusions, avoidance reactions, and PTSD symptom severity: A 4-year prospective study. *Journal of Traumatic Stress, 19*(4), 493–506.

Weathers, F. W., & Keane, T. M. (2007). The criterion a problem revisited: Controversies and challenges in defining and measuring psychological trauma. *Journal of Traumatic Stress, 20*(2), 107–121.

Wilson, M. (1993). DSM-III and the transformation of American psychiatry: A history. *American Journal of Psychiatry, 150*(3), 399–410.

Yehuda, R., & McFarlane, A. C. (1997). *Psychobiology of posttraumatic stress disorder*. New York Academy of Sciences.

Young, A. (1995). Reasons and causes for post-traumatic stress disorder. *Transcultural Psychiatric Research Review, 32*(3), 287–298.

Zatzick, D. F., Grossman, D. C., Russo, J., Pynoos, R., Berliner, L., Jurkovich, G., et al. (2006). Predicting posttraumatic stress symptoms longitudinally in a representative sample of hospitalized injured adolescents. *Journal of the American Academy of Child and Adolescent Psychiatry, 45*(10), 1188–1195.

Ziobrowski, H. N., Kennedy, C. J., Ustun, B., House, S. L., Beaudoin, F. L., An, X., et al. (2021). Development and validation of a model to predict posttraumatic stress disorder and major depression after a motor vehicle collision. *JAMA Psychiatry, 78*, 10.

The Recovered Memory Debate: Wins, Losses, and Creating Future Open-Minded Skeptics

Lawrence Patihis, Henry Otgaar, Steven Jay Lynn, Elizabeth F. Loftus, and Richard J. McNally

Scott O. Lilienfeld was among the most influential clinical psychological scientists and critics of pseudoscience in our time. An expert in the psychometric assessment of psychopathy, Scott's intellectual range extended far beyond this specialty. He was a prolific generalist who promoted a healthy skepticism about dubious clinical claims as embodied in his canonical edited volume *Science and Pseudoscience in Clinical Psychology* (Lilienfeld et al., 2003). His audience was as broad as his interests. He wrote for clinicians, researchers, and the public.

Scott was an influential critic of the claim that victims of trauma encode, consolidate, and then repress their memories of trauma precisely because they are so emotionally distressing (e.g., Lilienfeld & Loftus, 1998; Lilienfeld et al., 2003; Lilienfeld, 2007; Lilienfeld et al. 2008; Lynn et al., 2014; Lynn et al., in press; Otgaar et al., 2019). He was especially critical of the notion that hypnosis and other putative memory recovery methods could unlock supposedly repressed (or dissociated) memories without running the risk of fostering false memories of trauma. Finally, he and his colleagues developed the sociocognitive theory of dissociative identity disorder (DID) as an alternative to the trauma-based theory of this

L. Patihis (✉)
Portsmouth University, Portsmouth, UK
e-mail: Lawrence.Patihis@port.ac.uk

H. Otgaar
Catholic University of Leuven, Brussels, Belgium

Maastricht University, Maastricht, Netherlands

S. J. Lynn
Binghamton University (SUNY), Binghamton, NY, USA

E. F. Loftus
University of California, Irvine, Irvine, CA, USA

R. J. McNally
Harvard University, Cambridge, MA, USA

C. L. Cobb et al. (eds.), *Toward a Science of Clinical Psychology*,
https://doi.org/10.1007/978-3-031-14332-8_19

syndrome (Lilienfeld et al., 1999). Although some scholars, such as McHugh (2006, p. 129), proclaimed victory for critics of repressed memories of trauma in the so-called "Memory Wars" (Crews, 1995; Loftus, 2004), the debate over reports of repressed and recovered memories of trauma appears to continue, especially in Europe (e.g., Otgaar et al., 2019).

Scott was as critical of a cynical perspective that cavalierly dismissed ideas without giving them their due as he was of a mindset that credulously embraced claims absent any cogent evidence. Scott was humble; yet if he ever displayed a scintilla of pride, it was in his view of himself as an open-minded skeptic who carefully weighed strong claims against the evidence. He succeeded famously in this regard, as many authors of chapters in this volume attest.

In this chapter, we identify some of the wins and losses in the repressed memory debate from our perspective, contribute insight into misleading rhetoric employed in past losses, and look, with some conditional optimism, to the future. We describe the use of the motte-and-bailey technique of defending repressed memory theory in such a way that we hope will help improve our understanding of current debates and contentious issues. We outline the conditions under which future generations could continue to produce scientific skeptics with a rare mix of attributes that Scott so well exemplified: kindness, fearlessness, sophisticated quantitative skills, indefatigable energy, productivity, commitment to scientific methods, and a critical and thorough philosophy of science. We suggest that current trends in academia may have to be challenged for the concept of academic freedom to prevail and for the next generation of scientists to be able to speak freely and flourish in academic settings. We conclude with a call for those on both sides of the memory wars to be skeptical of their own beliefs and perspectives and to search for disconfirming evidence and objective truth.

The Memory Wars and Why They Matter

Pivotal to the memory wars are conflicts regarding the authenticity of so-called repressed memories—memories presumedly repressed to defend against the negative repercussions of trauma. These memories are purportedly inaccessible for years yet can be recovered with pristine accuracy in psychotherapy. On one side of the fray are those who generally accepted the existence of repressed memories and touted the importance of uncovering and processing them to cope successfully with the aftereffects of trauma (e.g., Blume, 1990; Freyd, 1994).

In contrast, scholars who question the existence of repressed memories, including the present authors, have expressed an alternative view (Loftus, 1993; Loftus & Davis, 2006; Lynn & Baltman, 2016; McNally, 2003a, b; Otgaar et al., 2019; Patihis et al., 2014). The notion of repression of memories is challenged by findings that traumatic memories are generally highly memorable and are at times intrusive and troubling, as in cases of posttraumatic stress disorder, rather than repressed or dissociated (McNally, 2003b). Repressed memory critics further questioned the accuracy of memories that were supposedly uncovered or de-repressed in psychotherapy and further expressed concerns about iatrogenic treatment effects produced by attempts at excavating such memories.

In research studies involving strong forms of suggestion, and depending on the conditions, about 30% to almost 50% of individuals report memories of a variety of autobiographical events that did not happen or had been previously denied by the participants (e.g., being bullied as a child, riding in a hot air balloon; see Scoboria et al., 2017, for a mega-analysis), rendering concerns about false recovered memories plausible and concerning (Otgaar et al., 2022). Researchers have also expressed concerns about resurgent belief in repressed memories among the public, mental health professionals, and potential jurists (see Otgaar et al., 2019; Patihis et al., 2014). As Patihis et al. (2014) observed and co-authored with Scott: "These differing beliefs can have profound consequences for clinical practice and the judicial system. For example, therapists who believe that traumatic memories can be repressed may develop treatment plans that differ dramatically from those developed by practitioners who do not hold this belief. In the courtroom beliefs about memory often determine whether repressed-memory testimony is admitted into evidence" (p. 520).

Perhaps even more importantly, individuals who come to mistakenly believe that they suffered terrible abuse during childhood, for example—based on memories they recover during therapy—can give credence to a narrative of a past that "never was," with potentially disturbing and destabilizing consequences. The memory wars spawned substantial concern regarding harms linked to therapy techniques geared to recover repressed memories (see Lilienfeld, 2007; Otgaar et al., 2019). In their review of evidence from research and legal cases, Otgaar et al. (2019) contend that the memory wars are alive and well "and may even be on the rise" (p. 1073). They further suggest that in recent years, the scientifically controversial concept of dissociative amnesia (integral to the diagnosis of dissociative identity disorder [DID]) has gained popularity as a way to denote a condition akin to memory repression (p. 1073). Accordingly, the concept of repression is intimately entwined with controversies regarding dissociative amnesia and DID. Although we will allude to the latter conditions, a full discussion of their link with repressed memory is beyond the scope of this chapter.

Wins for Skepticism

Since the 1990s, there have been some successes from our perspective in the memory wars. The first win was that the subject of repressed memory became widely discussed outside of psychoanalysis and the self-help community. Until the 1990s, it appeared that psychodynamic practitioners were informed by repression theory and existed in their own bubble, whereas psychological scientists generally did not comment much on the authenticity of repressed memories. However, many of those successes were likely invisible in that psychotherapy clients may not have known that they were spared such a fate or that they benefited from the movement to implement evidence-based therapies that do not rely on memory recovery.

Critiques of the putative evidence for repressed and recovered memories of trauma proved persuasive to many, and perhaps was the cause of a decline in legal cases involving claims of repressed memory, which peaked in 1994 (Lipton, 1999). The attorney and psychologist Christopher Barden (2016) commented that he observed a large decrease in DID legal cases that involved false memories. Kevin Felstead, of the British False Memory Society, estimates that the Society's caseload was about 260 per year in 1993, and today they deal with approximately 40 legal cases per year (Felstead, 2022). The US-based False Memory Syndrome Foundation was dissolved at the end of 2019, with a message that included "The need for the FMS Foundation diminished dramatically over the years" (FMSF, 2019). These examples may indicate a decrease in the number of memory recovery legal cases active in the USA and UK. Nevertheless, some of the current authors can attest that memory recovery legal cases still occur. Indeed, recent data from the Netherlands Expert Committee for Equivocal Sexual Abuse Allegations show between 2008 and 2020, 17% ($n = 88$) of the cases involved recovered memories (Nierop, 2022).[1]

We have witnessed notable successes in communicating the hazards of recovered memory therapy for the lay public. Major documentaries highlight these hazards and the possibility of false memories, such as the 2021 Showtime series *Buried*. In the USA, the television program *60 Minutes*, *Public Broadcasting Service's Frontline*, *National Public Radio*, and many more media venues have aired stories questioning the validity of repressed memories. In the UK, the BBC and many broadsheet newspapers have highlighted stories on the hazards of repressed memory recovery. Some researchers have given TED talks and TEDx talks on repressed memory and false memory themes (e.g., Loftus, 2013). In some circles, false memories have become a well-known hazard to avoid when processing trauma in psychotherapy.

Guidelines for psychologists have been changed for the better in some areas, too. The British Psychology Society Research Board Working Group (2008) came to nuanced conclusions, which included the possibility that childhood events recalled in adulthood can be accurate, but sometimes can be "highly inaccurate, and sometimes wholly false" (p. 11). For example, the British Psychological Society's Working Party on Recovered Memories in 1995 offered recommendations on recovered memories with some preliminary caution about the production of false memories (Andrews et al., 1995). The American Psychological Association's report on false and recovered memories came to an uneasy consensus that both accurate remembering and false memories were possible (Alpert, 1997). The Health Council of the Netherlands (2004) report on false and recovered memories also concluded

[1] This committee consists of investigative psychologists, sex crime investigators, and experts in memory, cognition, and psychopathology. The second author of this chapter is a member of this committee. The committee investigates cases involving, for example, recovered memories and claims of ritual abuse and provides advice to the Public Prosecution on what the next steps should be (e.g., stop the investigation).

that recovered memories could be false. At least the possibility of false memories was becoming more widely communicated in the field.

Guidelines in some court systems have also seen improvements. For example, New Jersey adopted a detailed and evidence-based set of juror instructions for eyewitness testimony cases (New Jersey *v.* Henderson, 2011), and hypnosis-augmented testimony was banned from the courtroom in that state in 2006 (State *v.* Moore, 2006). Memories retrieved via hypnosis have been deemed inadmissible in 27 states in the USA, and in only 3 states, it is admissible without preconditions such as when procedural guidelines (e.g., only one person present in the room) are followed. Repressed memory evidence has also been deemed inadmissible in some courts. The earlier mentioned Dutch expert committee has also been established to evaluate potential recovered memories cases and advise prosecutors whether a criminal investigation of abuse, for example, should be pursued (Nierop et al., 2021).

Losses for Skepticism

To balance these wins or partial wins, some losses are notable. Some have documented continued beliefs in the concept of repressed memory among the public and clinicians (Patihis et al., 2014; Otgaar et al., 2019), with data suggesting that these beliefs appear to translate to clinical practice, too (e.g., Patihis & Pendergrast, 2019).

In addition, dissociative amnesia is now deeply embedded in psychiatry's "bible" for mental disorders, the *Diagnostic and Statistical Manual of Mental Disorders* (*DSM-5*; American Psychiatric Association, 2013), as well in the *International Classification of Diseases* (ICD-11). The definition of dissociative amnesia in the *DSM-5* has the unfortunate side effect of legitimizing the dubious claim that traumatic memories can be stored yet blocked, only to be retrieved in pristine form years or decades later. This claim is based on repression theory and is presented in the guise of the different terminology of trauma and dissociation in arguably the most important book in psychology and psychiatry. Specifically, in the *DSM-5*, the diagnostic criteria on page 298, state that dissociative amnesia is:

> An inability to recall important autobiographical information, usually of a traumatic or stressful nature, that is inconsistent with ordinary forgetting. Note: Dissociative amnesia most often consists of localized or selective amnesia for a specific event or events; or generalized amnesia for identity and life history.

Accordingly, the *DSM* proposes that "dissociative amnesia most often consists of localized or selective amnesia for a specific event or events" (p. 298). Localized is described as a "failure to recall events during a circumscribed period of time" and selective is described as, "the individual can recall some, but not all, of the events during a circumscribed period of time" (p. 298). Both subtypes of dissociative amnesia are functionally indistinguishable from repressed memory (see Otgaar et al., 2019). The rarer subtype of generalized dissociative amnesia is "a complete loss of memory for one's life history" (p. 298), which is different from the alleged selective inability to recall a trauma. Even in the case of generalized dissociative amnesia, "dissociative" is suggestive of a psychological traumatic cause, when in fact it is extraordinarily difficult to rule out physical neurological problems and non-trauma environmental causes of forgetting (see Mangiulli et al., 2022). Dropping the word "dissociative" from the term dissociative amnesia in the *DSM-5* would thus improve the document and eliminate a term with connotations associated with a controversial and unproven theory. However, any such changes would have to be cautiously examined to identify potential unforeseen consequences. "Dissociative," when referenced in the *DSM-5*, legitimizes psychiatric folklore regarding dissociation that dates as far back as the nineteenth-century physicians/hypnotists such as Jean-Martin Charcot and Pierre Janet and persists to the present time (see Otgaar et al., 2019). The phrase "selective amnesia" would be much less suggestive of cause than the term "selective dissociative amnesia." "Generalized amnesia" is also arguably less laden with problematic theoretical baggage than "generalized dissociative amnesia," and so on. We hope these changes will be considered in future iterations of the *DSM*, along with corresponding added cautions noted in the text.

Controversy surrounding the retention of DID in the *DSM-5* represents another contested battle for skeptics who have been outnumbered in this arena. The use of the word "dissociative" has deep historical links to the dubious proposition that traumas are sequestered from working memory yet cause the diverse symptoms of DID (e.g., Prince, 1906). As researchers have contended that DID is a disorder of a person's *belief* in a fractured self (see Lynn et al., 2019, in press), the term "identity disorder" would be less theory-contaminated, more parsimonious (i.e., not requiring the construct of dissociation), and therefore preferable. Although some patients do report serious identity and memory problems, we recommend that clinicians in such cases keep an open mind about other possible causes, such as physical brain or neuronal problems, substance use, and environmental damage to the brain. This open-minded stance is preferable to assuming that uncorroborated reports of early childhood (ritualistic) abuse, for example, are the hidden cause of serious dissociative symptoms (Mangiulli et al., 2022). Such cautions regarding causal assumptions should be integrated into routine clinical practice to avoid unnecessary traumatization to those patients who suspect they harbor repressed memories of childhood trauma. In short, the iatrogenic recovery of purported repressed memories should be a concern in treating individuals who report dissociative symptoms, including reports of multiple identities.

Social media bubbles on the topics of dissociative amnesia, blocked trauma, and DID are also problematic. The reader is invited to type in "dissociative identity disorder" into YouTube to assess the magnitude of the problem. YouTube channels and Facebook groups on these topics have gathered millions of views that often feature accounts of bizarre and improbable recovered memories and/or strongly encourage self-diagnosis of DID. In these social media echo-chambers, nonsense and implausible claims flourish, and a disturbing disparity exists between the few people familiar with science-based portrayals of dissociative conditions and the millions of people who watch social media videos promoting repressed memories and multiple personalities. In this context, extreme expressions of credulity in social media comments sections for people claiming to harbor multiple personalities are potentially harmful. There is a need for responsible education and encouragement for consumers to participate in critical thinking about iatrogenic social media rabbit-holes on topics like DID.

The social influence of a burgeoning online culture is difficult to navigate and challenge insofar as some of the same individuals who mis-educate the public on social media platforms often simultaneously claim to be victims of terrible trauma. Direct confrontation of such miseducation on social media can thus be defended against with claims of personal offense, devaluation, and accusations of denying trauma victims' identity or even their existence. Dialogue can be quashed by confusing legitimate scientific inquiry regarding dissociative amnesia and DID with invalidating the reality, repercussions, or scope of child sexual abuse. To the extent that harmful suggestive "therapies" instantiate false narratives of familial abuse that fracture families and eventuate in legal actions against therapists for harmful practices, it depreciates the claims and suffering of survivors of actual childhood abuse and hampers much-needed efforts to raise awareness of childhood abuse and prevent its occurrence.

Another loss in the memory wars is that some journals continue to publish uncritical and unchallenged articles that advocate for the concept of trauma-induced dissociative amnesia. One prominent example is a recent issue of the *Journal of Trauma and Dissociation* in which multiple articles (2022, volume 23, issue 2) suggest, with scant credible evidence, that a political agenda motivates research on false memories (e.g., Cheit, 2022; Crook, 2022).

Threats to free speech in academia are also a disappointing loss that scientific skeptics have suffered in the last decade (O'Donohue & Fisher, 2022). Scott himself felt some foreshadowing of this loss decades earlier when he commented on the suppression of the Rind et al. (1998) meta-analysis on abuse and psychopathology. Scott also showed intellectual courage in his critique of the evidential merit of work on microaggressions (Lilienfeld, 2017, 2020). As Scott voiced heterodox ideas, he faced a vocal minority of critical social justice activists within the Society for Science in Clinical Psychology (see Pignotti, 2020). Unfortunately, such events could have a chilling effect on other individuals who are considering voicing courageous yet unpopular opinions. In some circumstances, academics who are outspoken in expressing skeptical views regarding controversial topics can benefit the public by calling attention to potentially iatrogenic psychological treatments and implausible, untested, and even nonsensical theories. Some of the current authors have also faced challenges due to changes that have limited academic freedoms of speech and inquiry.

The debate over repression, dissociative amnesia, and DID requires that academics know that they can speak freely on the issues without undue constraint, being targeted by *ad hominem* attacks or physical threats to their safety, or fear they will lose their academic positions. In the UK, for example, although there is a tradition of free speech and critical rationalism, tenure for academics was removed in 1988 (Education Reform Act, 1988). Nevertheless, the freedom of inquiry traditions of

British academia, as well as free speech clauses in various education acts, likely encouraged scholars to engage with contentious issues in the repressed memory debate. America has retained a tenure system and that might explain why some of the most direct criticisms of repressed memories were from American professors in the 1990s and 2000s (even then, some of those critics faced foreshadowing of so-called cancel culture). In the USA recently there is at least a perception that there has been a weakening of the free speech protections of those on the tenure track, and the perception now is that tenured positions no longer guarantee free speech on controversial issues. The Netherlands also has a tradition of free speech and an ethic that everything can and should be discussed, which may explain why resident scholars have also contributed to this topic. Similar observations are arguably relevant with respect to countries, such as New Zealand and Canada, where scholars have likewise contributed to the debate. As a link appears to exist between the conditions of free inquiry and valuable skepticism on the topic of repressed memories, we suggest that it is imperative to protect and reward such inquiry in the universities.

A potential example of how free speech restrictions might cause harm is when academics are hesitant to debunk social media DID bubbles that harm young people. Concerns about social media mobbing might also dissuade concerned experts from speaking freely in response to viral videos that promote self-misdiagnosis in thousands of young adults. Without guarantees of free speech protections, the debate will be dominated by those who misleadingly claim that repressed memory and DID skeptics, delegitimize or harm victims of childhood trauma. The misdirected insinuation that scientific skeptics do not empathize with or care about suffering clients has made it especially difficult to freely critique DID without risking online attacks and negative responses from others.

In fact, participants on the skeptical side in the memory wars do appreciate the potential aftereffects of genuine trauma or sexual abuse. The authors of this chapter have written with concern about the harmful effects of sexual abuse captured by diagnoses such as posttraumatic stress disorder and/or developed treatments or preventive programs related to sexual abuse and dissociation, thereby acknowledging the real and long-lasting effects of trauma and the experience of associated symptoms (e.g., Blackwell et al., 2004; Layman et al., 1996; Mohajerin et al., 2020). To be clear, what is at issue in terms of dissociation is not that people believe they have DID—they do, in that their experiences meet diagnostic formal criteria—but rather whether the genesis of their symptoms invariably resides in traumatic experiences. As Spanos (1994) and others (Lynn et al., 2019, 2022, in press) have pointed out, DID might have other causes such as role enactment, social influence (e.g., suggestive psychotherapeutic interventions, media influence), and cognitive (e.g., fantasy proneness, suggestibility, hyperassociation, failure of thought suppression) and affective (e.g., emotion dysregulation, avoidance of negative affect) factors. Informing people of such causes who have developed or are at risk of iatrogenic DID has great potential to help them escape pseudoscientific echo-chambers.

Another loss is the development of a motte-and-bailey argument technique among proponents of trauma–dissociation theory. The motte-and-bailey fallacy (named after the motte-and-bailey castle, see Fig. 1 is an argument where an

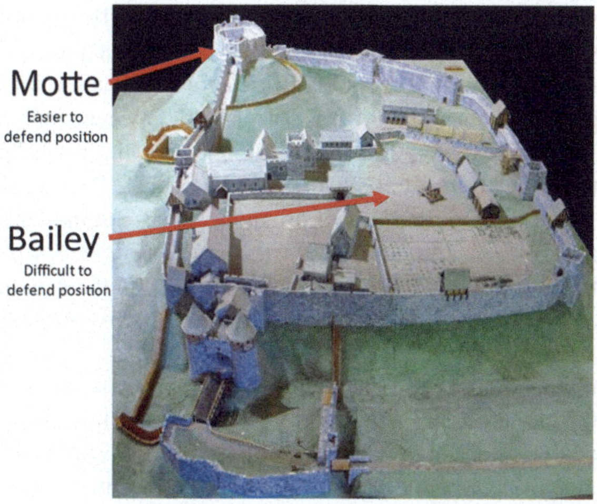

Fig. 1 An example of a fourteenth-century motte-and-bailey arrangement of Carisbrooke Castle on the Isle of Wight, Hampshire, UK. Creative Commons Licence: CC-BY-2.0

easy-to-defend position (the "motte") is used to obscure or direct attention away from a more controversial position (the "bailey"). It is a fallacious argument technique. While in the bailey the arguer advances the controversial position, but when challenged, they run up the motte into the castle and take an easy-to-defend position. Upon retreating to the motte, the arguer can claim that the bailey has not been refuted because the critic did not defeat the motte. The arguer may equate an attack on the bailey with an attack on the motte.

The analogy to the recovered memory debate is that advocates advance (as a battle force might advance) controversial ideas while out on the *bailey* (e.g., claims about dissociative amnesia, DID, extraordinary remembering via repressed memories, widespread ritualistic abuse). However, when challenged they run up into *motte* to the castle and adopt a much easier to defend position (e.g., that trauma correlates with dissociation, that memories of words can be suppressed, that DID is merely identity confusion). While out on the bailey, trauma and dissociative amnesia advocates have succeeded in embedding many of their ideas into culture, journals, books, the *DSM-5*, and the *ICD-11*. Entries in the *DSM-5* on dissociative amnesia and dissociative identity disorder hint at extraordinary claims such as the ability to accurately retrieve blocked memories, and the idea that people can *literally* (not figuratively) have multiple personalities that dwell inside a single brain. Yet when these claims are challenged, many trauma/dissociation advocates retreat to their motte. From this motte, they state that numerous studies have shown trauma is correlated with dissociation. Of course, the latter is the more defensible claim, although correlation does not necessarily signify causation.

From this motte, proponents may argue that there is evidence of suppression in Anderson and Green's (2001) "think/no-think" memory research. From the motte, some may claim that the idea that many people believe in unconscious repression is a red herring (e.g., Brewin et al., 2020). However, out on the bailey, larger claims are made. In court, trauma/dissociation theory proponents may state as expert witnesses that dissociative amnesia and DID involve recovered memories that should be treated credibly by the courts. Yet their peer-reviewed writings on the topic tend to revolve around the more defensible argument (from the motte) that past research has shown a correlation between traumatic experiences and the dissociative experiences scale (Dalenberg et al., 2012; Brand et al., 2017a, b; for critiques see Lynn et al., 2014; Merckelbach & Patihis, 2018).

Until scientific skeptics are more successful in identifying and naming the motte-and-bailey technique of trauma–dissociation theory proponents, skeptics will continue to fall into the trap of debating them in their motte: For example, debating the size of the correlation between trauma and dissociation, or debating whether telling a participant to forget a list of words leads to worse recall from that list. Skeptics might profitably invite trauma-centric theorists back out onto the bailey to debate the claim of complete memory blockages followed by extraordinary remembering that is proposed to be so accurate that people could be convicted based on repressed memories. Skeptics should invite trauma-centric theorists to debate whether dissociative identity disorder involves *literal* multiple personalities inside people's minds, or whether it is a delusional belief. Noticing the retreat to the motte in the coming years might improve the relevance and quality of the discussion of these important and controversial issues.

The Future: How to Create Open-Minded Skeptics

Scott Lilienfeld had a positive effect on the recovered memory debate in part due to a rare and extraordinary combination of traits and behaviors embedded in an academic climate that tolerated and often embraced his skeptical positions on controversial issues. His fair-minded, balanced, thoughtful arguments and impeccable scholarship were well equipped to tilt even some true believers or people "on the fence," regarding well-entrenched views, toward being more critical thinkers and considering alternative perspectives. Scott's ability to welcome and consider diverse opinions and change his own ideas also earned personal and professional respect in his mission to distinguish scientific from pseudoscientific claims.

Scott boldly applied a broad scientific toolkit to examine sensitive and controversial topics such as sexual abuse, the Rind et al. (1998) controversy, dissociative identity disorder, autism and facilitated communication, left-wing authoritarianism, and of course the repressed memory controversy. If he were alive today, he would, we predict, endeavor to help resolve the most painful and controversial topics that confront society.

There is a need for more skeptical scientists to follow in Scott's path, not only because of the losses in the memory wars that we recounted but also because the debate can impose a burden on scholars over years. Many critics may only engage *directly* in a limited number of battles or for a limited period on the topic before returning to their own research programs. For example, challenging the wording in the *DSM-5* will inevitably prove to be daunting, and individual researchers may only be able to devote direct engagement in such an immense, protracted, and consuming undertaking only a few times in their career. Accordingly, early-career scientists must ideally not only be dedicated to taking on challenges but also perceive that they have guaranteed free speech rights in academia, even before tenure, and during the time they still possess the desire and energy to address the most difficult and controversial topics. These circumstances present an immense challenge for academia because it can take years to acquire a sufficient understanding of all the deep roots of a controversial topic. Moreover, whether hard-nosed scientific critical thinkers would be attracted to and seek a career in a modern psychology department is another matter. Nevertheless, future skeptics, if retained in academia, have the potential to debunk pseudoscience inside psychology and thereby mitigate harmful practices in therapies worldwide.

The aforementioned ideas lead us to raise this question: What is required in academia to attract productive and brilliant scientific critical thinkers like Scott—and to sustain their motivation to address controversial topics? As discussed earlier, speech protection for academics is essential for one to tackle many controversial issues. Some free speech provisions are guaranteed in the education acts in the UK and the Netherlands, in the US constitution, and in some academic contracts. Nevertheless, in recent years some academics have reported dire consequences after speaking freely on controversial topics (see Foundation for Individual Rights in Education, 2021; Boghossian, 2021). This situation is potentially a problem for future scientists in the area of traumatic memory recovery, which is a controversial topic linked with highly personal and important societal issues: identity, child abuse, and sexual assault. Without the kind of free speech parameters that were in effect when Scott was an early-career scientist, it is uncertain whether emerging skeptical scientists will choose to join academia and whether they will be hired over more credulous candidates. It is also far from certain that they will choose to speak out on controversial pseudoscience in the future.

Funding is needed to retain future skeptical scientists in academia. Funding that prioritizes highly constrained and programmatic research conducted by prestigious or established researchers, rather than research that challenges basic assumptions or received scientific wisdom, can impede motivation to pursue important research contra to the status quo. We hope that promising scientific work will be supported generously that questions the validity of underlying premises, currently popular theories, and the genesis of symptoms related to controversial *DSM* diagnoses, including DID. Research on trending psychology topics and methods (e.g., neuroscience) likely influence both funding and hiring in tenure track jobs at prestigious universities, which poses a potential problem for investigators who wish to pursue topics that are not necessarily viewed as "cutting edge" or that could stir controversy. Theoretical and empirical initiatives regarding issues that are over 100 years old, such as pseudoscientific clinical practices, dissociative amnesia, and dissociative identity disorder, may well be harder to sell to funders and hiring committees.

We also suggest that toning down, if not eliminating, relational aggression and *ad hominem* arguments in psychology would potentially help retain science-oriented skeptics motivated to root out pseudoscience in the field. Relational aggression consists of *indirect* undermining of reputation, usually without the target present. It arises in socially competitive environments that breed a web of social influence in which the truth is secondary. Hard-nosed scientists will be more interested in what is true from first principles, rather than living in a conflict-laden web of social influence.

In addition, many scholars will likely be put off by *ad hominem* arguments in the publishing world and in academia, as the authors of this chapter have encountered. Scott eschewed such arguments, and his unique brand of skepticism facilitated his attempts to teach critical thinking and embrace an open-minded scientific mindset. Direct *ad hominem* attacks pose a major obstacle in (a) achieving the goal of disclosing evidence-based "truths" in the debate over recovered memories, (b) encouraging movements toward rapprochement across competing perspectives, and (c) engaging in potentially invaluable adversarial collaborations.

For people like Scott, the foundation of the American Psychological Society (APS; since renamed as the Association of Psychological Science) in 1988 provided essential oxygen for the scientific branch of psychology at the time, and for a few decades following was at the vanguard in advocating for clinical psychological science. We are concerned that if psychological organizations gravitate toward or endorse ideologically motivated ideas, political slogans, and arguments inspired by postmodernism and critical theory (see Pluckrose & Lindsay, 2020), it will put off potential scholars who value critical thinking. It would benefit the field if psychological organizations promoted the highest values of scientific inquiry and continued to apply and exemplify critical thinking to resist political and social pressures put upon them. Any attempts to stifle open inquiry can dampen the very dialogues essential to foment progress on scientific and societal fronts. On a brighter note, Scott was a member of the Heterodox Academy, and an attendee of its conferences, and it remains to be seen whether this organization becomes a new haven for critical thinkers in psychology.

Summary

In summary, we argue that the arena in which future combat in the memory wars takes place should be signposted and demarcated by markers of free speech, free thought, and open and civil discourse. As shown in the rise and fall of skepticism in Ancient Greece, and the Dark Ages, the struggle to defend the gains of the scientific method and the Enlightenment, and the postmodern and critical theory movement more recently (see Pluckrose & Lindsay, 2020), scientific skepticism and freethought can fade and lose ground if not valued and encouraged.

Prominent challenges that face skeptics of recovered memories span the inclusion of poorly validated categories in the *DSM-5* (American Psychiatric Association, 2013), which implicitly endorses attempts to recover purportedly dissociated memories, the rampant unconstrained viral nature of trauma and DID misinformation in social media bubbles, and the motte-and-bailey argument of traumagenic theorists.

Still, debates on false memories, recovered memory, dissociation, and dissociative amnesia should proceed with the assumption that scientific methods can and should be applied by skeptics and non-skeptics alike. Science is an evolving process that ideally, with accumulating evidence, weeds out claims that do not survive demanding tests. Moreover, as the physicist Richard Feynman noted, scientists should bend over backwards to prove themselves wrong.

Another challenge that skeptics face is to develop a research agenda with priorities that encompass the study of recovered memories and whether and how trauma impacts memory in and apart from psychotherapy. The following examples merely serve as suggestions but might surely be promising next steps. Specifically, future researchers could determine under what conditions memories that arise during or after psychotherapy are likely to be correct, incorrect, or of indeterminate accuracy. Relatedly, it will be important to acknowledge that memories are forgotten and remembered, and often morph and are recalled in different ways during quotidian living as well as in the consulting room. Researchers from competing camps could profit from the following: (a) clarifying the mediators and moderators of significant changes in memories and attributions associated with "recovered memories" and how they fit with pre-existing narratives and/or contribute to novel beliefs integral to personal identity; (b) examining how recovered memories may be perceived in divergent ways as a function of psychiatric diagnosis and personality characteristics; (c) evaluating the role of suggestion and demand characteristics in the emergence and appraisal of recovered memories; and (d) determining how memories take on particular salience and meaning, whether recovered or not. Developing different typologies of memories that are recovered (e.g., trauma vs. non-trauma-related; high vs. low arousal level; positive vs. negative valence) would also be important and fascinating to validate in the context of the initiatives mentioned. Given the fact that memories of unknown or unsubstantiated accuracy constantly surface and resurface, we suggest that informed consent procedures be routinely applied that acknowledge the possibility that false memories will arise during therapy, particularly when high-risk procedures (e.g., hypnosis) are considered or employed.

There are promising indications that at least some differences across competing views can be breached in certain arenas of conflict. For example, there is some degree of rapprochement across theoretical divides in the conceptualization of DID, which has been close to the epicenter of battles in the memory wars. For example, advocates of competing perspectives acknowledge that DID is related to self-understanding and that fantasy proneness may lead to inaccurate trauma reports, implying that recovered memories of trauma may not be accurate (see Lynn et al., 2019). Importantly, researchers have "failed to detect consistent objective evidence (e.g., behavioral tasks, event-related potentials) of distinct personalities segregated by impermeable amnesic barriers…" (Lynn et al., 2019, p. 3), buttressing the notion that DID involves a subjective sense of self.

Meanwhile, critics of repressed and recovered memories acknowledge the possibility that an unknown percentage of recovered memories will turn out to be accurate and corroborated, forgotten for a period and cued by current events, and only years later, for example, be interpreted as abuse (McNally, 2012). However, the index of suspicion regarding the accuracy of recovered memories should be particularly high when the memory (a) surfaces for the first time in psychotherapy or after learning about a trauma repression theory; (b) relates to a traumatic or highly emotional, ordinarily memorable event, which would likely be remembered (e.g., violent sexual assault); (c) is highly implausible (e.g., satanic ritual abuse); (d) is not corroborated or at variance with the reports of individuals who would be in a position to verify the occurrence of the event; and/or (e) is reported by a highly credulous consumer of social media relevant to memory recovery, dissociation, and/or dissociative amnesia.

The debate over trauma, repression, and memory has elicited considerable research, theoretical developments, and even, at times, productive dialogue. Whether adversarial collaborations would be profitable might depend on the situation. One of us (RJM) successfully moderated a civil debate between psychologists who disagree on whether memories of trauma tend to be especially fragmented or disorganized (McNally et al., 2022), prompted by an article by McNally (2022). Although this was not an empirical research adversarial collaboration, it nevertheless shows that people with sharply divergent views can clarify their points of agreement and disagreement when they share principles of reason and evidence. Such collaborations may be profitable under the constraints of the scientific method, using a disconfirming approach, investigating basic assumptions, and focusing on valuing singular precise constructs more than vague loose constructs. These adversarial collaborations could pertain to multiple fronts of the memory wars; they could center on topics such as (a) the nature and mechanisms of remembering and forgetting, (b) re-examining the assumptions, reliability, and validity of the dissociation concept, and (c) potentially harmful psychotherapies that elevate the risk of false recovered memories. Nonetheless, in the area of repressed and false memory, some adversarial efforts were unsuccessful in accusations going back and forth between different camps (Ceci & Williams, 2022; Clark et al., 2022).

We believe in the long and extraordinarily successful tradition of scientific skepticism. This approach posits that there is an objective truth, and that we should adapt to evidence with a very cautious understanding that cause can be difficult to establish in complex dynamic systems. This approach posits that humans are flawed, and that people need the scientific method to acknowledge, compensate for, and potentially mitigate confirmation and other ubiquitous biases, mental heuristics, and logical fallacies (see Lynn et al., Chap. 7, this volume). The approach is based on empiricism guided by careful examination of the wide breadth of cognitive and neurobiological research in memory. Such an approach has reduced harm in the world. Scott was an example of the type of beautiful mind this open-minded skepticism can shape. These habits of mind that are allied with this school of thought allow people like Scott, for a few fleeting but enlightened years, to discern some of the deeper meanings and workings of the world.

In conclusion, we hope that readers will look to Scott as an inspiring role model, as we do. He displayed remarkable intellectual clarity and courage in calling attention to the dark side of psychotherapy and the harms of pseudoscientific clinical practices. Scott engaged directly and indirectly, via his prolific writings, with individuals who expressed views that diverged sharply from his opinions. Yet we suspect that his kindness, empathy, and even-handed arguments encouraged some of his many readers to recognize, if not outright reject, pseudoscientific practices and adopt a more scientific mindset. Scott was keenly aware of the limitations of his knowledge, and he embodied the important trait of epistemic humility. While he expressed an unwavering commitment to the scientific method, he steadfastly questioned his own beliefs in his openness to novel ideas, discoveries, and emerging evidence as it accumulated. We believe that Scott would be pleased to learn something new about trauma and memory, regardless of whether it challenged or refuted his beliefs, and whether he ultimately was proven to be right or wrong. That is the kind of person and scientist that Scott O. Lilienfeld was and the person we miss dearly.

References

Alpert, J. L. (1997). Unsubstantiated claims of false memory and essential responsibilities. *American Psychologist, 52*(9), 987. https://doi.org/10.1037/0003-066X.52.9.987.a

American Psychiatric Association. (2013). *Diagnostic and statistical manual of mental disorders* (5th ed.). Author.

Anderson, M. C., & Green, C. (2001). Suppressing unwanted memories by executive control. *Nature, 410*(6826), 366–369.

Andrews, B., Morton, J., Bekerian, D. A., Brewin, C. R., Davies, G. M., & Mollon, P. (1995). The recovery of memories in clinical practice: Experiences and beliefs of British psychological society practitioners. *Psychologist, 8*(5), 209–214.

Barden, R. C. (2016). Memory and reliability: Developments and controversial issues. In P. Radcliffe, A. Heaton-Armstrong, G. Gudjonsson, & D. Wolchover (Eds.), *Witness Testimony in Sex Cases* (pp. 343–359). Oxford University Press.

Blackwell, L. M., Lynn, S. J., Vanderhoff, H., & Gidycz, C. (2004). Sexual assault revictimization: Toward effective risk-reduction programs. In L. J. Koenig, L. S. Doll, A. O'Leary, & W. Pequegnat (Eds.), *From child sexual abuse to adult sexual risk: Trauma, revictimization, and intervention* (pp. 269–295). American Psychological Association. https://doi.org/10.1037/10785-014

Blume, E. S. (1990). *Secret survivors: Uncovering incest and its aftereffects in women*. Wiley.

Boghossian, P. (2021). My university sacrificed ideas for ideology. So today I quit. [Letter]. *Common Sense*: Bari Weiss's Substack [Website]. https://bariweiss.substack.com/p/my-university-sacrificed-ideas-for?

Brand, B. L., Schielke, H. J., & Brams, J. S. (2017a). Assisting the courts in understanding and connecting with experiences of disconnection: Addressing trauma-related dissociation as a forensic psychologist, part I. *Psychological Injury and Law, 10*(4), 283–297.

Brand, B. L., Schielke, H. J., Brams, J. S., & DiComo, R. A. (2017b). Assessing trauma-related dissociation in forensic contexts: Addressing trauma-related dissociation as a forensic psychologist, part II. *Psychological Injury and Law, 10*(4), 298–312.

Brewin, C. R., Li, H., McNeilis, J., Ntarantana, V., & Unsworth, C. (2020). On repression, and avoiding red herrings. *Journal of Experimental Psychology: General, 149*(10), 2001–2004.

British Psychology Society Research Board Working Group. (2008, June). *Guidelines on memory and the law: Recommendations from the scientific study of human memory.* British Psychological Society.

Ceci, S. J., & Williams, W. M. (2022). The importance of viewpoint diversity among scientific team members. Comment on Clark et al. *Journal of Applied Research in Memory and Cognition, 11*(1).
Cheit, R. E. (2022). Hyping Hypnosis: The Myth That Made Capturing the Friedmans Persuasive. *Journal of Trauma & Dissociation, 23*(2), 152–164.
Clark, C., Costello, T., Mitchell, G., & Tetlock, P. (2022). Keep your enemies close: Adversarial collaborations will improve empirical accuracy. *Journal of Applied Research in Memory and Cognition, 11*(1), 1–18. https://doi.org/10.1037/mac0000004
Crews, F. C. (1995). *The memory wars: Freud's legacy in dispute. NY: New York Review of Books.*
Crook, L. (2022). The Power of False Memory Rhetoric. *Journal of Trauma & Dissociation, 23*(2), 148–151.
Dalenberg, C. J., Brand, B. L., Gleaves, D. H., Dorahy, M. J., Loewenstein, R. J., Cardeña, E., et al. (2012). Evaluation of the Evidence for the Trauma and Fantasy Models of Dissociation. *Psychological Bulletin, 138*(3), 550–588.
Education Reform Act. (1988). London, UK: Her Majesty's Stationary Office. https://www.legislation.gov.uk/ukpga/1988/40/contents
Felstead, K. (2022, April, 1). *Address at the British false memory society annual meeting*. Online virtual meeting.
FMSF. (2019). *False Memory Syndrome Foundation* [Website]. http://www.fmsfonline.org/
Foundation for Individual Rights in Education. (2021). *Scholars Under Fire: 2021 Year in Review.* https://www.thefire.org/research/publications/miscellaneous-publications/scholars-under-fire/scholars-under-fire-2021-year-in-review-full-text/
Freyd, J. J. (1994). Betrayal-trauma: Traumatic amnesia as an adaptive response to childhood abuse. *Ethics & Behavior, 4*, 307–329.
Health Council of the Netherlands. (2004). *Disputed memories. The Hague: Health Council of the Netherlands, publication no. 2004/02.* http://dx.doi.org.ezp-prod1.hul.harvard.edu/10.1037/0033-2909.125.5.507
Layman, M. J., Gidycz, C. A., & Lynn, S. J. (1996). Unacknowledged versus acknowledged rape victims: Situational factors and posttraumatic stress. *Journal of Abnormal Psychology, 105*(1), 124–131. https://doi.org/10.1037/0021-843X.105.1.124
Lilienfeld, S. O. (2007). Psychological treatments that cause harm. *Perspectives on Psychological Science, 2*(1), 53–70.
Lilienfeld, S. O. (2017). Microaggressions: Strong claims, inadequate evidence. *Perspectives on Psychological Science, 12*(1), 138–169.
Lilienfeld, S. O. (2020). Microaggression research and application: Clarifications, corrections, and common ground. *Perspectives on Psychological Science, 15*(1), 27–37.
Lilienfeld, S. O., & Loftus, E. F. (1998). Repressed memories and World War II: Some cautionary notes. *Professional Psychology: Research and Practice, 29*(5), 471–475.
Lilienfeld, S. O., Kirsch, I., Sarbin, T. R., Lynn, S. J., Chaves, J. F., Ganaway, G. K., & Powell, R. A. (1999). Dissociative identity disorder and the sociocognitive model: Recalling the lessons of the past. *Psychological Bulletin, 125*(5), 507–523.
Lilienfeld, S. O., Lohr, J. M., & Lynn, S. J. (2003). *Science and pseudoscience in contemporary clinical psychology*. Guilford.
Lilienfeld, S. O., Ruscio, J., & Lynn, S. J. (Eds.). (2008). *Navigating the mindfield: A guide to separating science from pseudoscience in mental health.* Prometheus Books.
Lipton, A. (1999). Recovered memories in the courts. In S. Taub (Ed.), *Recovered memories of child sexual abuse: Psychological, social, and legal perspectives on a contemporary mental health controversy* (pp. 165–210). Charles C. Thomas.
Loftus, E. F. (1993). The reality of repressed memories. *American Psychologist, 48*(5), 518–537.
Loftus, E. (2004). Dispatch from the (un) civil memory wars. *The Lancet, 364*, 20–21.
Loftus, E. F. (2013). *How reliable is your memory?* [Video]. TED Conferences. https://www.ted.com/talks/elizabeth_loftus_how_reliable_is_your_memory.

Loftus, E. F., & Davis, D. (2006). Recovered memories. *Annual Review of Clinical Psychology, 2*, 469–498.
Lynn, S. J., Aksen, D., Sleight, F., Polizzi, C., Moretti, L. S., & Medrano, L. A. (in press). Combating pseudoscience in clinical psychology: From the scientific mindset to busting myths, to prescriptive remedies. In C. Cobb, W. O'Donohue, & S. J. Lynn (Eds.), *Toward a science of clinical psychology: A tribute to the life and work of Scott O.* Springer.
Lynn, S. J., & Baltman, J. (2016). Recovered memories. In N. Naples (Ed.), *The Wiley Blackwell encyclopedia of gender and sexuality studies* (pp. 1–3). Wiley-Blackwell.
Lynn, S. J., Lilienfeld, S. O., Merckelbach, H., Giesbrecht, T., McNally, R. J., Loftus, E. F., et al. (2014). The trauma model of dissociation: Inconvenient truths and stubborn fictions. Comment on Dalenberg et al. (2012). *Directions in Psychological Science, 12*(1), 32–35.
Lynn, S. J., Maxwell, R., Merckelbach, H., Lilienfeld, S. O., van Heugten-van der Kloet, D., & Miskovic, V. (2019). Dissociation and its disorders: Competing models, future directions, and a way forward. *Clinical Psychology Review, 73*, 101755.
Lynn, S. J., Polizzi, C., Merckelbach, H., Chiu, C. D., Maxwell, R., van Heugten, D., & Lilienfeld, S. O. (2022). Dissociation and dissociative disorders reconsidered: Beyond sociocognitive and trauma models toward a transtheoretical framework. *Annual Review of Clinical Psychology, 18*.
Mangiulli, I., Otgaar, H., Jelicic, M., & Merckelbach, H. (2022). A critical review of case studies on dissociative amnesia. *Clinical Psychological Science, 10*(2), 191–211.
McHugh, P. R. (2006). *The mind has mountains: Reflections on society and psychiatry*. Johns Hopkins University Press.
McNally, R. J. (2003a). Recovering memories of trauma: A view from the laboratory. *Current Directions in Psychological Science, 12*(1), 32–35. https://doi.org/10.1111/1467-8721.01217
McNally, R. J. (2003b). *Remembering trauma*. The Belknap Press of Harvard University Press.
McNally, R. J. (2012). Searching for repressed memory. In R. F. Belli (Ed.), *True and false recovered memories: Toward a reconciliation of the debate* (Nebraska Symposium on Motivation) (Vol. 58, pp. 121–147). Springer.
McNally, R. J. (2022). Are memories of sexual trauma fragmented? *Memory, 30*(1), 26–30.
McNally, R. J., Berntsen, C., Brewin, C. R., & Rubin, D. C. (2022). Are memories of sexual trauma fragmented? A post publication discussion among Richard J. McNally, Dorthe Berntsen, Chris R. Brewin, and David C. Rubin. *Memory*. https://doi.org/10.1080/09658211.2022.2061135.
Merckelbach, H., & Patihis, L. (2018). Why "trauma-related dissociation" is a misnomer in courts: A critical analysis of Brand et al. (2017a, b). *Psychological Injury and Law, 11*(4), 370–376.
Mohajerin, B., Lynn, S. J., Bakhtiyari, M., & Dolatshah, B. (2020). Evaluating the unified protocol in the treatment of dissociative identify disorder. *Cognitive and Behavioral Practice, 27*(3), 270–289.
New Jersey v. Henderson. (2011). *A-8-08 (062218)*. https://law.justia.com/cases/new-jersey/supreme-court/2011/a-8-08-1-opn.html
Nierop, N. (2022, March). *Netherlands expert committee for equivocal sexual abuse allegations*. Presentation at the annual LEBZ meeting.
Nierop, N., van den Eshof, P., & Brandt, C. (2021). *A practical approach to sexual abuse allegations: Netherlands Expert Committee for Equivocal Sexual Abuse Allegations* (pp. 1–13). Psychiatry.
O'Donohue, W., & Fisher, J. E. (2022). Are illiberal acts unethical? APA's Ethics Code and the protection of free speech. *American Psychologist, 77*(8), 875–886. https://doi.org/10.1037/amp0000995
Otgaar, H., Howe, M. L., & Patihis, L. (2022). What science tells us about false and repressed memories. *Memory, 30*(1), 16–21.
Otgaar, H., Howe, M. L., Patihis, L., Merckelbach, H., Lynn, S. J., Lilienfeld, S. O., & Loftus, E. F. (2019). The return of the repressed: The persistent and problematic claims of long-forgotten trauma. *Perspectives on Psychological Science, 14*(6), 1072–1095.

Patihis, L., & Pendergrast, M. H. (2019). Reports of recovered memories of abuse in therapy in a large age-representative US national sample: Therapy type and decade comparisons. *Clinical Psychological Science, 7*(1), 3–21.
Patihis, L., Ho, L. Y., Tingen, I. W., Lilienfeld, S. O., & Loftus, E. F. (2014). Are the "memory wars" over? A scientist-practitioner gap in beliefs about repressed memory. *Psychological Science, 25*(2), 519–530.
Pignotti, M. (2020). *SSCPnet listserve controversy.* Potentially Harmful and Other Questionable Therapies [Website]. https://phtherapies.wordpress.com/2020/06/22/sscpnet-listserve-controversy/
Pluckrose, H., & Lindsay, J. (2020). *Cynical theories: How activist scholarship made everything about race, gender, and identity – And why this harms everybody.* Pitchstone Publishing.
Prince, M. (1906). Hysteria from the point of view of dissociated personality. *The Journal of Abnormal Psychology, 1*(4), 170–187. https://doi.org/10.1037/h0071515
Rind, B., Tromovitch, P., & Bauserman, R. (1998). A meta-analytic examination of assumed properties of child sexual abuse using college samples. *Psychological Bulletin, 124*(1), 22–53.
Scoboria, A., Wade, K. A., Lindsay, D. S., Azad, T., Strange, D., Ost, J., & Hyman, I. E. (2017). A mega-analysis of memory reports from eight peer-reviewed false memory implantation studies. *Memory, 25*(2), 146–163.
Spanos, N. P. (1994). Multiple identity enactments and multiple personality disorder: A sociocognitive perspective. *Psychological Bulletin, 116*(1), 143–165.
State v. Clarence M. Moore. (2006). *A-38-2003.* https://law.justia.com/cases/new-jersey/supreme-court/2006/a-38-03-doc.html

The Conundrum of Measuring Authoritarianism: A Case Study in Political Bias

Thomas H. Costello

Psychological measurement is ripe with the potential for bias. Measurement entails a myriad of degrees of freedom for the researcher (i.e., disclosed and undisclosed flexibility in decision-making), both in its methodological "nuts and bolts" (e.g., item wording) and concerning broader conceptual issues (e.g., namingf factors and constructs). Consequently, beginning in the early 1900s, with the advent of intelligence testing (Binet & Simon, 1916/1973; Stern, 1914), researchers, clinicians, and the lay public alike have extensively explored and debated the prospect of systematic cultural biases in psychological assessments (Reynolds & Suzuki, 2013). These investigations typically emphasize bias attributable to identity commitments, such as race, gender, class, and sexuality. Notwithstanding the well-established degree to which such identity commitments influence and distort research practices and conclusions (e.g., Gurven, 2018), far less attention has been devoted to ideological commitments, such as political, moral, and religious beliefs, which may too be a salient source of test bias (Honeycutt & Jussim, 2020).

In the wake of psychology's replication crisis, political bias, particularly, has been highlighted as a potentially important source of non-replicable research findings (e.g., Jussim et al., 2015), perhaps because the ratio of liberals to conservatives within social and personality psychology has been estimated from 8:1 to nearly 100:1 (Haidt, 2011; Inbar & Lammers, 2012; Langbert et al., 2016; von Hippel & Buss, 2017). Such a political tilt by itself may not be worrisome if scholars can maintain a reasonably objective stance toward politically tinged scientific claims that activate their congeniality bias, a variant of confirmation bias in which individuals are especially likely to accept assertions that accord with their broader worldviews (Hart et al., 2009). Still, in a survey of 506 members of the Society for

T. H. Costello (✉)
Department of Psychology, Emory University, Atlanta, GA, USA

C. L. Cobb et al. (eds.), *Toward a Science of Clinical Psychology*,
https://doi.org/10.1007/978-3-031-14332-8_20

Personality and Social Psychology, Inbar and Lammers (2012) found that a substantial proportion of left-leaning respondents were willing to discriminate against right-leaning applicants in hiring, symposia invitations, journal reviews, and grant reviews. This finding is consistent with past research suggesting that grant proposals and Institutional Review Board submissions are sometimes rejected due to their political implications (see Ceci & Williams, 2018, for a review). Duarte et al. (2015) argued that "the peer-review process likely offers much less protection against error when the community of peers is politically homogeneous…In this way, certain assumptions, theories, and findings can become the entrenched wisdom in a field…because they have consistently undergone less critical scrutiny" (p. 8) (cf. Reinero et al., 2019). Public health scholars similarly speak of "white hat bias," the propensity to favor scientific assertions that strike researchers as morally virtuous (Cope & Allison, 2009).

In the context of measurement, bias refers to a systematic difference in the correspondence between test scores and true scores as a function of a grouping variable (e.g., age, sex, education, political ideology), such that a test demonstrates differential validity across groups (Reynolds & Suzuki, 2013). Given that many commonly used psychological instruments are designed to measure political constructs (e.g., authoritarianism, system justification motives, prejudice), widespread political bias in measurement, if present in said popular measures, has far-reaching implications for political psychology (Charney, 2015; Harper, 2020; Honeycutt & Jussim, 2020; Reyna, 2017; Stanovich & Toplak, 2019; Wright, 2019). In the present chapter, we identify several potential sources of bias in political measures and, as an illustrative case example, explore the interactions among these different sources of bias in authoritarianism research. In focusing on a single construct, we hope to illustrate how test bias can, over decades, come to shape and define entire research literatures (Reyna, 2017).

Test Bias in Political Psychology

Van de Vijver and Tanzer (2004) have proposed a useful tripartite taxonomy of test bias (i.e., construct bias, method bias, and item bias). *Construct bias* stems from heterogeneity in a construct across groups, either at the level of conceptualization or in the construct's behavioral manifestations (e.g., item responses on a personality measure may reflect conscientiousness in one culture, whereas they reflect social desirability in another culture). Construct bias as a function of political ideology (i.e., differences in a construct across the political left and right) may be important to consider, as political constructs presumably differ across the political spectrum and may not exist in a "Platonic," value-neutral form (Harper, 2020). For instance, there are both conceptual and behavioral differences in authoritarianism across the political left and right (Costello et al., 2021). As noted by Harper (2020):

> The standardization of [self-reports] with regard to item wording necessitates a particular epistemological (and perhaps ideological) position to be embedded into the measures themselves ...in using such an approach to examine the manifestation of behavior that is politically- or ideologically-salient (e.g., authoritarian-like tendencies to suppress the expression of counter-ideological viewpoints), researchers are hamstrung with regard to developing ideologically-neutral measures that are standardized for all potential respondents. That is, if such a measure is ideologically-framed (e.g., the right-wing authoritarianism scale; Altemeyer, 1981), scores on the measure suggest that 'authoritarianism' is synonymous with the right wing of the political spectrum...However, in an ideologically-neutral version of such a measure it would be the case that agreeing with some items (i.e., those framed in a liberal-consistent direction) and disagreeing with others (i.e., those framed in a conservative-consistent direction) both mean the same thing, making standardization and score interpretation difficult processes (p. 12).

Developing complementary measures of political constructs tailored to specific political contexts (e.g., administering measures of left-wing authoritarianism [LWA] to leftists and measures of right-wing authoritarianism [RWA] to conservatives) is one promising strategy for addressing construct bias in political psychology (see Costello et al., 2021). Still, developing such parallel measures is quite complicated, as merely varying political content across otherwise identical items is unlikely to mitigate construct bias.

Construct bias can also occur for measures of political ideology (Everett, 2013). In the last 100 years alone, political movements have spanned such ideologies as anarchism (i.e., rejecting all involuntary, coercive forms of hierarchy), totalitarianism, communism, sortition (i.e., selection of political officials as a random sample from a larger pool of candidates), and radical centrism (i.e., call for fundamental reforms of institutions alongside a belief that genuine solutions require pragmatism). These heterogeneous ideologies are often combined in unintuitive ways that fall outside of the left–right spectrum (e.g., anarcho-communism vs. anarcho-capitalism, religious communism). Nevertheless, a large proportion of political psychology research has emphasized cognitive and personality differences between political liberals and conservatives in the United States, perhaps artificially reifying the left–right spectrum (Malka, 2020). Measures that fail to account for the vicissitudes of political ideology are vulnerable to construct bias.

Method bias describes methodological artifacts that arise from sampling, features of a measurement instrument, and/or test administration procedures. Psychological science has increasingly grappled with the degree to which overreliance on Western, Educated, Industrialized, Rich, and Democratic (WEIRD; Henrich et al., 2010) samples has distorted our understanding of fundamental psychological processes (e.g., Gurven, 2018). There is ample reason to suspect that such inattention to meaningful cultural variability also influences the measurement of political constructs. Indeed, coherent and stable ideological orientations may only exist among the 20–30% most knowledgeable, politically engaged individuals (Kalmoe, 2020), who are generally committed to their political identities and have a sense of which political positions they "should" endorse. Focusing predominantly on these individuals may artificially attenuate or accentuate political ideology's relations with external criteria, depending on the sample type. For instance, Houck and Conway III (2019), in a meta-analysis of relations between political ideology and integrative complexity (i.e., a propensity for adopting multiple perspectives when evaluating an issue and recognizing connections across divergent perspectives; Suedfeld et al., 1992), found that, among public officials, conservatives are less complex in their thinking than are political liberals ($r = -0.37$; 95% CI [−0.47 to −0.26]); in contrast, among private citizens, the same relation did not manifest ($r = -0.01$; 95% CI [−0.07 to 0.05]). This is but one instance from a growing body of evidence to suggest that relations between political conservatism and psychological variables vary considerably across cultures and contexts (Costello et al., in press). An overrepresentation of highly WEIRD, highly politically engaged samples in the literature may overstate ideology's relations with psychological variables for the general population.

Further, concerning method bias due to instrument characteristics, meta-analytic evidence suggests that political conservatives tend to score highly on self-report measures of cognitive rigidity, yet these left-differences are greatly diminished, or occasionally reversed, for performance-based measures of rigidity (Costello et al., in press; Van Hiel et al., 2016). Failing to account for bias due to sampling or mono-method bias may, therefore, falsely result in the appearance of political left–right differences.

Finally, *item bias* occurs when individuals with the same levels of a trait are not equally likely to endorse a given item (Van de Vijver & Leung, 1997). For example, "I often visit art museums," a commonly used openness to experience item, may well be a sound indicator of openness among liberals, who tend to live in cities and, therefore, have access to many museums. Among conservatives, however, who tend to live in sparsely populated areas, this item may function relatively poorly (see also Charney, 2015). As another example of item bias due to ideological commitments, Stanovich and Toplak (2019) found that religious individuals respond differently than non-religious individuals to Actively Openminded Thinking Scale (AOT; Stanovich & West, 1997) items that include the word "belief." Individuals with strongly held religious views generally take "belief" to mean "religious beliefs," whereas non-religious individuals generally take "belief" to mean "opinion." After removing the offending items, Stanovich and Toplak (2019) found that AOT-religiosity correlations were reduced from roughly $r = -0.60$ to roughly $r = -0.20$. By the same token, several critics of the Symbolic Racism Scale have argued that many items confound value judgments about meritocracy and hard work with racism (Redding, 2001; Reyna, 2017; Sniderman & Tetlock, 1986).

Theory-Ladenness

For many psychological variables, measurement is a foundational element of theory development, and vice versa (Loevinger, 1957). To assess latent or unobservable variables, such as depression or extraversion, one usually develops indicators (i.e., items on a self-report measure) that are, in theory, caused by the unobservable variable (Michell, 1997). To use an example from physics, heat cannot be directly observed, but heat causes mercury to expand, so one can assess temperature using a mercury thermometer.

As such, early self-report measures of psychological variables are often informed by a priori theories, without which the development of indicators would be mostly arbitrary (e.g., without a preliminary theory of depression, it would be challenging to construct potential items for a depression scale). Critically, these early measures can then be used to modify the theories on which these are based (Westen & Rosenthal, 2003). If, for example, a mercury thermometer described the temperature as −10 degrees Celsius on a hot summer day, one might conclude that the law of thermal expansion is incorrect and should be modified, the thermometer is poorly constructed and should be modified, or both. To reconcile this interdependence, the development of theory and measurement of variables that cannot be directly observed often proceeds iteratively and mutually, with theory shaping measurement and measurement, in turn, shaping theory. This process is known as construct validational bootstrapping or "exploratory test construction" (Tellegen & Waller, 2008).

The interdependence of theory and measurement limits opportunities to identify biases that are simultaneously embedded in a measure and the theory underlying said measure. Consider the perils of measuring temperature with a mercury thermometer during a test of the law of thermal expansion—problematically, the theoretical hypothesis under investigation is already presupposed as part of the measurement instrument. This apparent paradox can be resolved by adopting multimethod approaches (e.g., if one has calibrated a mercury thermometer against another thermometer that does not presuppose the law of thermal expansion, using a mercury thermometer in a test of the law of thermal expansion is less problematic; Franklin et al., 1989). Still, for measures of political constructs, theory-ladenness is rarely accounted for.

For instance, scholars have long theorized that political conservatives are more prejudiced than political liberals (e.g., Adorno et al., 1950), and, indeed, an impressive body of research, dating to the 1950s, has consistently found this to be the case (Hodson & Dhont, 2015). Nevertheless, emerging evidence suggests that these conservatism–prejudice relations are a function of bias in measures of prejudice (Crawford & Brandt, 2020). Specifically, psychologists have generally assessed only prejudice toward members of disadvantaged and/or low-status groups, who tend to be politically liberal. Conservatives score highly on such prejudice measures. Yet, measures of prejudice toward groups that tend to be politically conservative (e.g., rich people, Christians, businesspeople, the military) show the opposite effect—liberals are roughly as prejudiced toward these groups as conservatives are toward groups that tend to be liberal (Brandt & Crawford, 2019; Crawford, 2017). Hence, although researchers' apparent inclination to primarily study prejudice toward disadvantaged groups is understandable, doing so may have detracted from their ability to accurately understand the psychological processes underlying prejudice writ large.

A similar example of political bias can be found in tests of the "rigidity of the right" hypothesis, the notion that a constellation of interrelated psychological attributes comprising cognitive inflexibility; dogmatism; intolerance of ambiguity; needs for closure, order, and structure; and cognitive miserliness foster right-wing political attitudes (Jost et al., 2003). To avoid criterion contamination, a fair test of this hypothesis requires measures of cognitive rigidity that are free of explicit political content and vice versa. Yet a considerable proportion of tests of the model have used proxy measures of conservatism that rest on the theoretical assumption that conservatism is heavily imbued with rigidity. In Jost et al.'s (2003) seminal meta-analysis of the rigidity of the right model, for example, 60% of the studies assessed ideology using either the Fascism (F) Scale (Adorno et al., 1950), the Right-wing Authoritarianism Scale (Altemeyer, 1996), or the Conservatism (C) Scale (Wilson & Patterson, 1968). The F Scale is intended to assess "fascist receptivity at the personality level" (e.g., "Most of our social problems would be solved if we could somehow get rid of the immoral, crooked, and feebleminded people," "A person who has bad manners, habits, and breeding can hardly expect to get along with decent people"), but, because it is strongly correlated with political conservatism (cf. Lindgren, 2012), it has been used in many studies as a stand-in for political ideology. The Right-wing Authoritarianism Scale is intended to assess unquestioned reverence for authority, aggression toward outgroup members, and strict adherence to a set of socially conservative norms (e.g., "Our country desperately needs a mighty leader who will do what has to be done to destroy the radical new ways and sinfulness that are ruining us"). And the C Scale asks participants to indicate their support for "general attitudes concerning uncertainty avoidance" (Jost et al., 2003, p. 340), artistic movements that often involve ambiguity (e.g., jazz music, modernism), and specific social-political issues that carry authoritarian or prejudicial connotations (e.g., censorship, white superiority, church authority, women judges).

Hence, many reported positive associations between political conservatism and cognitive rigidity may merely reflect the covariance of different types of rigidity-related content (see Malka et al., 2017, pp. 119–121). Indeed, Jost (2017) meta-analytically estimated the overall relations between political conservatism, on the one hand, and dogmatism and cognitive/perceptual rigidity, on the other, to be $r = 0.51$ and $r = 0.38$, respectively. In contrast, after removing criterion-contaminated measures such as the F Scale, RWA Scale, and C Scale from the study pool (i.e., leaving only relatively "pure" measures of ideology, such as policy preferences or self-identification as a liberal vs. conservative), Costello et al. (in press) reported these same relations to be $r = 0.21$ and $r = 0.10$, suggesting that the inclusion of politically biased measures had distorted conclusions about left–right asymmetries.[1]

Hidden Invalidity

A growing chorus of authors have argued that a major but largely invisible cause of psychology's replication crisis is poor validity in measurement (e.g., Hussey & Hughes, 2020; Schimmack, 2019). After testing the structural validity of 15 widely used self-report measures in nearly 145,000 experimental sessions, Hussey and Hughes (2020) found that only 1 of the 15 measures demonstrated satisfactory internal consistency, test–retest reliability, factor model fit, and measurement invariance. The authors concluded that social and personality psychology relies on numerous structurally invalid measures, theorizing that this invalidity stems from "(a) the staggering degrees of freedom available to researchers when they assess the structural validity of their measures and (b) the fact that researchers are heavily motivated to conclude that their measures are valid in order to test their core hypotheses" (p. 16). Among the 14 structurally invalid measures were the RWA Scale, the Social Dominance Orientation Scale, the Protestant Work Ethic Scale, and the Belief in a Just World Scale, all of which are widely used in political psychology and broadly reflect efforts to capture the psychology of political conservatism. Therefore, the possibility that systematic structural invalidity is present in political psychology merits consideration in the context of political bias.

Furthermore, the construct validity of many measures in psychological science is unknown, at best, and questionable, at worst (Flake et al., 2017; Schimmack, 2019). Perhaps because robust construct validational investigations are time-consuming and resource-intensive, requiring multi-method tests of convergent and discriminant validity based on detailed theoretical models (Cronbach & Meehl, 1955), quantitative claims concerning the degree of validity demonstrated by popular measures are relatively rare (Westen & Rosenthal, 2003). This rarity is quite problematic, as valid measurement is necessary for replicability and, as such, governs the confidence that we can place in research findings. If measures are invalid, noisy, and/or systematically biased, the principle of "garbage in, garbage out" suggests that open science procedures (i.e., pre-registration, open data, and registered reports) may be insufficient to combat non-replicable or false findings. Further, robust tests of construct validity are perhaps our best check on problems stemming from theory-ladenness (Franklin et al., 1989).

[1] Moreover, these estimates do not account for content related to political conservatism that is present in popular measures of cognitive rigidity. The Gough-Sanford Rigidity Scale, for instance, includes items that almost certainly reflect social conservatism, such as "I never miss going to church." Future work using non-contaminated measures will be needed to better characterize the population effect size of these associations.

Authoritarianism: A Case Study in Political Bias

Given the interdependence of measurement and theory for many or most psychological constructs, systematic measurement bias carries broad implications. Over time, measurement bias may lead to questionable theoretical conclusions that appear to rest on a solid evidentiary foundation. Indeed, as noted by Reyna (2017), "because science is inherently incremental and iterative, [political bias in measurement] can skew future research on the topic, leading to biased perspectives that can dominate our thinking, and ultimately our field, over time" (accessed online). Merely detailing bias in items, self-report instruments, and individual studies, therefore, risks missing a forest of bias for its psychometric trees. With this in mind, let us take a "big picture" view of political bias in one of the oldest and most storied constructs in political psychology. Authoritarianism has been an object of psychological research for 70 years (e.g., Adorno et al., 1950), and debate concerning political bias in authoritarianism research has existed for nearly as long. Hence, the possibility of political bias in the authoritarianism literature merits exegesis.

A Brief History of Authoritarianism Research

Authoritarianism research can be traced to 1930s Germany, when and where a cohort of psychoanalysts and social scientists strove to understand the psychological processes underlying Hitler's appeal (Adorno et al., 1950; Fromm, 1941; Reich, 1933/1976). The earliest among them was Reich (1933), who asserted that submission to powerful figures is anxiolytic, followed by Fromm (1941), who argued that surrendering one's autonomy to authority fulfills fundamental psychological needs, especially a "simultaneous love for authority and hatred against those who are powerless" (p. 72).

It was not until Adorno et al.'s (1950) *The Authoritarian Personality* (TAP), however, that authoritarianism emerged as a central construct in political psychology. In the wake of World War II, TAP popularized the notion that susceptibility to totalitarianism and political conservatism is rooted in personality, positing that the principal attributes of authoritarianism are obsequiousness to authority figures and dominance toward subordinates, a superficially paradoxical pair of traits amounting to strict adherence to hierarchy. Seven additional traits were also alleged to accompany authoritarianism, including adherence to in-group norms, superstitiousness and fatalism, rigid thinking, exaggerated concern with toughness and power, and cynicism, as well as psychoanalytically oriented traits such as anti-intraception (i.e., a dislike of subjectivity, imaginativeness, tender-mindedness), projectivity, and sexual repression. To identify authoritarian individuals, Adorno et al. (1950) constructed the Fascism (F) Scale, a self-report measure of authoritarianism. Arguably the first scientific measure to bridge political behavior and psychology, the F Scale galvanized social science, serving as a point of genesis for an untold number of influential research findings.

F Scale scores manifested large correlations with what Adorno et al. termed "pseudo-conservative" ideology (i.e., aiming to abolish traditional American values and institutions while claiming to uphold and defend them). As Adorno et al. had predicted, authoritarianism seemed to be specific to the political right. Yet many authors soon objected to this claim of political specificity, in part because many real-world authoritarian regimes are left-wing. As noted by McClosky and Chong (1985):

> [T]he findings derived from the available research studies, and especially those using the F-Scale, do not correspond to what is obvious from even the most casual observation of actual political regimes of the far left and far right. No particular expertise is required to discern the striking similarities in political style, organization, and practice among, on the one side, such left-wing dictatorships as the Soviet Union, Communist China, East Germany, Cambodia under Pol Pot, Cuba under Castro, Albania, Bulgaria, Ethiopia and Angola; and on the other side, such right-wing dictatorships as Fascist Italy, Spain under Franco, Nazi Germany, Portugal under Salazar, Argentina (especially from 1976 to 1983), Uruguay, Zaire and Chile under Pinochet. One can cite, in addition, a number of highly repressive dictatorships in which left-wing and right-wing elements (or at least left-wing and right-wing rhetoric) are so heavily intermingled that even experts might find it difficult to decide whether to place them on the left or the right. Possible examples include Ghana, Libya under Khadaffi, Syria, Iraq and Iran under Khomeini. (p. 331)

Fromm (1950) similarly criticized Adorno et al. (1950) for ignoring authoritarians in the Soviet Union, "[who] will find a thousand and one reasons why Russian nationalism is not nationalism, why authoritarianism is democracy, why slave labor is designed to educate and improve anti-social elements…arguments used to explain racial or sexual prejudices are illustrations of the same rationalizing capacity" (p. 56). Shils (1954) raised a similar criticism, proposing that a companion to the F Scale be constructed, the R Scale ("R" being short for "Red"), to assess authoritarianism on the left. Eysenck (1954) sought to empirically establish value-neutral authoritarianism, which he conceptualized and measured as *tough-mindedness* (i.e., an attitudinal manifestation of extraversion comprising practicality, lack of sentimentality, and intractability). Rokeach (1960) also rejected the notion that authoritarianism is specific to political conservatives, conceptualizing the authoritarian personality as an identifiable species of general cognitive rigidity that lists toward absolutism in the face of ideological threat, which he termed *dogmatism*. Ray (1983), too, defined authoritarianism value-neutrally as *directivity* (i.e., the tendency to seek power and control others via socially sanctioned power). Despite these many attempts to understand authoritarianism in a value-neutral manner, none are used in contemporary political psychology. Critics dismissed tough-mindedness, dogmatism, and directivity as distinct from authoritarianism (Christie, 1991; Stone, 1980; Stone & Smith, 1993) and/or methodologically problematic (e.g., Billig, 1985; Duckitt, 1983; Sidanius, 1988; Stone, 1983; Ward, 1988).

Of course, TAP's methodology and conceptual minutiae are also considered largely obsolete. Indeed, the nine facets of authoritarianism outlined in TAP, and measured by the F Scale, were developed in an armchair fashion on the basis of

Freudian psychoanalysis, anti-positivism, and Marxist theory, and there is little evidence to suggest they offer a comprehensive or accurate description of authoritarianism writ large. Further, the F Scale is deeply psychometrically unsound and has been roundly criticized in the research literature, leading TAP to be called by one author "the most deeply flawed work of prominence in political psychology" (Martin, 2001, p. 1). Lindgren (2012) goes so far as to note that:

> Given that the F-Scale was designed to identify "pre-fascist" people (the "F" stands for "Fascism") and Altemeyer describes his RWA Scale as having a "Hitler end" (Altemeyer, 1996), one would expect the authoritarianism scales to include more items that would appeal to mid-twentieth century Nazis and fascists and fewer items that would probably be opposed by fascists. Adorno et al. (1950) did not include many of the primary aspects of fascism's appeal to non-Jewish, non-immigrant Germans, such as German fascism's collectivism, price controls, guaranteeing of jobs, environmentalism, supplanting of religion, appeal to youth, love of danger and struggle, hostility to the status quo, destruction of the traditional social class system (and its planned replacement with a new class structure based on race and performance), hostility to the traditional family, and so on. Other conservative beliefs that Nazis opposed, such as religion, are often coded as fascist in authoritarianism scales, particularly Altemeyer's…At its best, then, the Adorno F-Scale is an extraordinarily biased scale of Nazi-like tendencies. More realistically, some of the items in the F-Scale should be reverse coded (pp. 6–12).

Nevertheless, for all of its flaws, Adorno et al.'s descriptive account of authoritarianism remains largely intact in modern iterations of the construct. Nearly 70 years after TAP's publication, Adorno et al.'s claims that (a) the principal attribute of authoritarianism is strict adherence to hierarchy and (b) authoritarianism is exclusive to political conservatives have arguably become canonical (see Honeycutt & Jussim, 2020) elements of political psychology. Indeed, RWA's three constituent higher-order dimensions were directly adapted from TAP. In contrast, once robust debates concerning the possibility of LWA were effectively abandoned until quite recently.[2] This radical asymmetry across LWA and RWA, despite the empirical basis of both constructs being roughly equivalent in their unsoundness, may be a manifestation of repeated instances of political bias. Such bias has seemingly occurred not only at the level of measurement, but also in Adorno et al.'s original theory and methodology, and in the differing standards of rigor applied to papers championing right-wing vs. value-neutral and/or left-wing authoritarianism (see Jussim, 2019).

[2] Altemeyer (1996) also created the first published measure of LWA. He concluded that LWA is effectively non-existent after finding that subjects rarely scored above his scale's mid-point. Still, there is little reason to consider the scale's mid-point meaningful: Individuals who are high on a latent LWA construct would score well below the mid-point on a scale marked by levels of extreme item difficulty. Indeed, the LWA Scale contains numerous items such as "The conservative, right-wing Establishment will never give up its power peacefully, so a revolutionary movement is justified in using violence to crush it" (Altemeyer, 1996, p. 225), whereas even the most severe items on the RWA Scale are far less extreme in comparison (e.g., "There are many radical, immoral people in our country today, who are trying to ruin it for their own godless purposes, whom the authorities should put out of action)." Moreover, in constructing his LWA Scale, Altemeyer used only direct parallels of the three RWA dimensions. There is little reason to believe that RWA provides a sufficient account of authoritarianism writ large and, therefore, that LWA runs precisely parallel to RWA.

Identifying Political Bias in Authoritarianism Measures

Although anecdotal evidence cannot support a hypothesis, it may be sufficient to falsify a null hypothesis: if LWA exists, then authoritarianism is not entirely exclusive to the political right. Moreover, considering the numerous atrocities committed in the name of left-wing authoritarian regimes (e.g., the USSR, China, Cambodia, North Korea), certain anecdotes may carry more weight than others: if the prospect of LWA is unduly dismissed, we risk losing an opportunity to better understand the psychological antecedents of authoritarianism and political violence. It is with this in mind that I will add one further anecdote to the pile. Friedrich Engels, who, alongside Karl Marx, developed what is now known as Marxist theory, explicitly championed authoritarianism:

> …the anti-authoritarians demand that the political state be abolished at one stroke, even before the social conditions that gave birth to it have been destroyed. They demand that the first act of the social revolution shall be the abolition of authority. Have these gentlemen ever seen a revolution? A revolution is certainly the most authoritarian thing there is; it is the act whereby one part of the population imposes its will upon the other part by means of rifles, bayonets and cannon — authoritarian means, if such there be at all; and if the victorious party does not want to have fought in vain, it must maintain this rule by means of the terror which its arms inspire in the reactionists. Would the Paris Commune have lasted a single day if it had not made use of this authority of the armed people against the bourgeois? Should we not, on the contrary, reproach it for not having used it freely enough? (as quoted in Tucker, 1978, p. 733).

On an empirical front, Costello et al. (2021) recently explored and described left-wing authoritarianism's nature and structure in six samples. We sought to address questions concerning LWA's constituent features and how these features are organized by systematically deriving a new conceptualization of LWA. Beginning with a broad preliminary conceptualization of LWA, we used exploratory and empirical strategies of test construction to iteratively construct a measure of LWA with good content validity; refine our conceptualization based on the measure's structural and nomological validity; and update the measure to reflect these changes, repeating this process three times. We then evaluated LWA's relations with over 50 criterion variables, finding that the LWA Index manifested a highly similar pattern of relations to both right-wing authoritarianism's and social dominance orientation's pattern of relations with those same variables.

To reconcile these data with LWA's reputation as "the Loch Ness Monster [of political psychology]: an occasional shadow, but no monster" (Altemeyer, 1996, p. 216), let us first consider the outsized influence of Adorno et al.'s conceptualization of authoritarianism. By most standard definitions, political conservatism involves upholding the status quo and protecting the present hierarchy (Jost et al. 2013). Accordingly, Adorno et al.'s conceptualization of authoritarianism is fundamentally tied to and imbued with conservatism. Indeed, individuals who are disposed to (a) favor absolutist forms of government and (b) weaponize the *presently dominant* hierarchy to facilitate said absolutism (i.e., individuals who, per Adorno et al., are authoritarians), are necessarily also political conservatives. In contrast, individuals who are psychologically disposed to favor absolutist forms of government, but who believe that the dominant hierarchy should be overthrown (i.e., what might be considered left-wing authoritarians), do not fall within the scope of Adorno et al.'s conceptualization. Thus, from the outset, the construct of authoritarianism conflated conservatism and authoritarianism. Even critics of LWA have readily acknowledged such theory-ladenness. Stone (1980), who argued vehemently against the significance of LWA, wrote that "Almost by definition, [TAP] treated authoritarianism as a right-wing phenomenon. Had the F Scale not correlated with conservatism, something would have been wrong with its conceptualization" (p. 7). In other words, the F Scale (and RWA Scale) systematically differs in its validity across the political left and right and, as such, is an example of political bias.

In recent years, there have been several psychometrically sophisticated attempts to construct value-neutral measures of authoritarianism (e.g., Duckitt et al., 2010; Dunwoody & Funke, 2016) by eliminating item bias from the RWA Scale (e.g., references to religion, conservative norms). Yet given that conservatism is "baked in" to the RWA Scale's conceptualization of authoritarianism, offsetting item bias, alone, is not enough to mitigate political bias in authoritarianism measures. Indeed, parsing the RWA Scale's authoritarian wheat from its conservatism chaff may be nigh-impossible without alternative conceptualizations of authoritarianism if we assume, for the sake of illustration, that authoritarians on both the right and left are dogmatic, adherent to in-group norms, disposed toward social uniformity, aggressive and prejudiced against different others, and intolerant of opposing views, but that only authoritarians on the right are subservient to the *current* hierarchy.

Construct bias notwithstanding, hidden invalidity has also contributed to the paucity of research able to falsify the notion that authoritarianism is exclusive primarily to the political right. Rigorous tests of RWA's and LWA's relative merits presumably require measures of authoritarianism that do not presuppose core elements of Adorno et al.'s conceptualization. Further, fascistic and anti-democratic behaviors are, for the most part, rare among members of the general population in liberal democracies, limiting the feasibility of adopting a multi-method approach (e.g., comparing RWA's and LWA's ability to predict authoritarian behaviors). Indeed, to account for the lack of fascist behavior in the United States, the F Scale was designed to reflect "pre-fascist" traits (i.e., one's liability to support totalitarian regimes under the right conditions), which are sufficiently imprecisely defined as to border on unfalsifiable. Without stringent tests of construct validity that are independent of the theory on which a measure is based, seemingly robust, decades-old bodies of literature may be considerably less informative than they appear.

Moreover, construct validational examinations of the F Scale and RWA Scale have often used criterion-related measures that are imbued with conservatism content, such as measures of ethnocentrism, prejudice, threat sensitivity, and dogmatism (Costello et al., in press). Scholars have sometimes interpreted this shared conservatism variance to be evidence that authoritarianism is particular to the political right (e.g., Jost et al., 2003), but an alternative explanation is that these measures are biased in the same direction. The RWA Scale is also often used as a criterion-related variable in tests of newer measures' construct validity, potentially further perpetuating political bias (i.e., politically biased measures will presumably manifest larger relations with the RWA Scale than non-biased measures; consequently, biased measures will evince better construct validity than non-biased measures). In this manner, it is plausible that a vicious cycle of sorts has occurred, whereby political bias has been gradually woven into the nomological networks of political constructs. Robust tests of construct validity would serve to mitigate this sort of bias, but, as described previously, such tests are relatively rare.

Hence, from its very origins, the authoritarianism literature has suffered from pervasive political bias at the level of both theory and measurement and practice.

Recommendations to Reduce Political Bias in Measurement

Scientific procedures are useful largely for their ability to guard against confirmation bias, the natural human tendency to seek out evidence that supports one's prior beliefs and minimize evidence that runs counter to them (Hart et al., 2009; Nickerson, 1998; see also Lilienfeld et al., 2009). Scientists, being human, are not immune to bias. Evaluating our research and measurement tools with this spirit in mind may be the foremost means of mitigating measurement bias. Indeed, it is likely that political values and assumptions are embedded in many constructs not mentioned in the present chapter (Duarte et al., 2015), and we encourage researchers to carefully evaluate political measures before using them for research purposes.

More specifically, at the measure development stage, researchers should consider employing *political decentering*, a modification of *cultural decentering* (Werner & Campbell, 1970) whereby a measurement instrument is developed simultaneously by several researchers with different political perspectives, and only the common elements across the different versions are retained. At the analysis stage, researchers should conduct tests of measurement invariance across the political left and right. It may also be useful to examine whether respondents with different political ideologies respond anomalously to certain items. Differential item functioning analysis is used to investigate anomalous responding across cultures and could be easily adapted for political ideology (Zumbo, 1999). Finally, rigorous, structured, multi-method tests of construct validity, using phenotypically diverse criterion-related outcomes, may be one potent measure of countering test bias. To that end, Westen and Rosenthal's (2003) metrics for quantifying construct validity provide effect size estimates and significance tests of the degree to which an observed pattern of correlations between a measure of interest and relevant external criteria accords with a predicted pattern of correlations (see Furr & Heuckeroth, 2019, for implementation of these metrics in *R*).

We encourage future researchers to adopt these and other practices when developing and evaluating measures of political constructs. Above all, as scientists, there are few better safeguards against bias than diligently attempting to disprove our own hypotheses. So long as we have not "kicked the tires" of the measures we use, there is little reason to be confident that our research findings, be they favorable to our hypotheses or not, are anything other than interesting noise.

References

Adorno, T. W., Frenkel-Brunswik, E., Levinson, D. J., & Sanford, R. N. (1950). *The authoritarian personality*. Harper.

Altemeyer, B. (1981). *Right wing authoritarianism*. University of Manitoba Press.

Altemeyer, B. (1996). *The authoritarian specter*. Harvard University Press.

Billig, O. (1985). The lawyer terrorist and his comrades. *Political Psychology, 6*, 29–46.

Binet, A., & Simon, T. (1973). *The development of intelligence in children*. Arno. (Original work published 1916).

Brandt, M. J., & Crawford, J. T. (2019). Studying a heterogeneous array of target groups can help us understand prejudice. *Current Directions in Psychological Science, 28*, 292–298.

Ceci, S. J., & Williams, W. M. (2018). Socio-political values infiltrate the assessment of scientific research. In L. Jussim & J. Crawford (Eds.), *The politics of social psychology* (pp. 156–167). Routledge.

Charney, E. (2015). Liberal bias and the five-factor model. *Behavioral and Brain Sciences, 38*, e139.

Christie, R. (1991). Authoritarianism and related constructs. In J. P. Robinson & P. R. Shaver (Eds.), *Measures of personality and social psychological attitudes* (pp. 501–571). Academic Press.

Cope, M. B., & Allison, D. B. (2009). White hat bias: Examples of its presence in obesity research and a call for renewed commitment to faithfulness in research reporting. *International Journal of Obesity, 34*, 84–88.

Costello, T. H., Bowes, S. M., Stevens, S. T., Waldman, I. W., Tasimi, A., & Lilienfeld, S. O. (2021). Clarifying the structure and nature of left-wing authoritarianism. *Journal of Personality and Social Psychology, 122*, 135–170. https://doi.org/10.1037/pspp0000341

Costello, T. H., Bowes, S. M., Malka, A., Baldwin, M., Tasimi, A. (in press). Revisiting the rigidity-of-the-right hypothesis: A meta-analytic review. Journal of Personality and Social Psychology. *Advance online publication*. https://doi.org/10.1037/pspp0000446

Crawford, J. T. (2017). The politics of the psychology of prejudice. In *Politics of social psychology* (pp. 109–125). Psychology Press.

Crawford, J. T., & Brandt, M. J. (2020). Ideological (a) symmetries in prejudice and intergroup bias. *Current Opinion in Behavioral Sciences, 34*, 40–45.

Cronbach, L. J., & Meehl, P. E. (1955). Construct validity in psychological tests. *Psychological Bulletin, 52*, 281–302.

Conway III, L. G., Houck, S. C., Gornick, L. J., & Repke, M. A. (2018). Finding the Loch Ness monster: Leftwing authoritarianism in the United States. *Political Psychology, 39*(5), 1049–1067.

Duckitt, J. H. (1983). Directiveness and authoritarianism: Some research findings and a critical reappraisal. *South Africa Journal of Psychology, 13*, 10–12.

Duckitt, J., Bizumic, B., Krauss, S. W., & Heled, E. (2010). A tripartite approach to right-wing authoritarianism: The authoritarianism-conservatism-traditionalism model. *Political Psychology, 31*, 685–715.

Dunwoody, P. T., & Funke, F. (2016). The aggression-submission-conventionalism scale: Testing a new three factor measure of authoritarianism. *Journal of Social and Political Psychology, 4*, 571–600.

Duarte, J. L., Crawford, J. T., Stern, C., Haidt, J., Jussim, L., & Tetlock, P. E. (2015). Political diversity will improve social psychological science 1. *Behavioral and Brain Sciences, 38*.

Eysenck, H. J. (1954). The science of personality: Nomothetic. *Psychological Review, 61*(5), 339–342.

Everett, J. A. (2013). The 12 item social and economic conservatism scale (SECS). *PloS one, 8*(12), e82131.

Feynman, R. P. (1985). *Surely you're joking, Mr. Feynman: Adventures of a curious character*. Norton.

Flake, J. K., Pek, J., & Hehman, E. (2017). Construct validation in social and personality research: Current practice and recommendations. *Social Psychological and Personality Science, 8*, 370–378.

Franklin, A., Anderson, M., Brock, D., Coleman, S., Downing, J., Gruvander, A., et al. (1989). Can a theory-laden observation test the theory? *The British Journal for the Philosophy of Science, 40*, 229–231.

Fromm, E. (1941). *Escape from freedom*. Holt, Rinehart, & Winston.

Fromm, E. (1950). *Psychoanalysis and religion*. Yale University Press.

Furr, R. M., & Heuckeroth, S. (2019). The "quantifying construct validity" procedure: Its role, value, interpretations, and computation. *Assessment, 26*, 555–566.

Gurven, M. D. (2018). Broadening horizons: Sample diversity and socioecological theory are essential to the future of psychological science. *Proceedings of the National Academy of Sciences, 115*, 11420–11427.

Haidt, J. (2011, January). The bright future of post-partisan social psychology. In *Talk given at the annual meeting of the Society for Personality and Social Psychology*, San Antonio.

Harper, C. A. (2020, March 19). *Ideological measurement in social and personality psychological science*. https://doi.org/10.31234/osf.io/wpsje.

Hart, W., Albarracín, D., Eagly, A. H., Brechan, I., Lindberg, M. J., & Merrill, L. (2009). Feeling validated versus being correct: A meta-analysis of selective exposure to information. *Psychological Bulletin, 135*, 555–588.

Henrich, J., Heine, S. J., & Norenzayan, A. (2010). Most people are not WEIRD. *Nature, 466*, 29.

Hodson, G., & Dhont, K. (2015). The person-based nature of prejudice: Individual difference predictors of intergroup negativity. *European Review of Social Psychology, 26*, 1–42.

Honeycutt, N., & Jussim, L. (2020). A model of political bias in social science research. *Psychological Inquiry, 31*, 73–85.

Houck, S. C., & Conway, L. G., III. (2019). Strategic communication and the integrative complexity-ideology relationship: Meta-analytic findings reveal differences between public politicians and private citizens in their use of simple rhetoric. *Political Psychology, 40*, 1119–1141.

Hussey, I., & Hughes, S. (2020). Hidden invalidity among 15 commonly used measures in social and personality psychology. *Advances in Methods and Practices in Psychological Science, 3*, 166–184.

Inbar, Y., & Lammers, J. (2012). Political diversity in social and personality psychology. *Perspectives on Psychological Science, 7*, 496–503.

Jost, J. T. (2017). Ideological asymmetries and the essence of political psychology. *Political Psychology, 38*, 167–208.

Jost, J. T., Glaser, J., Kruglanski, A. W., & Sulloway, F. J. (2003). Political conservatism as motivated social cognition. *Psychological Bulletin, 129*(3), 339–375.

Jost, J. T., Federico, C. M., & Napier, J. L. (2013). Political ideologies and their social psychological functions. In *The Oxford handbook of political ideologies* (pp. 232–250)

Jussim, L. (2019, August 7). *Confirmation bias: Real bias or delegitimization rhetoric?* [Blog post]. Retrieved from https://www.psychologytoday.com/us/blog/rabble-rouser/201908/confirmation-bias-real-bias-or-delegitimization-rhetoric

Jussim, L., Crawford, J. T., Anglin, S., & Stevens, S. (2015). Ideological bias in social psychological research. In J. Forgas, K. Fiedler, & W. Crano (Eds.), *Sydney symposium on social psychology and politics* (pp. 91–109). New York, NY: Taylor & Francis.

Kalmoe, N. P. (2020). Uses and abuses of ideology in political psychology. *Political Psychology, 41*, 771–793.

Langbert, M., Quain, A. J., & Klein, D. B. (2016). Faculty voter registration in economics, history, journalism, law, and psychology. *Econ Journal Watch, 13*, 422–451.

Lilienfeld, S. O., Ammirati, R., & Landfield, K. (2009). Giving debiasing away: Can psychological research on correcting cognitive errors promote human welfare? *Perspectives on Psychological Science, 4*, 390–398.

Lindgren, J. T. (2012). *The centrist authoritarian. Available at SSRN*. https://ssrn.com/abstract=2029435 or https://doi.org/10.2139/ssrn.2029435
Loevinger, J. (1957). Objective tests as instruments of psychological theory. *Psychological Reports, 3*, 635–694.
Malka, A. (2020). A closer look at the ideological structuring of political attitudes. In E. Boreida, C. M. Federico, & J. M. Miller (Eds.), *At the forefront of political psychology: Essays in honor of John L.* Routledge.
Malka, A., Lelkes, Y., & Holzer, N. (2017). Rethinking the rigidity of the right model: Three suboptimal methodological practices and their implications. In *Politics of Social Psychology* (pp. 126–146). Psychology Press.
Martin, J. L. (2001). The authoritarian personality, 50 years later: What questions are there for political psychology? *Political Psychology, 22*, 1–26.
McClosky, H., & Chong, D. (1985). Similarities and differences between left-wing and right-wing radicals. *British Journal of Political Science, 15*(3), 329–363.
Michell, J. (1997). Quantitative science and the definition of measurement in psychology. *British Journal of Psychology, 88*, 355–383.
Nickerson, R. S. (1998). Confirmation bias: A ubiquitous phenomenon in many guises. *Review of General Psychology, 2*(2), 175–220.
Nilsson, A., & Jost, J. T. (2020). The authoritarian-conservatism nexus. *Current Opinion in Behavioral Sciences, 34*, 148–154.
Ray, J. J. (1983). Half of all authoritarians are left wing: A reply to Eysenck and Stone. *Political Psychology, 4*, 139–143.
Redding, R. E. (2001). Sociopolitical diversity in psychology: The case for pluralism. *American Psychologist, 56*, 205.
Reich, W. (1933). *The mass psychology of fascism*. Orgone Institute Press.
Reinero, D. A., Wills, J. A., Brady, W. J., Mende-Siedlecki, P., Crawford, J., & Van Bavel, J. J. (2019, February 7). *Is the political slant of psychology research related to scientific replicability?* https://doi.org/10.31234/osf.io/6k3j5
Reyna, C. (2017). Scale creation, use, and misuse: How politics undermines measurement. In *Politics of social psychology* (pp. 91–108). Psychology Press.
Reynolds, C. R., & Suzuki, L. (2013). Bias in psychological assessment: An empirical review and recommendations. In *Handbook of psychology, volume 10: Assessment psychology* (pp. 82–113). Wiley.
Rokeach, M. (1960). *The open and closed mind: Investigations into the nature of belief systems and personality systems*. Basic Books.
Schimmack, U. (2019, February 19). *The validation crisis in psychology*. https://doi.org/10.31234/osf.io/q247m
Shils, E. (1954). *Authoritarianism "right" and "left"*. Free Press.
Sidanius, J. (1988). Intolerance of ambiguity, conservatism, and racism: Whose fantasy, whose reality?: A reply to Ray. *Political Psychology, 9*, 309–316.
Skinner, B. F. (1953). *Science and human behavior*. Simon and Schuster.
Sniderman, P. M., & Tetlock, P. E. (1986). Symbolic racism: Problems of motive attribution in political analysis. *Journal of Social Issues, 42*, 129–150.
Stanovich, K. E., & Toplak, M. E. (2019). The need for intellectual diversity in psychological science: Our own studies of actively open-minded thinking as a case study. *Cognition, 187*, 156–166.
Stanovich, K. E., & West, R. F. (1997). Reasoning independently of prior belief and individual differences in actively open-minded thinking. *Journal of Educational Psychology, 89*, 342.
Stern, W. (1914). *The psychological methods of testing intelligence*. Warwick & York.
Stone, W. F. (1980). The myth of left-wing authoritarianism. *Political Psychology, 2*, 3–19.
Stone, W. F. (1983). Left and right in personality and ideology: An attempt at clarification. *The Journal of Mind and Behavior, 4*, 211–220.

Stone, W. F., & Smith, L. D. (1993). Authoritarianism: Left and right. In Strength and weakness (pp. 144–156). Springer, New York, NY.

Suedfeld, P., Tetlock, P. E., & Streufert, S. (1992). Conceptual/integrative complexity. In C. Smith (Ed.), *Motivation and personality: Handbook of thematic content analysis* (pp. 401–418). Cambridge University Press.

Tellegen, A., & Waller, N. G. (2008). Exploring personality through test construction: Development of the multidimensional personality questionnaire. In G. J. Boyle, G. Mathews, & D. H. Saklofske (Eds.), *Handbook of personality theory and testing: Vol II. Personality measurement and testing*. Sage.

Tucker, R. C. (1978). *The Marx-Engels reader*. W.W. Norton.

Van de Vijver, F., & Tanzer, N. K. (2004). Bias and equivalence in cross-cultural assessment: An overview. *European Review of Applied Psychology, 54*, 119–135.

Van de Vijver, F., & Leung, K. (1997). Methods and data analysis of comparative research. *Handbook of Crosscultural Psychology, 1*, 257–300.

Van Hiel, A., Onraet, E., Crowson, H. M., & Roets, A. (2016). The relationship between right-wing attitudes and cognitive style: A comparison of self-report and behavioural measures of rigidity and intolerance of ambiguity. *European Journal of Personality, 30*, 523–531.

Von Hippel, W., & Buss, D. M. (2017). *Do ideologically driven scientific agendas impede the understanding and acceptance of evolutionary principles in social psychology? Politics of social psychology* (pp. 17–35). Psychology Press.

Ward, D. (1988). A critic's defense of the criticized. *Political Psychology, 9*, 317–320.

Wilson, G. D., & Patterson, J. R. (1968). A new measure of conservatism. *British Journal of Social and Clinical Psychology, 7*(4), 264–269.

Werner, O., & Campbell, D. T. (1970). Translating, working through interpreters, and the problem of decentering. In *A handbook of method in cultural anthropology*. American Museum of Natural History.

Westen, D., & Rosenthal, R. (2003). Quantifying construct validity: Two simple measures. *Journal of Personality and Social Psychology, 84*, 608–618.

Wright, J. D. (2019, June 23*). Ideological bias in expert personality assessment of political figures: A commentary*. https://doi.org/10.31234/osf.io/8mn6w

Zumbo, B. D. (1999). *A handbook on the theory and methods of differential item functioning (DIF)*. National Defense Headquarters.

Experiences of Lifelong Learners in Clinical Psychology

Jason J. Washburn, Bethany A. Teachman, Gerald C. Davison, Brandon A. Gaudiano, Steve D. Hollon, J. Kim Penberthy, and Tara S. Peris

A Brief History of Lifelong Learning

The famous fantasy author, J. R. R. Tolkien, wrote that "[t]rue education is a kind of never ending story." Learning across the lifespan, particularly outside of formal education and training, acknowledges that knowledge, skills, and attitudes are in a constant state of change (London, 2012). Although the intentional pursuit of lifelong learning can likely be traced back to the start of recorded history, formal lifelong learning opportunities within professions and the sciences in wealthy, industrialized societies can be traced back to at least the 1800s (Shannon, 2015).

J. J. Washburn (✉)
Department of Psychiatry & Behavioral Sciences, Northwestern University, Chicago, IL, USA
e-mail: j-washburn@northwestern.edu

B. A. Teachman
Department of Psychology, University of Virginia, Charlottesville, VA, USA

G. C. Davison
Department of Psychology, University of Southern California, Los Angeles, CA, USA

B. A. Gaudiano
Department of Psychiatry & Human Behavior, Warren Alpert Medical School of Brown University, Providence, RI, USA

S. D. Hollon
Department of Psychology, Vanderbilt University, Nashville, TN, USA

J. K. Penberthy
Psychiatry and Neurobehavioral Sciences, University of Virginia School of Medicine, Charlottesville, VA, USA

T. S. Peris
Semel Institute for Neuroscience & Human Behavior, University of California Los Angeles, Los Angeles, CA, USA

C. L. Cobb et al. (eds.), *Toward a Science of Clinical Psychology*,
https://doi.org/10.1007/978-3-031-14332-8_21

Some have argued that Benjamin Franklin assembled the first formal lifelong learning club in the United States with the forming of the Junto in 1727 (Cartwright, 1945). The Junto, otherwise known as the Leather Apron Club, was a "club of mutual improvement" that required that "every member, in his turn, should produce one or more queries on any point of Morals, Politics, or Natural Philosophy" (Franklin, 1771, p. 72). Other systems followed the Junto in the United States, such as the Chautauqua and Lyceum movements, which offered opportunities for adults to hear debates and lectures. The Cooperative Extension System, which helped farmers and ranchers to adapt to changes and learn new technologies, and University Extensions, which offered lectures, correspondence work, special institutes, and short or "refresher" courses, were some of the first systems specifically aimed at changing the knowledge, skills, and attitudes of the workforce (Cartwright, 1945).

Lifelong learning in health service professions began at least 100 years ago in the United States. As early as 1906, the American Medical Association encouraged county medical societies to provide weekly educational programs (Manning & DeBakey, 2011). With the transformation of medical education in the United States from for-profit, proprietary trade schools to universities that embraced science and the biomedical model within medical education (Duffy, 2011; Flexner, 1910), the need for lifelong learning in medicine became even clearer. By the mid-nineteenth century, an organized approach to continuing medical education was introduced, acknowledging the need for physicians to keep pace with a quickly evolving science and the increasing complexity of medical practice (Murphy, 1951). As Franklin Murphy noted in the mid-1900s, "[t]he four formal years in medical school must be regarded as only the first four years of a 'forty-year medical educational experience'" (Murphy, 1951, p. 89).

In writing about lifelong training specifically within psychotherapy, Carol Whitaker (1960) famously stated as a "fact that training must continue or we die" (p. 151). Within psychology more broadly, lifelong learning is intended to build upon graduate education and training through engagement in formal learning opportunities that:

> (1) are relevant to psychological practice, education and science; (2) enable psychologists to keep pace with the most current scientific evidence regarding assessment, intervention, and education as well as important legal, statutory, or regulatory issues; and (3) allow psychologists to maintain, develop, and increase competencies in order to improve services to the public and enhance contributions to the profession (American Psychological Association [APA], 2015, p. 2).

As a discipline and profession that is based in science, lifelong learning sits firmly at the foundation of psychology.

Multiple Perspectives of Lifelong Learners

Lifelong learning is critical to both psychological science and the practice of health service psychology. The authors of this chapter worked closely with Dr. Scott Lilienfeld as part of a working group examining the *Issues in Professional Psychology Education*, which was sponsored by a collaboration of the Society for the Science of Clinical Psychology, the Society of Clinical Psychology, and the Society of Clinical Child and Adolescent Psychology. Dr. Lilienfeld hosted the meeting at Emory University in September 2017 and September 2018, and he proved to be the backbone for the group. Indeed, Dr. Lilienfeld's life work is an embodiment of the spirit of lifelong learning. He approached every endeavor with a remarkably creative and questioning mind. As a quintessential lifelong learner, Dr. Lilienfeld was skeptical of everything. With an open yet critical mind, Dr. Lilienfeld was always questioning the field of psychology and science. He evaluated and critiqued the extant literature, questioning theories and beliefs, and pushed us all to constantly do better.

In honor of his legacy, we lay bare in this chapter some of our own challenges in lifelong learning to highlight both the barriers and opportunities that can follow from viewing the receipt of the doctorate as only the start of the learning that makes the field of psychological science so dynamic and vibrant. The remainder of the chapter presents our experiences (the authors, all PhD-level clinical psychologists) as lifelong learners. These experiences include someone involved in helping to regulate lifelong learning for licensed clinical psychologists, a clinical researcher who has been humbled by the lives of the people he's researched, a clinical supervisor who has learned how to supervise over the length of her career, a clinical researcher juggling the limits of her statistical prowess, a clinician who has come to see the similarities in different theoretical orientations, a psychopathologist experiencing a radical change in their approach to conducting research, and an educator learning cultural humility.

The Experience of a Regulator of Lifelong Learning (J. Kim Penberthy)

Lifelong learning is built into the APA's *Ethical Principles of Psychologists and Code of Conduct*. Significantly, Standard 2.03 maintains that "psychologists undertake ongoing efforts to develop and maintain their competence." Not only are psychologists required to maintain competence, but Standard 2.04 stipulates that this learning must be "based upon established scientific and professional knowledge of the discipline" (APA, 2017, p.5). In addition to being an ethical imperative, lifelong learning is a regulatory imperative. Like many healthcare providers, clinical psychologists who are licensed to practice in the United States are also currently required to participate in lifelong learning in order to maintain licensure. Given that the purpose of licensing is to protect the public and the profession (Britt, 1939), regulating lifelong learning in the form of required continuing education (CE) serves to extend such protection beyond initial licensure. Regulation of lifelong learning in clinical psychology began in the 1950s when some states started to require CE credits for licensure renewals. The expansion of regulatory requirements for lifelong learning in health service psychology was slow; indeed, the field seemed reluctant to mandate lifelong learning (Buttars et al., 2021). In the 1970s, however, an increasing number of states began to mandate lifelong learning for license renewal. Eventually all states in the United States had such a mandate, with the final holdout, New York State, requiring lifelong learning starting in 2021 (Buttars et al., 2021).

While making lifelong learning obligatory for clinical psychologists in the form of required CE may be a reasonable plan, it also has some challenges. Although clinical psychologists may be driven to engage in lifelong learning to maintain their competence (VandeCreek et al., 1990), current evidence suggests that psychologists are more likely to engage in formal lifelong learning only when mandated to do so through regulatory requirements (Neimeyer et al., 2010; Neimeyer et al., 2009; Neimeyer et al., 2019). Moreover, research demonstrates that psychologists tend to pursue continuing education in a narrow content area, typically one that is already familiar to them (Taylor, et al., 2019). This author has been guilty of such. I focus much of my clinical work on assessing and treating persistent depressive disorders and often find myself drawn to CE in this specific area. This content area is in my "comfort zone," and I feel knowledgeable and competent in the assessment and therapeutic approaches. In limiting myself to CE in these familiar areas only, however, I miss learning opportunities in other areas, and gaps in my knowledge may emerge. Although it can be tempting to resist branching out to avoid the challenge and "discomfort" of new material, I have learned over time that it is important to intentionally try to avoid this pitfall and to become more comfortable being uncomfortable!

A second challenge regarding CE involves the actual content and implementation of training. Keeping up with the ever-growing scientific knowledge base in psychology may be one of the biggest challenges clinical psychologists face in meeting the ethical requirement of lifelong learning. Psychological research and best practices are ongoing and new data emerge daily. Given the rapidity by which psychological knowledge is generated, clinical psychologists may not be trained in current therapeutic interventions that have strong research support for their efficacy (Baker et al., 2008). They may be practicing outdated or ineffective therapies or using old and invalidated assessments (Neimeyer et al., 2014). Despite this, CE offerings that are intended to help promote new knowledge and skills may or may not be based upon quality research or taught by qualified professionals. A multitude of individuals and organizations provide CE courses to clinical psychologists (Walshok, 2012). State licensing boards as well as national professional organizations, including the APA, provide some level of oversight of these CE providers, such as specific scientific requirements for CE activities (Rabasco et al., 2021). However, a cottage industry of CE offerings includes a proportion of programs that are not based on scientific evidence, are taught in an ineffective manner, or are presented by unqualified individuals, and these programs still find their way to professionals looking for lifelong learning (Washburn et al., 2019). The motto "Buyer Beware" applies to those seeking CE, and psychologists are encouraged to not only investigate the quality of CE offerings but to also report poor quality or unsupported offerings to the appropriate organization. Better yet, offer high-quality CE yourself or join an organization that does! I have found that being part of the solution in lifelong learning is better than merely complaining about poor-quality CE. I joined the APA Continuing Education Committee in order to help facilitate ongoing high-quality, science-based CE in clinical psychology, and I continue to volunteer on the committee as an advisor while also leading the CE subcommittee for the Society of Clinical Psychology.

Another challenge in utilizing CE for lifelong learning is that it remains unclear if it actually helps improve or maintain competence in clinical psychology. In fact, there is little evidence that CE mandates result in psychologists improving their competencies in delivering the most effective and safe psychological services to the public (Babeva & Davison, 2017; Neimeyer et al., 2012). Although psychologists report learning new information and having more effective practices from required CE courses (Neimeyer et al., 2019), the issue of whether CE requirements have any impact on actual practice or whether they improve outcomes and decrease complaints to licensing boards remains an open question (Rothke et al., 2021). In contrast to other health service professions (Cervero & Gaines, 2015), rigorous research methodologies are yet to be fully implemented in examining the impact of required CE on the practice of clinical psychology. The positive news is that there is increasing research in the area of continuing education, effective pedagogy, and the importance of lifelong learning (as evidenced by this chapter!). Committees and interest groups have formed at APA and within clinical psychology to increase awareness of the need to examine and improve lifelong learning (Taylor et al., 2019). In addition, a special edition of the journal, *Professional Psychology: Research and Practice*, was published in 2019 devoted to the importance of science-based continuing and professional education for psychologists, including clinical psychologists. The challenges of lifelong learning invite opportunities for solutions and growth. Rapid changes in technology, information, and exponential research growth necessitate ongoing learning and the development of research about not only what we learn, but how we learn.

The Experience of a Questioning Expert (Brandon A. Gaudiano)

One of the topics that Scott Lilienfeld was working on toward the end of his career had to do with intellectual humility. Being intellectually humble means that we strive to be skeptical and aware of our own thinking biases, as well as to correct them whenever and wherever we find them (Lilienfeld et al., 2020). When I think about lifelong learning and the importance of intellectual humility, it reminds me of recent work that opened my eyes to some biases in my own ways of approaching research. This evolution in my thinking began while I was developing a video-based intervention featuring people with lived experience telling personal stories of how they managed their condition successfully. The intervention was designed to highlight principles of evidence-based treatment by mobilizing people's stories of struggle and recovery to help others currently suffering with depression (Gaudiano et al., 2019, 2020). Decidedly, this was a departure from my earlier intervention work, which could be characterized as rather traditional in terms of its focus and approach. I am a clinician who has worked with numerous clients and their family members to help them get better. I also am a human being who can relate to the various emotional and behavioral struggles that other affected individuals experience. However, I realized after collaborating more closely with mental health consumers from the ground up with the aforementioned video project that my past patients and research participants had not been my partners—at least in the truest sense of the word—when it came to my intervention work.

I can now look back at how the focus of my graduate training and early career had been somewhat myopic when approaching intervention research. The research process I was taught mostly followed a top-down model, logically focusing on identifying evidence-based principles of behavior change and developing efficacious strategies for facilitating this change. To be sure, this is a reasonable and fruitful process in its own right. However, the identified "patient" was never a formal member of my scientific team and now I can see how this was likely a detriment to my research.

In clinical psychology, we have long bemoaned the scientist–practitioner divide in the field, but what about the historically wider gulf represented by our scientist–patient divide? We know that service users' perspectives are important in all areas of healthcare, but mental health is perhaps even more personal and subjective than other forms of illness. Ultimately, perceptions and functioning are *the* important factors when it comes to determining successful outcomes for mental health problems. Thus, interventions must be sensitive to issues of acceptability, usability, and approachability, because psychotherapy requires that clients do most of the work themselves for progress to occur, and, even more importantly, so that this progress can be maintained. However, far too often (at least in my experience), the field has been overly focused on patients' perceived differences and deficits, rather than their much more salient similarities and strengths.

As healthcare professionals, we are limited in our perspectives because we usually only see the people who reach out to us for help to treat their identified problems. As Bowes et al. (2020) remind us, this is a *neglect of missing data* problem, in that we overlook the events that we do not know about, which then leads to the *clinician's illusion*, or the tendency for us to overestimate the chronicity and intractability of certain problems. However, millions of people regularly recover from common mental health problems in a variety of ways, and they are largely accomplishing this *without* formal professional help (Bischof et al., 2012). There is so much still to be learned by this natural recovery process, and yet we have barely scratched the surface in our psychotherapy or capitalized on it in intervention development research up to this point (van Weeghel et al., 2019). Has this neglect been part of the reason why we have seen potential ceiling effects for our evidence-based therapies over time (Fordham et al., 2021)? To answer this question, we would not only need to study the phenomenon of lived experience and natural recovery more systematically but also include patients at all levels of the research process to retain more of these valuable insights into human behavior. However, when I reflect on my own experience and training, at least until recently, much of the research I conducted involved patients only after the fact, and sometimes not at all in the development process.

One must also contend with the fact that the perspectives of patients are potentially just as biased as those of researchers. Nevertheless, both perspectives can be fruitful to examine if we deal with this issue explicitly. In addition, merely making interventions satisfying to patients will not by default make them more effective. One might find eating a donut more satisfying than eating a piece of fruit, but the latter objectively has more nutritional value than the former. Therefore, while satisfaction is an important aspect of any treatment that is designed to be voluntary and not compulsory, we also must combine these efforts with the best scientific understanding of the problem and its effective change strategies.

I want to readily acknowledge that incorporating the patient perspective into research and treatment is not a new approach: people have been doing this work in the field for decades to varying degrees. Support groups such as Alcoholics Anonymous and the mental health recovery movement have been driven by people with lived experience (Warner, 2010). National funding agencies such as the Patient-Centered Outcomes Research Institute (www.pcori.org) require patient and family involvement at all levels of the research endeavor, including in initial peer review, project funding selection, study implementation, and dissemination. In addition, recent movements within the field have spurred some clinicians and academics to publicly acknowledge their own struggles with mental health problems to reduce stigma (Varghese & Boyd, 2022). As the field continues to learn from the experiences of others as an overlooked context of discovery, I personally have learned a useful lesson: incorporating persons with lived experience into the research has helped me to gain new insights into how to do my work, be more compassionate, and hopefully make the findings more useful in the process.

The Experience of a Clinical Supervisor (Tara S. Peris)

Clinical supervision is a cornerstone of training for all mental health practitioners. The process of supporting, developing, and providing feedback to emerging therapists is essential to graduate training, and we are asked to track both supervision structure (individual versus group) and quantity (number of hours per supervisee) carefully over time. The requirement that we monitor and report supervision hours across different stages of training (pre- and post-doctoral) speaks to its importance both for guiding new therapists and for protecting patients and the public at large.

I received plenty of supervision in graduate school, but relatively little structured training about *how to be the supervisor*. Through my own clinical training, I encountered many clinical supervisors both within my doctoral program and outside of it. I learned from their interpersonal styles what I liked (and didn't) and what worked for me (and didn't) when learning to apply a new approach or work with a particular population. Although my clinical responsibilities and independence increased over time to the point where I offered mentorship and support to other students, there was no coursework or exposure to models of supervision. Doctoral and internship accreditation standards now require education in supervision models and practices; however, it seemed that the philosophy at that time was that you would learn by watching others supervise and then gradually jump in and find your way on your own.

As a postdoc and early career faculty member, my work began to involve more clinical trials methodology, where therapy practice was monitored more closely for fidelity and adherence. Through these research activities, my own approach to supervision grew more structured and systematic. It began to focus on therapist competency and measurement of learning outcomes, mainly because these needed to be documented as part of the clinical trials I was overseeing. However, my supervision still was not informed by any formal pedagogy on *how* to teach others what I knew. Worse, it rarely considered whether my approach was a good match for the student with whom I was working.

This shifted as my work began to encompass more clinical supervision within the predoctoral internship and the larger psychiatry department in which I work. The need for my own additional learning became clear as I started teaching child psychiatry fellows, residents, and social work interns in addition to psychology trainees. My supervision role required me to think more carefully about their varied training backgrounds and skill levels as well as the settings in which they were working (inpatient, outpatient, day treatment, etc.). It also placed me on training committees where I not only received peer supervision from other clinical supervisors but was exposed to the literature on approaches to clinical supervision, including models of supervision and the use of clinical supervision to support treatment dissemination (Bearman, 2021; Carlson et al., 2012).

Beyond beginning to familiarize myself with this literature, I have learned a great deal from my students, who approach their clinical training with a degree of savvy I never had. They are able to talk about bi-directional feedback in supervision, specific teaching techniques, and individual learning styles, and they approach these conversations as educated consumers with high standards and expectations. These conversations have pushed me to consider different supervision strategies and how to tailor them to the needs of individual students.

These conversations have also highlighted other areas in need of lifelong learning, particularly with respect to treating patients from diverse backgrounds. We assume our supervisors are competent inasmuch as they have the skills to teach their students how to assess and treat different mental health concerns. However, you can't teach what you don't know. My graduate training did not include exposure to LGBTQ+ interventions, and it involved guidance that is now wildly out of step (and indeed, potentially harmful) for Latinx and Black clients. In order to fulfill my responsibility as a supervisor, I've had to seek further training of my own regarding assessment of social determinants of health, case conceptualization, and evidence-based practice for different client populations.

It's still been a gradual process of self-reflection and questioning of my own knowledge and competence in the service of making sure I have something real (and effective) to teach in supervision. Although at times it is painful to recognize gaps (and errors) in my education, it's more often gratifying to learn something new and to see how far the field has come.

The Experience of a Researcher Who Needs a Statistical Upgrade (Bethany A. Teachman)

I do mobile assessments of anxiety in daily life using a mix of active and passive sensors (e.g., ecological momentary assessment surveys multiple times a day over a period of weeks, combined with GPS and accelerometer movement tracking), and direct a website that offers cognitive bias modification interventions to reduce anxious thinking patterns. Doing this kind of research can produce rich longitudinal datasets, but it is inevitably messy data with lots (and lots) of missingness and many data streams that are on different time scales and distinct frequency of measurement points that somehow need to be integrated to detect the signal amid the noise.

The statistics training that I received in graduate school was great but that was a long time ago. Thus, while my statistics knowledge is probably typical of most clinical faculty at my stage, the methods I was taught are not the optimal ones to manage the complexities of the datasets my team now routinely collects. I have struggled with how to address the gaps in my skills (I was not trained in R) and in my knowledge. To date, I have only found a partial solution—more of a Band-Aid than anything resembling an actual remedy. So, this is more of a confession than an evolution, but I hope it can at least serve as a chance to share a common challenge, raise a difficult question, and perhaps prompt me to do better.

The challenge is an obvious one. My students and collaborators routinely do analyses with our data that I am not capable of doing myself, raising concerns that I, as my students' advisor, am not well equipped to advise them on the analytic approach or to catch errors. Obtaining the desired knowledge and skills is not a simple task; almost all my graduate students do a quantitative minor to learn the complex dynamic and network modeling and machine learning approaches needed to optimally work with our data and answer the questions we want to ask. It's not simply a question of me sitting in on one course and getting caught up. I already feel like there are not nearly enough hours in the day to get done all the things I need to do, much less learn an entirely new statistics program and analytic methods.

I have tried to think about the priorities in this situation: (a) I want to ask our research questions in the best way we can, using whatever method has the greatest validity for the particular questions; (b) I want to be rigorous and do high-quality work, avoiding sloppy mistakes in our analyses, especially the ones that come from ignorance about the assumptions underlying an approach; (c) I want my students to get excellent training and feel well supported in pursuing their research, including when doing new analyses; (d) I want to feel confident that if my name is on a paper, I've contributed in a meaningful way and deserve authorship; and (e) I don't want gaps in my knowledge to ever hold my students back.

Given these priorities, the Band-Aid that I've developed over time involves working with exceptionally talented students who view learning new approaches as an exciting challenge. In other words, I have them teach me as much as I teach them. I also work very closely with collaborators in engineering and data science who have advanced analytic training so that they can serve as a secondary advisor on some of the analytic pieces. We also routinely invite one of our fantastic quantitative faculty or advanced graduate students to be a co-author on papers, so I advise on all the conceptual pieces, study design and implementation, and other components, while a more quantitatively focused collaborator advises on the analytic approach. I am fortunate that my students also help each other a lot, so we routinely have lab meetings where one student reviews the analyses they've done or are planning, and others raise questions and make suggestions. In addition, the norm in our lab is to preregister the studies so that the hypotheses and analytic plan are laid out prior to conducting analyses. This helps to ensure we're taking the time to really think through whether the selected analytic approach is the right way to ask the questions. It also pushes us to figure out which tests are exploratory, and which are confirmatory, and then interpret them accordingly, recognizing the different assumptions associated with each (e.g., differences in the need to correct for multiple tests). It also makes our thought process and analytic plans available for others to review.

This approach generally works insofar as we are able to be productive, collaborate with lots of fantastic people, and not shy away from using sophisticated analytic approaches to ask our questions. Yet I call it a Band-Aid approach because I routinely face a difficult question: do I know enough to be an effective advisor for a given paper? Are my gaps in knowledge and skills in this area leading us to make mistakes that I should be helping to catch as the advisor? In other words, how much is it appropriate to expect others to cover for your gaps? Where is the line between setting up win–win relationships with collaborators—where it's not only okay, but also quite efficient and sensible, that they provide expertise you don't have—and shirking my responsibility as a primary advisor to understand the analytic methods we use more deeply? I think it's not an either–or answer. I would like to deepen my statistics knowledge and feel better equipped to provide feedback on the analytic sections of our papers, but I don't think it makes sense for me to dedicate the kind of time that would be needed for me to develop the expertise that my quantitatively focused collaborators have developed over many years.

For now, I ask a lot of questions to my students and collaborators, so I feel I understand why we're making the analytic choices we're making and why we're interpreting the results the way we are. The questions probably get annoying sometimes but, this way, at least I feel I can stand by the work, raise some useful questions and checks, and explain it to others (e.g., if I'm asked a question at a presentation). I hope to carve out more time to find a better balance between being a lifelong learner and lifelong collaborator. I had planned on my last sabbatical to carve out an hour each week to watch a statistics tutorial on YouTube or read a relevant paper, which I did for a couple of weeks, but then COVID-19 happened and, like so many others, any extra time I had planned on was out of the window as we scrambled to manage full-time school at home for our children, and the many challenges that arose at work. Here is hoping the next sabbatical will get me a little closer!

The Experience of a Cognitive Behavior Therapist as a Phenomenologist (Gerald C. Davison)[1]

- There is nothing either good or bad, but thinking makes it so. (Shakespeare, *Hamlet*, act II, scene 2)
- The mind is its own place, and in itself Can make a Heav'n of Hell, a Hell of Heav'n. (Milton, *Paradise Lost*, line 247)
- [People] are disturbed not by things, but by the view they take of them. (Epictetus, Greek philosopher, first century AD)
- We tell ourselves stories in order to live. (Didion, *The White Album*, 1979).

My lifelong learning is due primarily to my lifelong teaching. That is, by having the responsibility and the privilege of teaching psychosocial intervention and assessment to scores of graduate students and postdocs over nearly six decades, I have had to continuously examine my thinking and actions while doing clinical work, in particular by explaining to my students what guides my long-term strategies and my short-term tactics. My many patients over the years have also afforded me the opportunity, indeed, have required me, to examine my clinical problem-solving. Through these experiences, readings, and spirited discussions with colleagues and students over the years, I have come to appreciate the humanistic–existential essence of cognitive behavior therapy (CBT) in ways that initially surprised me.

As an early proponent of including cognition in behavior therapy (Davison, 1966), I became convinced that people like George Kelly (1955), Julian Rotter (Rotter, 1954), and Jerome Bruner (Bruner et al., 1956) were correct in their basic belief that the way people construe their world is a major—if not *the* major—determinant of their feelings and behavior. This does not gainsay the importance of how people *behave* overtly toward others, for social interactions are very important is how one thinks, feels, and behaves. But the principal focus is on cognition—both conscious and unconscious.

[1] Portions of Dr. Davison's section are adapted from a chapter written by him in O'Donohue, W., & Masuda, A. (Eds.), (in press). *Behavior Therapy: First, Second, and Third Waves*. Springer.

Cognitive behavior therapists focus on how their patients perceive the world. It is not what impinges on us from the outside that controls our behavior—the assumption, based almost entirely on experiments with non-human species, that guided behavior therapy in the 1950s to the mid-1960s. Rather, our feelings and behavior are determined by how we view the world. Similarly, a central thesis of phenomenologist therapists like Carl Rogers and Fritz Perls is that clients must be understood from their own frame of reference, from their phenomenological world, for it is this experience of the world that determines how they conduct their lives.[2]

In my view, cognitive behavior therapy (CBT) is at its core phenomenological. As such, we CBTers are in agreement with humanistic–existential therapists. CBT also shares the humanistic–existential assumption that people have free will and are therefore capable of change as well as responsible for their actions and the consequences of those actions. To be sure, the techniques used by cognitive behavior therapists are quite different from those of the followers of Rogers and Perls. But as students of psychotherapy and of human nature, we should not allow these surface differences to blind us to the conceptual links between the two approaches.

In recent years, I have been teaching a first year required PhD course in the University of Southern California's clinical science program entitled "Clinical Interviewing and Professional Issues." For much of the semester, we practice Rogerian interviewing, something that, in my halcyon graduate school days at Stanford, was ignored or even derogated as an unnecessary element of the so-called "insight therapies" (London, 1963), the *bêtes noires* of the brave new world of behavior therapy. Things changed for me while spending much of my second year sitting in on numerous clinical sessions conducted by Arnold Lazarus. I began to see the undesirability and untenableness of the myopic view of early behavior therapy through the hundreds of hours I spent sitting in sessions with him (Lazarus, 1971). I came to see that what he called "the nonspecifics" were really not *non*-specific at all, rather they involved mostly the kind of empathic listening that is the foundation of Carl Rogers's work. I began to appreciate these strategies as a way both to establish a trusting working relationship with the patient and, most importantly, as a means to get relevant information that was essential to designing and implementing a cognitive–behavioral intervention. Empathic listening helps fill out the familiar functional–analytic framework for determining what Bandura (Bandura, 1969) called the "controlling variables" necessary for devising and implementing a science-based intervention.

But it is more complicated and more powerful than that.

The phenomenological core of humanistic and existential therapies is, I believe, evident in the fact that Rogers and his followers did not restrict their empathic work to what is obvious in the client's verbal and nonverbal expressions. This was spelled out more clearly for me in Gerald Egan's "The Skilled Helper" (Egan, 1975). Here's an example I have used often in my teaching of both undergraduates and graduate students:

---

[2]The concept of phenomenology in psychology shares some useful resemblances to that concept in philosophy but may not be identical. As used here, the term refers to the way people *structure* their experience and not to the Wundtian concept of "pure experience," uncluttered by the constructive categories that are discussed in this section.

> Client: I don't know what's going on. I study hard, but I just don't get good marks. I think I study as hard as anyone else, but all of my efforts seem to go down the drain. I don't know what else I can do.
>
> Counselor A: You feel frustrated because even when you try hard you fail [primary empathy].
>
> Counselor B: It's depressing to put in as much effort as those who pass and still fail. It gets you down and maybe even makes you feel a little sorry for yourself [advanced empathy]. (Egan, 1975, p. 135)

At the primary empathic level, the therapist accepts what the patient is saying, understands it, and communicates to the person that it is appreciated and respected. But at the advanced or what I see as the interpretive level, the therapist offers something new, a perspective that he or she hopes is more productive and implies new modes of action. At the beginnings of CBT, we called this cognitive restructuring.

Bear in mind that therapists operating both within a humanistic–existential framework and a cognitive–behavioral one assume that the client views things in an unproductive way, as evidenced by the psychological distress that has brought the client into therapy. The client-centered therapist—like the CBTer—operating within a phenomenological perspective, *must* have as a crucial goal moving the client from his or her present phenomenological world to another one, hence the importance of the advanced-empathy or interpretation stage. *Since the core belief of both the humanists and cognitive–behavioral clinicians is that people's emotions and actions are determined by how they construe themselves and their surroundings—by their phenomenology—those who are dysfunctional or otherwise dissatisfied with their present mode of living are in need of a new phenomenology*. From the very outset, then, all phenomenological therapies—including CBT—strive to move the client from an unproductive phenomenology to one that is *different from* what they had when they began treatment. Merely to reflect back to clients their current phenomenology cannot in itself bring therapeutic change. *A new phenomenology must be acquired.*

Thus, the core of CBT is essentially the same as all the phenomenological therapies—what matters most is how people construe their world. And in one way or another, cognitive behavior therapists try to change the patient's maladaptive phenomenology to a more useful, more productive one. This is quite different from original behavior therapy, whereby the person responds to stimuli and is either reinforced or not. That is an oversimplified picture of course but it is not inaccurate. What Rotter, Kelly, Ellis, Beck, Mischel, Bandura, and Goldfried and I (Goldfried & Davison, 1976) brought into the picture was the centrality of how patients view the world, the meaning they attach to what is going on in and around themselves. The defining feature of the CBT paradigm has always been that these constructions of the world—e.g., Ellis's irrational beliefs, Beck's schemata and cognitive biases—determine the person's emotional and behavioral reactions and must be altered to improve their lives.

Many of my CBT colleagues may object to being in bed with theoreticians and therapists whom we often have actively derogated. But at the end of the day, I believe that is where we have found ourselves since at least the late-1960s, with the seeds of this paradigmatic shift being discernible in the writings of people not usually regarded as part of the CBT family (e.g., George Kelly and Julian Rotter).

The foregoing is most assuredly not new to today's cognitive behavior therapy. And that is the point, for these ideas and practices were either poo-pooed by behavior therapy's leading lights in the 1950s and 1960s or were assigned to the realm of "clinical know-how" or "non-specifics," which was intellectually honest but not conducive to a thoroughgoing analysis of psychosocial assessment and intervention.

The Experience of an Evolving Psychopathologist (Steven D. Hollon)

Lifelong learning implies that our ideas are open to change. My fascination with depression led me to devote my career to understanding the nature and treatment of this most prevalent of the psychiatric disorders. What I knew with great certainty based on both professional expertise and personal experience was that depression was a miserable experience that robbed life of its pleasures and that sapped one's striving to succeed. My perspective at this time was that it was clearly a psychiatric disorder and maybe even a disease.

A little over a decade ago, I gave a collegial reading to an article by an evolutionary biologist that I met socially and his psychiatric colleague who considered depression to be an adaptation that evolved to serve a function. Most evolutionary biologists consider depression to be an evolved adaptation (like pain or anxiety) and not a "disease" or even a "disorder." Andrews and Thompson argued that the function that depression evolved to serve was rumination. I thought the argument was specious and clearly wrong, arguing that rumination is a symptom of depression and possibly even a maintaining cause. Despite my disagreements, I thought the arguments were coherent and the scholarship impressive, so I encouraged the authors to submit it to *Psychological Review*, the premier outlet for theoretical pieces in psychology.

The authors followed my advice, and the article was accepted (Andrews & Thomson, 2009). At the core of their argument was the notion that it is adaptive to think thoughtfully and carefully when you have a complex interpersonal problem to resolve. Specifically, the authors argued that depression evolved to promote rumination and note that energy is transferred to the cortex in a manner that does not occur in related "depression-like" syndromes like infection or starvation (Andrews et al., 2015). In our ancestral past, being ostracized from the group would likely lead to death. A lone primate would be picked off by predators or starve and the situation would be even more dire for a female caring for an infant. It is notable that women are twice as likely to get depressed as men and that gender difference first emerges in adolescence when reproductive capacity first comes online. If some interpersonal problem developed, one would have to resolve the issue or risk being driven from the troop. Depression promotes careful analysis of the causes of the problem, eventually leading to a solution that preserves their group membership (Andrews et al., 2020). More than just a symptom of depression, rumination was seen as the function that depression evolved to serve in that it helped our ancestors survive long enough to become our ancestors.

The implications for psychopathology are broader still. To an evolutionary biologist, most syndromes marked by high levels of affect distress are neither "diseases" (in which the brain is broken) nor "disorders" (in which the distress serves no useful purpose), but rather serve to coordinate the kind of "whole body response" (integrated patterns of cognition, physiology, and behavior) to specific types of challenges that were most likely to lead to a successful resolution in our ancestral past. Anxiety coordinates response to threat, anger coordinates response to challenge, and pain coordinates the avoidance of tissue damage. From the perspective of evolutionary biology, these painful affects "hurt," but they kept our ancestors alive. The tipping point for me came when Andrews gave me an article by Crook and colleagues that demonstrated how pain facilitated survival (Crook et al., 2014). In that 2 × 2 design, quartets of squids were either maimed (one of their swimmers was cut off) or not, either under anesthesia or not, and then placed in a tank with a hungry sea bass. Those squids that had not been maimed were most likely to survive, but those that had been maimed under anesthesia were more likely to be eaten than those that were maimed without. The reason was that the latter started their evasive maneuvers sooner than those that had not been maimed or than those that had been maimed but did not feel the pain. The moral of the story is that pain may hurt, but it keeps you alive.

Even after decades of thinking about depression as a disorder, I largely became a convert to this new way of thinking (Hollon, 2020). That is not to say that some instances of strong negative affect may not represent psychiatric diseases or disorder; the mechanisms underlying any adaptation can break down and cease to function in the way they were evolved to serve. Pain serves a function that helps keep us alive, as shown by the shorter lifespans of people born with congenital analgesia (Nagasako et al., 2003), but a breakdown in that mechanism can lead to the experience of pain (neuropathy) in the absence of any tissue damage. It is likely that the low prevalence/highly heritable psychotic disorders like bipolar I or the schizophrenias represent breakdowns in evolved adaptations that become manifest across the course of development in response to life stress (Syme & Hagen, 2020). (It is worth noting that heredity is not destiny; even identical twins are only about 50% concordant for bipolar I or schizophrenia.) It also is worth noting that those high prevalence/modest heritability common mental "disorders" that have negative affect at their core like nonpsychotic depression and anxiety—what evolutionary biologists would consider evolved adaptations—are at least as well treated by psychosocial interventions as with medications, and often with an enduring effect that medications lack. In contrast, the highly heritable/low prevalence severe mental disorders—what evolutionary biologists would consider true neurodevelopmental disorders or diseases—are best treated with medications (Hollon et al., 2021). There is no reason why an evolved adaptation cannot be treated if it causes undue distress, but it is a principle of evolutionary medicine that any treatment that facilitates the function that the adaptation evolved to serve is to be preferred over one that merely anesthetizes the pain. I now teach a course on depression in which I lay out all the things I was wrong about a decade ago. Even a psychopathologist can evolve.

The Experience of a Humbled Educator (Jason J. Washburn)

I have been involved at some level in antiracist education and training for the last two decades. This interest developed out of a more foundational desire for what is now referred to as equity, diversity, inclusion, and social justice. My interest in these areas was sparked by my early exposure to naked racism, sexism, heterosexism, ableism, and anti-Semitism. As a child growing up in a largely homogenous and privileged household and community, I was surrounded by adults and peers that espoused both blatant and conspicuous "isms," as well as more subtle expressions of stereotypes and prejudice. I am someone who holds multiple intersecting privileges, bestowed upon me because I live in, benefit from, and contribute to structures and systems that are built upon White supremacy and other forms of oppression. Explicit racism is part of my paternal lineage, as evidenced by my paternal grandfather being found with a KKK membership card in his wallet at the time of his death.

I chose a different path than my paternal grandfather. Although my father could have easily passed along to me his substantial "isms," he pointedly told me as a child that I had a choice: I could be like him, or I could be different. I chose different. As an undergraduate student, I initially worked toward understanding my privilege as a cisgender male, becoming the first male member of our university's women's student union during a time of substantial antifeminist sentiment (Faludi, 1991). In graduate school, I was drawn to understanding my role as White cisgender male. During a visit to Elmina Castle in Ghana, I read a gravestone that extolled the virtues of one of the commanders of the slave castle. I began to wonder what people would think of me 200 years from now. After returning from Ghana, I was invited to join a sociology professor in creating a new course titled *White Studies and Eradicating White Racism* (Manley et al., 2008; Washburn et al., 2003), which introduced me to concepts such as aversive and implicit racism (Dovidio & Gaertner, 2004). These formative experiences during my undergraduate and graduate education ultimately led to a persistent interest in antiracist education and training.

My work in antiracist education and training resulted in a strong awareness of my own biases and prejudices. Given my upbringing, I held a vast repository of ism-related thoughts and feelings. Using my antiracist training, however, I was able to at least partly identify and challenge those thoughts and feelings, actively working to manage discriminatory behavioral responses. In other words, I attempted to modulate my proclivity to engage in microaggressions (Sue & Spanierman, 2020). Although the concept, theory, and research on microaggressions have been hotly debated (e.g., Freeman & Stewart, 2021; Lilienfeld, 2017; Sue, 2017; Syed, 2021; Williams, 2020), I was personally aware that I was capable of acting on stereotyped thoughts and prejudicial feelings, even in spite of myself.

Given my self-awareness around these issues, I held a level of confidence about my ability to monitor and manage vulnerabilities to engaging in discriminatory behavior. My confidence, however, was shaken when I was challenged by a former student who shared with me that they believed I had treated them differently because of their race. I was surprised by this feedback and sought to better understand it; however, in doing so, I did everything wrong.

In hindsight, I believe my (over)confidence in my self-awareness worked against me. With my childhood training in -isms, I have "slipped" more times than I can remember in my life; however, I was under the impression that I was mostly aware of those errors. Even when I wasn't immediately aware of them, I *thought* that I quickly acknowledged my offenses when it was brought to my attention. In this situation, however, I didn't see my lapse. As much as I tried, I couldn't understand my former student's perspective. I fervently reviewed my actions, as well as interrogated my thoughts and feelings related to or leading up to those actions, but I just couldn't see it! That was when the problems started. In trying to understand my lapse or error, I began to interrogate my former student rather than myself. I asked them multiple questions in a desperate attempt to better understand the situation, yet my line of questions only served to communicate skepticism or disbelief of their experience. I became entrenched in my position that I had done nothing wrong and expressed bewilderment regarding their experience.

Despite over two decades of personal and professional work in anti-ism work, it was clear that my learning was not over. No level of education or training could keep me free from my own emotional and cognitive biases. In my desire to defend myself, I become overconfident, arrogant, and interpersonally dominant (Feist, 2006). In other words, I had lost my sense of humility. Although humility can be challenging to define (Davis et al., 2010; Lilienfeld & Bowes, 2021), it is increasingly considered an important construct in psychological science and practice. Cultural humility holds a particularly central role in the development of multicultural competencies (Vasquez & Johnson, 2022). From a cultural humility perspective, I failed to maintain a relational stance with my former student that was other-oriented, non-superior, and curious about how their lived experience and intersectional identities influenced their perspective (Hook et al., 2013; Raque et al., 2021).

I also had failed from an intellectual humility perspective. Lilienfeld and Bowes (2021) define intellectual humility as a "trait reflecting an awareness of one's intellectual limitations and propensity toward biases" (p. 450). Ironically, by being overconfident of my own sense of self-awareness, I lost track of my limitations and was blind to my cognitive biases. It wasn't until my former student reminded me that I hadn't shown any sign of care or concern for how this was making them feel that I suddenly realized that my response had been about me and my sense of self, that I wasn't respecting their perspective or opinion, that I wasn't willing to revise my perspective in response to their perspective, and that I was being overly confident about self-awareness (Krumrei-Mancuso & Rouse, 2016). In other words, humility was absent.

Lilienfeld and Bowes (2021) argue for a Meliorist position when considering the human condition. Pragmatist philosopher, Charles S. Peirce, defined Meliorism as "the doctrine that the world is neither the worst nor the best possible, but that it is capable of improvement: a mean between theoretical pessimism and optimism" (Pierce, 1889, p. 3697). As "unabashed Meliorists," Lilienfeld and Bowes (2021) propose that while we, as humans, remain vulnerable to cognitive biases that inevitably result in frequent errors with real-world consequences, we have an enduring capacity to improve—through debiasing techniques and other means—toward increased rationality. Specifically, they write that "humans are inherently fallible, but that with concerted education and training, they may be able to become more aware of their cognitive limitations and, ideally, come to implement means of compensating for them" (p. 463). As a fallible clinical psychologist and member of the human species, I will continue to embrace humility in a never-ending effort to learn throughout my life.

Conclusion

The experiences presented in this chapter provide a snapshot of the diversity of lifelong learning of clinical psychologists. In research and in clinical practice, the authors of this chapter found themselves evolving in response to a developing science and a growing field. Although each clinical psychologist approached their lifelong learning in different ways, they all focused on changing what they did in response to their lifelong learning. As demonstrated by the experiences provided in this chapter, lifelong learning is not a passive exercise but instead an active process of adaptation.

When asked about what advice he would give to somebody seeking an academic career in psychology. Dr. Lilienfeld responded with the following:

> Be sure that you are madly in love with science and want to spread that love to others, both by conducting research and by teaching. Be sure that you are willing to work very hard, and that you don't see a sharp distinction between your work and your play. If you find psychological research to be laborious, you don't want to go into academia. In contrast, if you find it to be enormously fun and fulfilling, you may want to consider it. Also, learn to develop a thick skin and not to take criticism personally. Academia is a great life, but it requires the ability to benefit from constructive feedback. (Lilienfeld, n.d.)

Psychologists who embrace constructive feedback, and consider it with a dash of skepticism and a large helping of humility, will inevitably stay madly in love with their science. As lifelong learners, we can learn a lot from Dr. Lilienfeld.

References

Andrews, P. W., & Thomson, J. A., Jr. (2009). The bright side of being blue: Depression as an adaptation for analyzing complex problems. *Psychological Review, 116*, 620–654. https://doi.org/10.1037/a0016242

Andrews, P. W., Bharwani, A., Lee, K. R., Fox, M., & Thomson, J. A., Jr. (2015). Is serotonin an upper or a downer? The evolution of the serotonergic system and its role in depression and the antidepressant response. *Neuroscience and Biobehavioral Reviews, 51*, 164–188. https://doi.org/10.1016/j.neubiorev.2015.01.018

Andrews, P. W., Maslej, M. M., Thomson, J. A., Jr., & Hollon, S. D. (2020). Disordered doctors or rational rats? Testing adaptationist and disorder hypotheses for melancholic depression and their relevance for clinical psychology. *Clinical Psychology Review, 82*, 101927. https://doi.org/10.1016/j.cpr.2020.101927

APA. (2015). *Standards and criteria for approval of sponsors of continuing education for psychologists*. https://www.apa.org/about/policy/approval-standards.pdf

APA. (2017). *Ethical principles of psychologists and code of conduct* (2002, amended effective June 1, 2010, and January 1, 2017). https://doi.org/10.1037/0003-066X.57.12.1060

Babeva, K. N., & Davison, G. C. (2017). A review and critique of continuing education. *The Behavior Therapist, 40*(1), 4–9.

Baker, T. B., McFall, R. M., & Shoham, V. (2008). Current status and future prospects of clinical psychology: Toward a scientifically principled approach to mental and behavioral health care. *Psychological Science in the Public Interest, 9*(2), 67–103.

Bandura, A. (1969). Principles of behavior modification. *Holt, Rinehart, & Winston.*

Bischof, G., Rumpf, H.-J., & John, U. (2012). Natural recovery from addiction. In H. Shaffer, D. A. LaPlante, & S. E. Nelson (Eds.), *APA addiction syndrome handbook: Recovery, prevention, and other issues* (Vol. 2, pp. 133–155). APA. https://doi.org/10.1037/13750-006

Bearman, S. K. (2021) Introduction to special issue: clinical supervision in implementation science. *The Clinical Supervisor 40(1), 1–7.* https://doi.org/10.1080/07325223.2021.1911900

Bowes, S. M., Ammirati, R. J., Costello, T. H., Basterfield, C., & Lilienfeld, S. O. (2020). Cognitive biases, heuristics, and logical fallacies in clinical practice: A brief field guide for practicing clinicians and supervisors. *Professional Psychology: Research and Practice, 51*(5), 435–445. https://doi.org/10.1037/pro0000309

Britt, S. H. (1939). Association reports: Report of committee on legislation, Board of Affiliates of the a.a.a.P. *Journal of Consulting Psychology, 3*(4), 123–127. https://doi.org/10.1037/h0050028

Bruner, J. S., Goodnow, J. A., & Austin, G. A. (1956). *A study of thinking*. Wiley.

Buttars, E. M., Taylor, J. M., & Neimeyer, G. J. (2021). Continuing education in professional psychology: Exploring the translation of learning into practice. *Professional Psychology: Research and Practice, 52*(6), 627–634. https://doi.org/10.1037/pro0000398

Carlson, L., Rapp, C. A., & Eichler, M.S. (2012) The Experts Rate: Supervisory Behaviors That Impact the Implementation of Evidence-Based Practices. *Community Mental Health Journal, 48(2), 179–186.* https://doi.org/10.1007/s10597-010-9367-4

Cartwright, M. A. (1945). The history of adult education in the United States. *The Journal of Negro Education, 14*(3), 283–292.

Cervero, R. M., & Gaines, J. K. (2015). The impact of CME on physician performance and patient health outcomes: An updated synthesis of systematic reviews. *Journal of Continuing Education in the Health Professions, 35*(2), 131–138.

Crook, R. J., Dickson, K., Hanlon, R. T., & Walters, E. T. (2014). Nociceptive sensitization reduces predation risk. *Current Biology, 24*(10), 1121–1125. https://doi.org/10.1016/j.cub.2014.03.043

Davison, G. C. (1966). Differential relaxation and cognitive restructuring in therapy with a paranoid schizophrenic or paranoid state. *Proceedings of the 74th Annual Convention of the American Psychological Association*. APA.

Davis, D. E., Worthington, E. L., Hook, J. N. (2010). Humility: Review of measurement strategies and conceptualization as personality judgment. *The Journal of Positive Psychology, 5(4), 243–252.* https://doi.org/10.1080/17439761003791672

Dovidio, J. F., & Gaertner, S. L. (2004). Aversive racism. In M. P. Zanna (Ed.), *Advances in experimental social psychology* (Vol. 36, pp. 1–51). Academic Press.

Duffy, T. P. (2011). The Flexner report – 100 years later. *Yale Journal of Biology and Medicine, 84*(3). https://doi.org/10.5116/ijme.4cb4.85c8

Didion, J. (2009). The White Album. Simon and Schuster.

Egan, G. (1975). *The skilled helper*. Brooks/Cole.

Faludi, S. (1991). *Backlash: The undeclared war against American women.* Crown Publishing Group.

Feist, G. J. (2006). *The psychology of science and the origins of the scientific mind.* Yale University Press.

Fordham, B., Sugavanam, T., Edwards, K., Stallard, P., Howard, R., das Nair, R., Copsey, B., Lee, H., Howick, J., Hemming, K., & Lamb, S. E. (2021). The evidence for cognitive behavioural therapy in any condition, population or context: A meta-review of systematic reviews and panoramic meta-analysis. *Psychological Medicine, 51*(1), 21–29. https://doi.org/10.1017/S0033291720005292

Flexner A. (1910). Medical Education in the United States and Canada: A Report To the Carnegie Foundation For the Advancement of Teaching. The Carnegie Foundation for the Advancement of Teaching.

Franklin, B. (1771). Autobiography and other writings.

Freeman, L., & Stewart, H. (2021) *Toward a Harm-Based Account of Microaggressions. Perspectives on Psychological Science, 16(5), 1008–1023.* https://doi.org/10.1177/17456916211017099

Gaudiano, B. A., Davis, C. H., Miller, I. W., & Uebelacker, L. A. (2019). Development of a storytelling video self-help intervention based on acceptance and commitment therapy for major depression: Open trial results. *Behavior Modification, 43*(1), 56–81. https://doi.org/10.1177/0145445517738932

Gaudiano, B. A., Davis, C. H., Miller, I. W., & Uebelacker, L. (2020). Pilot randomized controlled trial of a video self-help intervention for depression based on acceptance and commitment therapy: Feasibility and acceptability. *Clinical Psychology & Psychotherapy, 27*(3), 396–407. https://doi.org/10.1002/cpp.2436

Goldfried, M. R., & Davison, G. C. (1976). *Clinical behavior therapy*. Holt, Rinehart & Winston.

Hollon, S. D. (2020). Is cognitive therapy enduring or antidepressant medications iatrogenic? Depression as an evolved adaptation. *American Psychologist, 75*(9), 1207–1218. https://doi.org/10.1037/amp0000728

Hollon, S. D., Andrews, P. W., Keller, M. C., Singla, D. R., Maslej, M. M., & Mulsant, B. (2021). Combining psychotherapy and medications: It's all about the squids and sea bass (at least for nonpsychotic patients). In M. Barkham, W. Lutz, & L. G. Castonguay (Eds.), *Handbook of psychotherapy and behavior change* (7th ed., pp. 705–738). Wiley.

Hook, J. N., Davis, D. E., Owen, J., Worthington, E. L., & Utsey, S. O. (2013). Cultural humility: Measuring openness to culturally diverse clients. *Journal of Counseling Psychology, 60*(3), 353–366. https://doi.org/10.1037/a0032595

Kelly, G. A. (1955). *The psychology of personal constructs*. Norton.

Krumrei-Mancuso, E. J., & Rouse, S. V. (2016). The development and validation of the comprehensive intellectual humility scale. *Journal of Personality Assessment, 98*(2), 209–221. https://doi.org/10.1080/00223891.2015.1068174

Lazarus, A. A. (1971). *Behavior therapy and beyond*. McGraw-Hill.

Lilienfeld, S. O. (2017). Microaggressions: Strong claims inadequate evidence. *Perspectives on Psychological Science, 12*(1), 138–169.

Lilienfeld, S. O. (n.d.). *Interview with Dr. Scott Lilienfeld.* https://www.all-about-psychology.com/scott-lilienfeld.html

Lilienfeld, S. O., & Bowes, S. M. (2021). Intellectual humility: Ten key questions. In P. Graf & D. J. A. Dozois (Eds.), *Handbook on the state of the art in applied psychology* (pp. 449–468). Wiley.

Lilienfeld, S. O., Bowes, S. M., Costello, T. H., & Strother, A. (2020, March/April). Intellectual humility: A guiding principle for the skeptical movement. *Skeptical Inquirer,44*(5), 32–37. Retrieved from: https://skepticalinquirer.org/2020/09/intellectual-humility-a-guiding-principle-for-the-skeptical-movement/

London, P. (1963). *The modes and morals of psychotherapy*. Holt, Rinehart & Winston.

London, M. (2012). Lifelong learning: Introduction. In M. London (Ed.), *the Oxford handbook of lifelong learning* (pp. 1–16). https://doi.org/10.1093/oxfordhb/9780195390483.013.0013

Manley, T., Washburn, J. J., & Howliski, F. (2008). Teaching about white racism in the United States: Does it make a difference? In T. Fong (Ed.), *Handbook of research methods in ethnic studies* (pp. 427–449). AltaMira Press.

Manning, P. R., & DeBakey, L. (2011). Lifelong medical education: Past, present, future. In D. K. Wentz (Ed.), *Continuing medical education: Looking Back, planning ahead* (pp. 17–18). Dartmouth College Press.

Manley, T., Washburn, J.J., & Howliski, F. (2008). Teaching about White racism in the United States: Does it make a difference? In T. Fong (Ed.), Handbook of Research Methods in Ethnic Studies (pp. 427-449). Lanham, MD: AltaMira Press.

Murphy, F. D. (1951). The concept of continuation education in medicine. *California Medicine, 74*(2).

Nagasako, E. M., Oaklander, A. L., & Dworkin, R. H. (2003). Congenital insensitivity to pain: An update. *Pain, 101*(3), 213–219. https://doi.org/10.1016/s0304-3959(02)00482-7

Neimeyer, G. J., Taylor, J. M., & Wear, D. M. (2009). Continuing education in psychology: Outcomes, evaluations, and mandates. *Professional Psychology: Research and Practice, 40*(6), 617–624. https://doi.org/10.1037/a0016655

Neimeyer, G. J., Taylor, J. M., & Philip, D. (2010). Continuing education in psychology: Patterns of participation and perceived outcomes among mandated and nonmandated psychologists. *Professional Psychology: Research and Practice, 41*(5), 435–441. https://doi.org/10.1037/a0021120

Neimeyer, G. J., Taylor, J. M., & Cox, D. R. (2012). On hope and possibility: Does continuing professional development contribute to ongoing professional competence? *Professional Psychology: Research and Practice, 43*(5), 476–486. https://doi.org/10.1037/a0029613

Neimeyer, G. J., Taylor, J. M., Rozensky, R. H., & Cox, D. R. (2014). The diminishing durability of knowledge in professional psychology: A second look at specializations. *Professional Psychology: Research and Practice, 45*(2), 92–98. https://doi.org/10.1037/a0036176

Neimeyer, G. J., Taylor, J. M., Zemansky, M. F., & Rothke, S. E. (2019). Exploring the impact of continuing education mandates: A longitudinal look. *Professional Psychology: Research and Practice, 50*(3), 168–175. https://doi.org/10.1037/pro0000242

Peirce, C. S. (1889). Meliorism. In W. Whitney (Ed.), *Century dictionary and cyclopedia* (Vol. 5, p. 3697). The Century.

Rabasco, A., McKay, D., Washburn, J. J., Teachman, B. A., Gaudiano, B. A., & Davison, G. C. (2021). Standards for professional psychology continuing education sponsors: A comparative analysis of health service professions. *Professional Psychology: Research and Practice, 52*(1), 21–27. https://doi.org/10.1037/pro0000364

Raque, T. L., Mitchell, A. M., Coleman, M. N., Coleman, J. J., & Owen, J. (2021). Addressing racial equity in health psychology research: An application of the multicultural orientation framework. *American Psychologist, 76*(8), 1266–1279. https://doi.org/10.1037/amp0000888

Rothke, S. E., Neimeyer, G. J., Taylor, J. M., & Zemansky, M. F. (2021). Do CE mandates impact the number of CE providers and licensing board complaints? A longitudinal look. *Ethics & Behavior, 31*(7), 463–474. https://doi.org/10.1080/10508422.2020.1847112

Rotter, J. B. (1954). *Social learning and clinical psychology*. Prentice-Hall.

Shannon, D. W. (2015). A selective look at the history and practice of continuing education. In D. W. Shannon & R. Wiltenburg (Eds.), *Centennial conversations: Essential essays in professional, continuing, and online education* (pp. 3–14). University Professional and Continuing Education Association.

Sue, D. W. (2017). Microaggressions and "evidence": Empirical or experiential reality? *Perspectives on Psychological Science, 12*(1), 170–172. https://doi.org/10.1177/1745691616664437

Sue, D. W., & Spanierman, L. B. (2020). *Microaggressions in everyday life* (2nd ed.). Wiley.

Syed, M. (2021). *The Logic of Microaggressions Assumes a Racist Society. Perspectives on Psychological Science, 16(5), 926–931.* https://doi.org/10.1177/1745691621994263

Syme, K. L., & Hagen, E. H. (2020). Mental health is biological health: Why tackling "diseases of the mind" is an imperative for biological anthropology in the 21st century. *American Journal of Physical Anthropology, 171*, 87–117. https://doi.org/10.1002/ajpa.23965

Taylor, J. M., Neimeyer, G. J., Bedwell, J. S., Leach, M. M., Liese, B. S., Minniti, A., Penberthy, J. K., Philip, D., Segura, M. E., & Simonian, S. J. (2019). Continuing education in psychology: Preferences, practices, and perceived outcomes. *Professional Psychology: Research and Practice, 50*(2), 70–76. https://doi.org/10.1037/pro0000223

van Weeghel, J., van Zelst, C., Boertien, D., & Hasson-Ohayon, I. (2019). Conceptualizations, assessments, and implications of personal recovery in mental illness: A scoping review of systematic reviews and meta-analyses. *Psychiatric Rehabilitation Journal, 42*(2), 169–181. https://doi.org/10.1037/prj0000356

VandeCreek, L., Knapp, S., & Brace, K. (1990). Mandatory continuing education for licensed psychologists: Its rationale and current implementation. *Professional Psychology: Research and Practice, 21*(2), 135–140. https://doi.org/10.1037/0735-7028.21.2.135

Varghese, F. P., & Boyd, J. E. (2022). Clinicians with lived experience of mental illness: Introduction to a special section on prosumers, in honor of the late Dr. Fredrick J. Frese III. *Psychological Services, 19*(1), 1–5. https://doi.org/10.1037/ser0000613

Vasquez, M. J. T., & Johnson, J. D. (2022). *Multicultural therapy: A practice imperative*. APA.

Walshok, M. L. (2012). Reinventing continuing higher education. *Continuing Higher Education Review, 76*, 38–53.

Warner, R. (2010). Does the scientific evidence support the recovery model? *The Psychiatrist, 34*(1), 3–5.

Washburn, J. J., Manley, T., & Howliski, F. (2003). Teaching on racism: Tools for consultant training. *Journal of Educational and Psychological Consultation, 14*(3&4), 387–399. https://doi.org/10.1207/s1532768xjepc143&4_10

Washburn, J. J., Lilienfeld, S. O., Rosen, G. M., Gaudiano, B. A., Davison, G. C., Hollon, S. D., Otto, M. W., Penberthy, J. K., Sher, K. J., Teachman, B. A., Peris, T., & Weinand, J. (2019). Reaffirming the scientific foundations of psychological practice: Recommendations of the Emory meeting on continuing education. *Professional Psychology: Research and Practice, 50*(2), 77–86. https://doi.org/10.1037/pro0000235

Whitaker, C. A. (1960). The on-going training of the psychotherapist. In N. P. Dellis & H. K. Stone (Eds.), *The training of psychotherapists* (pp. 151–168). Louisiana State University Press.

Williams, M. T. (2020). Microaggressions: Clarification, evidence, and impact. *Perspectives on Psychological Science, 15*(1), 3–26. https://doi.org/10.1177/1745691619827499

Index

C. L. Cobb et al. (eds.), *Toward a Science of Clinical Psychology*,
https://doi.org/10.1007/978-3-031-14332-8

SPRINGER NATURE

GPSR Compliance

The European Union's (EU) General Product Safety Regulation (GPSR) is a set of rules that requires consumer products to be safe and our obligations to ensure this.

If you have any concerns about our products, you can contact us on ProductSafety@springernature.com

In case Publisher is established outside the EU, the EU authorized representative is:

Springer Nature Customer Service Center GmbH
Europaplatz 3
69115 Heidelberg, Germany

The manufacturer's authorised representative in the EU is Springer Nature Customer Service Centre GmbH, Europaplatz 3, 69115 Heidelberg, Germany. If you have any concerns regarding our products, please contact ProductSafety@springernature.com

Printed and bound by CPI Group (UK) Ltd, Croydon, CR0 4YY
01/10/2026
02225893-0015